Soft Tissue Tumors of the Skin

Steven D. Billings
Rajiv M. Patel • Darya Buehler
Editors

Soft Tissue Tumors of the Skin

Springer

Editors
Steven D. Billings
Department of Anatomic Pathology
Cleveland Clinic
Cleveland, OH
USA

Darya Buehler
Department of Pathology and
Laboratory Medicine
University of Wisconsin–Madison
Madison, WI
USA

Rajiv M. Patel
Departments of Pathology and
Dermatology
University of Michigan Medical Center
Ann Arbor, MI
USA

ISBN 978-1-4939-8810-5 ISBN 978-1-4939-8812-9 (eBook)
https://doi.org/10.1007/978-1-4939-8812-9

Library of Congress Control Number: 2018960891

This Springer imprint is published by the registered company Springer Science+Business Media, LLC part of Springer Nature.
The registered company address is: 233 Spring Street, New York, NY 10013, U.S.A.

Preface

Soft tissue pathology is arguably the most challenging area in dermatopathology. Cutaneous soft tissue tumors are relatively rare, have significant histologic overlap, and yet encompass a remarkable morphological diversity of entities. This book is our effort to provide a comprehensive, but succinct and well-illustrated, survey of soft tissue tumors and the non-mesenchymal mimics that may present in the skin. In this work, we emphasize the clinicopathologic features, differential diagnosis, and important diagnostic pitfalls encountered with these lesions. We hope that our undertaking will be a useful and practical resource for daily sign-out.

Cleveland, OH, USA — Steven D. Billings
Ann Arbor, MI, USA — Rajiv M. Patel
Madison, WI, USA — Darya Buehler

Acknowledgment

We would like to thank all of our teachers in pathology, but especially Drs. Sharon Weiss, Andrew L. Folpe, John Goldblum, and Brian Rubin. Not only did they teach us soft tissue pathology but also the mentorship and wisdom they have provided has shaped our careers and practice. We are tremendously grateful to our contributing authors, Drs. Andrew L. Folpe, Karen J. Fritchie, Reena Singh, Youran Zou, and Aaron M. Udager, without whom, this book would not have been possible. We would also like to thank Dr. Paul Weisman of the University of Wisconsin for valuable editorial insights on select chapters and Lisa Stephens of the ePathology Department of the Cleveland Clinic for her expert assistance with many of the figures in the book. We would also like to thank Drs. Carly Elston, Cody Carter, Grace Wang, and Joseph Zahn for their critical proofreading of the chapters.

Contents

Contributors

Steven D. Billings, MD Department of Pathology, Cleveland Clinic, Cleveland, OH, USA

Darya Buehler, MD Pathology and Laboratory Medicine, University of Wisconsin School of Medicine and Public Health, Madison, WI, USA

Andrew L. Folpe, MD Department of Laboratory Medicine and Pathology, Mayo Clinic, Rochester, MN, USA

Karen J. Fritchie, MD Mayo Clinic, Department of Laboratory Medicine and Pathology, Division of Anatomic Pathology, Rochester, MN, USA

Rajiv M. Patel, MD Department of Pathology, University of Michigan Medical School, Ann Arbor, MI, USA

Reena Singh, MD Department of Pathology, Oregon Health and Science University School of Medicine, Portland, OR, USA

Aaron M. Udager, MD, PhD Department of Pathology, University of Michigan Medical School, Ann Arbor, MI, USA

Introduction and General Approach

1

Steven D. Billings and Rajiv M. Patel

Abstract

Soft tissue tumor is a difficult area in dermatopathology. Although some soft tissue tumors like dermatofibromas are commonly encountered, many are rare. Therefore dermatopathologists and pathologists are often unfamiliar with relevant diagnostic criteria or even a method for approaching these challenging cases. This chapter will provide an introduction to the assessment of cutaneous soft tissue tumors, focusing on broad concepts.

It is almost universal that soft tissue tumors pose some of the most difficult challenges in the realm of dermatopathology. There is significant histologic and immunophenotypic overlap between entities, and given their relative rarity, dermatopathologists and pathologists are often unfamiliar with key diagnostic criteria. This book is our attempt to help clarify this difficult subject and provide some guidance in the approach to this area. We concentrate on cutaneous lesions, and this is therefore not an all-encompassing tome on soft tissue tumors. It is meant to be a practical book that is useful in everyday sign-out, and we hope you find it so.

Similar to inflammatory dermatopathology, it is important to recognize growth patterns and the cellular constituents of a given lesion. Low-magnification observation is critical to the evaluation of the overall growth pattern. The first thing that should be assessed is circumscription. Is the tumor circumscribed or infiltrative? As a general rule, although admittedly there are many exceptions, circumscription favors benignity, while an infiltrative growth pattern favors malignancy. With regard to circumscribed tumors, one should also assess whether the tumor has a true capsule (e.g., schwannoma) (Fig. 1.1) or pseudocapsule (e.g., angiomatoid fibrous histiocytoma) (Fig. 1.2), or lacks a capsule, but remains relatively circumscribed (e.g., dermatofibroma) (Fig. 1.3). For infiltrative tumors, the pattern of infiltration can also be informative. For example, does the tumor have a diffuse pattern of infiltration (e.g., dermatofibrosarcoma protuberans) (Fig. 1.4)? Does it infiltrate along cutaneous structures like subcutaneous septa (e.g., myxofibrosarcoma and variants of nodular fasciitis) (Fig. 1.5a, b)?

After assessing circumscription, one should determine the growth pattern, with the caveat that some tumors may exhibit a variety of different patterns. The principle ones encountered are

S. D. Billings (✉)
Department of Pathology, Cleveland Clinic, Cleveland, OH, USA
e-mail: billins@ccf.org

R. M. Patel
Department of Pathology, University of Michigan Medical School, Ann Arbor, MI, USA

S. D. Billings et al. (eds.), *Soft Tissue Tumors of the Skin*,
https://doi.org/10.1007/978-1-4939-8812-9_1

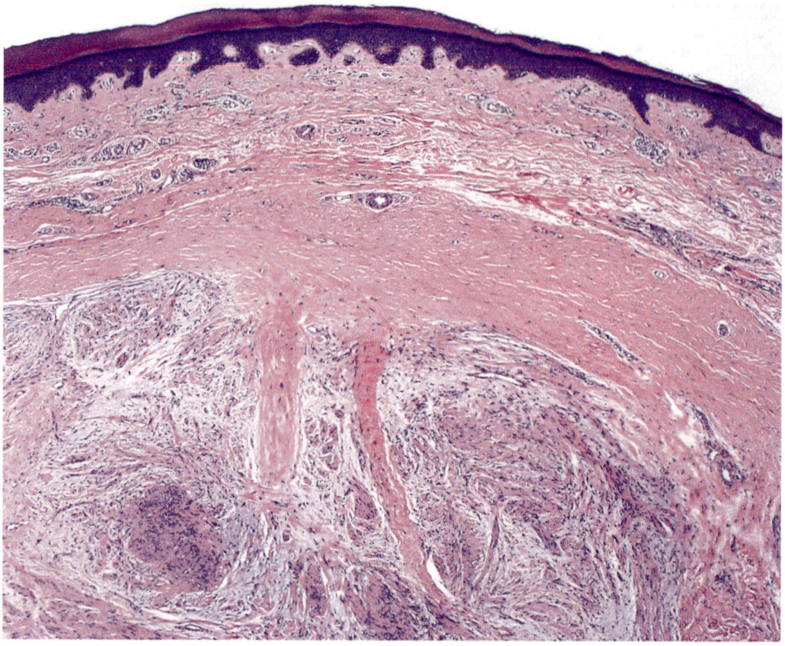

Fig. 1.1 Schwannoma with distinct fibrous capsule

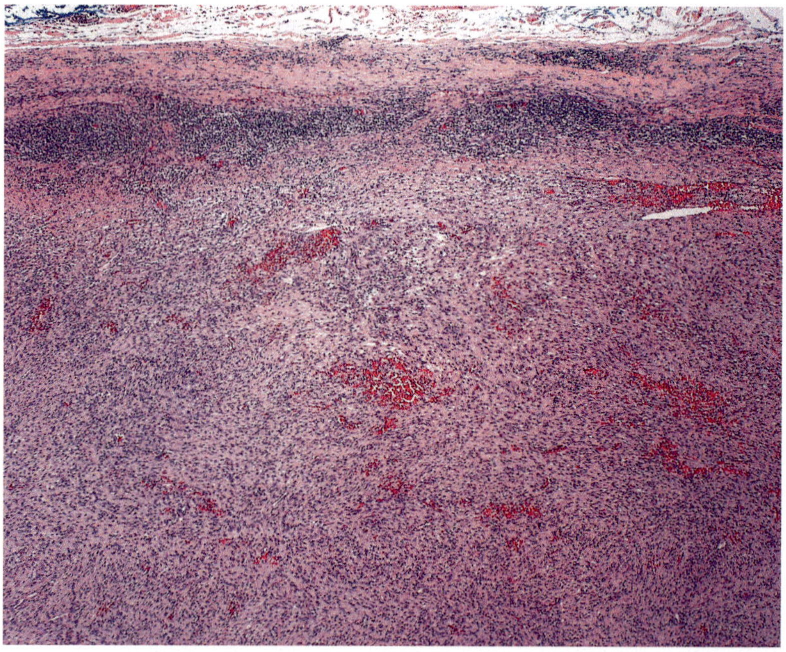

Fig. 1.2 Condensed fibrous tissue representing a pseudocapsule surrounding an angiomatoid fibrous histiocytoma

fascicular, sheet-like, nested, random (cells separated by stroma but arranged in no definitive pattern), and vasoformative. Fascicles are defined as organized, cohesive arrangements of spindled cells. Within the fascicular growth pattern, there are several subtypes: storiform (Fig. 1.6), irregular-to-swirling fascicles (Fig. 1.7a, b), short fascicles (Fig. 1.8), and long fascicles (Fig. 1.9). The storiform pattern, defined as a pinwheel-like arrangments of spinlded cells, is characteristic of dermatofibrosarcoma protuberans and, to a lesser extent, dermatofibroma. Irregular-to-swirling

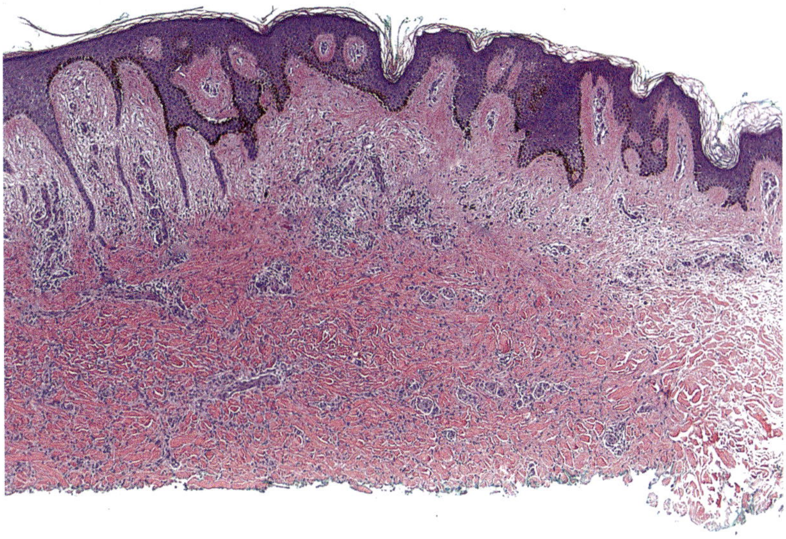

Fig. 1.3 Low-power image demonstrating relative circumscription of a dermatofibroma

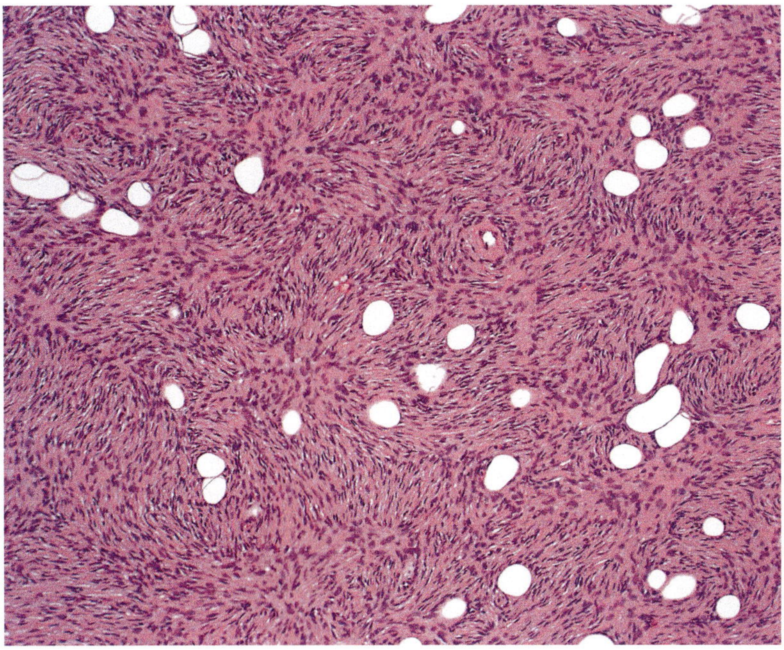

Fig. 1.4 Dermatofibrosarcoma protuberans diffusely infiltrating subcutaneous fat

fascicles are less cohesive than the tight architecture of the storiform pattern and are seen in entities such as nodular fasciitis and perineurioma. Short fascicles are composed of short parallel arrangements of spindled cells and may be seen in such entities as spindle cell lipoma. Longer fascicles are seen in superficial fibromatosis, and smooth muscle tumors, among others. The sheet-like growth pattern is one in which there is a diffuse, solid proliferation of tumor cells without an otherwise organized growth pattern (Fig. 1.10). This is often encountered in tumors with a round cell or epithelioid morphology (e.g., glomus tumor). The nested growth pattern is characterized by tumors with smaller, solid aggregates of tumor cells separated by interven-

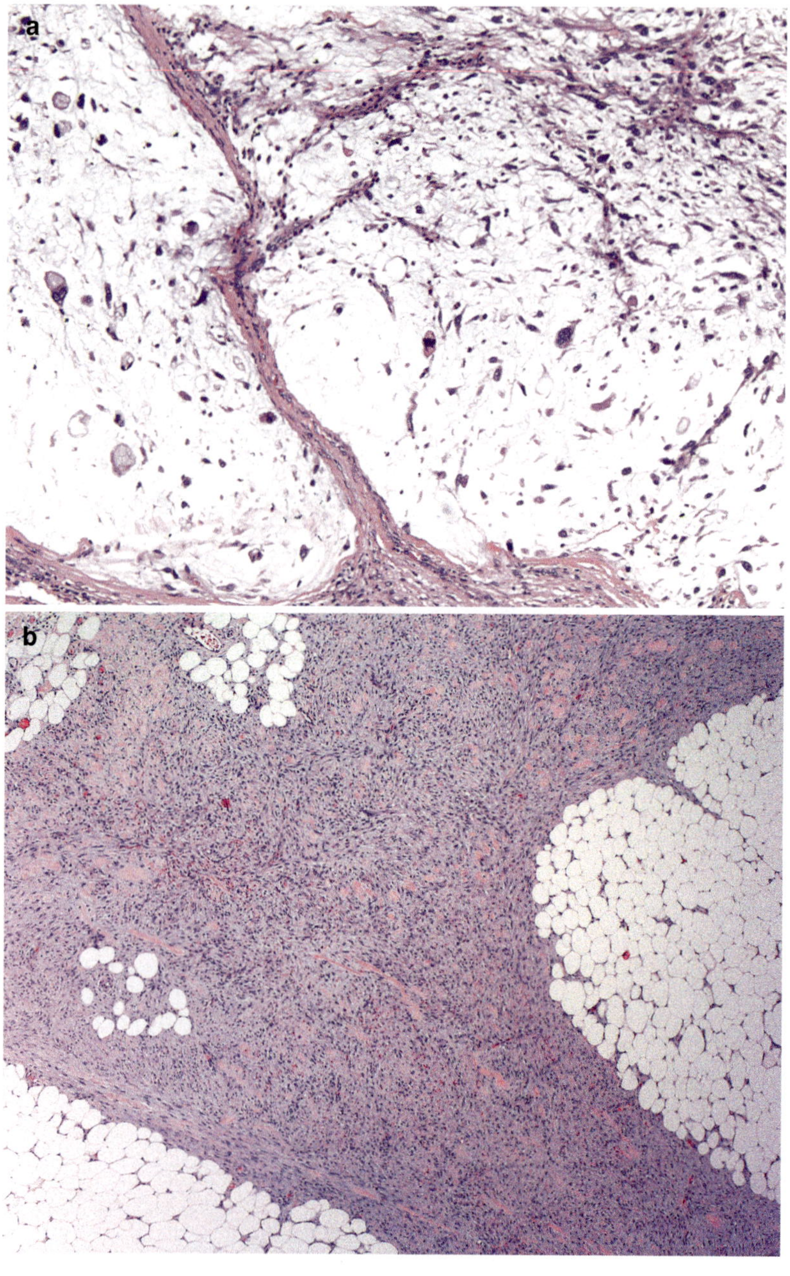

Fig. 1.5 (**a**). Myxofibrosarcoma is an infiltrative tumor that frequently extends along fibrous septa of the subcutis. (**b**). Nodular fasciitis extending along subcutaneous septa

ing stroma (Fig. 1.11). This pattern can be seen in a variety of entities, both benign and malignant (e.g., cellular neurothekeoma and epithelioid sarcoma). The random pattern is often seen in tumors where the stroma is the predominant feature, and the constituent cells generally lack an organized architecture (e.g., neurofibroma) (Fig. 1.12). Finally, tumors may have a vasoformative growth pattern in which neoplastic cells form multicellular endothelial-lined vascular channels that may recapitulate normal vessels (e.g., hemangioma) or be architecturally complex (e.g., angiosarcoma) (Fig. 1.13) (Table 1.1). It is important to remember that many tumors can have a combination of growth patterns, and that those described are mostly intended to serve

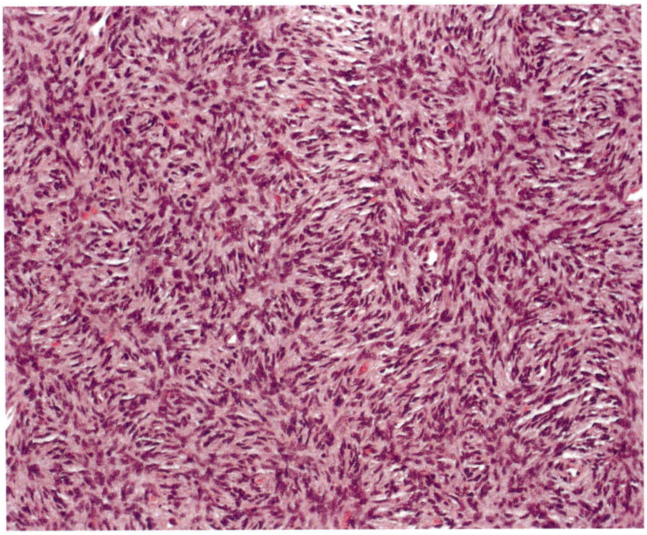

Fig. 1.6 The storiform pattern is characterized by spindled cells arranged in a pinwheel architecture, classically seen in dermatofibrosarcoma protuberans

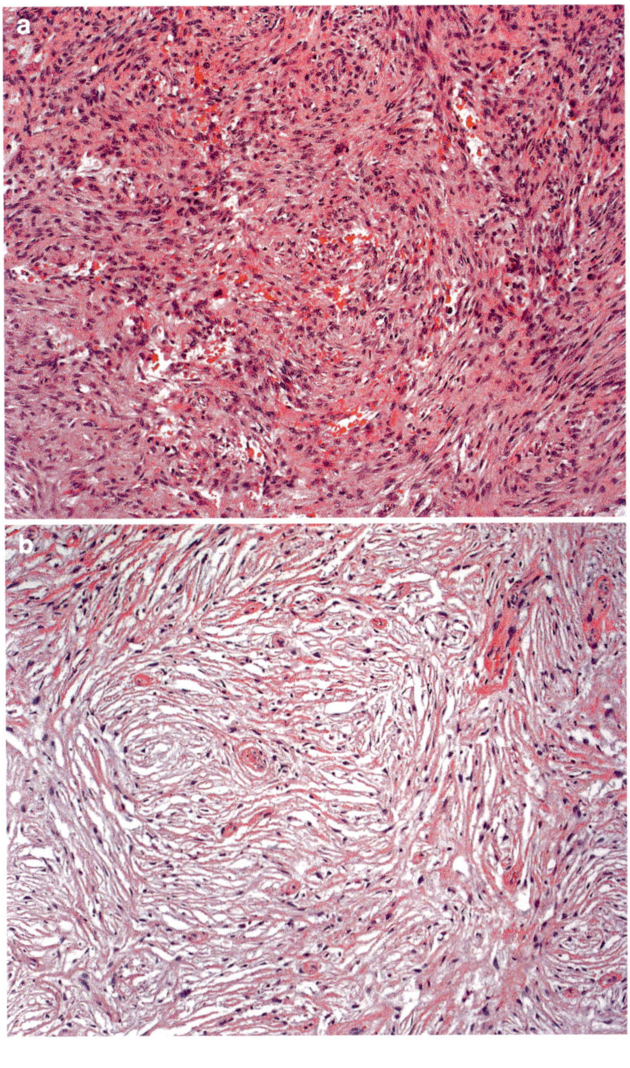

Fig. 1.7 Irregular-to-swirling fascicles of spindled cells are another common growth pattern illustrated in this figure in a case of nodular fasciitis (**a**) and perineurioma (**b**)

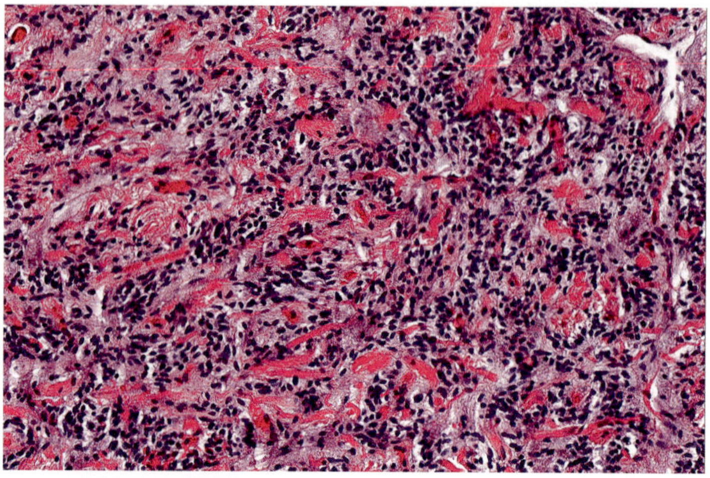

Fig. 1.8 In some tumors, the fascicles are relatively short. This is a case of a fat-free spindle cell lipoma with short fascicles of spindled cells that have been likened to a "school of fish"

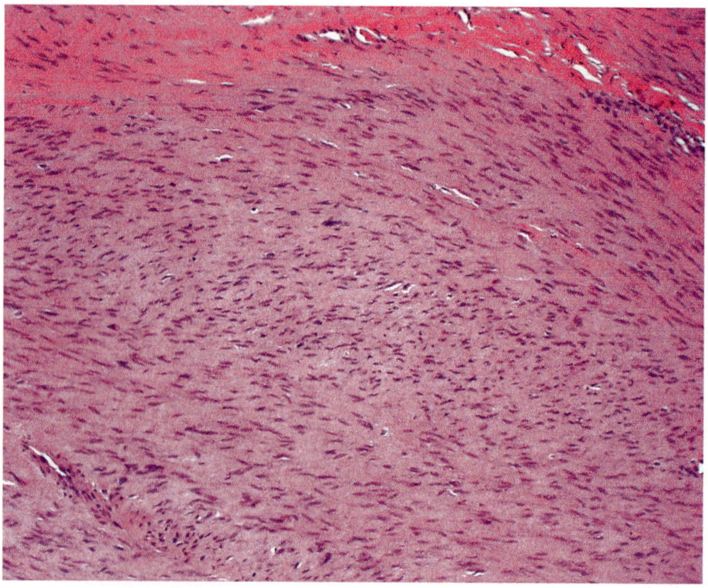

Fig. 1.9 In some cases the fascicles are relatively long, as in plantar fibromatosis

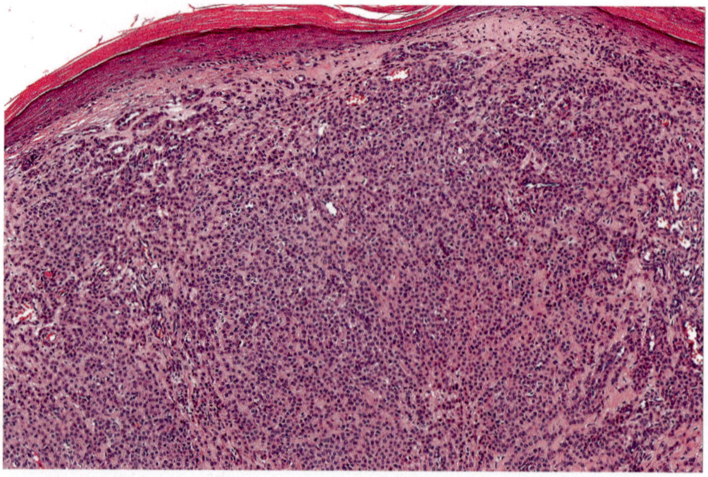

Fig. 1.10 Sheet-like growth without a distinctive pattern in a glomus tumor

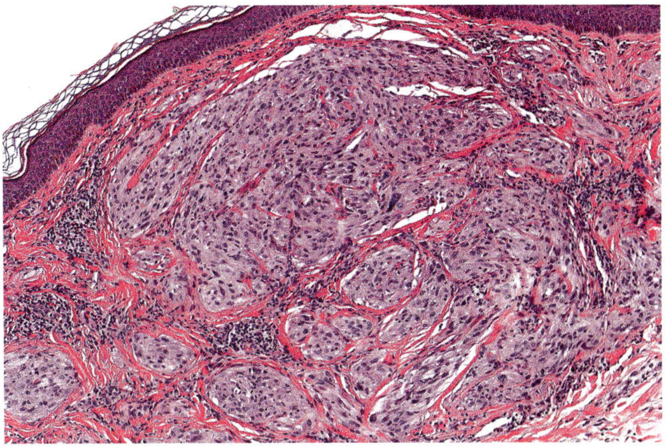

Fig. 1.11 Nested pattern characterized by discrete aggregates of tumor cells, as seen in cellular neurothekeoma

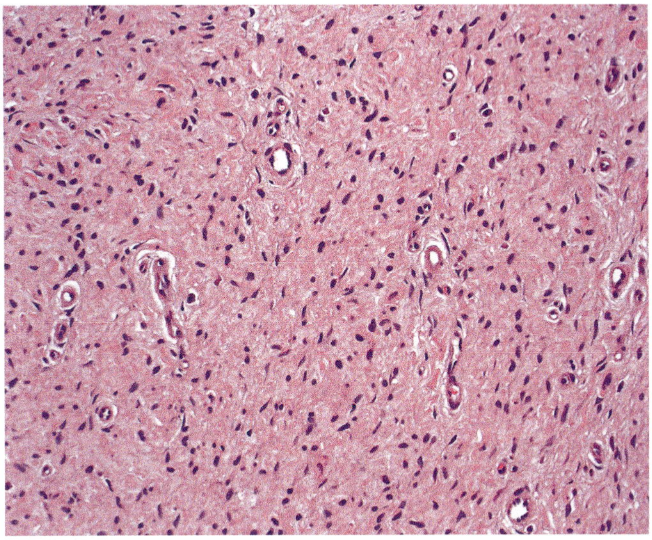

Fig. 1.12 The random pattern is usually seen in tumors with abundant stroma and relatively low cellularity, as in this neurofibroma

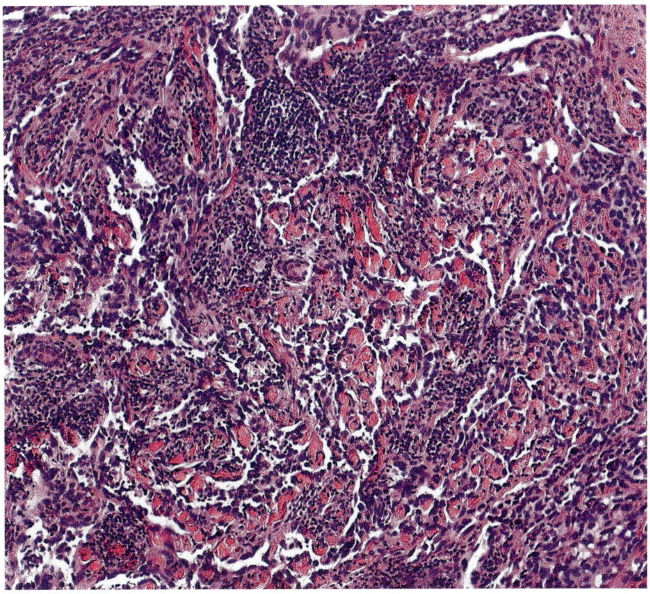

Fig. 1.13 The vasoformative pattern can closely resemble normal vessels or be architecturally complex, as in angiosarcoma

as a guide for the histopathologic evaluation of a given lesion.

Also included in the low-magnification evaluation is the determination of the overall cellularity of a lesion. Is the tumor uniformly or variably cellular, hypercellular or hypocellular or both (Fig. 1.14)?

Table 1.1 Growth patterns of cutaneous soft tissue tumors

Circumscribed
Nonencapsulated
True capsule
Pseudocapsule
Infiltrative
Fascicular
Storiform
Irregular to swirling
Short
Long
Sheet-like
Solid proliferation with little intervening stroma
Nodular
Nests and nodules of tumor separated by stroma
Random
Tumor separated by stroma with no definitive growth pattern
Vasoformative
Tumor cells form vascular channels lined by endothelial cells
Resemble normal vessels
Architecturally complex
Stroma
Collagenous
Myxoid
Both collagenous and myxoid

Another critical low-magnification assessment includes the nature of the tumor stroma. Does the tumor intercalate between native collagen bundles of the dermis like a dermatofibroma (Fig. 1.15) or make its own stroma (Fig. 1.16)? Is the stroma collagenous (Fig. 1.17), myxoid (Fig. 1.18), or a combination of collagenous and myxoid stroma (Fig. 1.19) (Table 1.1)?

With the circumscription, growth pattern, cellularity, and nature of the stroma established, cytologic features are then assessed at higher magnification. One should determine the cellular morphology: spindled, stellate, round cell, or epithelioid. Most mesenchymal lesions have a spindled morphology, being composed of cells with elongated nuclei, typically with bipolar cytoplasmic processes (Fig. 1.20). Some may have multiple cytoplasmic cellular processes imparting a stellate configuration (Fig. 1.21). In tumors with a round cell morphology, cells have round nuclei and less cytoplasm (Fig. 1.22). Epithelioid morphology is characterized by cells with round to oval nuclei and relatively abundant cytoplasm, resembling epithelial cells (Fig. 1.23) (Table 1.2).

Nuclear atypia is defined by size and shape, hyperchromasia, presence or absence of large nucleoli, and amount of pleomorphism. An open chromatin pattern and absent-to-small nucleoli are common in benign tumors (Fig. 1.24). Nuclear enlargement, hyperchromasia, prominent nucleoli, and pleomorphism are more common in malignant processes, with notable exceptions (e.g., atypical fibrous histiocytoma). It should be noted that some

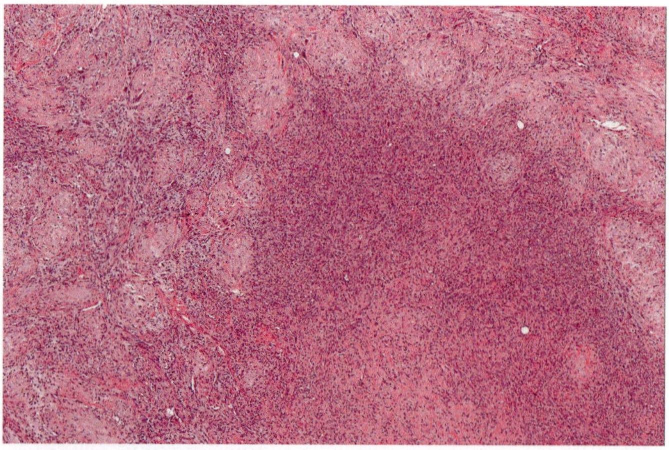

Fig. 1.14 Cellularity can be uniform or variable. This myofibroma has distinctly hypercellular and hypocellular areas

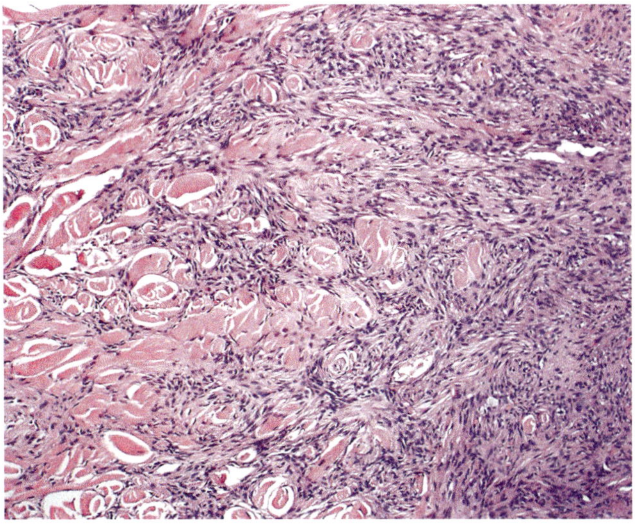

Fig. 1.15 Some tumors do not make their own stroma. This image illustrates the neoplastic cells of a dermatofibroma intercalating between collagen bundles of the reticular dermis

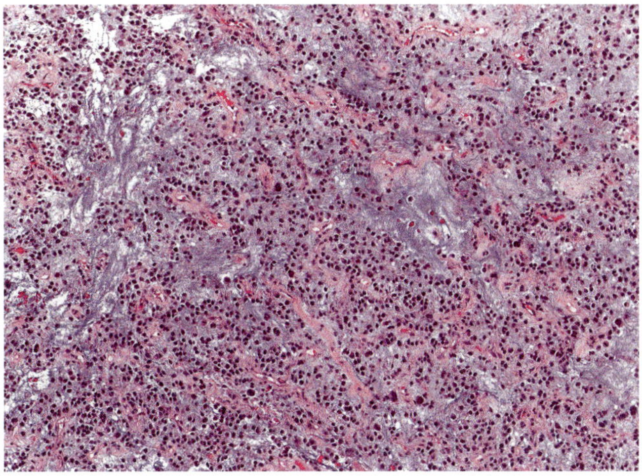

Fig. 1.16 Some tumor cells make their own stroma like the chondromyxoid matrix in this myoepithelioma

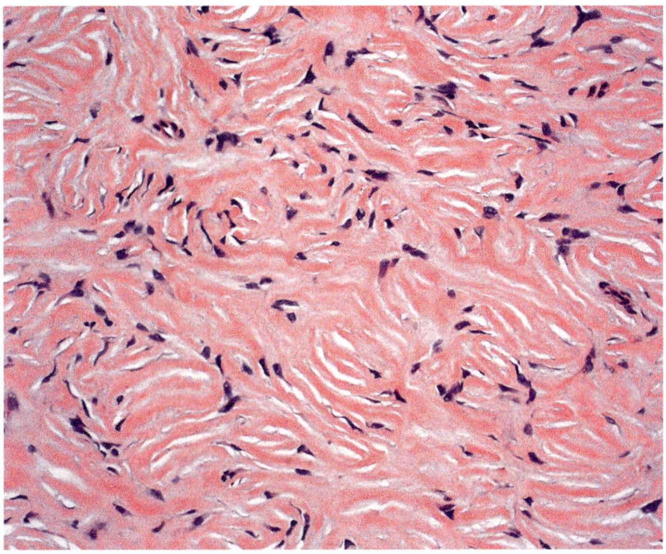

Fig. 1.17 Some tumors have a prominent collagenous stroma like this collagenous fibroma (storiform collagenoma)

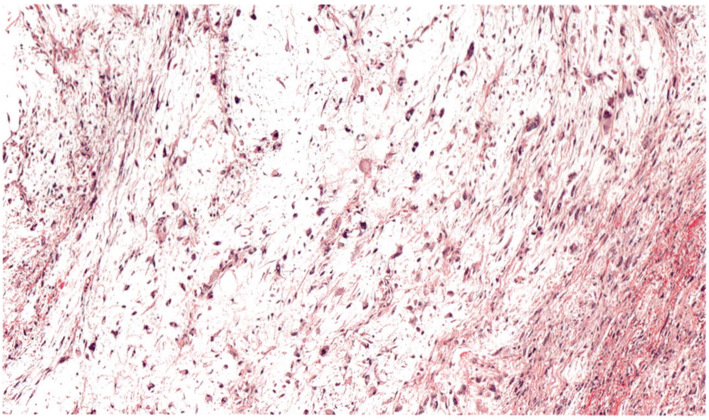

Fig. 1.18 Some tumors have a prominent myxoid stroma, as in this myxofibrosarcoma

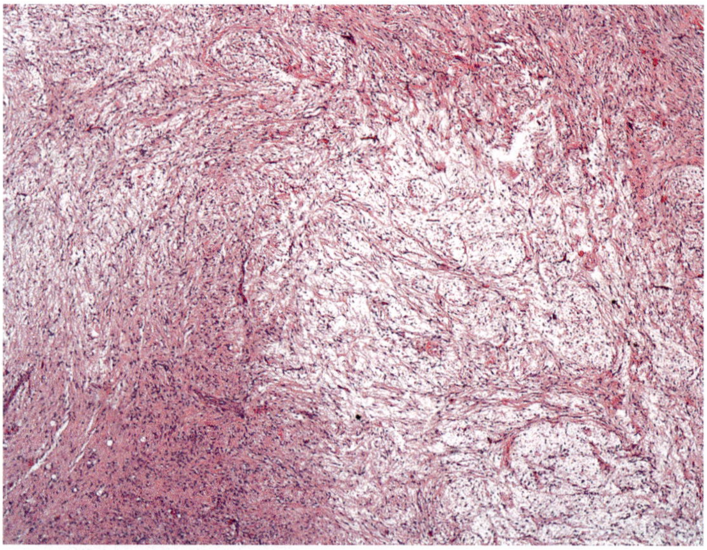

Fig. 1.19 Other tumors have a combination of collagenous and myxoid stroma, as in low-grade fibromyxoid sarcoma

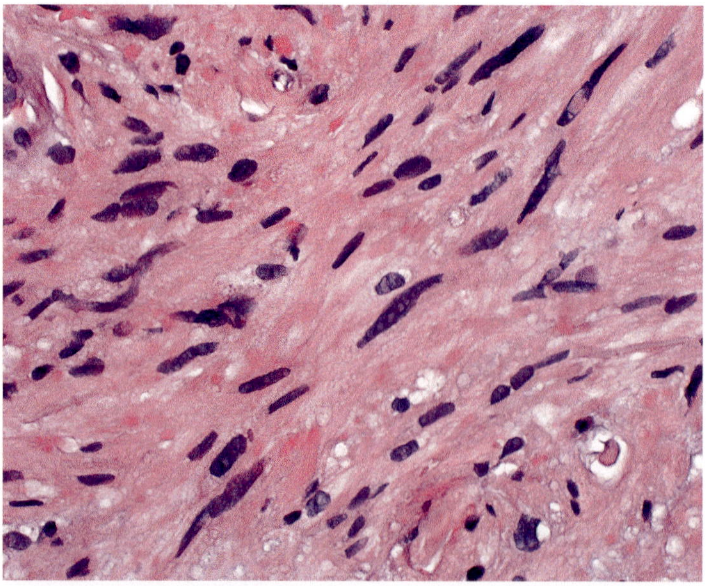

Fig. 1.20 Spindled cells of a leiomyoma with elongated nuclei and bipolar cytoplasmic processes

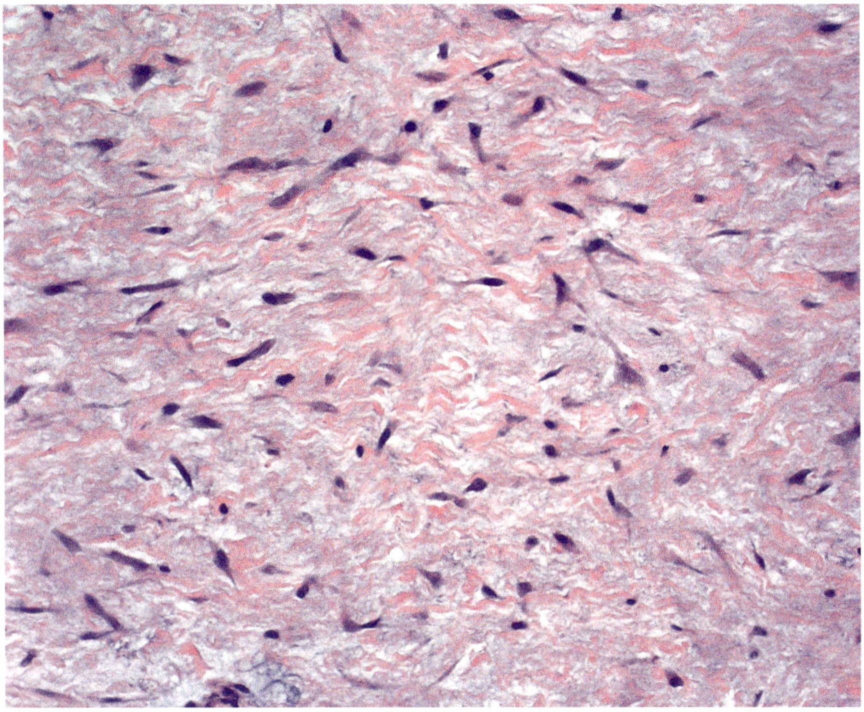

Fig. 1.21 Some tumors have stellate cells with multiple cytoplasmic processes. Tumors with stellate cells often have admixed spindled cells, as in this desmoplastic fibroblastoma

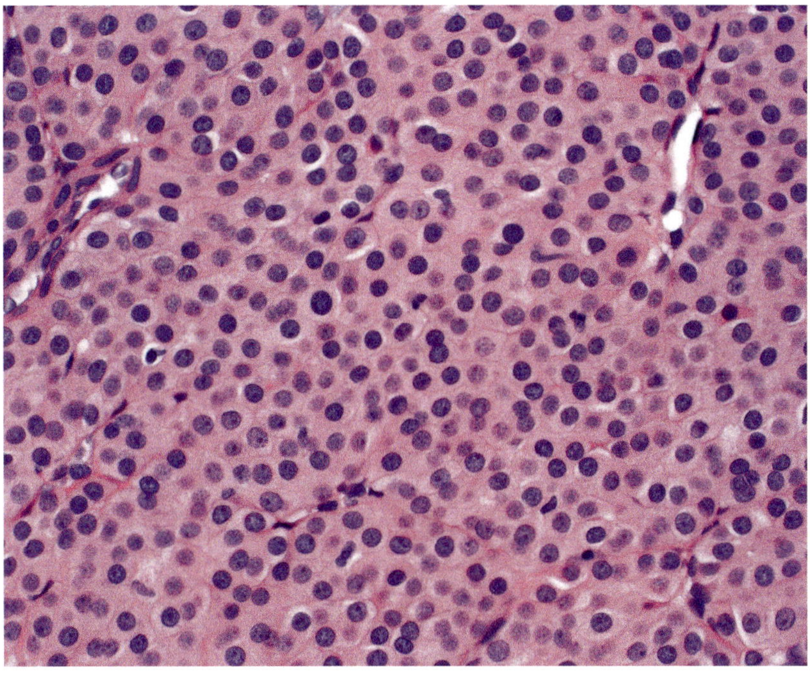

Fig. 1.22 Round cell morphology is characterized by uniform cells with round nuclei and less cytoplasm, as in this case of glomus tumor

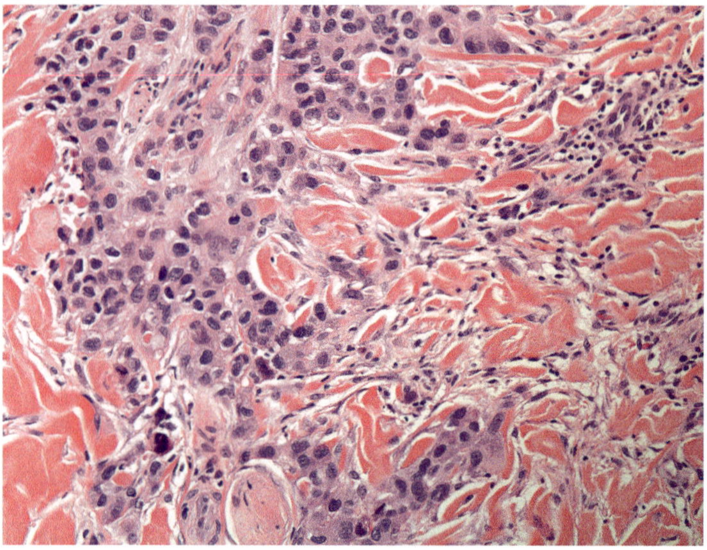

Fig. 1.23 Tumor cells with epithelioid morphology usually have round to oval nuclei with relatively abundant cytoplasm, as in this epithelioid sarcoma

Table 1.2 Cytologic features

General categories
Spindle cells
Stellate cells
Round cells
Epithelioid cells
Nuclear features
Spindled vs oval vs round
Chromatin pattern
Nucleoli
Pleomorphism
Size
Size

tumors may have significant atypia but lack nuclear pleomorphism (e.g., Ewing sarcoma) (Fig. 1.25). Pleomorphism is defined as the variability in size and shape between tumor cells in a given lesion (e.g., atypical fibroxanthoma) (Fig. 1.26). As a general rule, nuclear atypia and pleomorphism are features of malignancy, again with notable exceptions (e.g., pleomorphic fibroma).

Mitotic activity, atypical mitotic figures, and necrosis are also features more common in malignancies, but can occur in benign tumors, such as cellular fibrous histiocytoma, which may have frequent mitoses and sometimes tumor necrosis.

Assessment of the above histologic features allows the formulation of a histologic differential diagnosis. In the assessment of the differential diagnosis, the clinical presentation also needs to be considered. Some neoplasms have a strong predilection for certain locations (e.g., clear cell sarcoma) or certain age groups (e.g., fibrous hamartoma of infancy). These factors influence the approach to a given case. Just remember that tumors do not read textbooks; there are always exceptions to any stated "rule." Finally, in some cases, correlation with radiologic imaging results may be extremely useful (e.g., superficial biopsies of myxofibrosarcoma).

Only after a solid differential diagnosis has been constructed should one consider the possibility of confirmatory ancillary diagnostic testing. We have encountered many consult cases in which an extensive battery of unnecessary immunohistochemical stains was performed on a challenging case. After an exhaustive and inconclusive work-up, these cases are often then referred for consultation. This scenario is problematic. The shotgun approach to ancillary diagnostic testing runs the risk of exhausting the precious diagnostic tissue in the block, as many of these specimens are small shave or punch biopsies. Whenever one orders a diagnostic test, the result should be expected to confirm or refute clinical suspicion or answer a specific question. For example, there is absolutely no reason to order a vimentin stain in the assessment of cutaneous soft tissue tumors. Essentially

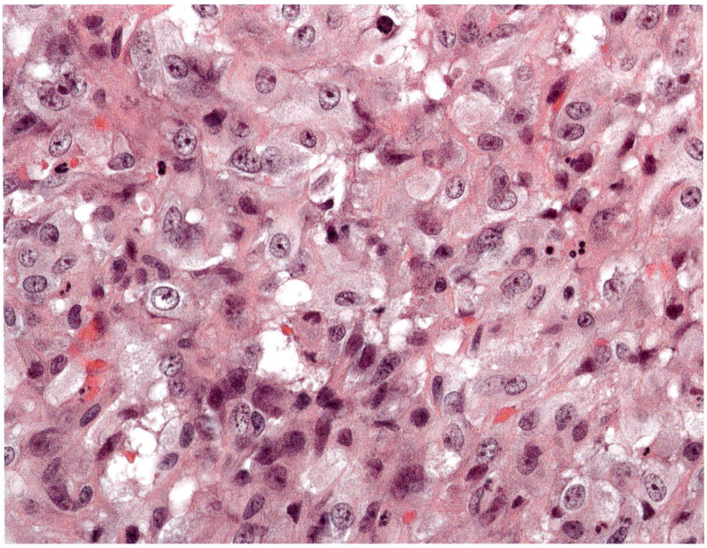

Fig. 1.24 Cutaneous epithelioid angiomatous nodule with uniform nuclei with open chromatin and small nucleoli

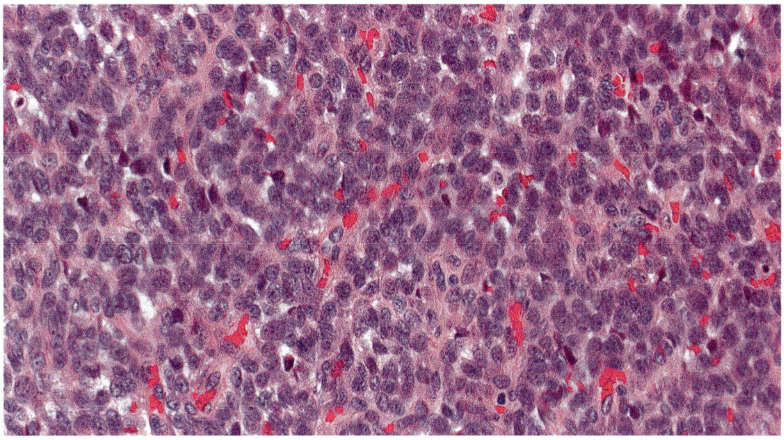

Fig. 1.25 Ewing sarcoma with uniform but atypical hyperchromatic nuclei

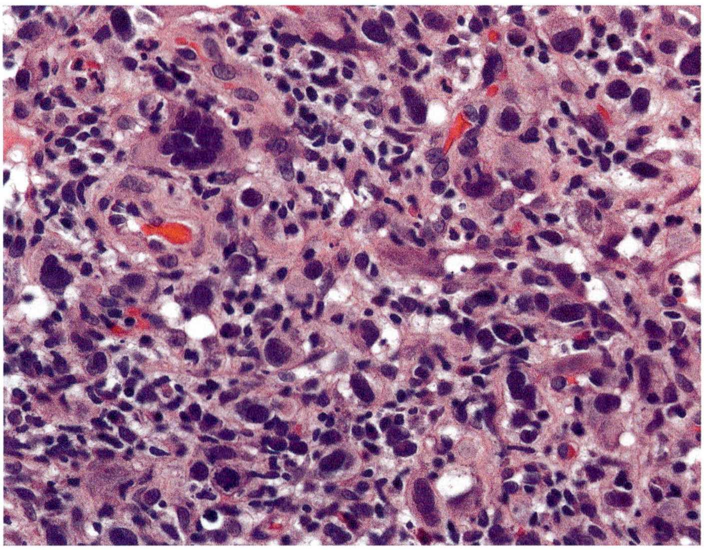

Fig. 1.26 Hyperchromatic and pleomorphic tumor cells of an atypical fibroxanthoma

Table 1.3 FNCLCC grading

FNCLCC grading	Score
Mitotic count: In the most mitotically active area, ten successive high-power fields (HPF) at 400× magnification = 0.1734 mm^2 using 40× objective	1: 0–9 mitoses/10HPF 2: 10–19 mitoses/10HPF 3: >20 mitoses/10HPF
Tumor necrosis: Evaluated on gross examination and validated with histologic sections	0: No necrosis 1: <50% necrosis 2: ≥50% necrosis
Tumor differentiation	1: Closely resembles normal adult mesenchymal tissue 2: Sarcomas for which histologic typing is certain 3: Undifferentiated sarcomas or those of uncertain type
Histologic grade	Grade 1: total score 2,3 Grade 2: total score 4,5 Grade 3: total score 6,7,8

all mesenchymal tumors and their mimics are positive for this marker. Therefore utilizing this stain only results in the depletion of diagnostic material and adds no diagnostic or prognostic value.

For certain malignant soft tissue tumors, grading is an important aspect of tumor assessment. We utilize the FNCLCC grading system (Table 1.3).

With these introductory comments completed, we hope that you find this book a useful aid in approaching cutaneous soft tissue tumors in your daily work.

Selected References

1. Billings SD, Folpe AL. Cutaneous and subcutaneous fibrohistiocytic tumors of intermediate malignancy: an update. Am J Dermatopathol. 2004;26(2):141–55.
2. Coindre JM. Grading of soft tissue sarcomas: review and update. Arch Pathol Lab Med. 2006;130(10):1448–53.
3. Goldblum J, Weiss S, Folpe A, editors. Enzinger and Weiss's soft tissue tumors. Philadelphia: Elsevier; 2013.
4. Mentzel T. Cutaneous mesenchymal tumours: an update. Pathology. 2014;46(2):149–59.
5. Patel RM, Billings SD. Cutaneous soft tissue tumors that make you say, "oh $*&%!". Adv Anat Pathol. 2012;19(5):320–30.

2 Ancillary Diagnostic Tests in the Diagnosis of Cutaneous Soft Tissue Neoplasms

Andrew L. Folpe

Abstract

This chapter will cover selected applications of immunohistochemistry (IHC) in the diagnosis of soft tissue tumors of the skin. This section will emphasize applications of IHC to common differential diagnoses in cutaneous soft tissue pathology, including (1) pleomorphic spindle cell tumors; (2) epithelioid malignant neoplasms; (3) monomorphic spindle cell tumors; (4) "fibrohistiocytic" or "histiocytoid" lesions; (5) small, round blue cell tumors; and (6) adipocytic tumors. It is not possible in this relatively brief section to provide a detailed discussion of each antigen or of every rare soft tissue tumor that may occasionally be seen in the skin, and the reader is referred to the relevant chapters in this book for more detailed discussions of specific entities.

It cannot be overemphasized that IHC is an *adjunctive* diagnostic technique to traditional morphologic methods in cutaneous soft tissue pathology, as in any other area of surgical pathology. The diagnosis of some soft tissue tumors does not generally require IHC (e.g., adipocytic tumors), and IHC should in almost all instances not be relied upon to distinguish benign from malignant tumors (e.g., the distinction of nodular fasciitis from leiomyosarcoma). Additionally, specific markers do not exist for certain mesenchymal cell types and their tumors, and a subset of soft tissue tumors defies classification, even with exhaustive IHC and ultrastructural and genetic study. There are also an increasing number of instances where molecular genetic testing may be more useful for selected differential diagnoses than are IHC tests. Table 2.1 summarizes the most widely used IHC markers for the diagnosis of cutaneous soft tissue tumors and their sarcoma diagnosis. Table 2.2 provides an overview of markers expressed by specific common tumor types.

Basic Principles of Diagnostic Immunohistochemistry

Attention to Positive and Negative Internal Controls

It cannot be overemphasized that all IHC slides must be evaluated for appropriate staining of normal tissues for the antigen in question. Because specimen fixation is the single greatest variable in IHC, internal positive and negative controls are much more important than are external controls, whether those external controls are placed on the same glass slide or not. Thankfully, the skin is rich in normal internal positive controls for the vast majority of antigens (see Table 2.1).

A. L. Folpe (✉)
Department of Laboratory Medicine and Pathology, Mayo Clinic, Rochester, MN, USA
e-mail: folpe.andrew@mayo.edu

S. D. Billings et al. (eds.), *Soft Tissue Tumors of the Skin*,
https://doi.org/10.1007/978-1-4939-8812-9_2

Table 2.1 Commonly used immunohistochemical markers in sarcoma diagnosis

Antigen	Expressed in
Keratins	Carcinomas, epithelioid sarcoma, synovial sarcoma, some angiosarcomas and leiomyosarcomas, mesothelioma, rhabdoid tumor, myoepithelial tumors
Desmin	Benign and malignant smooth and skeletal muscle tumors
Glial fibrillary acidic protein	Gliomas, some schwannomas, myoepithelial tumors
Smooth muscle actin	Benign and malignant smooth muscle tumors, myofibroblastic tumors and pseudotumors, myoepithelial tumors
Caldesmon	Benign and malignant smooth muscle tumors
Myogenic nuclear regulatory proteins (myogenin, MyoD1)	Rhabdomyosarcoma
S-100 protein	Melanoma, benign and malignant peripheral nerve sheath tumors, cartilaginous tumors, normal adipose tissue, Langerhans cells, myoepithelial tumors
SOX10	Melanoma, benign and malignant peripheral nerve sheath tumors, myoepithelial tumors
Epithelial membrane antigen	Carcinomas, epithelioid sarcoma, synovial sarcoma, perineurioma, meningioma, anaplastic large-cell lymphoma, some low-grade fibromyxoid sarcoma
CD31	Benign and malignant vascular tumors, histiocytes
CD34	Benign and malignant vascular tumors, solitary fibrous tumor, epithelioid sarcoma, dermatofibrosarcoma protuberans
STAT6	Solitary fibrous tumor
CD99 (MIC2 gene product)	Ewing sarcoma/primitive neuroectodermal tumor, some rhabdomyosarcomas, some synovial sarcomas, lymphoblastic lymphoma
CD45 (leukocyte common antigen)	Non-Hodgkin lymphoma
TdT	Lymphoblastic lymphoma
CD30	Anaplastic large-cell lymphoma, embryonal carcinoma
CD68 and CD163	Macrophages, fibrohistiocytic tumors, granular cell tumors, various sarcomas, melanomas, carcinomas
Melanosome-specific antigens (HMB-45, Melan-A, tyrosinase, microphthalmia transcription factor)	Melanoma, PEComa, clear cell sarcoma, melanotic schwannoma
Claudin-1	Perineurioma
Mdm2 and CDK4	Well-differentiated liposarcoma
Glut-1	Perineurioma, infantile hemangioma
SMARCB1 (INI1)	Expression lost in extrarenal rhabdoid tumor, epithelioid sarcoma, epithelioid malignant peripheral nerve sheath tumor, malignant myoepithelioma
TLE1	Synovial sarcoma
WT-1 (carboxy-terminus)	Desmoplastic small round cell tumor

Table 2.2 Commonly evaluated antigens and their normal positive internal controls in the skin

Antigen	Normal positive internal control in the skin
Pan-keratin and low-molecular-weight cytokeratins	Suprabasal keratinocytes and adnexae
High-molecular-weight cytokeratins	Basal keratinocytes
S100 protein	Melanocytes, Langerhans cells, nerves, myoepithelial cells
Melanocytic markers (e.g., HMB-45, Melan-A, MiTF, tyrosinase)	Dermal melanocytes (may be HMB-45 negative)
Smooth muscle actins	Pilar smooth muscle
Desmin	Pilar smooth muscle
Endothelial markers (e.g., CD31, CD34, FLI-1, ERG)	Endothelial cells

Attention to detail is critical here, as is, for example, not uncommon to see instances in which "pan-keratin" antibodies fail to label only basal keratinocytes, a phenomenon which may result in the misdiagnosis of high-molecular-weight keratin-positive sarcomatoid squamous cell carcinoma as "atypical fibroxanthoma" (Fig. 2.1a–c). Evaluation of negative controls simply involves ascertaining that tissues that do not express an antigen are negative. Inappropriate staining of negative controls is most often the result of inappropriate antibody concentration and/or excessive epitope retrieval.

Evaluation of all Pieces of Tissue on the Entire Slide and Careful Discrimination of Neoplastic from Nonneoplastic Cell Populations

A surprising number of cases are referred in consultation because the referring pathologist simply overlooked the most relevant IHC findings, such as a small focus of keratin or HMB-45-positive cells in a sarcomatoid carcinoma or melanoma, respectively. Similarly, it is critical to evaluate IHC studies at close enough magnification in order to determine whether staining is present in the neoplastic cells themselves or in a background population of nonneoplastic cells (e.g., misinterpretation of smooth muscle actin-positive myofibroblasts in desmoplastic melanoma as evidence of a myofibroblastic tumor or misinterpretation of CD31-positive intralesional histiocytes in carcinoma as "epithelioid angiosarcoma").

The Use of a Panel of Immunostains, Including Both Expected Positives and Negatives for All of the Entities in the Histologic Differential Diagnosis

The routine use of a small, carefully selected panel is time- and cost-effective and greatly eliminates the potential for misdiagnosis owing to anomalous expression of antigens (e.g., keratin expression in melanoma or angiosarcoma).

Epithelial Markers

Keratins

IHC to detect keratin expression is the most common way to detect epithelial differentiation, especially in the differential diagnosis of sarcomatoid squamous cell carcinoma, but also in some mesenchymal tumors with epithelioid morphology (e.g., epithelioid sarcoma and myoepitheliomas).

The skin serves as a superb control tissue for the evaluation of keratin expression, as each epithelial cell type present within the skin expresses unique keratins, as detailed in Table 2.3. The keratins (also known as cytokeratins) are a family of 20 intermediate filament proteins, whose expression is largely restricted to epithelial cells (although certain mesenchymal cell types, such as endothelium and smooth muscle, also routinely express keratins). Keratins can be thought of as individual cytokeratins (e.g., K 7, K 20), as acidic and basic pairs (e.g., K 8/18), or as "low"- and "high"-molecular-weight keratins. It is important to realize that the division of the keratins into low- and high-molecular weights is quite arbitrary, and it is more useful to think of the low-molecular-weight keratins as those of simple epithelia, such as simple ductules, and the high-molecular-weight keratins as those of complex epithelia, such as the urothelium or epidermis.

Pathologists most often consider keratins in terms of the antibodies used to identify them. The most widely used pan-keratin antibody is probably still the AE1/AE3 cocktail. AE1 recognizes the acidic keratins 10, 14, 15, 16, and 19, whereas AE3 recognizes the basic keratins 1, 2, 3, 4, 5, 6, and 8. Both antibodies recognize a mixture of high- and low-molecular-weight keratins, and there is no value in running them independently. So-called "wide-spectrum" keratin antibodies, such as the OSCAR mAb and a variety of polyclonal antibodies, potentially have somewhat broader keratin coverage than does the AE1/AE3 cocktail, although this is laboratory dependent. For example, the OSCAR mAb seems in most laboratories to perform as a more sensitive version of CAM 5.2, without coverage of high-molecular-weight keratins. MNF116 is another broad-spectrum keratin antibody that recognizes

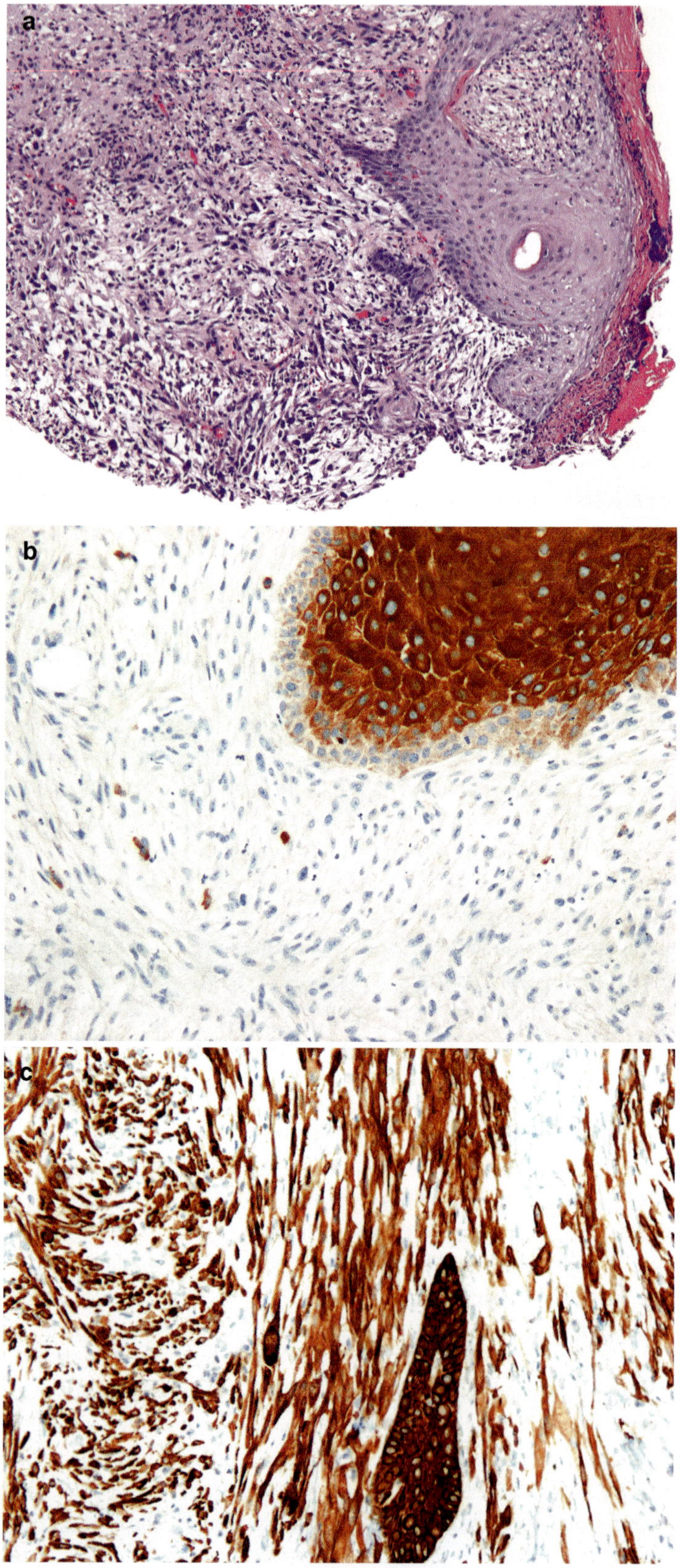

Fig. 2.1 Sarcomatoid squamous cell carcinoma (**a**). This case was referred in consultation with a suggested diagnosis of "atypical fibroxanthoma," because the outside pan-keratin immunostains (AE1/AE3) were negative. Close inspection, however, showed that the normal basal cells showed weak to absent staining (**b**), suggesting a false-negative study. Immunohistochemistry for keratins 5/6 was strongly positive in the tumor, confirming the diagnosis of sarcomatoid squamous cell carcinoma (**c**)

Table 2.3 Cytokeratin expression in normal skin

Cell type	Cytokeratins expressed
Suprabasal keratinocytes	1, 10, (11)
Basal keratinocytes	5 and 14
Hair shaft	5, 6, (14), 15, 16, 17
Eccrine ductular cells	7, 8, 17, 18, 19
Eccrine myoepithelial cells	5, 6, 14

keratins 5, 6, 8, 17, and 19. The most widely used low-molecular-weight keratin antibodies are CAM 5.2 (CK 8, 18, 19) and 35BH11 (CK 8 and 18). Almost all laboratories use the high-molecular-weight keratin antibody 34BE12 (CK 1, 5, 10, 14/15), also known as "cytokeratin 903," and keratin 5/6 antibodies are also widely utilized.

As mentioned previously, pan-keratin antibodies (e.g., AE1/3) frequently do not highlight the higher-molecular-weight keratins as well. As a general rule, IHC for keratins primarily plays a role in the diagnosis of sarcomatoid squamous cell carcinomas and a few mesenchymal tumors, such as epithelioid sarcoma.

Epithelial Membrane Antigen (EMA)

EMA is best thought of as a "second-line" epithelial marker. EMA is neither as specific nor as sensitive as are various keratin antibodies in the diagnosis of sarcomatoid carcinoma, epithelioid sarcoma, and other cutaneous soft tissue tumors with epithelial marker expression, such as myoepithelioma. EMA is, however, still the most useful marker for the diagnosis of perineurial tumors.

p63 and p40

The *p63* gene is a member of the *p53* gene family but does not appear to be involved in tumor suppression. p63 protein expression is routinely present in keratinocytes, as well as myoepithelial cells in the skin. Although p63 expression is a relatively sensitive marker of sarcomatoid carcinoma of various sites, including sarcomatoid squamous cell carcinoma, it can also be seen in soft tissue myoepithelial tumors, cellular neurothekeomas, soft tissue perineuriomas, Ewing sarcoma, diffuse-type giant cell tumor, giant cell tumors of soft tissue and bone, and other soft tissue tumors. p40 is an isoform of p63 whose expression is almost entirely limited to squamous carcinoma. Regrettably, p40 is usually negative in sarcomatoid squamous cell carcinoma.

Nerve Sheath Markers

S100 Protein

IHC for S100 protein is primarily used in the diagnosis of spindle cell melanoma and nerve sheath tumors of schwannian origin. Although S100 protein is a highly sensitive marker of in these entities, it should be kept in mind that it is by no means specific for melanoma or nerve sheath tumors. Expression may be seen in non-melanoma/non-nerve sheath tumors such as synovial sarcoma, rhabdomyosarcoma, leiomyosarcoma, myoepithelioma, adipocytic tumors, chondrocytic tumors, ossifying fibromyxoid tumor, and chordoma. In contrast to spindled melanomas, which are typically diffusely S100 protein-positive, S-100 protein expression in malignant peripheral nerve sheath tumors tends to be weaker and patchier (Fig. 2.2a and b). Malignant peripheral nerve sheath tumors are exceedingly rare in the skin, and one should be very reluctant to make this particular diagnosis. Regrettably, the distinction of very subtle, hypocellular desmoplastic melanomas from neurofibromas may not be possible by IHC methods alone. It should always be remembered that S100 protein is also present in Langerhans cells; intratumoral Langerhans cells should be rigorously distinguished from positive tumor cells.

Approximately 2–3% of melanomas, particularly "small-cell" melanomas of the sinonasal tract and metastatic melanomas, are negative for S-100 protein (and SOX10). Obviously, in such cases additional immunostaining for a melanosome-specific marker such as HMB-45 or Melan-A is essential for arriving at the correct diagnosis.

SOX10

SOX10 is a transcription factor involved in neural crest development and differentiation of neural crest cells into melanocytic and schwannian lineages. SOX10 is expressed by >85% of melanomas and clear cell sarcomas, essentially all schwannomas and neurofibromas, and 30% of malignant peripheral nerve sheath tumors. SOX10 expression is also common in myoepithelial tumors. In general, other S100 protein-positive tumors are SOX10-negative. The sensitivity of SOX10 for spindle cell melanoma is roughly comparable to that of S100 protein, although there are occasional cases in which one or the other may show more robust immunoreactivity (Fig. 2.2c).

Claudin-1

The claudins are a family of approximately 20 proteins involved in tight junction structure and permeability. Various claudins are differentially expressed in different normal tissue types and tumors. Claudin-1 expression appears to be limited to perineurial cells, and claudin-1 is a useful adjunctive marker of perineuriomas, present in 20–90% of perineuriomas, but not in other tumors in this differential diagnosis, such as neurofibromas, schwannomas, low-grade fibromyxoid sarcomas, etc.

GLUT-1

GLUT-1 is the erythrocyte-type glucose transporter protein. Expression of GLUT-1 protein is a consistent feature of normal perineurial cells and perineurial tumors. However, GLUT-1 expression is by no means specific for perineurial tumors, as it is frequently upregulated in ischemic foci within tumors (i.e., adjacent to necrosis). As with claudin-1, GLUT-1 is best used as an adjunct to EMA immunostaining, rather than as a standalone marker. Among vascular tumors, expression of GLUT-1 protein is seen in essentially all rapidly involuting juvenile capillary hemangiomas, but not in kaposiform hemangioendothelioma.

Melanocyte Specific Markers

HMB-45

Monoclonal antibody HMB-45 identifies the Pmel 17 gene product, gp100. The gp100 antigen is a premelanosomal protein, and as such HMB45 is melanosome-specific, but not melanoma-specific. HMB45 is positive in roughly 85% of conventional melanomas but is almost never positive in spindle cell/desmoplastic melanoma (Fig. 2.2d). HMB45 immunoreactivity is also commonly present in other melanosome-containing tumors, such

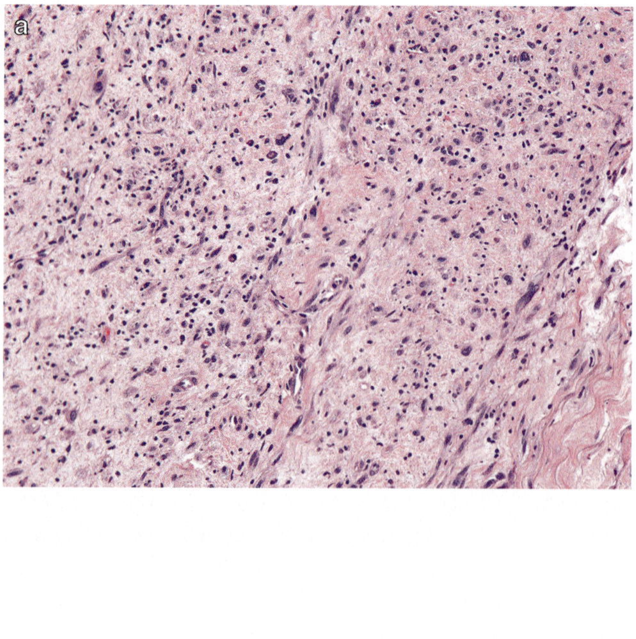

Fig. 2.2 Desmoplastic malignant melanoma (**a**), showing diffuse, strong immunoreactivity for S100 protein (**b**) and SOX10 (**c**). HMB45, Melan-A, tyrosinase, and MiTF were negative in this tumor, as is typically the case (**d**)

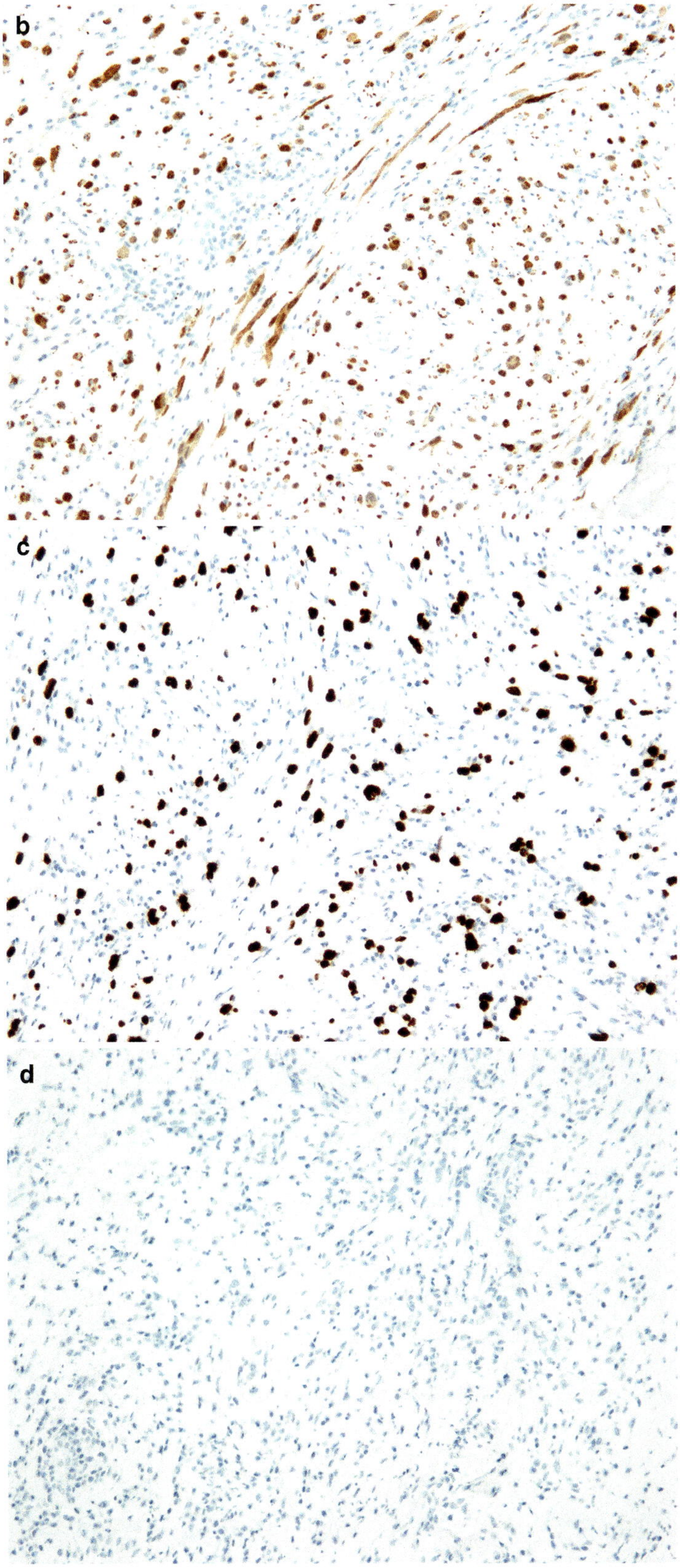

Fig. 2.2 (continued)

as perivascular epithelioid cell tumors and malignant melanotic schwannian tumors (Fig. 2.3a–c).

Melan-A

Melan-A, the product of the *MART-1* gene, is a component of the premelanosomal membrane. In general, the sensitivity and specificity of Melan-A are quite similar to those of HMB45. For unknown reasons, some melanomas express HMB45 but not Melan-A and vice versa. Melan-A is more often positive in resting melanocytes and nevi. The widely used A103 clone to Melan-A also shows reproducible cross-reactivity with an unknown epitope present in steroid-producing tumors and is useful in the diagnosis of adrenal cortical tumors, for instance.

Tyrosinase

Tyrosinase is an enzyme involved in the synthesis of melanin. Antibodies to tyrosinase have a sensitivity and specificity that are roughly equivalent to that of HMB-45 and Melan-A.

Microphthalmia Transcription Factor

Microphthalmia transcription factor (MiTF), the product of the microphthalmia (*MITF*) gene, is a transcription factor critical for melanocyte development. MiTF is expressed in essentially all resting melanocytes and nevi. MiTF is expressed in over 90% of epithelioid melanomas; spindle cell melanomas are less often positive (40%), and true desmoplastic melanomas are very infrequently positive (<5%). MiTF is also expressed in nearly all clear cell sarcomas and in PEComas of all types (Fig. 2.3d). However, MiTF expression is not limited to melanocytic tumors and may be seen in cellular neurothekeomas, leiomyosarcomas, atypical fibroxanthomas, atypical lipomatous neoplasms, and very rare carcinomas. MiTF is best used for the confirmation of S100 protein/SOX10-positive, HMB-45/Melan-A/tyrosinase-negative tumors suspected of being melanomas.

Markers of Smooth and Skeletal Muscle

Desmin

Desmin is the intermediate filament protein associated with both smooth and skeletal muscle differentiation. Desmin expression is much less common in myofibroblastic lesions. Desmin is the most sensitive marker of skeletal muscle tumors, present in nearly 100% of rhabdomyosarcomas of all subtypes and rhabdomyomas. Desmin is a considerably less sensitive marker of tumors of smooth muscle, as it is frequently negative in normal vascular smooth muscle and in tumors derived from such cells. Desmin expression is not, however, specific for myogenic tumors and may be seen in Ewing sarcoma, desmoplastic small round cell tumors, mesenchymal chondrosarcomas, mesothelial tumors, tenosynovial giant cell tumors, ossifying fibromyxoid tumors, angiomatoid fibrous histiocytomas, schwannomas, and melanoma.

Smooth Muscle Actin

Smooth muscle actin isoforms (most often identified with the 1A4 clone) are expressed by essentially all benign and malignant smooth muscle tumors, in glomus tumors and other "myopericytic" tumors such as myopericytoma and myofibroma, and in myofibroblastic lesions such as nodular fasciitis (Fig. 2.4). Smooth muscle actins are also often present in tumors showing myoepithelial differentiation, such as mixed tumors and myoepitheliomas. In general, myofibroblasts show expression of smooth muscle actin only at the periphery of their cytoplasm in a so-called "tram-track" pattern; this is in contrast to the uniform cytoplasmic expression in smooth muscle. One pitfall to be aware of with the use of the 1A4 mAb is aberrant nuclear cross-reactivity, a phenomenon sporadically encountered in many laboratories. Nuclear 1A4 immunoreactivity should not be taken as evidence of smooth muscle differentiation in any tumor.

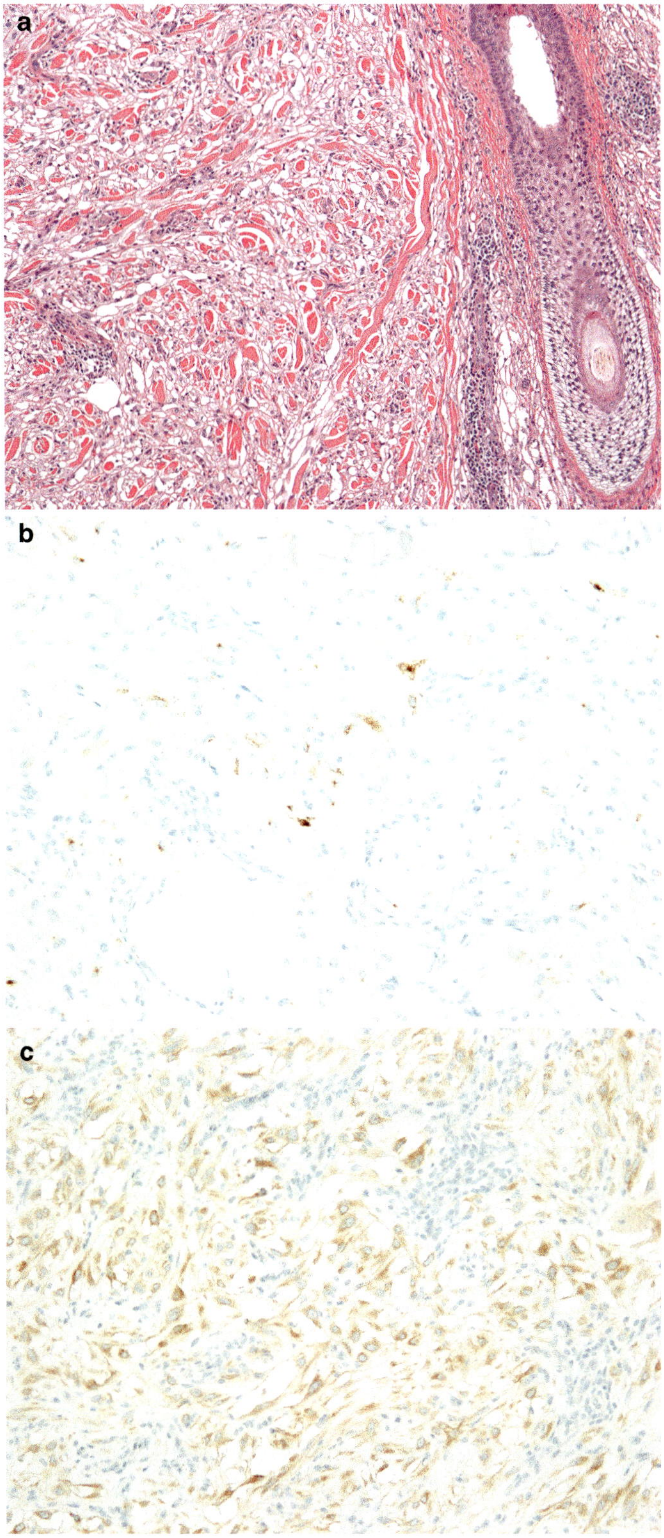

Fig. 2.3 Dermal perivascular epithelioid cell tumor (PEComa) (**a**), showing focal immunoreactivity with HMB45 (**b**) and more extensive expression of smooth muscle actins (**c**) and MiTF (**d**)

Fig. 2.3 (continued)

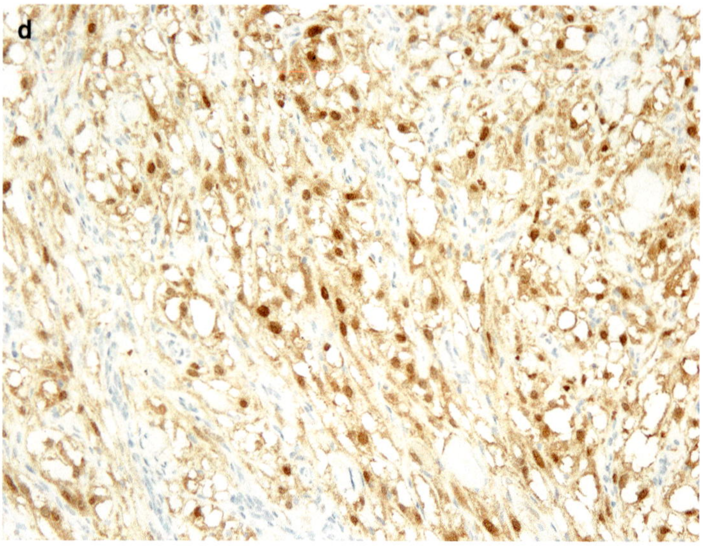

MyoD1 and Myogenin

MyoD1 and myogenin, members of the basic helix-loop-helix family of DNA-binding myogenic nuclear regulatory proteins, are responsible for activation of genes encoding structural proteins such as desmin during embryonic skeletal muscle differentiation. Both MyoD1 and myogenin are expressed by >95% of rhabdomyosarcomas of all types; alveolar rhabdomyosarcomas tend to express very high levels of myogenin and comparatively less MyoD1, whereas embryonal and spindle cell/sclerosing rhabdomyosarcomas often show the opposite pattern. Expression of MyoD1 and myogenin are highly specific for rhabdomyoblastic differentiation, although it is important to keep in mind that they may be expressed in tumors showing heterologous rhabdomyoblastic differentiation, such as squamous cell carcinoma, melanoma, and Merkel cell carcinoma (Fig. 2.5).

H-Caldesmon

Heavy caldesmon is a calcium-binding protein involved in the regulation of smooth muscle contractility. Although the sensitivity of h-caldesmon for smooth muscle tumors is lower than that of smooth muscle actin, h-caldesmon is not expressed by myofibroblastic tumors. H-Caldesmon expression is frequently present in glomus tumors. H-Caldesmon is generally best used for the distinction of poorly differentiated smooth muscle tumors from myofibroblastic tumors, rather than as a first-line marker of smooth muscle cells.

Endothelial Markers

CD31

CD31 is the single best currently available marker of endothelial differentiation, expressed in >90% of angiosarcomas, hemangioendotheliomas, hemangiomas, and Kaposi sarcoma (Fig. 2.6). Other than exceptional carcinomas, CD31 expression is not seen in almost any non-endothelial tissue or tumor, including melanoma. CD31 is, however, commonly expressed by macrophages and platelets. Large numbers of CD31-positive macrophages are routinely present in various malignant neoplasms, and great care should be taken not to mistake these as evidence of focal expression by the tumor cells themselves. CD31 expression in macrophages is distinctly granular and somewhat weak, as compared with the intense, “linear” membrane staining of the endothelium (Fig. 2.7).

CD34

CD34 is cell adhesion molecule expressed on hematopoietic stem cells, endothelium, the interstitial cells of Cajal, and dendritic cells present in the dermis, around blood vessels, and in the nerve sheath. CD34 is expressed in more than 90% of vascular tumors and is a particularly sensitive marker of Kaposi sarcoma. However, CD34 expression is wholly non-specific for vascular tumors and may be seen in dermatofibrosarcoma protuberans, solitary fibrous tumors, malignant peripheral nerve sheath tumors, spindle cell lipomas, and epithelioid sarcomas, among others. CD34 should not be used as a sole endothelial marker.

Podoplanin (D2-40)

Several different markers have been proposed to more specifically identify lymphatic endothelium, including podoplanin (D2-40) and Prox1. Expression of podoplanin is regulated by the homeobox gene *PROX1* and is normally seen in lymphatic endothelial cells, glomerular

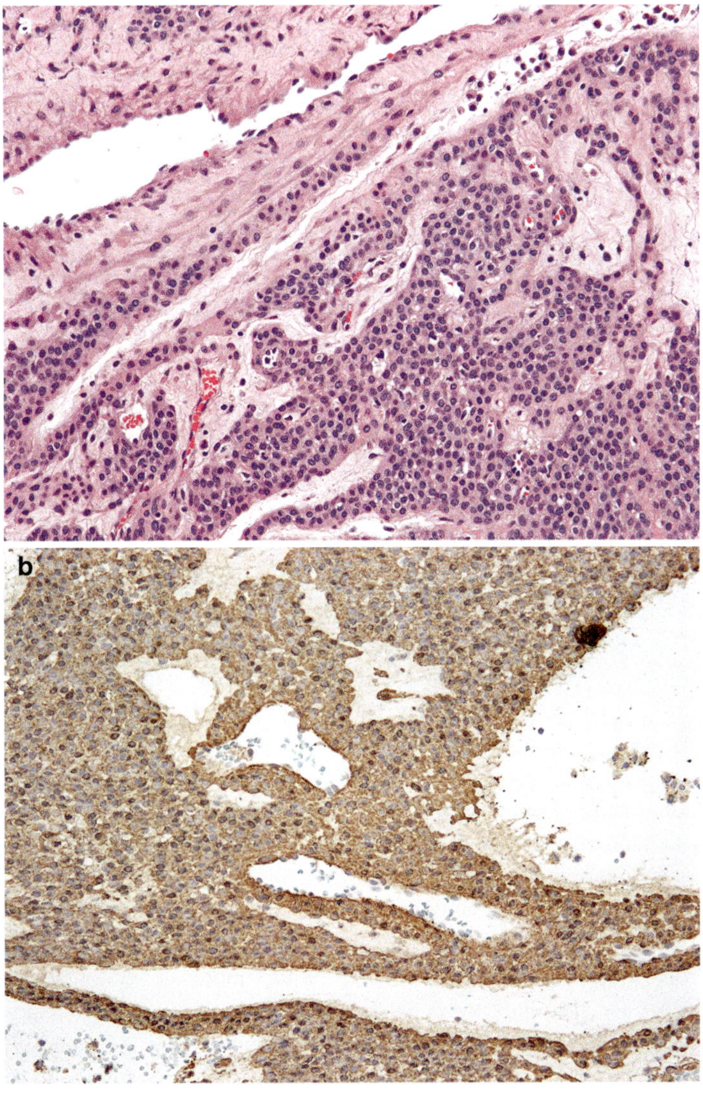

Fig. 2.4 Glomus tumor (**a**) showing diffuse expression of smooth muscle actins (**b**) and caldesmon (**c**). Glomus cells are also typically uniformly invested by collagen IV, as shown here (**d**)

Fig. 2.4 (continued)

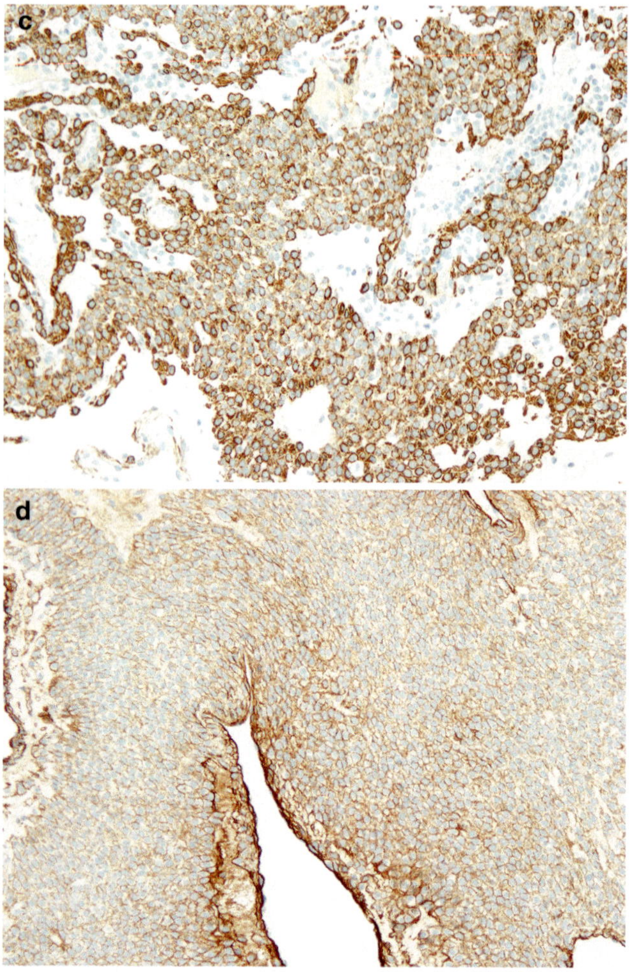

podocytes, choroid plexus epithelium, type 1 alveolar cells, osteoblasts, and mesothelial cells. Regrettably, podoplanin expression is present in a wide variety of endothelial tumors, including those without obvious features of lymphatic differentiation, and in many different types of mesenchymal, germ cell, and glial neoplasms. Similarly, Prox1expression does not appear to be confined to lymphatic-type endothelium or even to endothelial tumors. Thus, although antibodies to podoplanin and Prox1 may occasionally be of some value in the identification of certain lymphatic proliferations, they generally play little role in the diagnosis of endothelial tumors more generally. Certainly these markers have no role in the differential diagnosis of cutaneous spindle cell tumors.

FLI1 and ERG

FLI1 and ERG are members of the ETS family of transcription factors and represent the best *nuclear* markers of endothelial differentiation. Both FLI-1 and ERG are positive in >95% of endothelial neoplasms of all types. It is important to recognize that FLI1 and ERG are not specific markers of endothelial differentiation, as they may also be present in Ewing sarcoma, a variety of carcinomas, and rare melanomas, mesotheliomas, and hematolymphoid neoplasms. FLI1 and ERG have not been reported in spindle cell melanomas, sarcomatoid squamous carcinomas or AFX/SUDPS, although relatively few cases have been studied. FLI-1 and ERG are helpful in the differential diagnosis of epithelioid forms of angiosarcoma

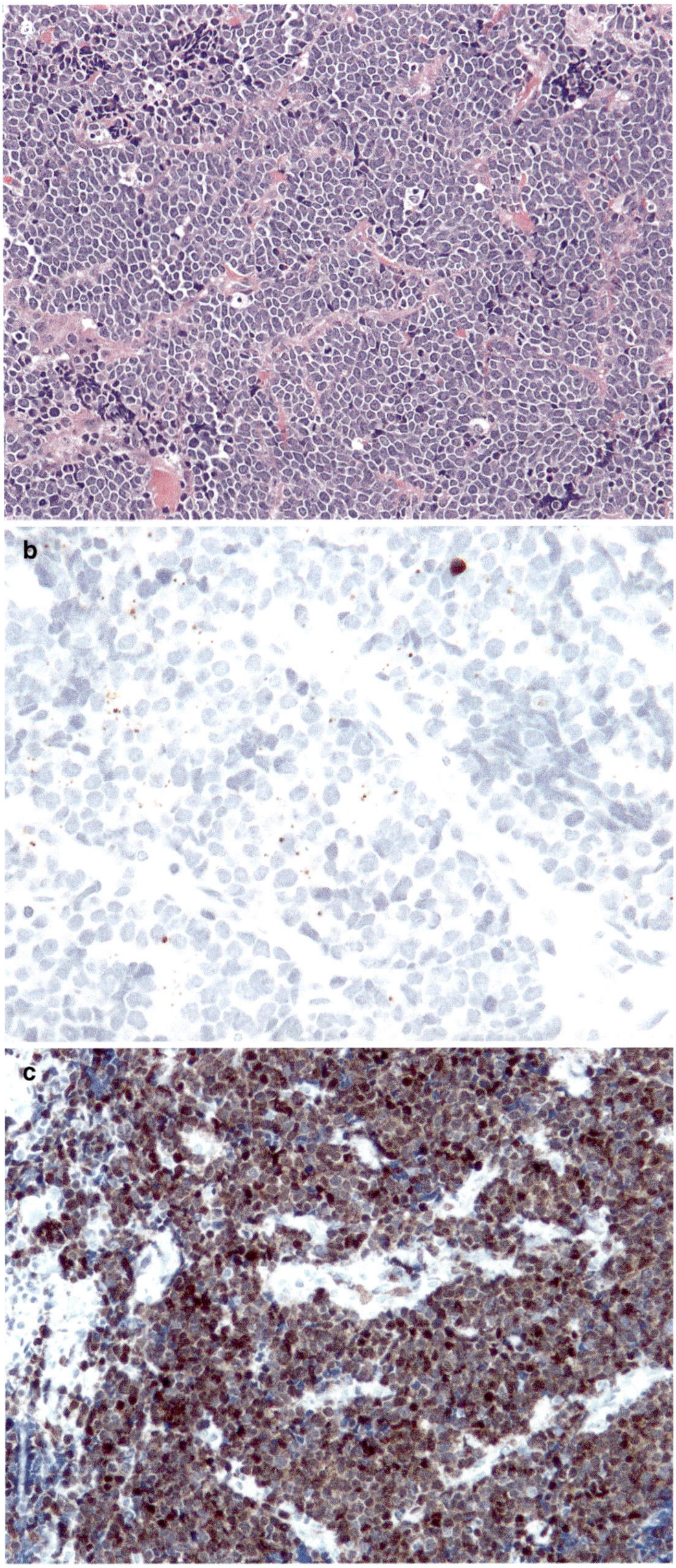

Fig. 2.5 Merkel cell carcinoma, (**a**), showing "dot-like" expression of keratin 20 (**b**) and diffuse expression of Merkel cell polyomavirus large T antigen (**c**). This case also showed aberrant expression of skeletal muscle markers, including desmin (not shown) and myogenin (**d**)

Fig. 2.5 (continued)

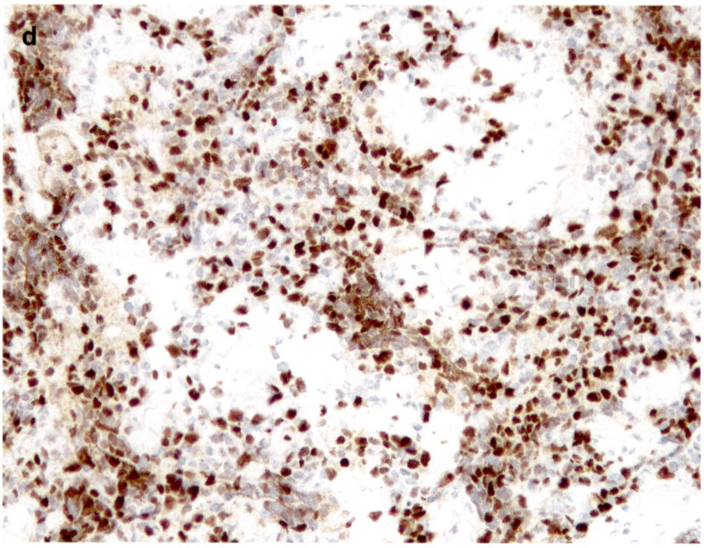

from epithelioid sarcoma, which is usually (but not always) negative for both markers. Although FLI1 and ERG are very useful markers, they are best used in combination with CD31 and a panel of other relevant markers and should not be used as one's sole endothelial marker.

vWF (Factor VIII)

The von Willebrand factor (vWF) was the first endothelium-specific marker employed in diagnostic immunohistochemical studies. vWF is the least sensitive of the vascular markers, positive in only 50–75% of vascular tumors. Although vWF expression is, in theory, absolutely specific for vascular tumors, technical problems limit its usefulness. vWF is not only produced by endothelial cells but circulates in the serum; and it therefore can be found often in zones of tumor necrosis and hemorrhage. In general, CD31, FLI1, and ERG are superior endothelial markers.

Histiocytic Markers (CD68, CD163, CD11c, CD4)

Antibodies to CD68 continue to be used by many pathologists as a marker of histiocytic differentiation; CD68 represents an entirely non-specific lysosomal antigen. Although macrophages contain large numbers of lysosomes (accounting for their CD68 expression), lysosomal accumulation may also be seen in a very large number of non-histiocytic tumors, including (but not limited to) granular cell tumors and granular cell variants of melanoma, carcinoma, angiosarcoma, and undifferentiated pleomorphic sarcoma. Thus, CD68 is an exceptionally non-specific marker. In particular, CD68 expression in a spindle cell neoplasm does not imply "fibrohistiocytic" differentiation. CD163, CD11c, and CD4 represent much more lineage-restricted markers of histiocytes and their tumors, including solitary (juvenile) xanthogranuloma (Fig. 2.8).

ALK

Expression of ALK is characteristic of epithelioid fibrous histiocytoma and is not seen in other variants of fibrous histiocytoma or in various epithelioid neoplasms that may mimic EFH (Fig. 2.9).

Markers that Are Generally of Little Value

Vimentin

Vimentin, an intermediate filament protein, is expressed in all mesenchymal cells and in virtually all mesenchymal tumors and is of minimal

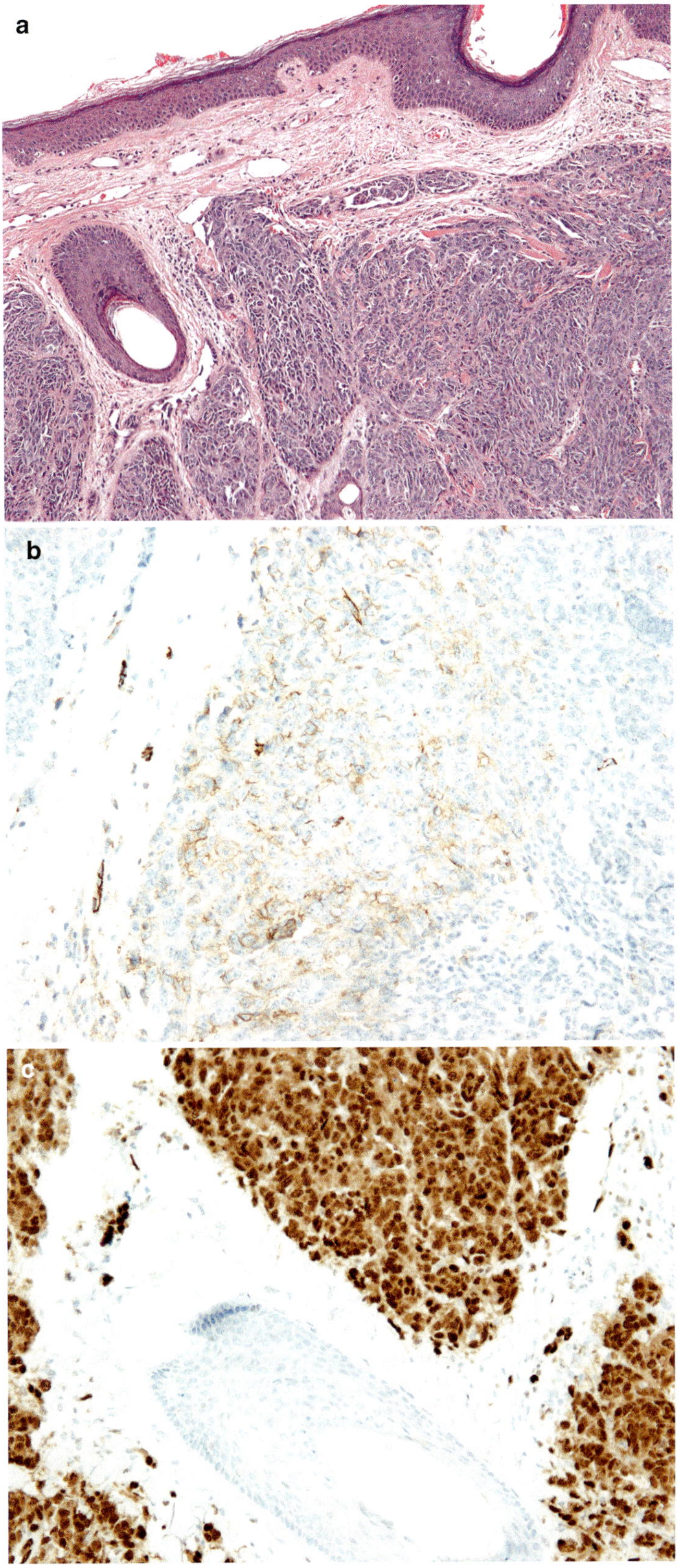

Fig. 2.6 Poorly differentiated angiosarcoma (**a**) with membranous expression of CD31 (**b**), intense nuclear immunoreactivity for ERG protein (**c**), and more limited expression of FLI1 protein (**d**)

Fig. 2.6 (continued)

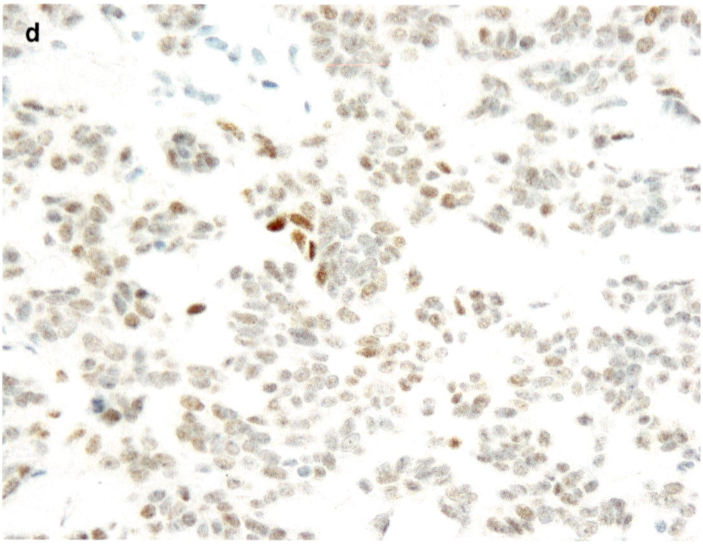

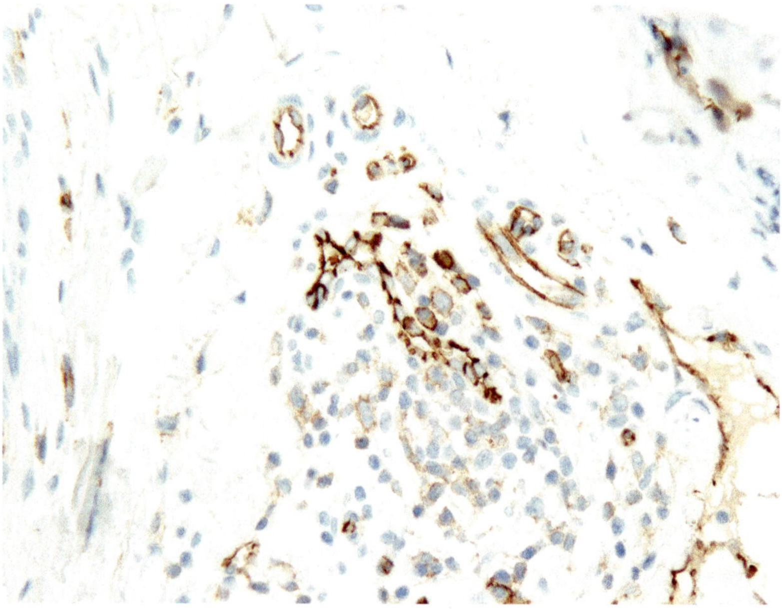

Fig. 2.7 CD31 expression is not confined to endothelial cells, and is also routinely present in macrophages, as shown here. CD31 expression in macrophages tends to be weaker and more granular than expression in endothelial cells. It is important not to mistake CD31-positive macrophages for tumor cells in a non-endothelial neoplasm

value in identifying particular tumors. Vimentin expression is also of little value in the immunohistochemical distinction of carcinomas from sarcomas. Vimentin immunoreactivity has been touted as a good marker of tissue preservation. However, vimentin expression, similar to that of all the intermediate filaments, is rather hardy and may remain present in tissues in which all other immunoreactivity has been lost. In general, there is no value in performing vimentin immunostains on any spindle cell neoplasm.

PGP9.5

PGP9.5 is an ubiquitin carboxyl terminal hydrolase originally identified in neurons and initially thought to be neuron-specific. However,

PGP9.5 expression is in fact essentially "ubiquitous" among tumors. Despite claims to the contrary, there is really no role for PGP9.5 immunohistochemistry in the diagnosis of dermal soft tissue tumors, in particular in the differential diagnosis of nerve sheath tumors and neurothekeoma.

Putative Markers of Atypical Fibroxanthoma and/or Superficial Undifferentiated Pleomorphic Sarcoma (CD99, CD10, Procollagen, CD34)

The dermatopathology literature is replete with studies examining the relative value of markers such as CD99, CD10, procollagen, and CD34 in the diagnosis of atypical fibroxanthoma (AFX) and in its distinction from superficial undifferentiated pleomorphic sarcoma (SUPS). Despite their widespread usage, none of these markers is useful in this differential diagnosis or in the distinction of AFX/SUPS from other pleomorphic spindle cell malignancies. Expression of all of these markers can be seen in both AFX and in SUPS and in many other spindle cell malignancies that may mimic these tumors. In the appropriate morphological context, however, expression of CD10 in combination with MiTF is characteristic of cellular neurothekeoma (Fig. 2.10).

Applications of Immunohistochemistry and Fluorescence In Situ Hybridization in Various Differential Diagnoses in Cutaneous Soft Tissue Pathology

IHC in the Evaluation of Cutaneous Pleomorphic Spindle Cell Tumors

This is one of the most common differential diagnoses in cutaneous soft tissue pathology and in most instances relates to the distinction of nonmesenchymal tumors (e.g., sarcomatoid squamous cell carcinoma and spindle cell melanoma) from atypical fibroxanthoma/superficial undifferentiated pleomorphic sarcoma (AFX/SUPS). Particularly in the setting of significant sun damage, this differential diagnosis may also include spindled forms of angiosarcoma. Rarely, other pleomorphic spindle cell tumors, such as leio-

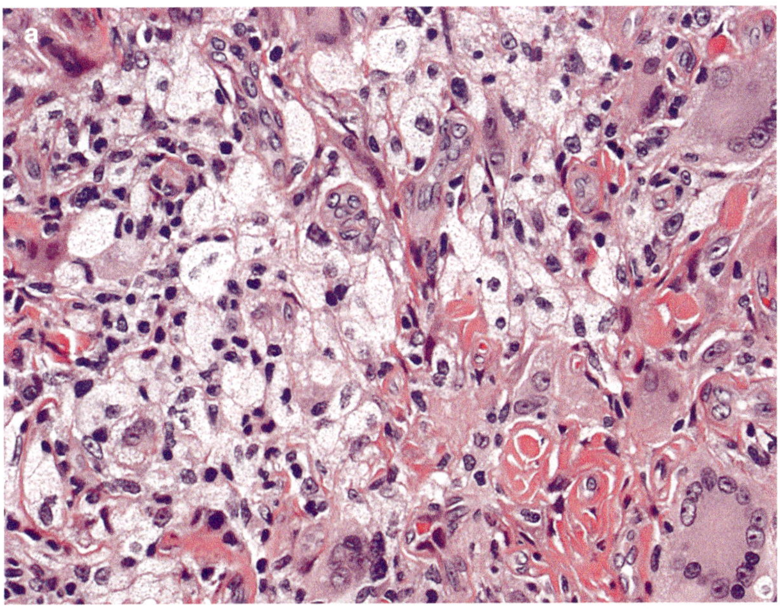

Fig. 2.8 Lipidized solitary xanthogranuloma (**a**), showing diffuse expression of the histiocyte-restricted markers CD163 (**b**) and C11c (**c**)

Fig. 2.8 (continued)

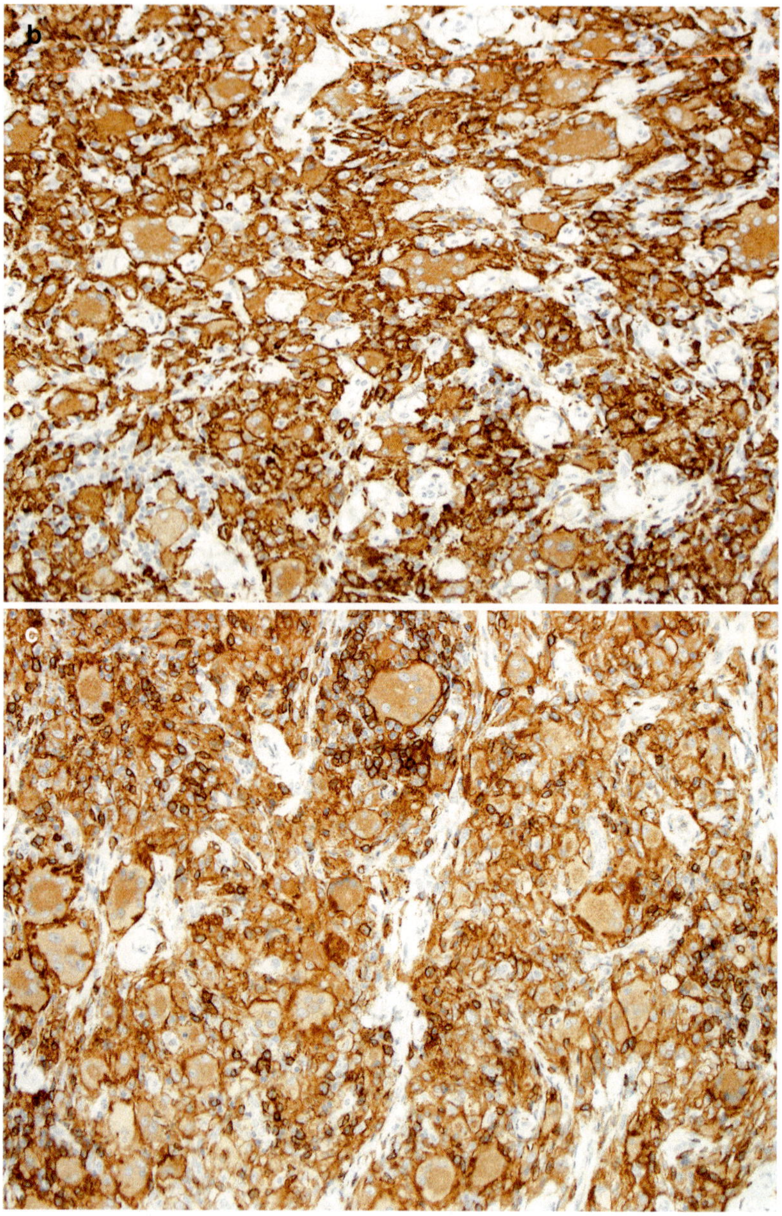

myosarcoma, rhabdomyosarcoma, pleomorphic liposarcoma, and osteosarcoma, may enter this differential diagnosis.

Table 2.4 lists a small panel of immunostains that may be helpful in this differential diagnosis, with their expected patterns of immunoreactivity in common and less common pleomorphic spindle cell tumors of the skin. In general, the differential diagnosis of these tumors is fairly straightforward, with expression of keratins in sarcomatoid squamous cell carcinoma, expression of S100 protein and SOX10 in spindle cell melanoma, expression of endothelial markers such as CD31/FLI1/ERG in spindled angiosarcoma, and absent expression of all relevant markers in AFX/SUPS. Essentially all spindle cell tumors in any anatomical location are vimentin-positive, and vimentin plays no role in this differential diagnosis.

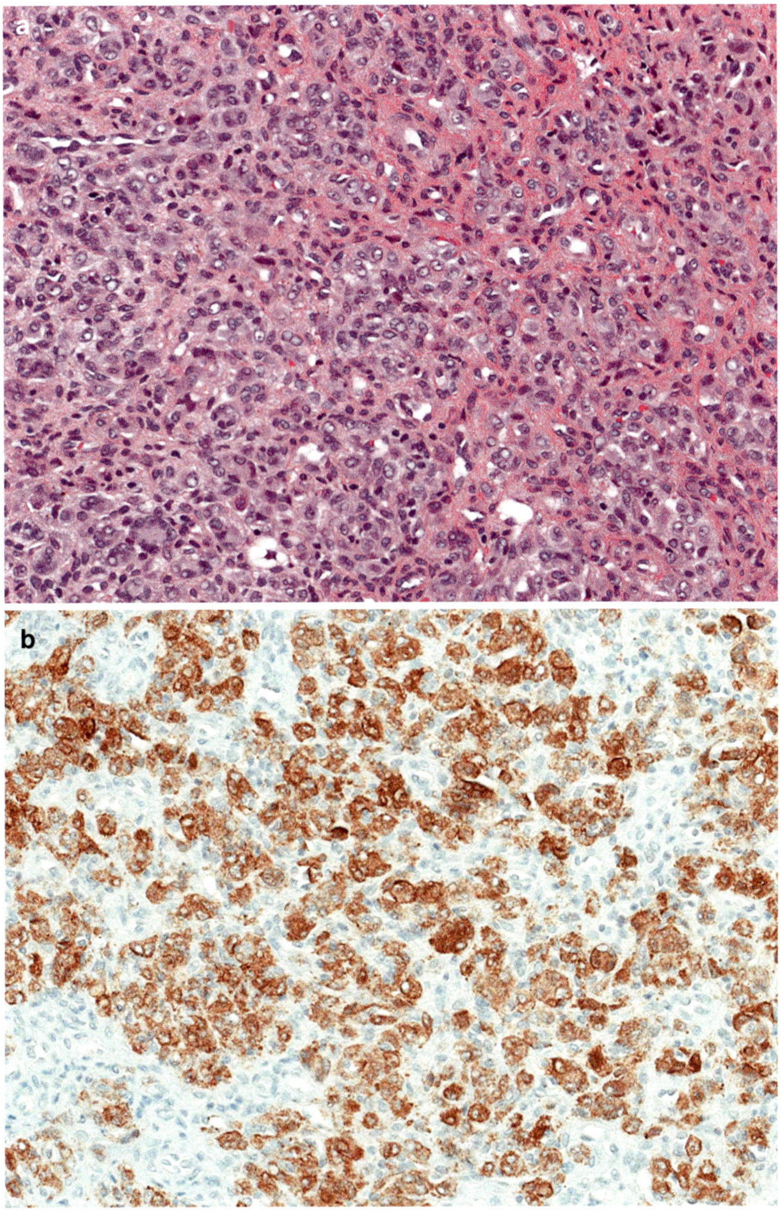

Fig. 2.9 Epithelioid fibrous histiocytoma (**a**) showing diffuse expression of ALK protein (**b**)

Leiomyosarcoma

It is important to keep in mind that the overwhelming majority of primary cutaneous leiomyosarcomas (also referred to as "atypical intradermal smooth muscle tumors" because of their superb prognosis) are very well-differentiated, non-pleomorphic lesions. Thus, leiomyosarcoma does not generally enter into the differential diagnosis of pleomorphic spindle cell tumors of the skin, except when a metastatic lesion from a soft tissue, visceral, or gynecologic primary tumor is a consideration. Antibodies to smooth muscle actin isoforms (e.g., the 1A4 mAb) represent the most sensitive markers of smooth muscle differentiation, although they are also routinely expressed by a variety of other cutaneous tumors, including myofibroblastic proliferations and neoplasm, cellular fibrous histiocytomas, glomus tumors, myoepithelial tumors, and cellular neurothekeomas. Antibodies to caldesmon and myosin heavy chain represent more specific markers of smooth muscle differentiation than do smooth muscle actins, although they are expressed by a smaller percentage of leiomyosarcomas, in particular poorly differentiated tumors. Glomus tumors are also routinely caldesmon-positive, and myosin heavy chain may be expressed by myoepithelial tumors. Although antibodies to desmin are used in many laboratories as "screening" markers for leiomyosarcoma, desmin expression is actually frequently absent in normal vascular smooth muscle and in tumors derived from it. Desmin is a much better screening marker for tumors of skeletal muscle differentiation.

Atypical Fibroxanthoma/Superficial Undifferentiated Pleomorphic Sarcoma (AFX/SUPS)

AFX typically presents as a rapidly growing mass in a sun-exposed region of an older adult. The diagnosis of AFX should be reserved for small (<1–1.5 cm) lesions that are confined to the dermis and which are completely visualized. The prognosis for larger tumors and tumors showing involvement of the subcutis is considerably worse, and such lesions should be labeled SUPS or pleomorphic dermal sarcoma. Histologically, most AFX are undifferentiated, pleomorphic spindle cell tumors, although relatively monomorphic variants do exist. In younger patients, and in non-sun-exposed skin, AFX/SUPS should be rigorously distinguished from atypical fibrous histiocytomas.

AFX/SUPS is a histologic and immunohistochemical diagnosis of exclusion. There are no markers or combinations of markers that establish the diagnosis of AFX/SUPS. The lesional cells of AFX must be negative for keratins (using more than one keratin antibody), S100 protein, and SOX10 (Fig. 2.11). Limited expression of smooth muscle actins, indicative of myofibroblastic differentiation, is acceptable, but caldesmon/desmin expression is not seen. AFX commonly contains S100 protein-positive Langerhans cells, CD31-positive endothelial cells and macrophages and Factor XIIIa-positive dendritic cells, and these must be carefully distinguished from the neoplastic cells. Despite their historical labeling as "fibrohistiocytic" neoplasms, AFX/SUPS have no relationship to true histiocytic tumors, and IHC for markers such as CD68 and CD163 plays no role in their differential diagnosis. CD68, in

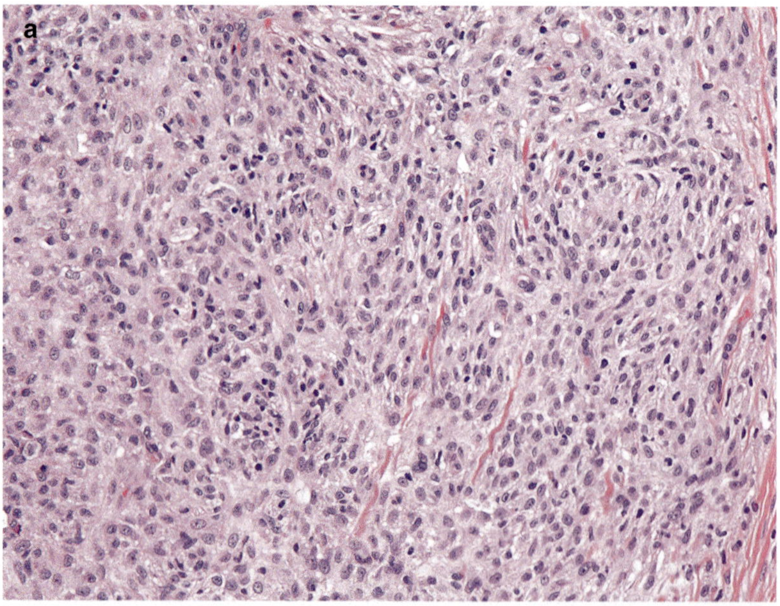

Fig. 2.10 Cellular neurothekeoma (**a**). Although there are no specific markers of cellular neurothekeoma, co-expression of CD10 (**b**) and MiTF (**c**) is a characteristic in the appropriate morphological context

Fig. 2.10 (continued)

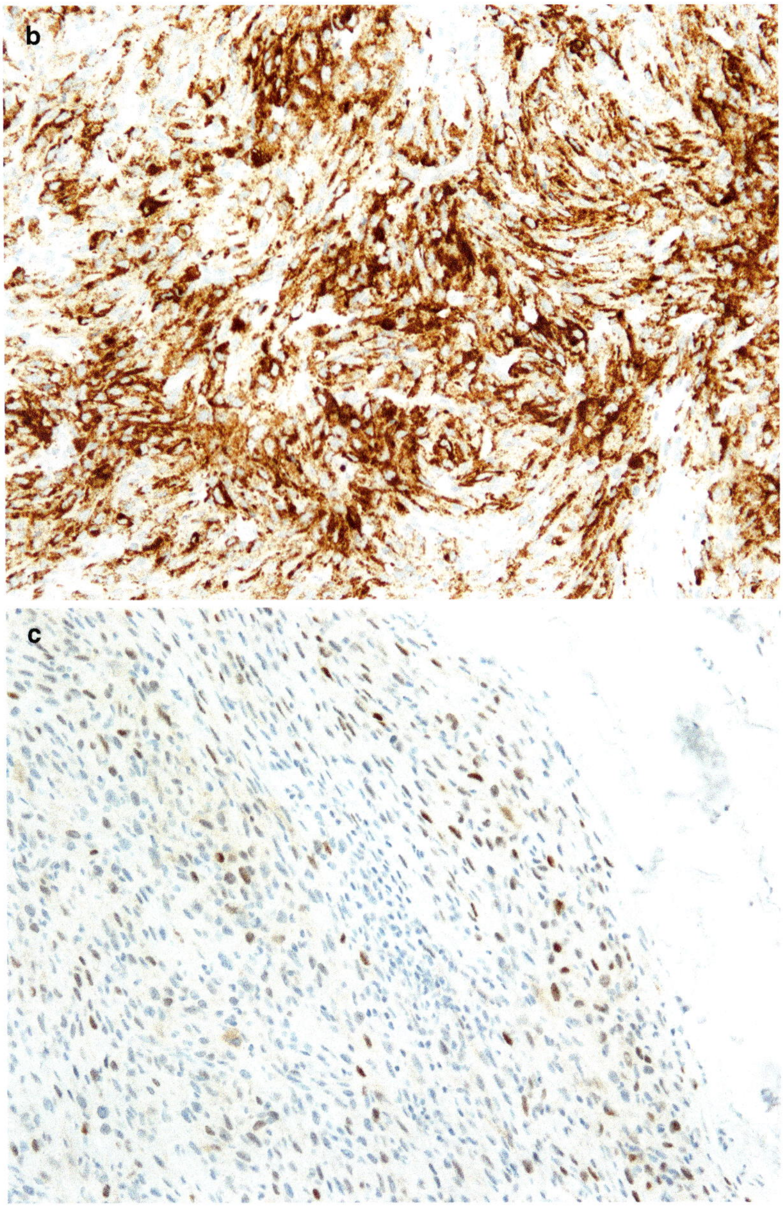

Table 2.4 IHC panel for the evaluation of pleomorphic spindle cell neoplasms

Antigen	CA	Melanoma	AS	LMS	RMS	AFX/SUDPS
Keratin	Positive	Variable	Variable	Variable	Negative	Negative
S-100 protein and/or SOX10	Negative	Positive	Negative	Negative	Negative	Negative
Smooth muscle actin	Negative	Negative	Negative	Positive	Negative	Variable
Desmin	Negative	Variable	Negative	Variable	Positive	Negative
CD31	Negative	Negative	Positive	Negative	Negative	Negative

AFX/SUDPS atypical fibroxanthoma/superficial undifferentiated pleomorphic sarcoma, *AS* angiosarcoma, *CA* carcinoma, *LMS* leiomyosarcoma, *RMS* rhabdomyosarcoma

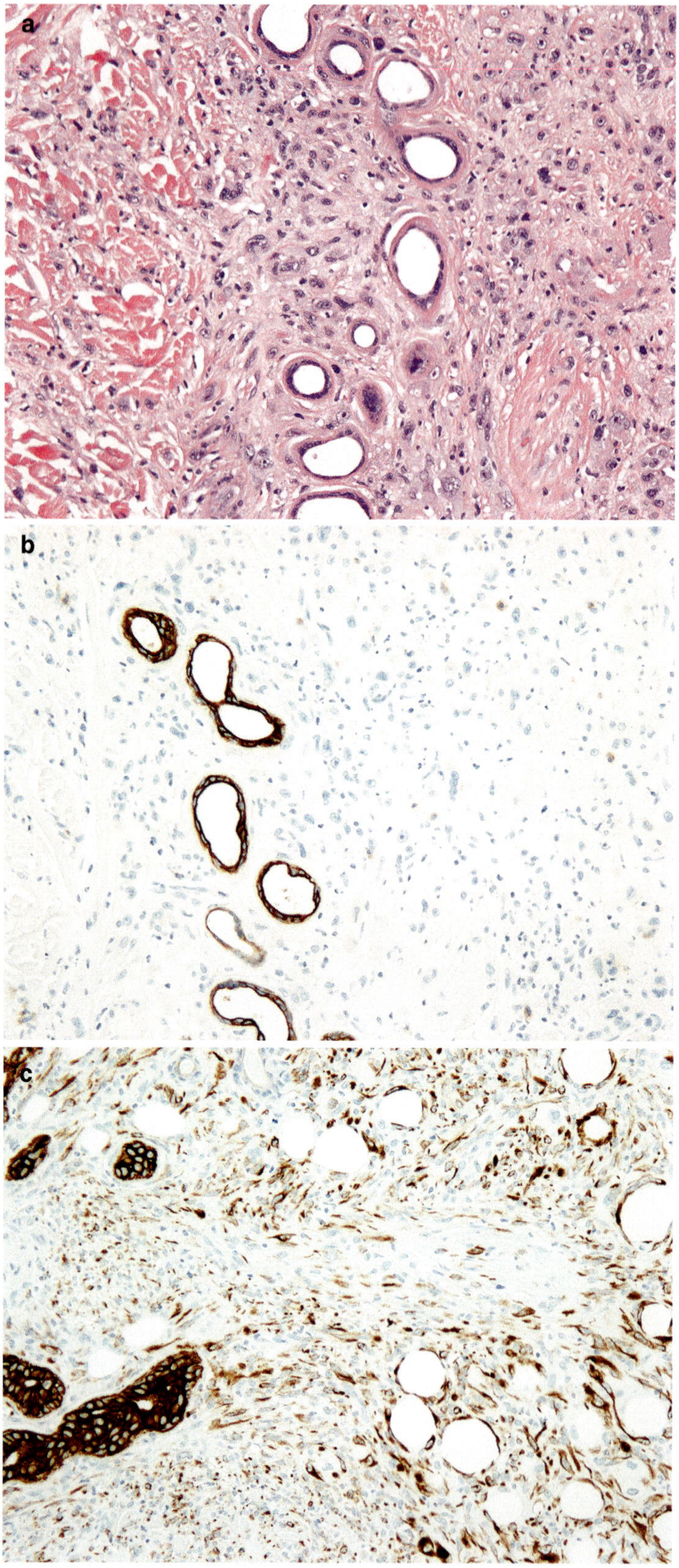

Fig. 2.11 The diagnosis of atypical fibroxanthoma must be one of exclusion, rendered only after a comprehensive panel of immunostains has excluded other possibilities. This malignant spindle cell tumor (**a**) was submitted in consultation as "atypical fibroxanthoma," with negative immunostains for melanoma-associated markers, markers of muscle differentiation, and keratins (using the AE1/AE3 antibodies) (**b**). However, it was strongly positive with the OSCAR keratin antibody (**c**) and represents a sarcomatoid squamous cell carcinoma

particular, is a non-specific marker of lysosomes and may be expressed by essentially any tumor type. There is no role for CD99, CD10, procollagen, or CD34 in this differential diagnosis.

Other Rare Pleomorphic Spindle Cell Sarcomas that May Involve the Skin

Essentially any pleomorphic sarcoma may occasionally present as a tumor involving the skin. For many of these tumors, IHC is not of value, as diagnosis depends on the identification of specific histologic features (e.g., pleomorphic lipoblasts in pleomorphic liposarcoma, osteoid in extraskeletal osteosarcoma). Exceptionally rare pleomorphic rhabdomyosarcomas involving the skin show expression of the specific markers of skeletal muscle differentiation, myogenin, and MyoD1, in addition to desmin.

IHC in the Differential Diagnosis of "Monomorphic" Spindle Cell Cutaneous Tumors

For practical purposes, the differential diagnosis of relatively monomorphic spindle cell tumors involving the skin centers around the distinction of dermatofibrosarcoma protuberans (DFSP) from cellular forms of benign cellular fibrous histiocytoma (CFH) (dermatofibroma). Other tumors that can be included in this differential diagnosis include predominantly spindled forms of solitary (juvenile) xanthogranuloma (SXG), dermatomyofibroma (DMF), low-grade fibromyxoid sarcoma (LGFMS), and perineurioma. Table 2.5 illustrates a panel of immunostains that may be helpful in some of these diagnoses.

DFSP, CFH, and Related Lesions

Despite the massive literature that exists on the immunohistochemical distinction of DFSP from CFH, this seems to us a fairly straightforward distinction. DFSP consists of a rather monomorphic proliferation of slender, lightly eosinophilic spindled cells with darkly staining nuclei, which grow in a diffusely infiltrative fashion into the subcutaneous fat and in almost all instances show intense, diffuse expression of CD34. Although pigmented forms of DFSP (Bednar tumor) may contain intermixed S100 protein and Melan-A-positive melanocytes, the great majority of DFSP lack other intermixed cell types showing expression of markers such as actins, CD163, etc. In contrast, CFH tends to consist of more variable, plumper spindled cells, occasionally with admixed siderophages and foamy macrophages. Involvement of the subcutaneous fat is typically quite limited in CFH and is often accompanied by lymphoid aggregates. By IHC, the lesional cells of CFH are negative for CD34, although nonneoplastic CD34-positive cells are often found adjacent to the tumor cells, sometimes forming a rim around the deep border of the tumor (Fig. 2.12). Although many pathologists believe that CFH should be Factor 13A-positive, this is in fact not the case. Large series of CFH have shown absent Factor 13A expression in up to 70% of CFH, and our own experience suggests that this figure may be much higher, if only Factor 13A expression by the lesional cells themselves is considered. The most characteristic feature of CFH, immunohistochemically, is the presence of multiple cell populations, including Factor 13A, CD34, S100 protein, and CD68-positive cells. Many CFH show limited myofibroblastic differentiation in the form of smooth muscle actin expression in a "tram-track" pattern; this should not be misinterpreted as evidence of "leiomyosarcoma," particularly as CFH may show mitotic figures and foci of necrosis. In exceptional instances, demonstration of the DFSP-associated molecular events, rearrangements, and amplification of *PDGFB* may be helpful in the definitive diagnosis of DFSP.

The morphological features of CFH also overlap to a degree with those of SXG. IHC may be quite helpful in the diagnosis of SXG, as these lesions typically display diffuse, strong immunoreactivity for Factor 13A in the neoplastic cells themselves, in addition to co-expression of histiocytic markers, including CD163, CD45, CD11c,

Table 2.5 Screening panel for selected monomorphic spindle cell tumors of the skin

Antigen	DFSP	BFH	SXG	PN	LGFMS
CD34	Positive	Variable[a]	Negative	Variable	Rare
Factor XIIIa	Negative	Variable[a]	Positive	Negative	Negative
CD163	Negative	Variable[a]	Positive	Negative	Negative
EMA	Negative	Negative	Negative	Positive	Variable
MUC4	Negative	Negative	Negative	Negative	Positive

BFH benign fibrous histiocytoma (dermatofibroma), *DFSP* dermatofibrosarcoma protuberans, *LGFMS* low-grade fibromyxoid sarcoma, *PN* perineurioma, *SXG* solitary (juvenile) xanthogranuloma

[a]BFH most often shows an admixture of CD34, Factor 13A, and CD163-positive cells, but close inspection often shows the lesional cells to be negative for all tested markers

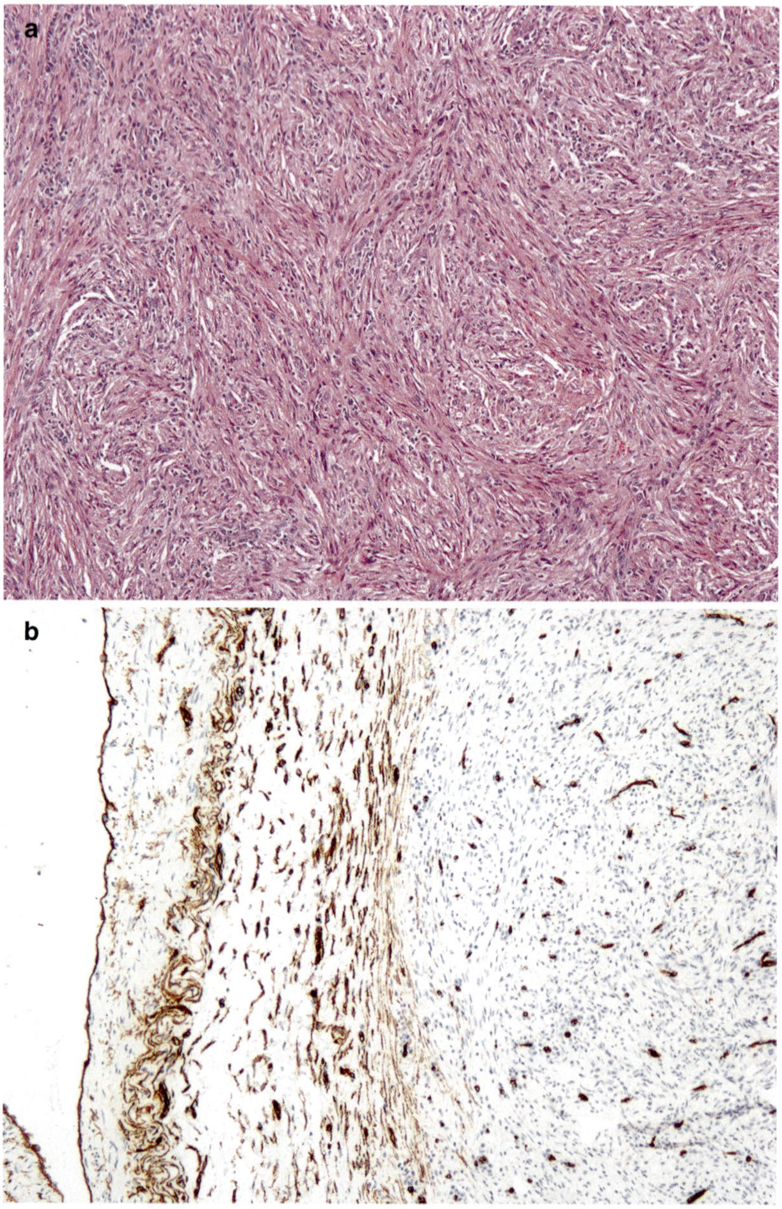

Fig. 2.12 Cellular benign fibrous histiocytoma (**a**). Although the lesional cells themselves are negative for CD34, a surrounding rim of CD34-positive spindled cells is often present (**b**). This should not be interpreted as evidence of “progression” to dermatofibrosarcoma protuberans

CD4, and CD31 (Fig. 2.13). Again, although CFH often contain cell populations that express Factor 13A or histiocytic markers, the lesional cells tend to be negative for both.

DMF may also resemble CFH, although the tumor cells tend to grow in fascicles oriented parallel to the overlying epidermis, and generally lack the cytologic variability of CFH. Despite their name, fewer than 30% of DMF express smooth muscle actins, and IHC generally does not play a large role in this diagnosis. DMF most often show a purely fibroblastic phenotype, with expression only of vimentin.

LGFMS and Perineurioma

Although LGFMS is typically thought of as a deeply situated soft tissue sarcoma of adults, it may occur in superficial locations including the skin, particularly in children. The morphological features of LGFMS in the skin are similar to those of deeply seated tumor, with markedly hypocellular, heavily collagenized zones, juxtaposed to more cellular myxoid nodules, often showing a whorling growth pattern and a well-developed, arborizing vasculature. Until very recently, IHC played little role in the diagnosis of LGFMS. However, it is now understood that nearly 100% of LGFMS are MUC4-positive, a finding that correlates extremely well with the presence of the LGFMS-specific *FUS-CREB3L2/CREB3L1* gene fusions (Fig. 2.14). IHC for MUC4 may thus serve as an excellent surrogate to molecular genetic studies (*FUS* FISH) in the diagnosis of LGFMS.

Approximately 40% of LGFMS also express epithelial membrane antigen (EMA), a finding that may cause confusion with perineurioma, especially as the morphological features of these two tumors overlap to a degree. In addition to EMA, perineuriomas typically show some combination of CD34, claudin-1, and GLUT1 expression, markers not expressed by LGFMS (Fig. 2.15). Expression of claudin-1, a tight junction-related protein, and GLUT1, a glucose transported molecule, in perineuriomas likely reflects the normal role of the perineurial cell in the establishment of the blood-nerve barrier. Expression of these markers, and absent expression of S100 protein and SOX10, also helps to distinguish perineuriomas from other nerve sheath tumors, such as schwannoma, solitary circumscribed neuroma, and neurofibroma.

IHC in the Differential Diagnosis of Epithelioid Malignant Cutaneous Tumors

The differential diagnosis of epithelioid malignancies in the skin is relatively broad and includes various types of carcinoma, melanoma, hematolymphoid tumors, and sarcomas, including epithelioid angiosarcoma, epithelioid sarcoma, malignant myoepithelioma (myoepithelial carcinoma), epithelioid malignant peripheral nerve sheath tumor, and other very rare sarcomas. Discussions of the immunophenotypes of the many different types of carcinoma that may involve the skin are beyond the scope of this chapter, as is a discussion of hematolymphoid tumors. Table 2.6 details a relatively small panel of IHC markers that may be of value in the differential diagnosis of malignant epithelioid tumors involving the skin.

Epithelioid Sarcoma and Epithelioid Endothelial Tumors

The distinction of epithelioid sarcoma from primary cutaneous carcinomas of various types, in particular squamous cell carcinoma, may be challenging and is of great clinical significance. Like squamous cell carcinoma, epithelioid sarcoma typically expresses keratins of both low- and high-molecular-weight types. Expression of keratin 5/6 is not, however, generally seen in epithelioid sarcoma. Squamous carcinomas may also express vimentin, particularly when they have at least some spindled morphology, and the presence of vimentin co-expression is not a specific feature of epithelioid sarcoma. In contrast, expression of CD34 is not a feature of carcinomas and is present in roughly 60% of epithelioid sarcomas. The most

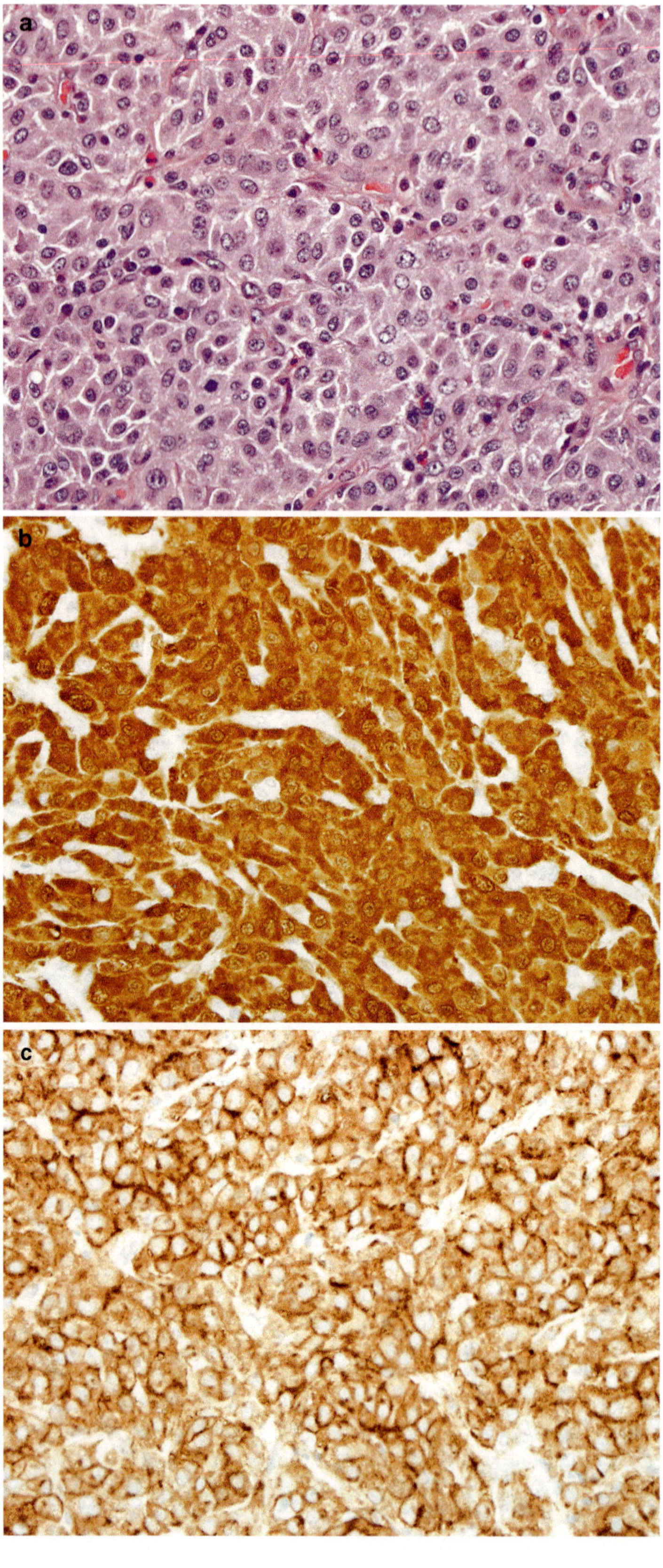

Fig. 2.13 Non-lipidized solitary xanthogranuloma (**a**), with intense immunoreactivity for Factor 13A in the tumor cells (**b**). Histiocytic markers, such as CD4, were also positive (**c**)

useful IHC marker for the distinction of epithelioid sarcoma from carcinoma is loss of expression of the SMARCB1 (INI1) tumor suppressor gene product. Loss of SMARCB1 is seen in approximately 90% of epithelioid sarcomas and is not a feature of the squamous cell carcinoma or of the overwhelming majority of other common human epithelial neoplasms (Fig. 2.16). Loss of SMARCB1 expression in epithelioid sarcoma typically is the result of *SMARCB1* gene deletion.

Loss of expression of SMARCB1 is also useful in the distinction of epithelioid sarcoma (especially those showing "pseudovascular" changes) from epithelioid endothelial tumors, in particular angiosarcoma. Epithelioid endothelial tumors that enter the differential diagnosis of epithelioid sarcoma include epithelioid angiosarcoma, epithelioid hemangioma, epithelioid hemangioendothelioma, and epithelioid sarcoma-like/pseudomyogenic hemangioendothelioma. Although all of these lesions may show keratin expression (and sometimes CD34), they all show normal (retained) expression of SMARCB1. Epithelioid hemangiomas and epithelioid sarcoma-like/pseudomyogenic hemangioendotheliomas frequently express FOSB protein, reflecting the *FOS* gene rearrangements and *SERPINE1-FOSB* fusions seen in these entities, respectively (Fig. 2.17). Epithelioid hemangioendotheliomas typically express CAMTA1 protein, resulting from the *WWTR1-CAMTA1* fusions that define this entity (Fig. 2.18).

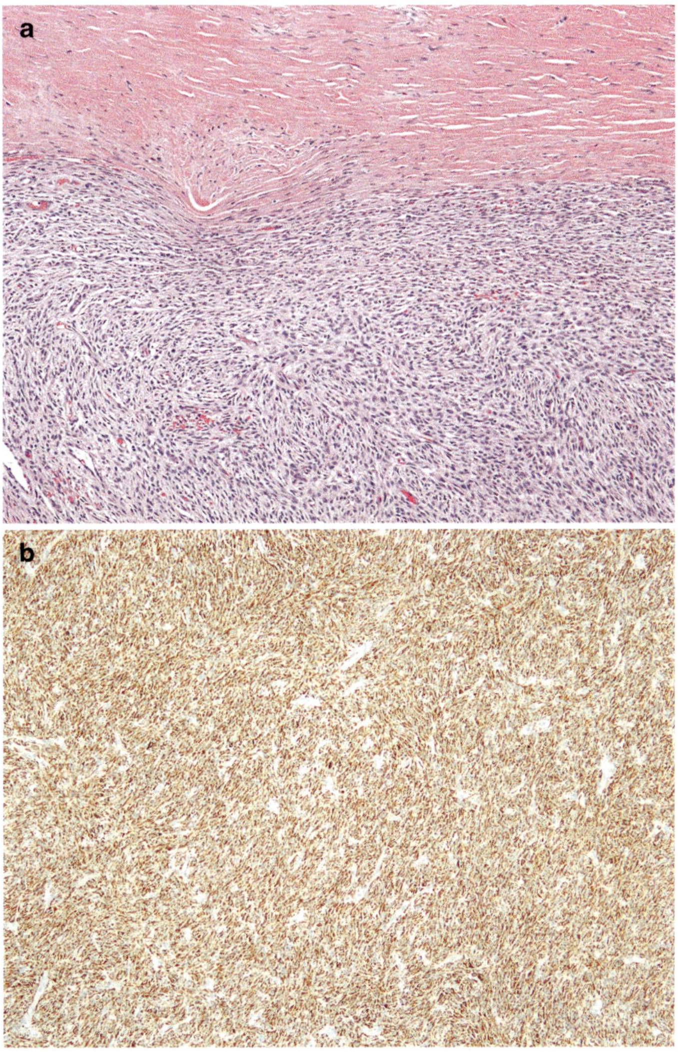

Fig. 2.14 Low-grade fibromyxoid sarcoma (**a**) with diffuse expression of MUC4 (**b**)

Melanoma

As noted above, almost all melanomas show strong expression of S100 protein and SOX10. Expression of S100 protein can be seen in some carcinomas, but usually not squamous cell carcinoma, whereas SOX10 expression seems to be limited to carcinomas showing some myoepithelial differentiation. The specific markers of melanocytic differentiation (HMB45, Melan-A, tyrosinase, MiTF) are positive in roughly 85% of epithelioid melanomas; individual cases may be positive for one or more than one of these markers.

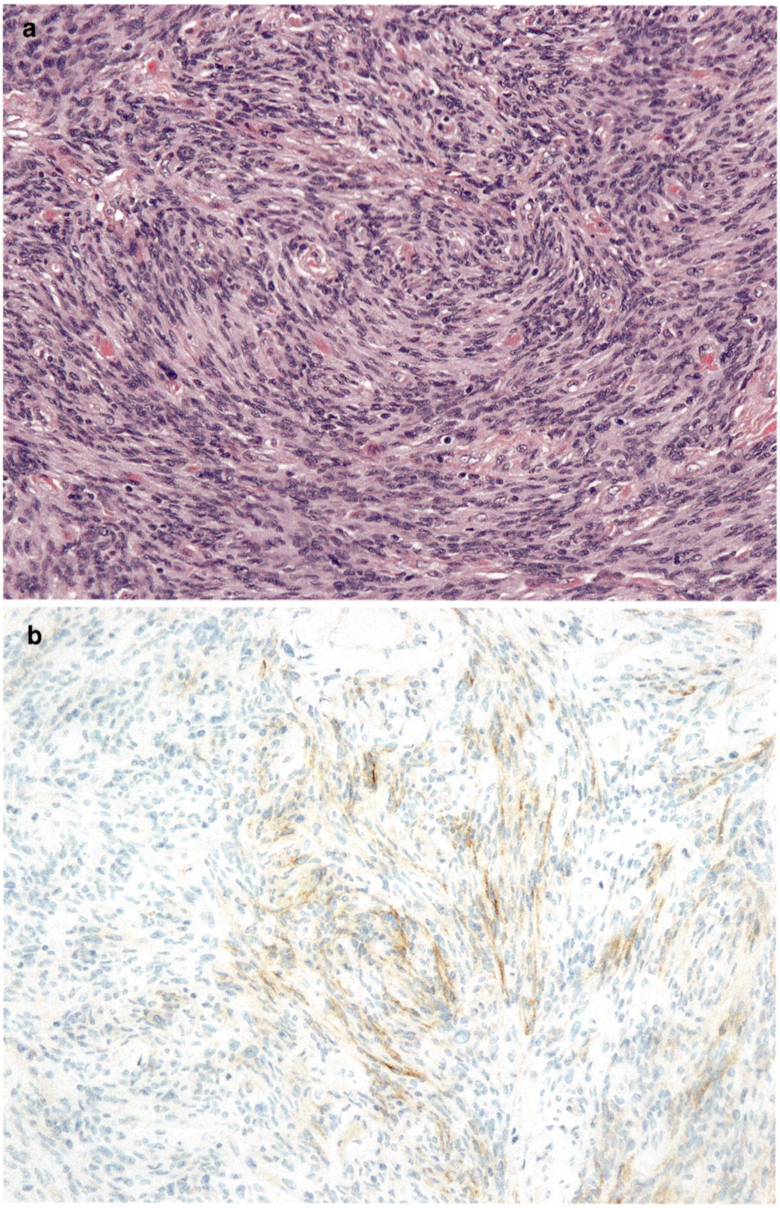

Fig. 2.15 Perineurioma (**a**) showing focal expression of epithelial membrane antigen (**b**). EMA expression may be limited in perineuriomas, and confirmation of this diagnosis may require immunostains for other perineurial markers, such as claudin-1 (**c**) or GLUT1

Fig. 2.15 (continued)

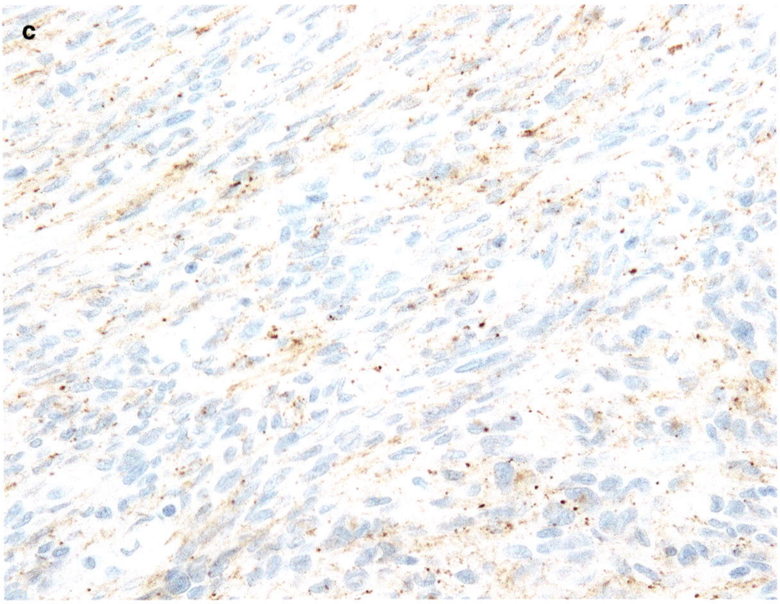

Table 2.6 Screening panel for epithelioid neoplasms

Antigen	CA	Melanoma/E-MPNST	Lymphoma	Myoepithelioma	ES	EAS
Keratin	Positive	Variable in melanoma, negative in E-MPNST	Negative	Negative	Positive	Variable
S-100 protein/ SOX10	Negative	Positive	Negative	Variable	Negative	Negative
CD45	Negative	Negative	Positive in conventional B and T cell lymphomas, negative in most ALCL	Negative	Negative	Negative
CD30	Negative	Negative	Negative in most conventional B and T cell lymphomas, positive in ALCL	Positive	Negative	Negative
CD31	Negative	Negative	Negative	Negative	Negative	Positive
SMARCB1 (INI1)	Normal	Normal in melanoma; lost in 50% of EMPNST	Normal	Lost in 50%	Lost in 90%	Normal

ALCL anaplastic large cell lymphoma, *CA* carcinoma, *EAS* epithelioid angiosarcoma, *E-MPNST* epithelioid malignant peripheral nerve sheath tumor, *ES* epithelioid sarcoma

Aberrant expression of intermediate filament proteins in epithelioid melanoma represents a significant diagnostic pitfall, in particular keratin expression (Fig. 2.19). Aberrant keratin expression may be seen in up to 40% of otherwise-typical epithelioid melanomas, in particular with the AE1/AE3 keratin antibodies. Melanomas may also show aberrant expression of desmin, neurofilament protein, and GFAP in smaller percentages of cases. Aberrant expression of neuro-

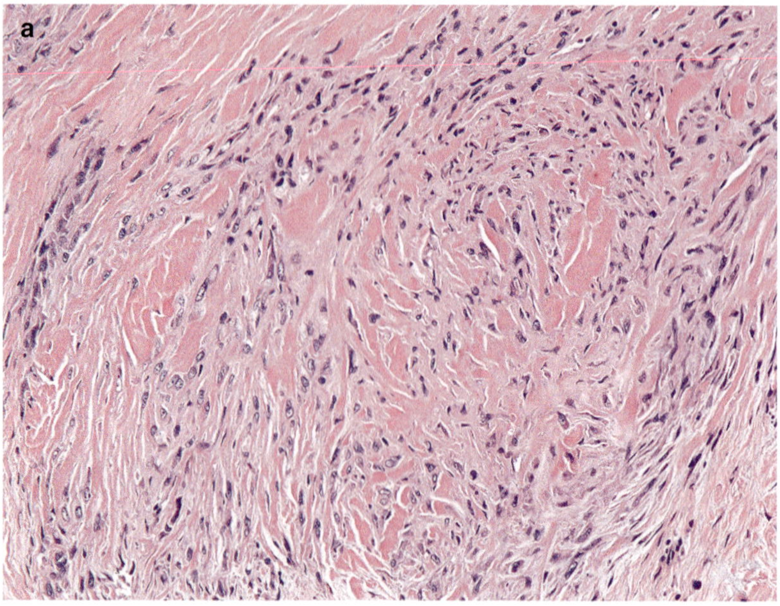

Fig. 2.16 Epithelioid sarcoma (**a**), positive for keratins (**b**). Although keratin expression in epithelioid sarcoma may cause confusion with carcinoma, loss of expression of SMARCB1 (INI1) is seen in >90% of epithelioid sarcomas (**c**) and is not a feature of the overwhelming majority of carcinomas

endocrine markers, such as synaptophysin, may also be seen potentially resulting in confusion with various neuroendocrine tumors. Application of a panel of IHC markers, to include S100 protein, SOX10, and specific melanoma markers, is the key to the recognition of melanomas with aberrant intermediate filament protein and/or neuroendocrine marker expression.

Epithelioid melanomas may also be confused with epithelioid malignant peripheral nerve sheath tumors (EMPNST) and with clear cell sarcoma (CCS). Although both EMPNST and CCS typically present as more deeply situated soft tissue masses, they may involve the skin on occasion or rarely present as primary dermal neoplasms. EMPNST are almost always strongly and diffusely positive for S100 protein, in contrast to other types of MPNST, which typically show only patchy and weak expression (Fig. 2.20). EMPNST characteristically show abundant collagen IV expression surrounding nests of cells, a feature not generally seen in melanoma. Unlike melanomas and CCS, which also show diffuse S100 protein expression, EMPNST are negative for melanocytic markers such as HMB45, Melan-A, and tyrosinase. Approximately 50% of EMPNST show loss of SMARCB1 expression, a finding that may be of value in their differential diagnosis with melanoma and CCS, both of which show retained expression of this protein. There are no IHC markers that distinguish melanoma and CCS; definitive diagnosis of CCS in the skin requires demonstration of the CCS-associated *EWSR1-ATF1/CREB1* gene fusions (Fig. 2.21).

Myoepithelial Tumors

The diagnosis of myoepithelial tumors in the skin and soft tissues is challenging, as these lesions may show a broad morphological spectrum, ranging from predominantly myxoid and reticulated tumors, mimicking extraskeletal myxoid chondrosarcoma, to solid, epithelioid, and rhabdoid lesions, closely resembling carcinoma, proximal-type epithelioid sarcoma, or rhabdoid tumor. Morphologically benign soft tissue myoepithelial tumors typically co-express epithelial

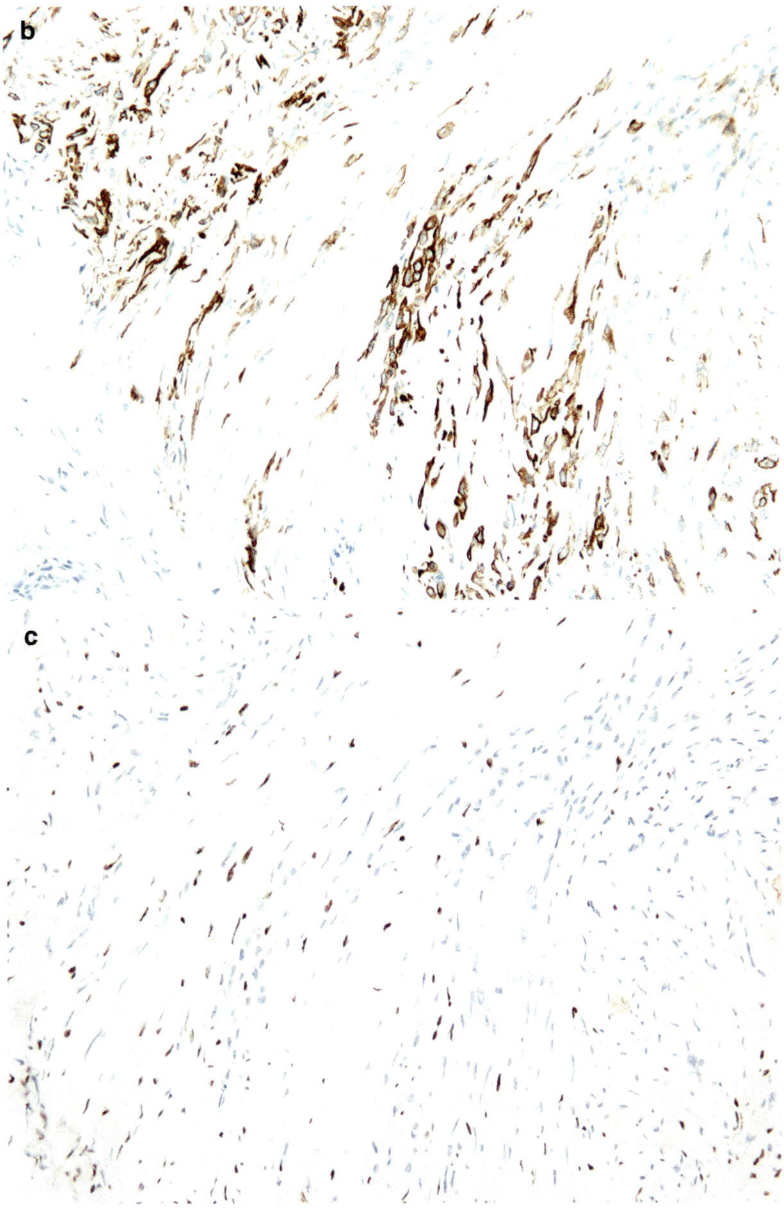

Fig. 2.16 (continued)

markers (e.g., keratins, EMA) and S100 protein/SOX10 and express other myoepithelial markers (e.g., muscle actins, calponin, glial fibrillary acidic protein, and p63) in up to 50% of cases (Fig. 2.22). IHC is less helpful in the diagnosis of myoepithelial carcinomas, as epithelial marker and S100 protein expression may be extremely limited (or even absent). It is generally (but not universally) accepted that expression of muscle actins *alone* in the appropriate morphological setting is sufficient for the diagnosis of myoepithelial carcinoma. SMARCB1 loss by IHC is seen in approximately 50% of myoepithelial carcinomas. Genetically, soft tissue myoepitheliomas are characterized in approximately 45% of cases by *EWSR1* gene rearrangements with a variety of different fusion partners, findings not seen in carcinoma or epithelioid sarcomas.

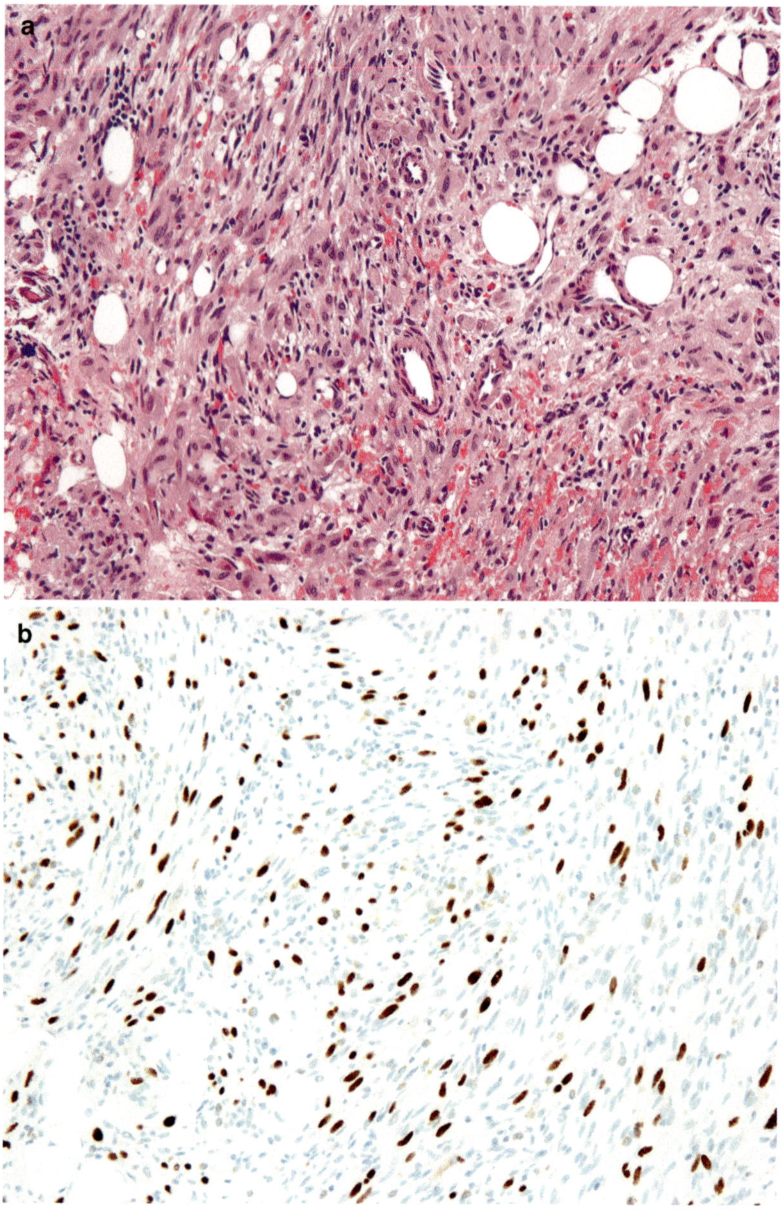

Fig. 2.17 Epithelioid sarcoma-like (pseudomyogenic) hemangioendothelioma (**a**) showing nuclear immunoreactivity for FOSB protein (**b**), indicative of the entity-defining *SERPINE1-FOSB* fusion

IHC in the Differential Diagnosis of Tumors Composed of Small, Round Cells

The differential diagnosis for tumors composed chiefly of small, round cells in the skin is quite broad, and different than in other soft tissue locations. Whereas in non-cutaneous soft tissue locations this differential diagnosis tends to center on lesions such as Ewing sarcoma, alveolar rhabdomyosarcoma, poorly differentiated synovial sarcoma, desmoplastic round cell tumor, mesenchymal chondrosarcoma, neuroblastoma, and the "Ewing-like" sarcomas defined by *CIC* or *BCOR* rearrangements, these tumors are quite rare in the skin. In the skin, tumors of small, round cells much more often represent carcinoma (e.g., Merkel cell carcinoma), small-cell melanoma, hematolymphoid tumors, and sometimes glomus tumors (includ-

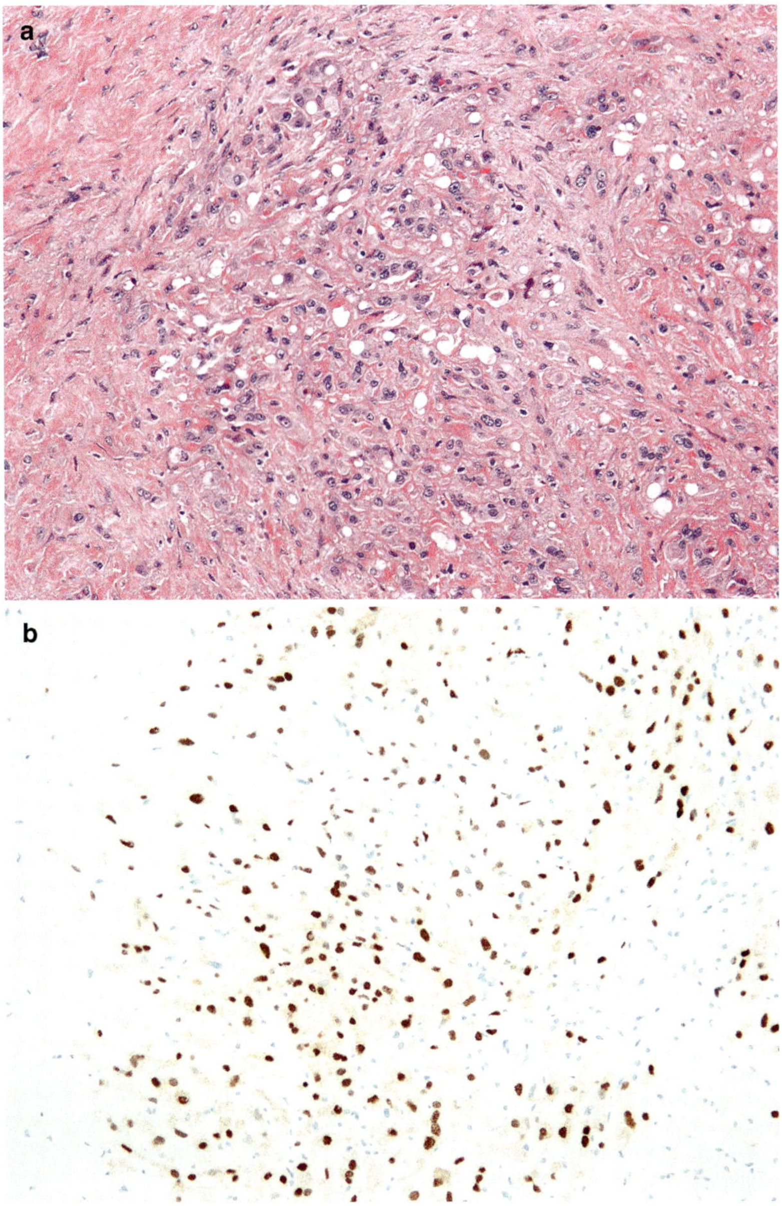

Fig. 2.18 Epithelioid hemangioendothelioma (**a**), with nuclear expression of CAMTA1 protein (**b**). CAMTA1 immunohistochemistry serves as a useful surrogate for molecular genetic studies to identify the EHE-specific *WWTR1-CAMTA1* gene fusion

ing malignant glomus tumors). Applications of IHC to the differential diagnosis of hematolymphoid tumors in the skin are outside of the focus of this chapter. Table 2.7 presents a screening panel of antibodies and the expected results for these tumors. The results of this panel dictate what additional studies are needed to confirm a specific diagnosis. In some instances, the best additional tests may be molecular genetic studies, rather than IHC.

Comments on Specific Round Cell Tumors

Merkel cell carcinomas will typically label for keratin 20 in addition to low molecular weight keratins, often in a distinctive "dot-like" pattern. Synaptophysin, chromogranin A, and CD56 are almost always positive as well. Antibodies to Merkel cell polyomavirus may also be helpful in confirming this diagnosis.

Fig. 2.19 Epithelioid malignant melanoma (**a**), showing expression of S100 protein (**b**). This tumor was also positive for other melanocytic markers, such as HMB45. Robust aberrant expression of keratins was present in this tumor, a potential diagnostic pitfall (**c**)

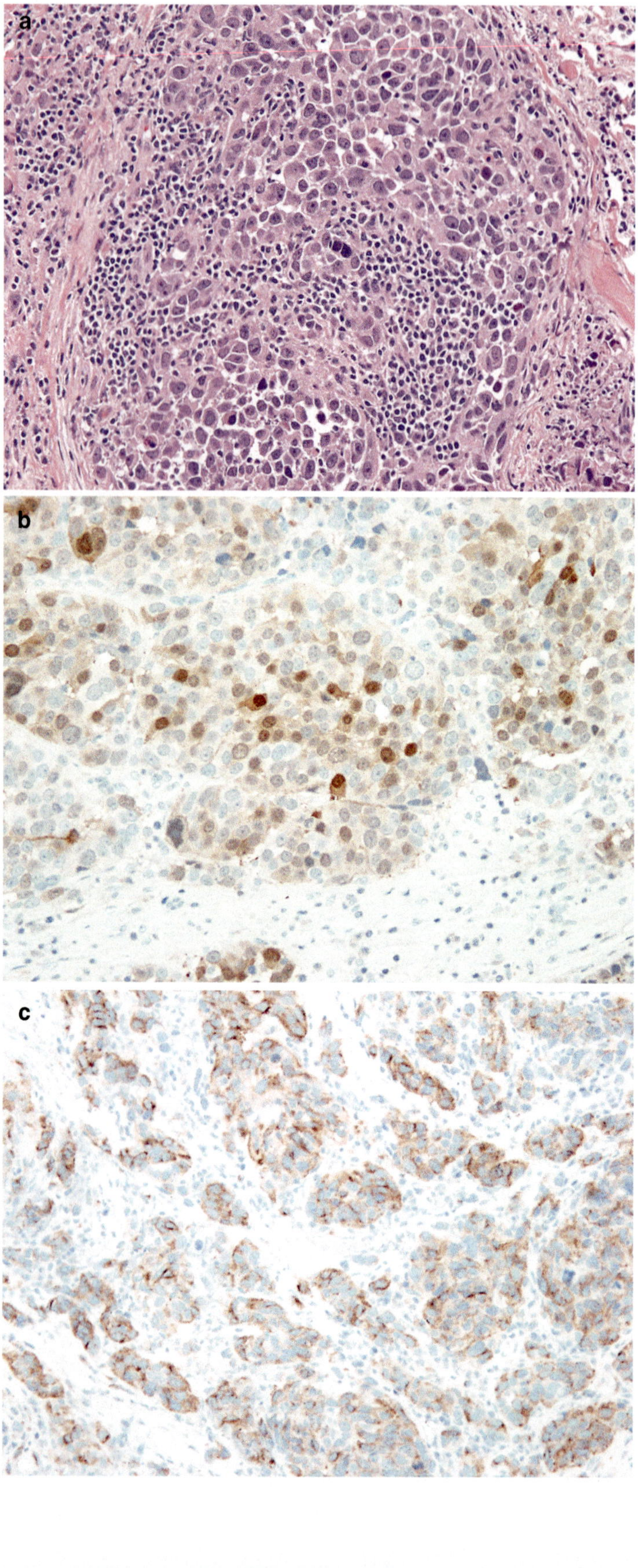

As noted previously, small-cell melanomas may show a deceptive S100 protein/SOX10-negative, HMB45/Melan-A-positive phenotype, and the absence of S100 protein/SOX10 does not exclude this diagnosis. Aberrant expression of keratins, desmin, and/or neuroendocrine markers may be particularly treacherous in small-cell melanomas.

Lymphoblastic lymphoma may be CD45-negative and CD99/FLI-1-positive, which can easily result in a misdiagnosis as Ewing sarcoma. TDT may be critical in arriving at the correct

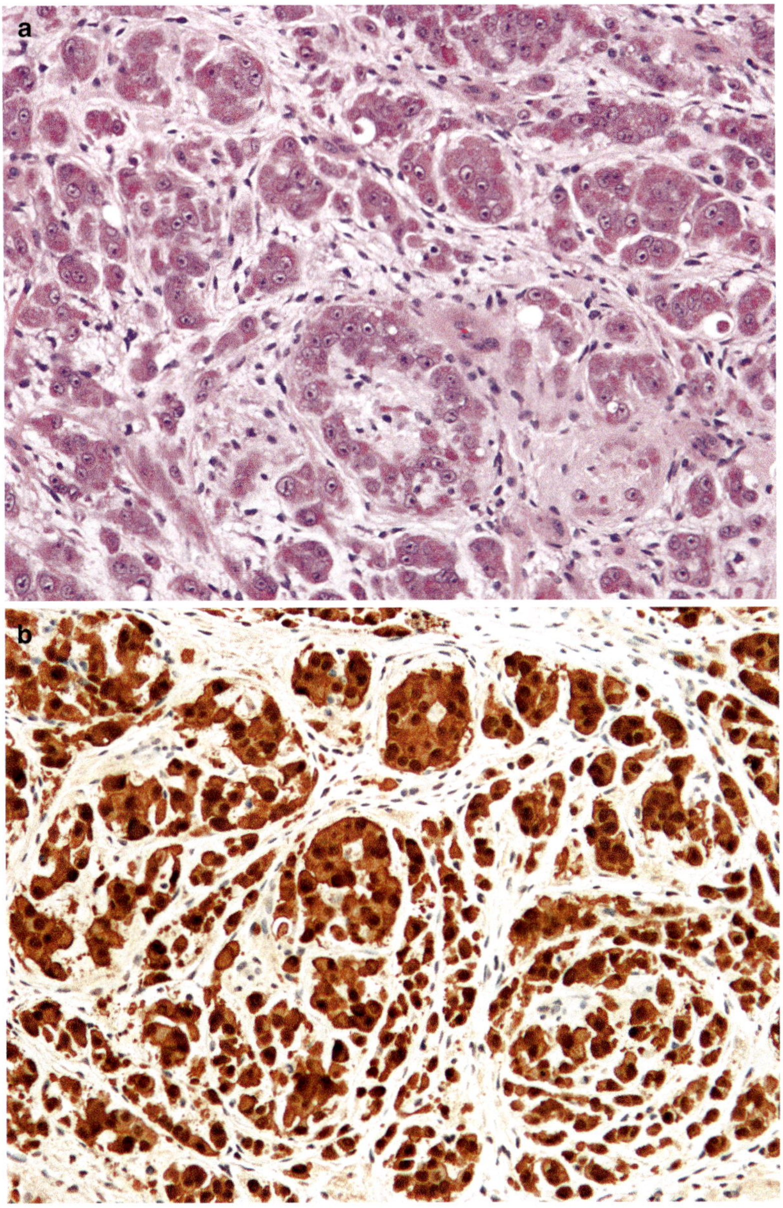

Fig. 2.20 The morphological features of epithelioid malignant peripheral nerve sheath tumor (**a**) overlap significantly with those of melanoma, and both tumors are typically strongly positive for S100 protein (**b**). However, >50% of epithelioid malignant peripheral nerve sheath tumor also show loss of SMARCB1 expression (**c**), a finding not seen in melanoma

Fig. 2.20 (continued)

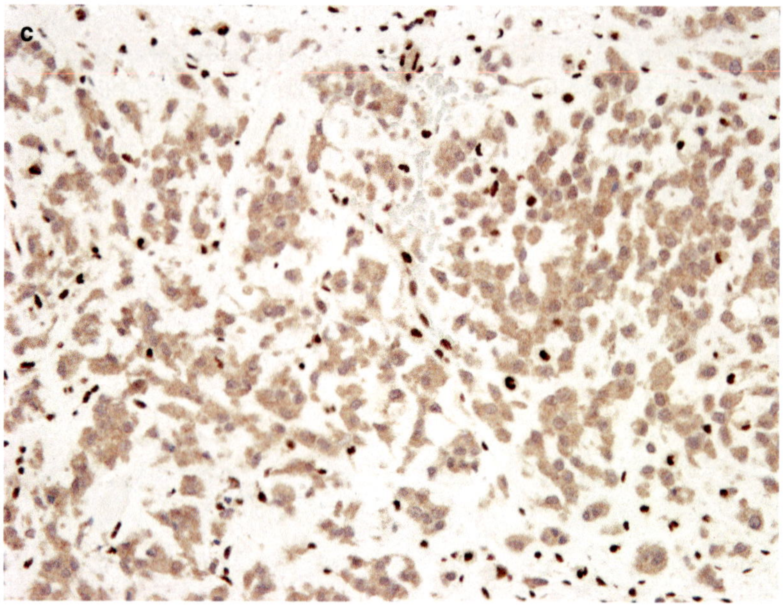

diagnosis. Anaplastic large-cell lymphomas, including the small-cell variant, may also be CD45-negative. CD30 is useful here. Myeloid markers should be performed for suspected myeloid malignancies.

Ewing sarcoma usually shows diffuse, membranous expression of CD99 in the absence of expression of other markers. CD99 is, however, a very non-specific marker, expressed by many different "small, round cell tumors." Roughly 20% of Ewing sarcoma show aberrant keratin expression, and rare cases show focal desmin expression. FLI1 and ERG protein expression may be helpful, but are also not specific. Over 95% of Ewing sarcoma show the *EWSR1-FLI1* or *EWSR1-ERG* fusion genes, detectable by RTPCR or FISH. In the appropriate morphological and immunohistochemical context, detection of *EWSR1* rearrangement alone by FISH is supportive. Very rare Ewing sarcoma shows *FUS* rearrangements, however.

Alveolar rhabdomyosarcoma will express desmin in addition to myogenin and MyoD1. Myogenin expression is typically strong and diffuse in alveolar RMS. Many alveolar RMS show aberrant expression of keratins and neuroendocrine markers, such as synaptophysin and CD56. Demonstration of the alveolar RMS-specific *PAX3/PAX7-FOXO1A* fusions by FISH or RT-PCR is confirmatory.

In poorly differentiated synovial sarcoma, keratin expression may be patchy or absent in some cases. EMA and high-molecular-weight keratins may be positive in such cases. CD34 expression is not seen in synovial sarcomas. Uniform, strong, nuclear expression of TLE1 protein is strongly suggestive of poorly differentiated synovial sarcoma and is a useful screening test. Cases showing only TLE1 expression should be confirmed with molecular tests for the *SSX1/2/4-SS18* fusions, either by RTPCR or FISH.

Desmoplastic small round cell tumors characteristically co-express keratins, desmin and vimentin. Carboxy-terminus WT1 antibodies can assist in confirmation of this diagnosis but are not widely available. The WT1 antibodies used in most laboratories are to the amino-terminus end and are not useful for this purpose. Definitive diagnosis may require demonstration of the *EWSR1-WT1* fusion gene by molecular means.

Glomus tumors show an identical phenotype to normal glomus cells, with expression of smooth muscle actin and caldesmon, but not desmin. Abundant pericellular collagen IV

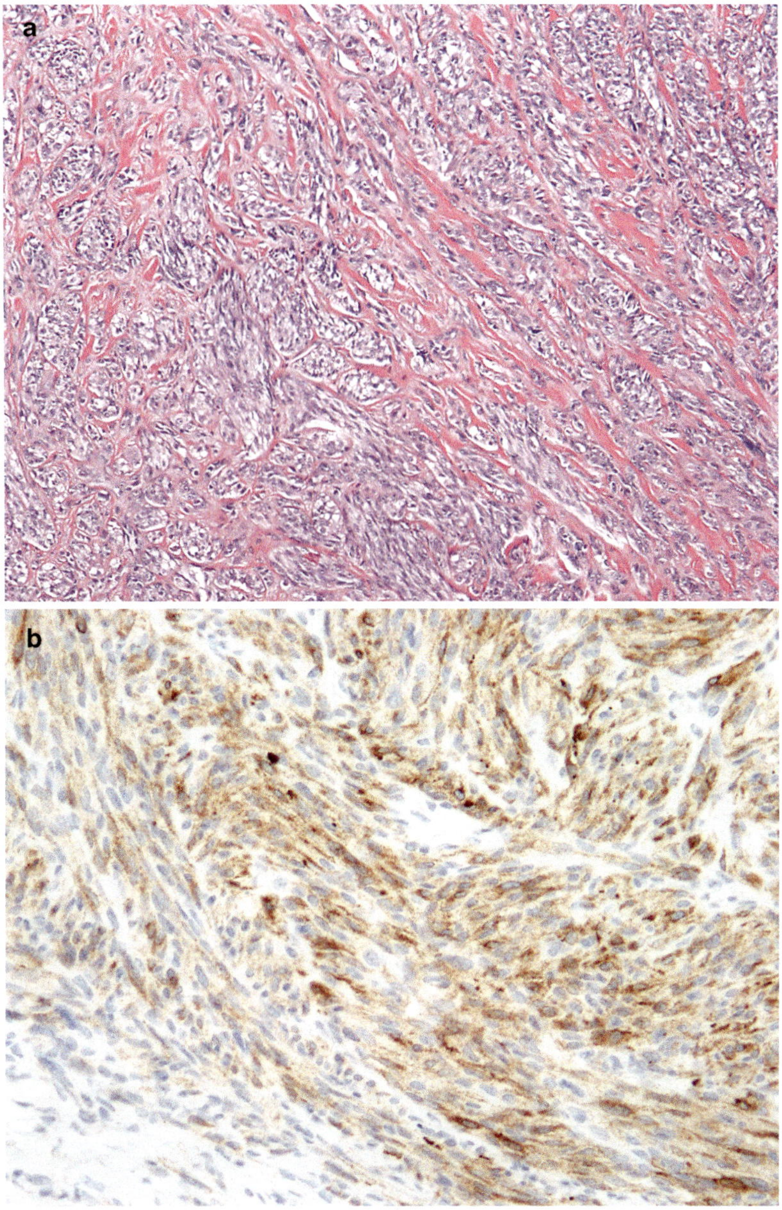

Fig. 2.21 The morphological features of clear cell sarcoma (**a**) are also very similar to those of melanoma. Unfortunately, there are no immunohistochemical markers that distinguish clear cell sarcoma from melanoma, as both are typically positive for S100 protein, SOX10, and more specific markers such as HMB45 (**b**). Molecular testing for the clear cell sarcoma-specific *EWSR1-ATF1* fusion may be required to make this distinction in some cases

expression is a characteristic of glomus tumors. Malignant glomus tumors show the same immunophenotype as do benign glomus tumors but may be extremely difficult to recognize in the absence of a pre-existing benign glomus tumor. Although antibodies to smooth muscle actins are not generally part of the panel of immunostains used to evaluate "small, round cell tumors" in extracutaneous sites, they may be very helpful in the skin.

Other Application of IHC in Cutaneous Mesenchymal Tumors

Adipocytic Tumors

Primary adipocytic tumors of the skin are uncommon, and most are easily diagnosed by morphology alone. The distinction of cutaneous spindle cell/pleomorphic lipoma (SCL/PL) from

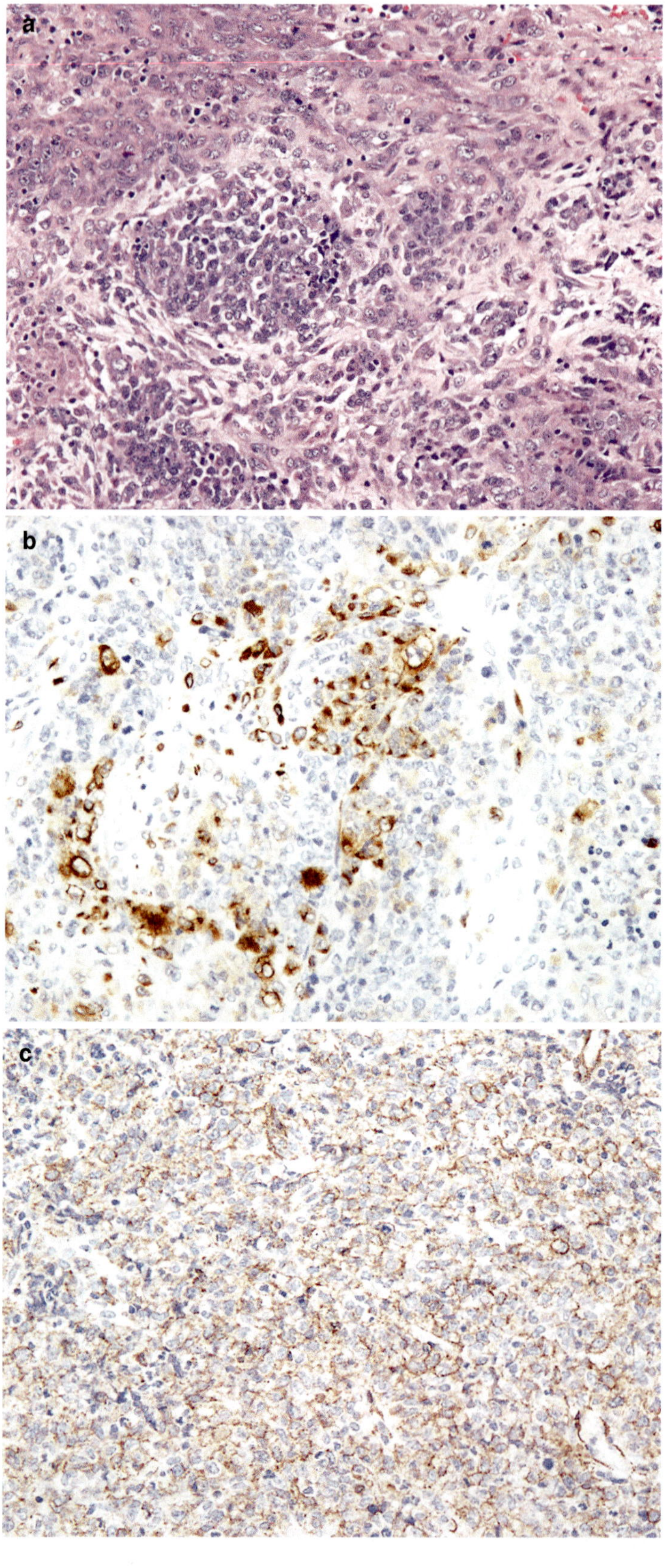

Fig. 2.22 Malignant myoepithelioma (**a**), showing co-expression of keratins (**b**) and smooth muscle actins (**c**)

superficial atypical lipomatous tumor (well-differentiated liposarcoma) (ALT) can at times be challenging, however. At the genetic level, SCL/PL show *RB* gene deletions, with loss of expression of Rb protein. This finding is not seen in ALT, which show instead amplification of the *MDM2* and *CDK4* genes, with overexpression of these proteins. In problematic cases, IHC for RB protein and MDM2 protein may be helpful in distinguishing SCL/PL from ALT. It should be noted that the lipid-laden histiocytes present in fat necrosis are also frequently MDM2 protein-positive, a potential pitfall in the distinction of this nonneoplastic process from ALT.

Atypical Vascular Lesions and Angiosarcomas Arising After Therapeutic Irradiation

In patients who have received therapeutic irradiation (usually, but not always, for breast cancer), the distinction of atypical vascular lesions (AVL) from well-differentiated angiosarcoma may be extremely difficult. Recent data indicates that postirradiation angiosarcoma frequently shows amplification of the *MYC* gene, with overexpression of MYC protein, whereas AVL lack these findings (Fig. 2.23). Demonstration of strong, uniform MYC protein expression in the nuclei of

Table 2.7 Screening panel for small, blue, round cell tumors

Antibody to	Merkel cell carcinoma	Melanoma	Lymphoma	ES	RMS	PDSS
Keratin	Positive	Variable	Negative	Variable	Rare	Positive
Keratin 20	Positive	Negative	Negative	Negative	Negative	Negative
Merkel cell polyoma virus	Positive	Negative	Negative	Negative	Negative	Negative
S-100 protein/SOX10	Negative	Positive	Negative	Variable	Rare	Variable
CD45	Negative	Negative	Positive	Negative	Negative	Negative
TdT	Variable	Negative	Positive	Negative	Negative	Negative
Desmin	Negative	Variable	Negative	Rare	Positive	Negative
CD99	Negative	Negative	Variable	Positive	Variable	Positive

ES Ewing sarcoma, *PDSS* poorly differentiated synovial sarcoma, *RMS* rhabdomyosarcoma, *SCCA* small-cell carcinoma

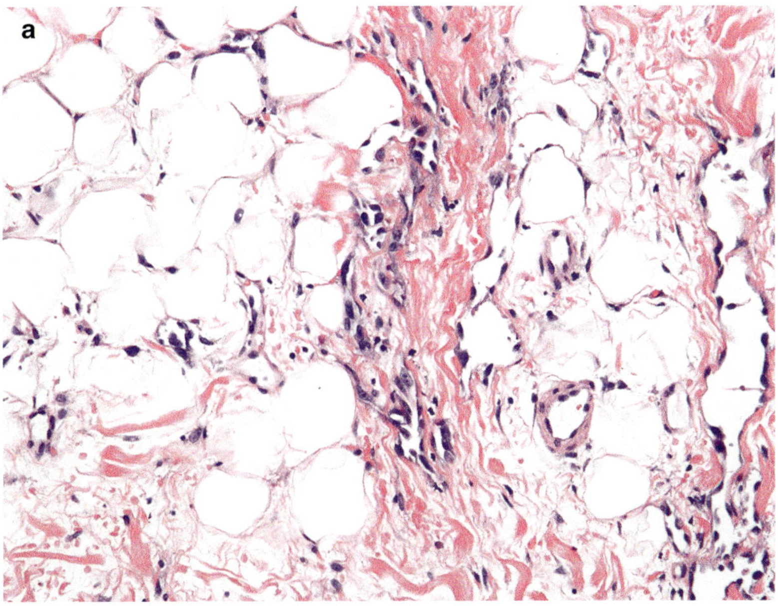

Fig. 2.23 Postirradiation angiosarcoma of the skin of the breast (**a**). Strong nuclear immunoreactivity for MYC protein was present (**b**), further supporting classification of this tumor as angiosarcoma, as opposed to an atypical vascular lesion following irradiation

Fig. 2.23 (continued)

endothelial cells lining the vascular channels in question may be helpful in confirming a diagnosis of angiosarcoma in selected cases, although caution is urged in interpreting this finding. This is because some cases may show MYC staining as the result of polysomy of chromosome 8, rather than MYC gene amplification, and because this immunostain can be difficult to interpret or may label only scattered endothelial cells. There may be some benefit in performing both MYC IHC and FISH for *MYC* amplification. It is important to keep in mind that *MYC* amplification is not a feature of primary cutaneous angiosarcoma, and MYC IHC is not helpful in this setting.

Selected References

1. Adhikari LA, McCalmont TH, Folpe AL. Merkel cell carcinoma with heterologous rhabdomyoblastic differentiation: the role of immunohistochemistry for Merkel cell polyomavirus large T-antigen in confirmation. J Cutan Pathol. 2012;39(1):47–51.
2. Alomari AK, Glusac EJ, McNiff JM. p40 is a more specific marker than p63 for cutaneous poorly differentiated squamous cell carcinoma. J Cutan Pathol. 2014;41(11):839–45.
3. Azumi N, Battifora H. The distribution of vimentin and keratin in epithelial and nonepithelial neoplasms. A comprehensive immunohistochemical study on formalin- and alcohol-fixed tumors. Am J Clin Pathol. 1987;88(3):286–96.
4. Bacchi CE, Bonetti F, Pea M, Martignoni G, Gown AM. HMB-45. A review. Appl Immunohistochem. 1996;4(2):73–85.
5. Barnoud R, Sabourin JC, Pasquier D, Ranchere D, Bailly C, Terrier-Lacombe MJ, et al. Immunohistochemical expression of WT1 by desmoplastic small round cell tumor: a comparative study with other small round cell tumors. Am J Surg Pathol. 2000;24(6):830–6.
6. Bishop JA, Montgomery EA, Westra WH. Use of p40 and p63 immunohistochemistry and human papillomavirus testing as ancillary tools for the recognition of head and neck sarcomatoid carcinoma and its distinction from benign and malignant mesenchymal processes. Am J Surg Pathol. 2014;38(2):257–64.
7. Bridge JA. The role of cytogenetics and molecular diagnostics in the diagnosis of soft-tissue tumors. Mod Pathol. 2014;27(Suppl 1):S80–97.
8. Brown DC, Theaker JM, Banks PM, Gatter KC, Mason DY. Cytokeratin expression in smooth muscle and smooth muscle tumours. Histopathology. 1987;11(5):477–86.
9. Busam KJ, Jungbluth AA. Melan-A, a new melanocytic differentiation marker. Adv Anat Pathol. 1999;6(1):12–8.
10. Cassidy M, Loftus B, Whelan A, Sabt B, Hickey D, Henry K, et al. KP-1: not a specific marker. Staining of 137 sarcomas, 48 lymphomas, 28 carcinomas, 7 malignant melanomas and 8 cystosarcoma phyllodes. Virchows Arch. 1994;424(6):635–40.

11. Dei Tos AP, Wadden C, Calonje E, Sciot R, Pauwels P, Knight JC, et al. Immunohistochemical demonstration of glycoprotein p30/32(MIC2) (CD99) in synovial sarcoma: a potential cause of diagnostic confusion. Appl Immunohistochem. 1995;3(3):168–73.
12. Doyle LA, Moller E, Dal Cin P, Fletcher CD, Mertens F, Hornick JL. MUC4 is a highly sensitive and specific marker for low-grade fibromyxoid sarcoma. Am J Surg Pathol. 2011;35(5):733–41.
13. Doyle LA, Fletcher CD, Hornick JL. Nuclear expression of CAMTA1 distinguishes epithelioid hemangioendothelioma from histologic mimics. Am J Surg Pathol. 2016;40(1):94–102.
14. Fanburg-Smith JC, Miettinen M. Angiomatoid "malignant" fibrous histiocytoma: a clinicopathologic study of 158 cases and further exploration of the myoid phenotype. Hum Pathol. 1999;30(11):1336–43.
15. Fetsch JF, Laskin WB, Hallman JR, Lupton GP, Miettinen M. Neurothekeoma: an analysis of 178 tumors with detailed immunohistochemical data and long-term patient follow-up information. Am J Surg Pathol. 2007;31(7):1103–14.
16. Folpe AL. MyoD1 and myogenin expression in human neoplasia: a review and update. Adv Anat Pathol. 2002;9(3):198–203.
17. Folpe AL. Selected topics in the pathology of epithelioid soft tissue tumors. Mod Pathol. 2014;27(Suppl 1):S64–79.
18. Folpe AL, Kwiatkowski DJ. Perivascular epithelioid cell neoplasms: pathology and pathogenesis. Hum Pathol. 2010;41(1):1–15.
19. Folpe AL, Chand EM, Goldblum JR, Weiss SW. Expression of Fli-1, a nuclear transcription factor, distinguishes vascular neoplasms from potential mimics. Am J Surg Pathol. 2001;25(8):1061–6.
20. Folpe AL, Goldblum JR, Rubin BP, Shehata BM, Liu W, Dei Tos AP, et al. Morphologic and immunophenotypic diversity in Ewing family tumors: a study of 66 genetically confirmed cases. Am J Surg Pathol. 2005;29(8):1025–33.
21. Fox MD, Billings SD, Gleason BC, Moore J, Thomas AB, Shea CR, et al. Expression of MiTF may be helpful in differentiating cellular neurothekeoma from plexiform fibrohistiocytic tumor (histiocytoid predominant) in a partial biopsy specimen. Am J Dermatopathol. 2012;34(2):157–60.
22. Gleason BC, Fletcher CD. Myoepithelial carcinoma of soft tissue in children: an aggressive neoplasm analyzed in a series of 29 cases. Am J Surg Pathol. 2007;31(12):1813–24.
23. Gray MH, Rosenberg AE, Dickersin GR, Bhan AK. Cytokeratin expression in epithelioid vascular neoplasms. Hum Pathol. 1990;21(2):212–7.
24. Guillou L, Wadden C, Kraus MD, Dei Tos AP, Fletcher CDM. S-100 protein reactivity in synovial sarcomas – a potentially frequent diagnostic pitfall. Immunohistochemical analysis of 100 cases. Appl Immunohistochem. 1996;4(3):167–75.
25. Henderson SA, Torres-Cabala CA, Curry JL, Bassett RL, Ivan D, Prieto VG, et al. p40 is more specific than p63 for the distinction of atypical fibroxanthoma from other cutaneous spindle cell malignancies. Am J Surg Pathol. 2014;38(8):1102–10.
26. Hill DA, Pfeifer JD, Marley EF, Dehner LP, Humphrey PA, Zhu X, et al. WT1 staining reliably differentiates desmoplastic small round cell tumor from Ewing sarcoma/primitive neuroectodermal tumor. An immunohistochemical and molecular diagnostic study. Am J Clin Pathol. 2000;114(3):345–53.
27. Hornick JL, Fletcher CD. Myoepithelial tumors of soft tissue: a clinicopathologic and immunohistochemical study of 101 cases with evaluation of prognostic parameters. Am J Surg Pathol. 2003;27(9):1183–96.
28. Hornick JL, Fletcher CD. Cutaneous myoepithelioma: a clinicopathologic and immunohistochemical study of 14 cases. Hum Pathol. 2004;35(1):14–24.
29. Hornick JL, Fletcher CD. Soft tissue perineurioma: clinicopathologic analysis of 81 cases including those with atypical histologic features. Am J Surg Pathol. 2005;29(7):845–58.
30. Hung YP, Fletcher CD, Hornick JL. FOSB is a useful diagnostic marker for pseudomyogenic hemangioendothelioma. Am J Surg Pathol. 2017;41(5):596–606.
31. Jagdis A, Rubin BP, Tubbs RR, Pacheco M, Nielsen TO. Prospective evaluation of TLE1 as a diagnostic immunohistochemical marker in synovial sarcoma. Am J Surg Pathol. 2009;33(12):1743–51.
32. Jo VY, Fletcher CD. p63 immunohistochemical staining is limited in soft tissue tumors. Am J Clin Pathol. 2011;136(5):762–6.
33. Karamchandani JR, Nielsen TO, van de Rijn M, West RB. Sox10 and S100 in the diagnosis of soft-tissue neoplasms. Appl Immunohistochem Mol Morphol. 2012;20(5):445–50.
34. Kosemehmetoglu K, Vrana JA, Folpe AL. TLE1 expression is not specific for synovial sarcoma: a whole section study of 163 soft tissue and bone neoplasms. Mod Pathol. 2009;22(7):872–8.
35. Mentzel T, Dei Tos AP, Sapi Z, Kutzner H. Myopericytoma of skin and soft tissues: clinicopathologic and immunohistochemical study of 54 cases. Am J Surg Pathol. 2006;30(1):104–13.
36. Mentzel T, Schildhaus HU, Palmedo G, Buttner R, Kutzner H. Postradiation cutaneous angiosarcoma after treatment of breast carcinoma is characterized by MYC amplification in contrast to atypical vascular lesions after radiotherapy and control cases: clinicopathological, immunohistochemical and molecular analysis of 66 cases. Mod Pathol. 2012;25(1):75–85.
37. Miettinen M. Immunoreactivity for cytokeratin and epithelial membrane antigen in leiomyosarcoma. Arch Pathol Lab Med. 1988;112(6):637–40.
38. Miettinen M, Fanburg-Smith JC, Virolainen M, Shmookler BM, Fetsch JF. Epithelioid sarcoma: an immunohistochemical analysis of 112 classical and variant cases and a discussion of the differential diagnosis. Hum Pathol. 1999;30(8):934–42.
39. Miettinen M, Wang ZF, Paetau A, Tan SH, Dobi A, Srivastava S, et al. ERG transcription factor as an

immunohistochemical marker for vascular endothelial tumors and prostatic carcinoma. Am J Surg Pathol. 2011;35(3):432–41.
40. Miller K, Goodlad JR, Brenn T. Pleomorphic dermal sarcoma: adverse histologic features predict aggressive behavior and allow distinction from atypical fibroxanthoma. Am J Surg Pathol. 2012;36(9):1317–26.
41. Mohamed A, Gonzalez RS, Lawson D, Wang J, Cohen C. SOX10 expression in malignant melanoma, carcinoma, and normal tissues. Appl Immunohistochem Mol Morphol. 2013;21(6):506–10.
42. Nonaka D, Chiriboga L, Rubin BP. Sox10: a pan-schwannian and melanocytic marker. Am J Surg Pathol. 2008;32(9):1291–8.
43. Palla B, Su A, Binder S, Dry S. SOX10 expression distinguishes desmoplastic melanoma from its histologic mimics. Am J Dermatopathol. 2013;35(5):576–81.
44. Rangdaeng S, Truong LD. Comparative immunohistochemical staining for desmin and muscle-specific actin. A study of 576 cases (see comments). Am J Clin Pathol. 1991;96(1):32–45.
45. Romano RC, Carter JM, Folpe AL. Aberrant intermediate filament and synaptophysin expression is a frequent event in malignant melanoma: an immunohistochemical study of 73 cases. Mod Pathol. 2015;28(8):1033–42.
46. Rossi S, Orvieto E, Furlanetto A, Laurino L, Ninfo V, Dei Tos AP. Utility of the immunohistochemical detection of FLI-1 expression in round cell and vascular neoplasm using a monoclonal antibody. Mod Pathol. 2004;17(5):547–52.
47. Sandell RF, Carter JM, Folpe AL. Solitary (juvenile) xanthogranuloma: a comprehensive immunohistochemical study emphasizing recently developed markers of histiocytic lineage. Hum Pathol. 2015;46(9):1390–7.
48. Truong LD, Rangdaeng S, Cagle P, Ro JY, Hawkins H, Font RL. The diagnostic utility of desmin. A study of 584 cases and review of the literature (see comments). Am J Clin Pathol. 1990;93(3):305–14.
49. Ud Din N, Zhang P, Sukov WR, Sattler CA, Jenkins SM, Doyle LA, et al. Spindle cell lipomas arising at atypical locations. Am J Clin Pathol. 2016;146(4):487–95.
50. van de Rijn M, Rouse R. CD34: a review. Appl Immunohistochem. 1994;2(2):71–80.
51. Wang NP, Marx J, McNutt MA, Rutledge JC, Gown AM. Expression of myogenic regulatory proteins (myogenin and MyoD1) in small blue round cell tumors of childhood. Am J Pathol. 1995;147(6):1799–810.
52. Watanabe K, Kusakabe T, Hoshi N, Saito A, Suzuki T. h-Caldesmon in leiomyosarcoma and tumors with smooth muscle cell-like differentiation: its specific expression in the smooth muscle cell tumor. Hum Pathol. 1999;30(4):392–6.
53. Weiss SW, Langloss JM, Enzinger FM. Value of S-100 protein in the diagnosis of soft tissue tumors with particular reference to benign and malignant Schwann cell tumors. Lab Investig. 1983;49(3):299–308.

3 Mimics of Cutaneous Mesenchymal Tumors

Darya Buehler, Rajiv M. Patel, and Steven D. Billings

Abstract

This chapter briefly describes reactive or neoplastic mimics of primary cutaneous mesenchymal neoplasms that are commonly encountered by dermatopathologists and can lead to misinterpretation as a primary soft tissue tumor, especially sarcoma. A comprehensive review of these lesions is beyond the scope of this chapter; rather, we focus our discussion on helpful histologic clues, diagnostic pitfalls, and useful ancillary tests. The entities reviewed in this chapter and their clinically important mesenchymal tumor mimics are listed in Table 3.1.

D. Buehler (✉)
Pathology and Laboratory Medicine, University of Wisconsin School of Medicine and Public Health, Madison, WI, USA
e-mail: buehler2@wisc.edu

R. M. Patel
Department of Pathology, University of Michigan Medical School, Ann Arbor, MI, USA

S. D. Billings
Department of Pathology, Cleveland Clinic, Cleveland, OH, USA

Palisading Necrobiotic Granulomas: Granuloma Annulare and Rheumatoid Nodule

Clinical Features

Cutaneous granuloma annulare presents as one or a crop of reddish to skin-colored papules that tend to spread peripherally usually forming a ring-like arrangement. It occurs sporadically in a broad age range. Disseminated forms may occur in patients with hepatitis C and HIV or as a paraneoplastic syndrome. Deep granuloma annulare typically presents as subcutaneous nodules in the head and neck or lower limbs of children and young adults. Rheumatoid nodules develop as subcutaneous masses in patients with seropositive rheumatoid arthritis and tend to occur over bony prominences, such as the elbows and hands, or rarely the lungs. Both lesions are benign. Granuloma annulare and rheumatoid nodules are very important histologic mimics of distal-type epithelioid sarcoma (Table 3.1).

Pathologic Features

Granuloma annulare and rheumatoid nodule display similar histologic features, namely, palisading necrobiotic granulomas. The center of the granuloma contains necrobiotic material consist-

S. D. Billings et al. (eds.), *Soft Tissue Tumors of the Skin*,
https://doi.org/10.1007/978-1-4939-8812-9_3

Table 3.1 Important histologic mimics of primary cutaneous mesenchymal tumors

Mimic	Soft tissue counterpart
Necrobiotic granulomas *Granuloma annulare* *Rheumatoid nodule*	Distal-type epithelioid sarcoma
Sarcomatoid carcinoma including spindle cell squamous cell carcinoma	Hypertrophic scar Spindle cell and pleomorphic sarcoma Atypical fibrous histiocytoma
With heterologous differentiation	Osteosarcoma Rhabdomyosarcoma Angiosarcoma
Spindle cell melanoma	Malignant peripheral nerve sheath tumor
	Cellular schwannoma
	Clear cell sarcoma
Desmoplastic melanoma	Malignant peripheral nerve sheath tumor
	Neurofibroma
	Hypertrophic scar
	Spindle cell sarcoma
Cellular blue nevus	Clear cell sarcoma
Massive localized lymphedema	Atypical lipomatous tumor/well-differentiated liposarcoma
Silicone granuloma	Atypical lipomatous tumor/well-differentiated liposarcoma, pleomorphic liposarcoma
Acroangiodermatitis	Kaposi sarcoma
	Angiosarcoma
Mycobacterial spindle cell pseudotumor	Inflammatory myofibroblastic tumor
	Deep benign fibrous histiocytoma
	Fascicular spindle cell sarcomas
Erythema elevatum diutinum	Nodular fasciitis
	Storiform/collagenous fibroma
	Myofibroblastic sarcoma
Metastatic clear cell carcinoma	Cutaneous perivascular epithelioid cell tumor (PEComa)
Florid reactive periostitis/fibro-osseous pseudotumor of digit	Osteosarcoma
Bizarre parosteal osteochondromatous proliferation (BPOP)	Chondrosarcoma
	Osteosarcoma
	Soft tissue chondroma
Crystal-storing histiocytosis	Granular cell tumor
	Mycobacterial spindle cell pseudotumor
	Xanthogranuloma
	Rosai-Dorfman disease

ing of altered collagen bundles and mucin in the case of granuloma annulare and fibrin and necrotic debris in rheumatoid nodule; this necrobiotic material is surrounded by a palisade of spindled to epithelioid CD68- and CD163-positive histiocytes (Fig. 3.1a–d). Mucin within the necrobiotic granulomas of granuloma annulare can be highlighted by colloidal iron or Alcian blue special stains (Fig. 3.2). A perivascular lymphocytic inflammatory infiltrate is often present. Deep granuloma annulare typically lacks multinucleated giant cells, but they may be present in rheumatoid nodules. The subtler interstitial variant of granuloma annulare shows infiltration of dermal collagen by spindled histiocytes and dermal mucin deposits without broad zones of necrobiosis. The necrobiotic zones in rheumatoid nodules tend to be more eosinophilic in quality due to the presence of predominantly fibrin and collagen fibers and, to a lesser degree, mucin deposition in comparison to granuloma annulare, but there is substantial overlap between these lesions. They may be difficult to distinguish from one another in the absence of a corroborating

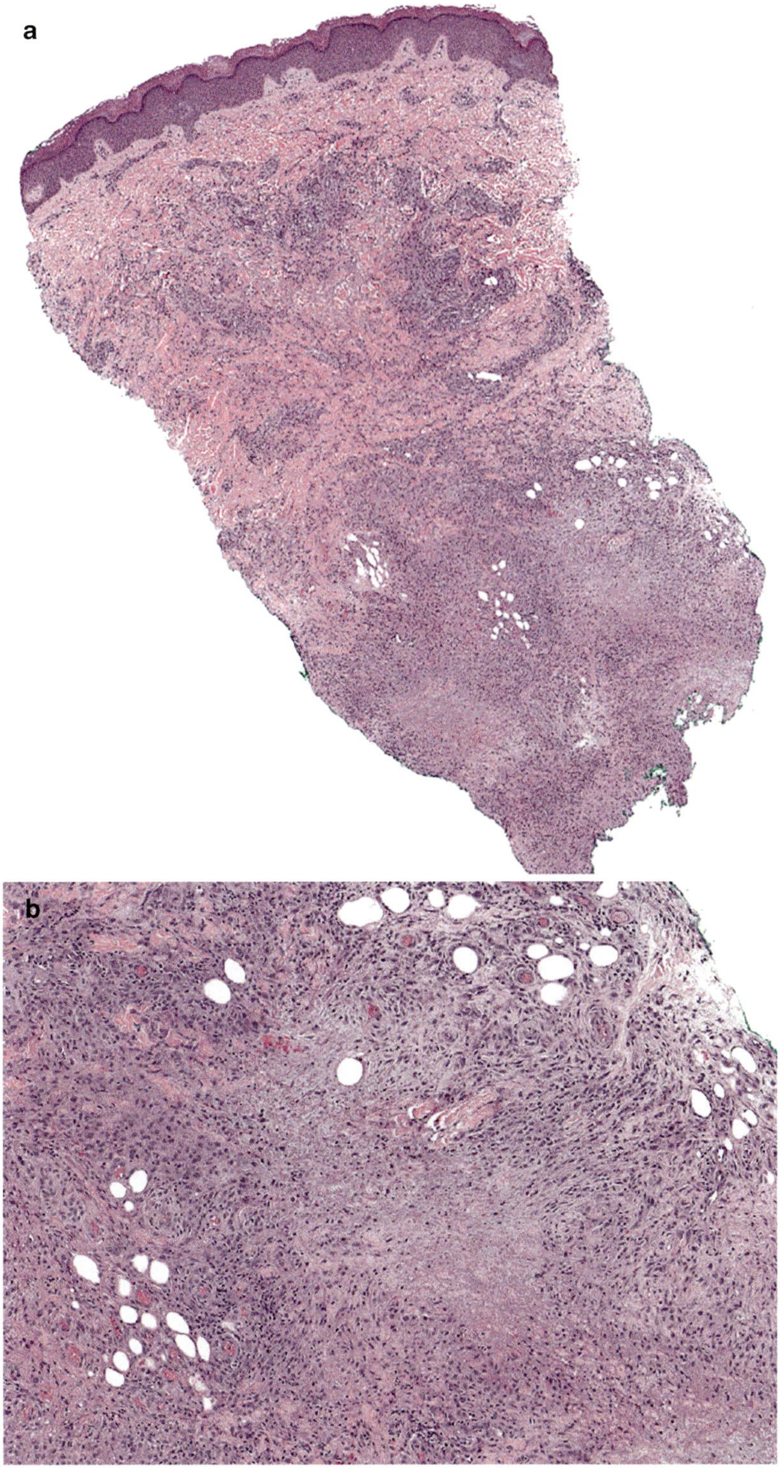

Fig. 3.1 Granuloma annulare and rheumatoid nodule. (**a**). Granuloma annulare: Coalescing granulomatous nodules in the dermis. (**b**). Granuloma annulare: Necrobiotic material in the center is surrounded by a palisade of spindled to epithelioid, cytologically banal histiocytes. (**c** and **d**). Rheumatoid nodule: palisading granuloma surrounding necrotic debris and fibrin

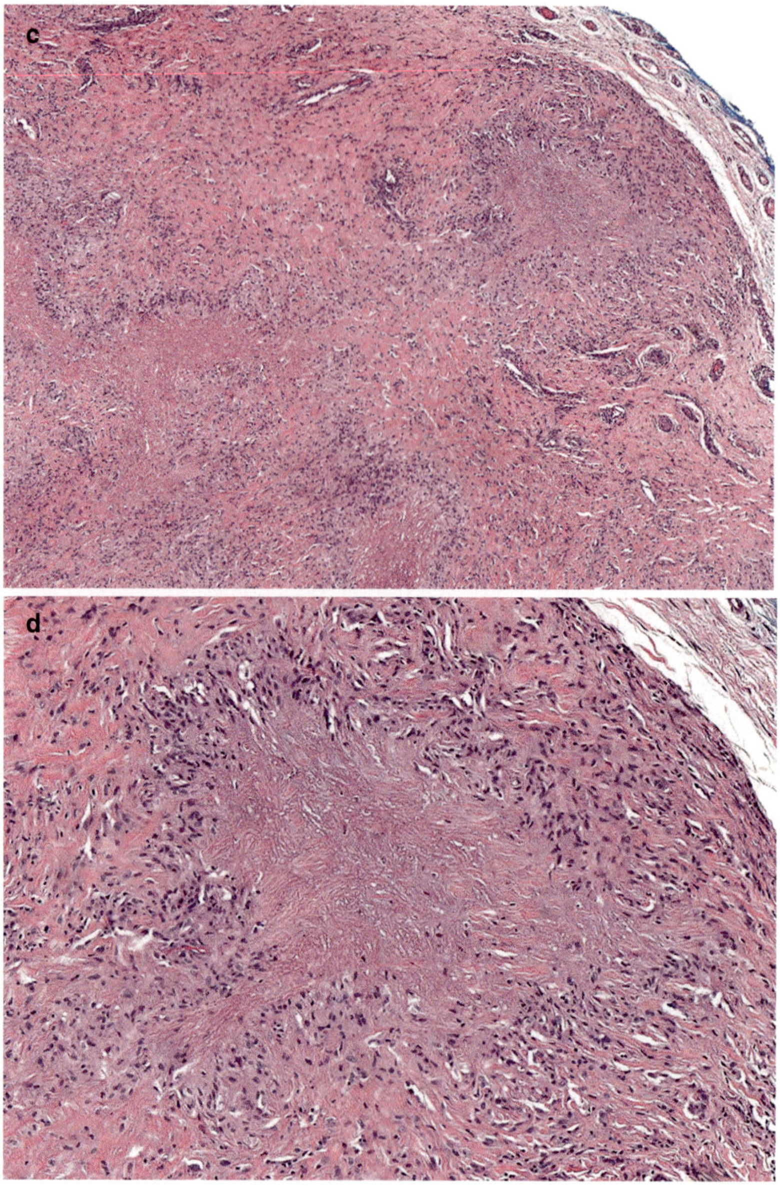

Fig. 3.1 (continued)

clinical history of rheumatoid arthritis for rheumatoid nodule. Key pathologic features of granuloma annulare and rheumatoid nodule are presented in Table 3.2.

Differential Diagnosis

Granuloma annulare and rheumatoid nodule can be mistaken for distal-type epithelioid sarcoma. The latter also presents as single or multiple infiltrative dermal or subcutaneous nodules with ill-defined margins. These nodules often surround a zone of central geographic necrosis or fibrosis with a palisaded arrangement of tumor cells at the periphery, resembling a necrobiotic granuloma. The most helpful histologic feature is identification of nuclear atypia, which is at least focally present in distal-type epithelioid sarcoma, but is not seen in the benign histiocytes and fibroblasts of granuloma annulare and rheumatoid nodule. The constituent cells of epithelioid sar-

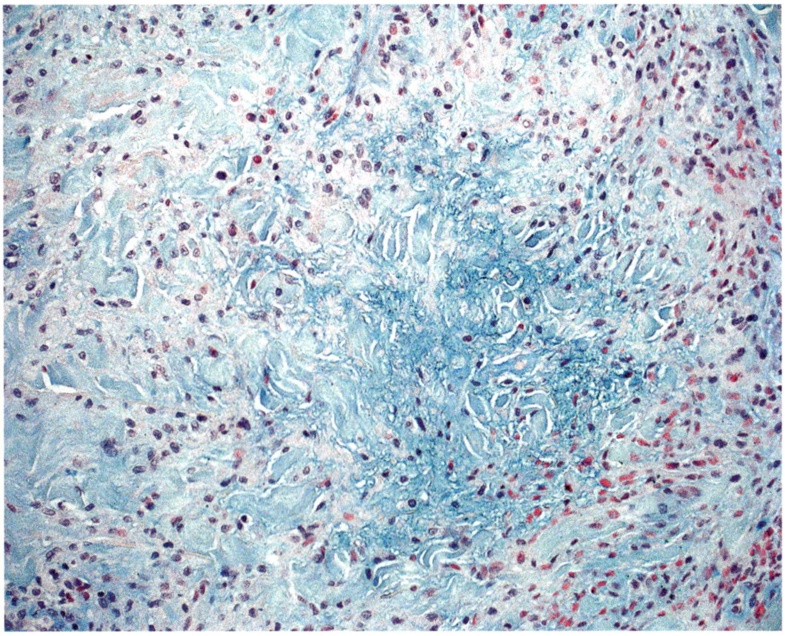

Fig. 3.2 Granuloma annulare. Alcian blue stain demonstrates abundant mucin in the necrobiotic zone

Table 3.2 Key pathologic features: granuloma annulare and rheumatoid nodule

Zone of necrobiosis surrounded by spindled to epithelioid histiocytes
Necrobiotic material is composed of fibrin, mucin deposits, and collagen
No significant cytologic atypia or mitotic activity
The histiocytes are positive for CD68 and CD163 and negative for cytokeratins, EMA, and melanocytic markers

coma also have prominently eosinophilic "hard" cytoplasm, unlike the histiocytes in granuloma annulare and rheumatoid nodule. Histiocytes in the nonneoplastic granulomatous proliferations express CD68 and CD163 and, unlike epithelioid sarcoma, lack cytokeratin and EMA immunoreactivity and retain nuclear INI1 expression.

Non-mesenchymal Spindle Cell Neoplasms that Mimic Primary Cutaneous Soft Tissue Lesions

Non-mesenchymal neoplasms with spindle cell morphology outnumber primary mesenchymal tumors in all locations and generally must be considered before a diagnosis of a primary mesenchymal neoplasm, especially sarcoma, is rendered. In the skin and subcutis, the most common non-mesenchymal spindle cell neoplasms are spindle cell (sarcomatoid) squamous cell carcinoma and spindle cell and desmoplastic melanoma.

Sarcomatoid Carcinoma

Clinical Features

Sarcomatoid carcinoma (also referred to as carcinosarcoma or metaplastic carcinoma) is a neoplasm composed of malignant epithelial and mesenchymal elements. In the skin, sarcomatoid carcinoma most often occurs in a background of squamous cell carcinoma and, rarely, basal cell carcinoma, adnexal carcinomas (spiradenocarcinoma, porocarcinoma, trichilemmal carcinoma, etc.), and Merkel cell carcinoma. Occasionally, it may present as cutaneous metastases from visceral sites, like sarcomatoid renal cell or pulmonary carcinoma. Most primary tumors occur in the head and neck, trunk, or upper arms of middle-aged to elderly adult patients. Spindle cell squamous cell carcinoma (unassociated with radiation) is a subtype of sarcomatoid squamous cell carcinoma, which tends to affect sun-damaged skin in elderly patients. In contrast to other sarcomatoid carcinomas, it is associated with relatively indolent behavior and low rate of nodal and systemic metastases. Desmoplastic squamous cell carcinoma is associated with a densely collagenous scar-like stroma and tends to behave aggressively, as do adnexal carcinosarcomas. Cutaneous sarcomatoid carcinomas are usually treated with surgery.

Pathologic Features

The mesenchymal component in sarcomatoid carcinomas usually consists of a dermal prolif-

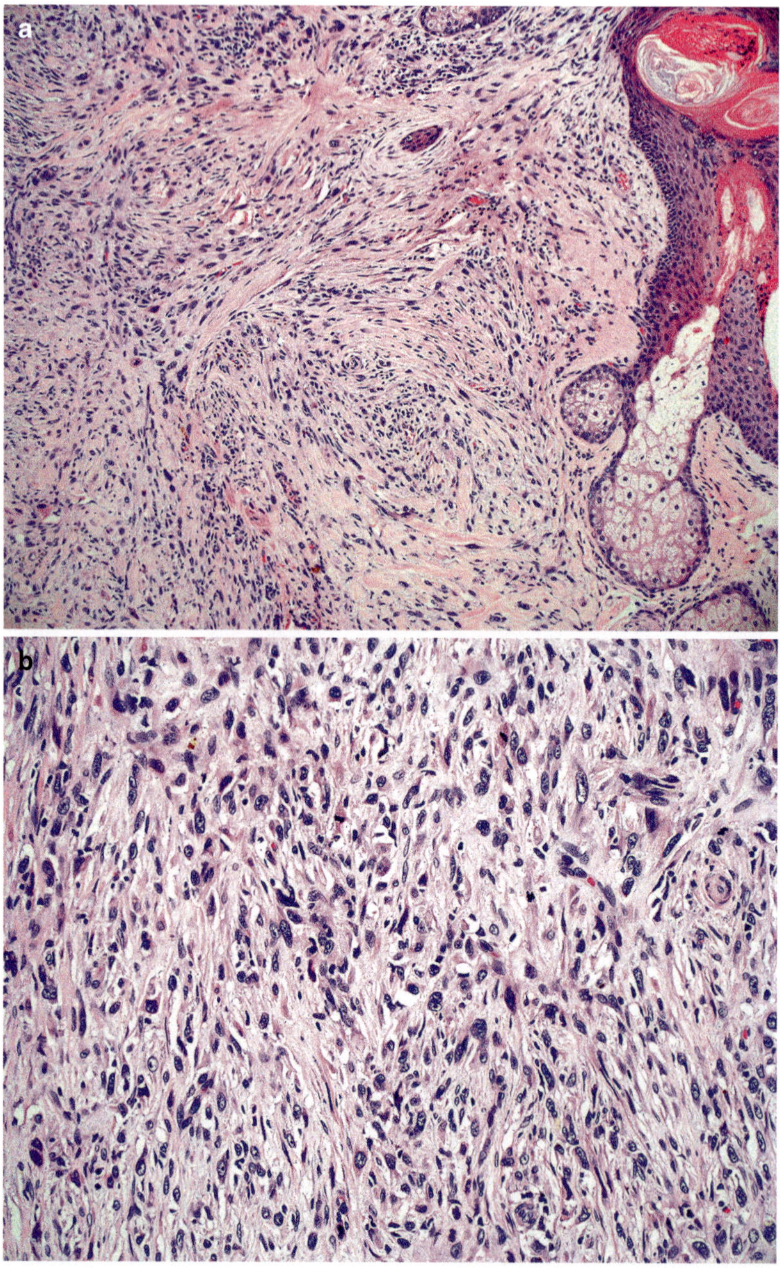

Fig. 3.3 Spindle cell squamous cell carcinoma. (**a**). Dermal proliferation of undifferentiated spindle cells arranged in vague fascicles or storiform growth pattern resembling atypical fibroxanthoma and pleomorphic dermal sarcoma. (**b**). Nuclear atypia, pleomorphism, and mitotic activity are apparent

eration of undifferentiated spindle cells arranged in sheets, vague fascicles, or a storiform growth pattern mimicking atypical fibroxanthoma and pleomorphic dermal sarcoma (Fig. 3.3a, b). There is a variable degree of nuclear atypia, pleomorphism, and mitotic activity. Modestly cellular examples with mild atypia and an extensively collagenous stroma (desmoplastic squamous cell carcinoma) may mimic a hypertrophic scar (Fig. 3.4a–b). Perineural and vascular invasions are very helpful features for establishing the diagnosis in mildly atypical cases. Rarely, tumors with heterologous osteosarcomatous, chondrosarcomatous, myogenic (smooth or skeletal muscle), or angiosarcomatous elements may be encountered. Osteosarcomatous heterologous differentiation is most common and differs from benign metaplastic ossification by the presence of immature, lace-like osteoid deposits and markedly atypical, mitotically active spindled or epithelioid stromal cells (Fig. 3.5). The overlying epidermis may show squamous cell carci-

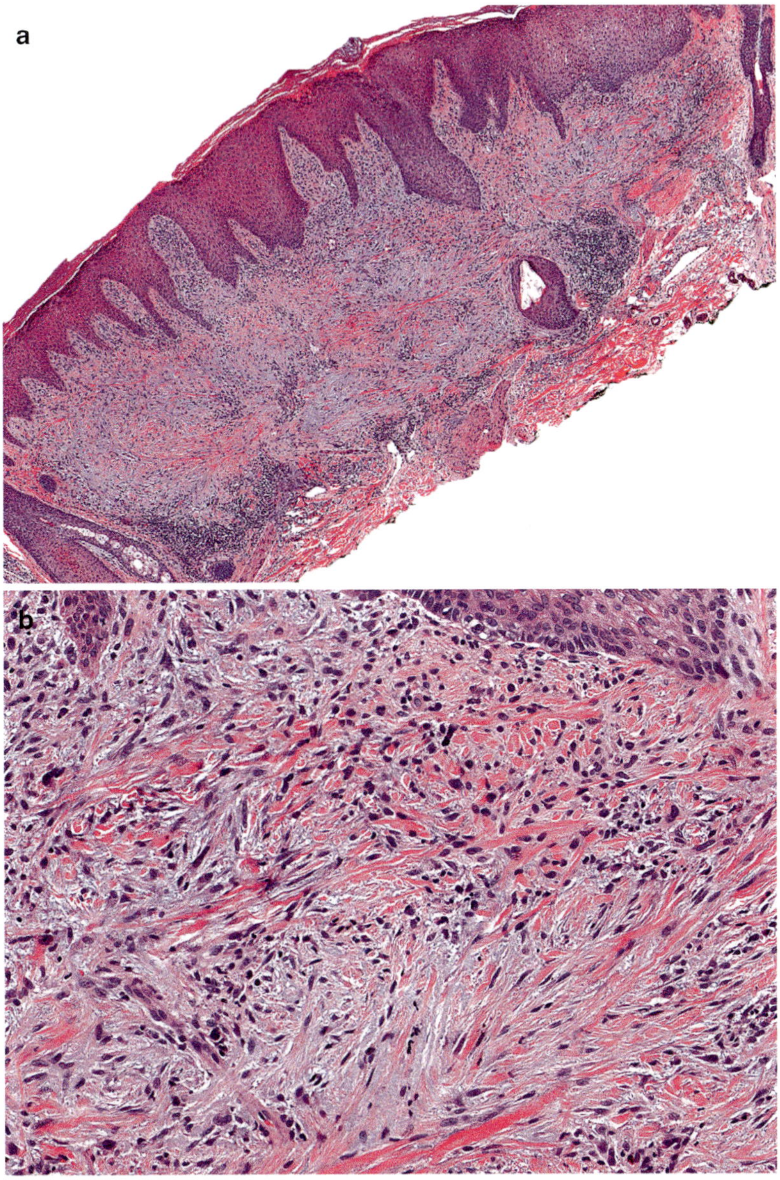

Fig. 3.4 Desmoplastic squamous cell carcinoma. (**a**). This example is shows low cellularity resembling a scar at low power. Inflammatory aggregates are present at the periphery. (**b**). Scattered atypical spindle cells in fibrous stroma

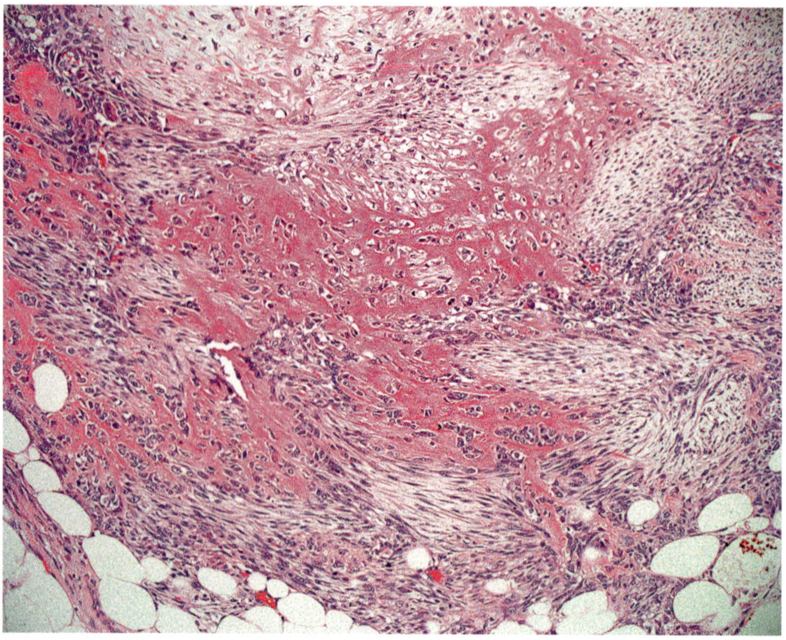

Fig. 3.5 Sarcomatoid squamous cell carcinoma with heterologous osteosarcomatous differentiation. Spindle cells transition to zones of malignant-appearing lace-like osteoid mimicking osteosarcoma

noma in situ or features of actinic keratosis, but often there is no obvious precursor disease. By immunohistochemistry, the spindle cell areas in cutaneous sarcomatoid carcinoma often express a variety of cytokeratins, including broad-spectrum (AE1/AE3 and MNF116) and high-molecular-weight cytokeratins such as CK5/6 or 34betaE12 and p63 and EMA (Fig. 3.6a, b). We usually apply a panel including a broad-spectrum cytokeratin, a high-molecular-weight cytokeratin, and an S100 protein. In selected cases, EMA, p63, SMA, desmin, CD34, and vascular markers CD31 and ERG may be used as well. Key pathologic features of sarcomatoid carcinoma are presented in Table 3.3.

Differential Diagnosis

Sarcomatoid carcinoma needs to be distinguished from spindle cell and desmoplastic melanoma, atypical fibroxanthoma, and pleomorphic dermal sarcoma (superficial undifferentiated pleomorphic sarcoma). Recognition of an epithelial component, oftentimes at the edge of the lesion, and overlying surface dysplasia/carcinoma in situ are useful clues to the diagnosis. However, many sarcomatoid carcinomas lack epithelial changes and require a high index of suspicion. Any expression of cytokeratins, even if focal, is helpful in supporting the diagnosis of sarcomatoid carcinoma. The finding of p63 expression alone must be interpreted with caution and should not be used as the sole evidence of epithelial differentiation, as many primary mesenchymal neoplasms can express this marker (usually focally). Sarcomatoid carcinomas with heterologous elements need to be distinguished from primary or metastatic extraosseous osteosarcoma, chondrosarcoma, leiomyosarcoma, and rhabdomyosarcoma, all of which are rare in the skin, and angiosarcoma. Myogenic, vascular makers and SATB2 (marker of osteoblastic differentiation) can help to identify the heterologous component, but the key to the correct diagnosis is proving an epithelial origin for the tumor. Desmoplastic squamous cell carcinoma closely mimics a hypertrophic scar but, in contrast to the latter, usually diffusely expresses cytokeratins and p63. Cytokeratin expression together with p63 positivity strongly supports a diagnosis of sarcomatoid squamous or sarcomatoid adnexal carcinoma in our experience. Desmoplastic and spindle cell melanomas express S100 protein and SOX10 in nearly every case, while expression of cytokeratins is exceptional.

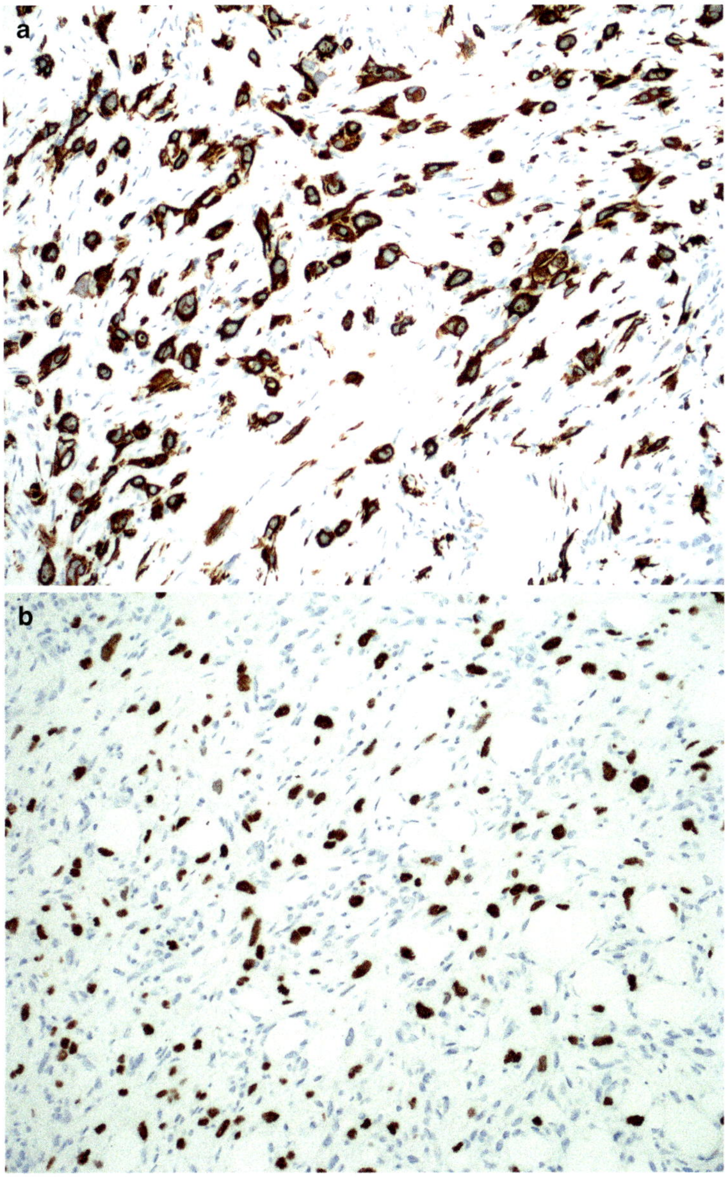

Fig. 3.6 Spindle cell squamous cell carcinoma. (**a**). Immunohistochemical staining for CK5/6 (**a**) and p63 (**b**) supports epithelial origin of the spindle cells

Table 3.3 Key pathologic features: sarcomatoid carcinoma

Most often in the background of cutaneous squamous cell carcinoma
Spindle to pleomorphic fibroblastic cells resembling dermal pleomorphic sarcoma or atypical fibroxanthoma
Surface dysplasia/carcinoma in situ or epithelial component may be focal or absent
Desmoplastic squamous cell carcinoma has mild atypia and abundant densely collagenized stroma resembling a scar, an important pitfall
Any expression of cytokeratin is helpful to prove epithelial differentiation

Spindle Cell, Desmoplastic, and Dedifferentiated Melanoma

Clinical Features

Spindle cell melanoma can occur anywhere in the body and is often identified at metastatic sites. Desmoplastic melanoma is a variant of spindle cell melanoma with a predilection to arise on sun-damaged skin of the head and neck of older individuals. Neurotropism (a growth pattern within

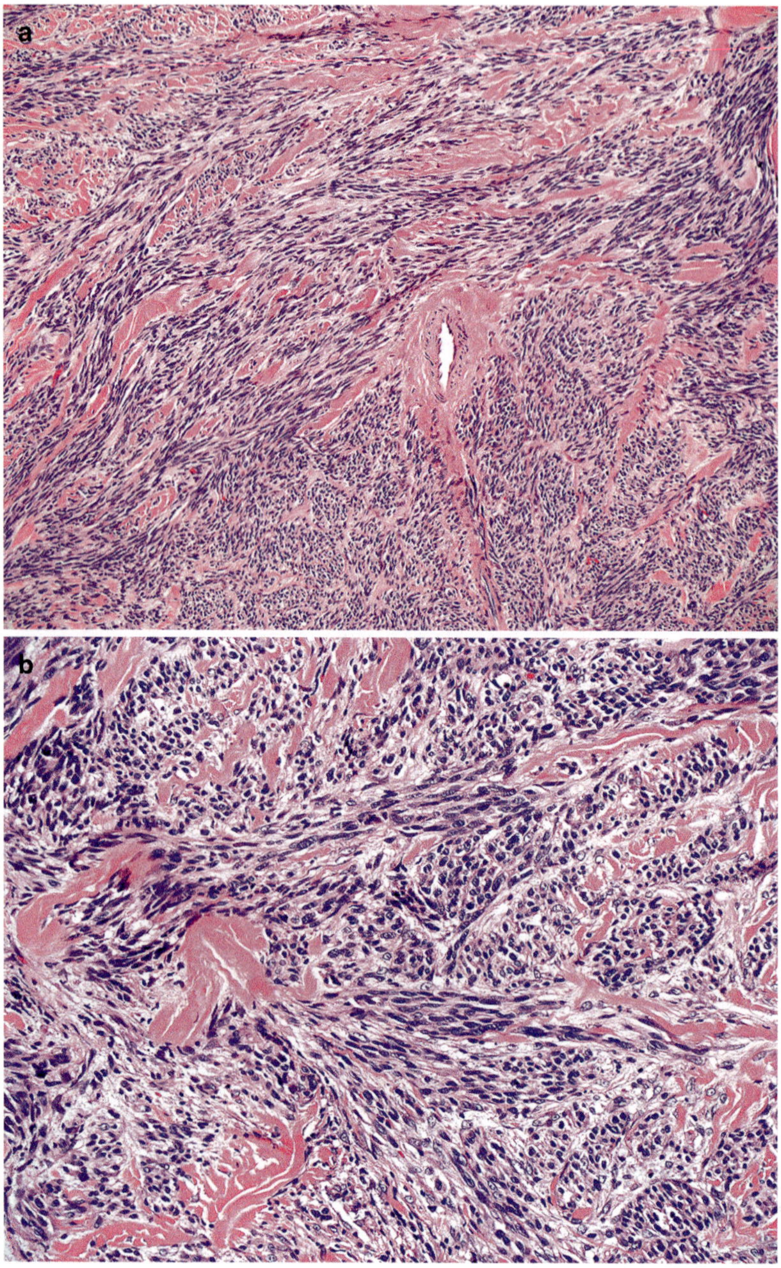

Fig. 3.7 Spindle cell melanoma. (**a**). Uniform, densely cellular fascicles and nests of spindle cells infiltrating between dermal collagens. (**b**). The tumor cells have atypical oval nuclei with vesicular chromatin, variably prominent nucleoli and amphophilic cytoplasm

and around nerves away from the main tumor mass) and frequent local recurrences are also common. The prognosis of desmoplastic melanoma is superior to that of spindle cell and conventional melanoma subtypes. Dedifferentiated or sarcomatoid melanoma is an aggressive variant often identified at metastatic sites that lacks morphologic features or diagnostic immunohistochemical evidence of melanocytic differentiation. This tumor essentially has an undifferentiated spindle cell sarcoma phenotype or displays divergent differentiation like rhabdomyosarcoma.

Pathologic Features

Spindle cell melanomas are composed of relatively uniform densely cellular fascicles and nests

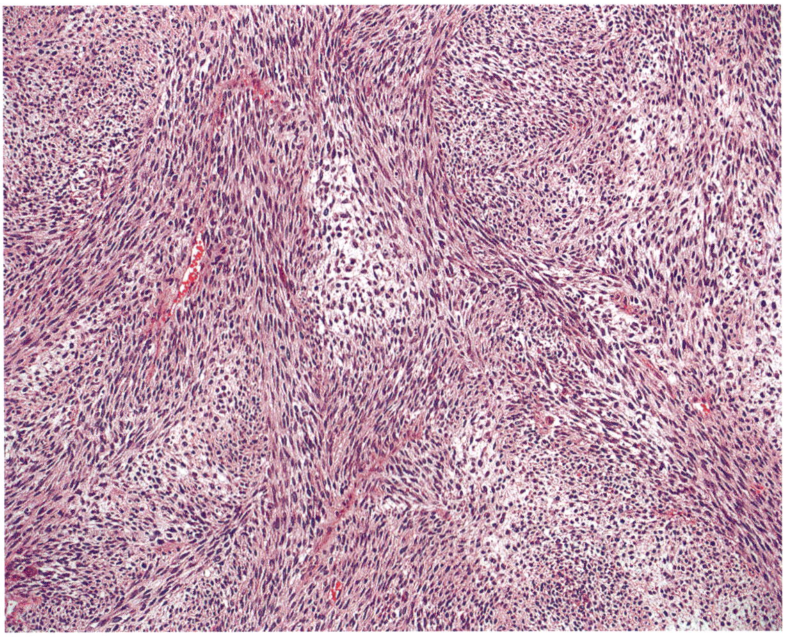

Fig. 3.8 Metastatic spindle cell melanoma. This example shows monotonous intersecting fascicles and myxoid stroma and resembles malignant peripheral nerve sheath tumor

of mitotically active spindle cells with oval nuclei, vesicular chromatin, variably prominent nucleoli, and usually amphophilic cytoplasm. The nests of tumor cells may be separated by thin fibrous bands like those seen in clear cell sarcoma (Fig. 3.7). While nuclear atypia is obvious in most cases, marked nuclear pleomorphism is not a typical feature of spindle cell melanoma. Inflammatory infiltrates and lymphoid aggregates at the periphery of the lesion are common. At primary sites, spindle cell melanoma often coexists with melanoma with more conventional epithelioid morphology and may be associated with a junctional in situ component and pagetoid spread. It may appear entirely spindled at metastatic sites, such as lymph nodes (Fig. 3.8). Desmoplastic melanoma is characterized by modest cellularity and vague fascicles of spindle cells embedded in an abundant, densely collagenous stroma and displays a highly infiltrative growth pattern (Fig. 3.9a, b). Cytologically, desmoplastic melanoma may be deceptively bland (Fig. 3.10). Neurotropism is especially common in desmoplastic melanoma (Fig. 3.11). Both spindle cell and the desmoplastic melanoma are typically amelanotic. By immunohistochemistry, tumor cells are usually strongly and diffusely positive for S100 and SOX10, but they tend to lack expression of other melanocytic markers such as Melan-A, HMB45, and tyrosinase, which are positive in less than 10% of cases. Dedifferentiated melanoma lacks diagnostic immunophenotypic evidence of true melanocytic differentiation and is instead characterized by phenotypic plasticity and frequently expresses cytokeratins and myogenic markers like desmin, SMA, and myogenin. A component of adjacent conventional melanoma may be the only way to recognize dedifferentiated melanoma on routine histologic sections. V600E *BRAF* is the most common mutation type in spindle cell melanoma (approximately 30% of spindle cell and 5% of desmoplastic melanoma), while *NRAS* and *KIT* mutations are very rare. Key pathologic features of the above melanoma subtypes are presented in Table 3.4.

Differential Diagnosis

Spindle cell melanoma mimics a variety of fascicular spindle cell sarcomas, most notably conventional malignant peripheral nerve sheath tumor (MPNST), cellular schwannoma, and clear cell sarcoma. Superficial MPNST (discussed in Chap. 10) and desmoplastic/spindle cell melanoma might be especially difficult to distinguish

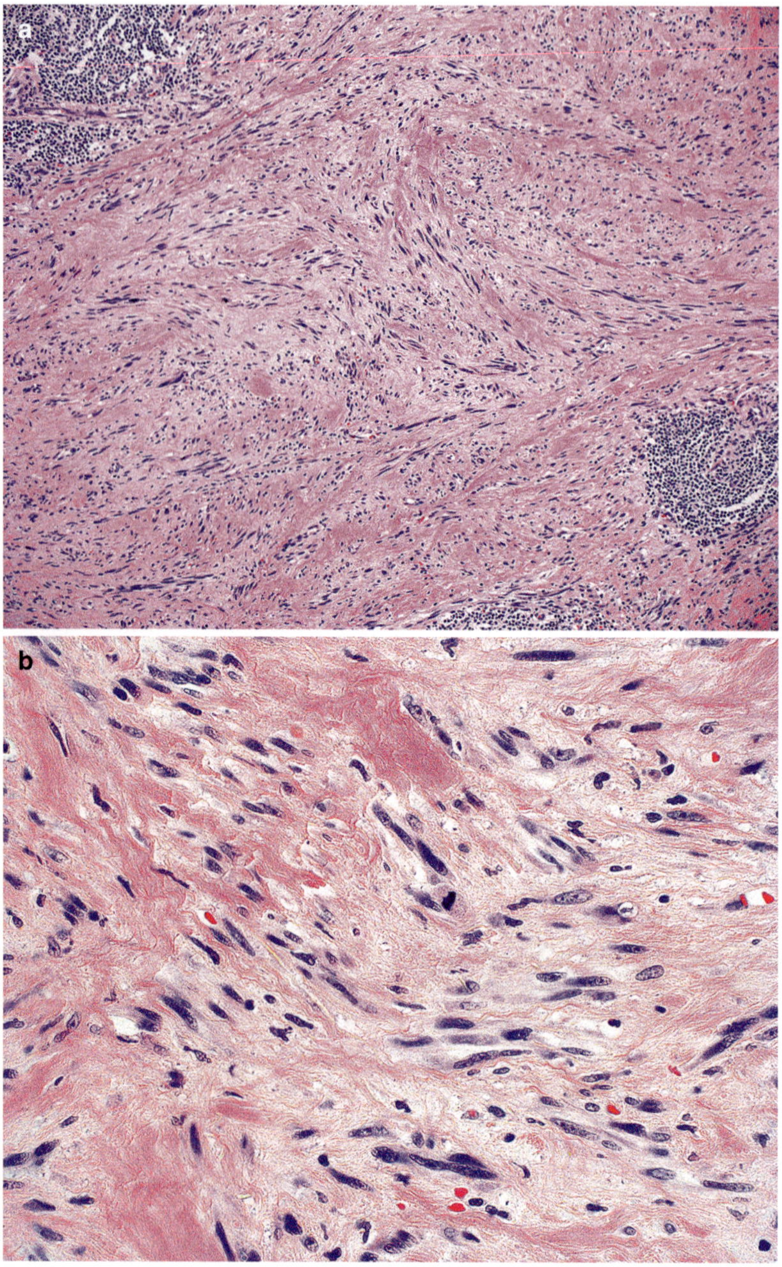

Fig. 3.9 Desmoplastic melanoma. (**a**). Modestly cellular infiltrative spindle cell neoplasm in a densely collagenous background with peripheral lymphoid aggregates. (**b**). Atypical mitotically active spindle cells with oval nuclei and variable nucleoli

on morphologic grounds alone. The pattern of S100 protein and SOX10 expression is very helpful in this case. Most spindle cell and desmoplastic melanomas are strongly and diffusely positive for both markers (over 95%), whereas S100 protein expression is usually focal or negative in conventional MPNSTs, and SOX10 expression is seen in approximately 50–70% of cases. Complete loss of H3K27 methylation, a useful diagnostic marker of MPNST, is not helpful in this context as up to 37% of all melanomas and up to 25% of desmoplastic melanomas display loss of H3K27me. Cellular schwannomas (discussed in Chap. 10) usually present as deep-seated retroperitoneal or mediastinal masses, rather than cutaneous tumors, and, along with densely cellular

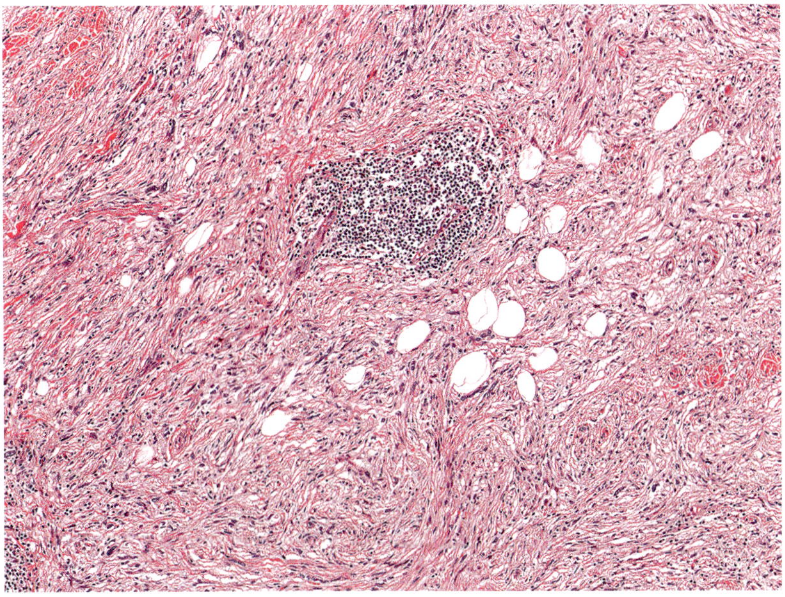

Fig. 3.10 Desmoplastic melanoma. This example resembles benign fibrous histiocytoma (dermatofibroma). Tumor cells are arranged in a storiform growth pattern, and there is only mild nuclear atypia

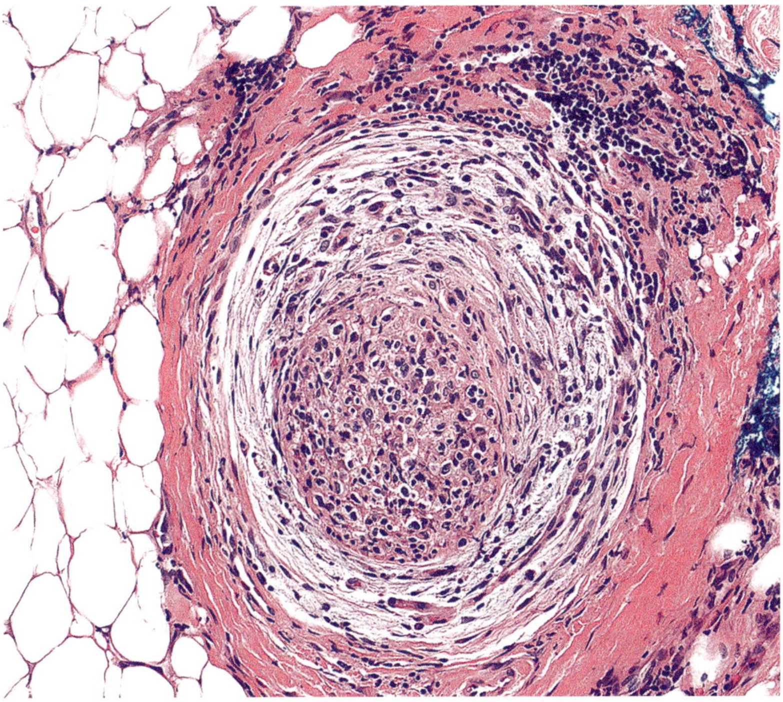

Fig. 3.11 Desmoplastic melanoma exhibiting peri- and intraneural growth pattern away from the main tumor mass (neurotropism)

fascicles of schwannian cells, usually demonstrate hyalinized vessels, foci of palisading, and aggregates of foamy histiocytes, features not seen in spindle cell melanoma. A nested growth pattern is not typical of cellular schwannoma. These tumors share common genetic pathways involving *NF1*, *RAS*, and *TSC* mutations and have some overlapping patterns of copy number gains and losses, but in our experience, some of the copy number variants can be used to distinguish nerve sheath tumors from melanoma and benign nerve sheath tumors from low-grade (well-differentiated)

Table 3.4 Key pathologic features: spindle cell, desmoplastic, and dedifferentiated melanoma

Spindle cell melanoma
Nests and fascicles of mitotically active spindle cells with oval nuclei, vesicular chromatin, and variably prominent nucleoli
The nests may be separated by fibrous bands
Inflammatory aggregates at the periphery
Desmoplastic melanoma
Ill-defined scar-like infiltrative growth pattern
Nests and vague fascicles of deceptively bland spindle cells in abundant densely collagenized stroma
Inflammatory aggregates at the periphery
Neurotropism is common
Strong, diffuse expression of S100 protein and SOX10, negative for Melan-A, HMB45, or tyrosinase
Dedifferentiated (sarcomatoid) melanoma lacks expression of all melanocytic markers

MPNST. Clear cell sarcoma (discussed in Chap. 12) may be virtually indistinguishable from spindle cell melanoma by morphology and immunoprofile, including the possibility of a junctional component and pagetoid intraepidermal spread (so-called epidermotropic clear cell sarcoma), and often requires confirmatory molecular testing for *EWSR1* gene rearrangement.

Desmoplastic melanoma may be mistaken for a hypertrophic scar, fibromatosis, or neurofibroma. Helpful diagnostic clues for distinguishing desmoplastic melanoma from hypertrophic scar include nesting of tumor cells, lack of vertically oriented vessels, and diffuse immunoreactivity for S100 protein and SOX10. We maintain a high index of suspicion for both desmoplastic melanoma and desmoplastic squamous cell carcinoma when encountering a stellate-shaped irregular scar-like lesion in sun-damaged skin. Superficial and desmoid-type fibromatoses lack nested architecture, show a distinctive pattern of uniform, gaping vessels with perivascular lymphocytes, and lack expression of S100 protein and SOX10. Desmoplastic melanomas with neurotropism resemble neurofibromas but can be distinguished based on their greater degree of nuclear atypia and patchy chronic inflammatory infiltrate, which are not typical of neurofibromas, and the more diffuse pattern of staining with S100 protein and p53 expression of the latter. Spindle cell, desmoplastic, and especially dedifferentiated melanomas with loss of melanocytic markers may be difficult to distinguish from primary cutaneous undifferentiated spindle cell sarcoma and other pleomorphic dermal spindle cell neoplasms. In our experience, meticulous examination of the tumor periphery is especially helpful in these challenging cases, as it may reveal recognizable precursor melanoma.

Cellular Blue Nevus

Clinical Features

Cellular blue nevi most commonly present in young adult patients, as small nodules on the buttock or sacrococcygeal region, followed by the scalp, face, and extremities. Cellular blue nevi are usually intensely pigmented blue-black nodules but may be amelanotic. This is a benign melanocytic lesion that may mimic a spindle cell sarcoma, which is cured by simple excision.

Pathologic Features

Cellular blue nevus classically has a circumscribed pushing border and is composed of a biphasic population of pigmented dendritic melanocytes and spindled to oval melanocytes with clear-to- lightly eosinophilic cytoplasm and nuclei with fine chromatin and small nucleoli (Fig. 3.12). Rare hypopigmented or amelanotic forms have little to no pigmented dendritic melanocytes (Fig. 3.13). Occasional multinucleated wreath-like giant cells may be present. Cellular blue nevus is positive for S100 protein, SOX10, and HMB45, as well as other melanocytic markers, such as MiTF, Melan-A, and tyrosinase. Key pathologic features of cellular blue nevus are presented in Table 3.5.

Differential Diagnosis

Cellular blue nevus may be confused with clear cell sarcoma. Clear cell sarcoma typically presents in the foot/ankle region, is more infiltrative, has more pronounced nuclear atypia, and lacks the pigmented dendritic cells seen in most

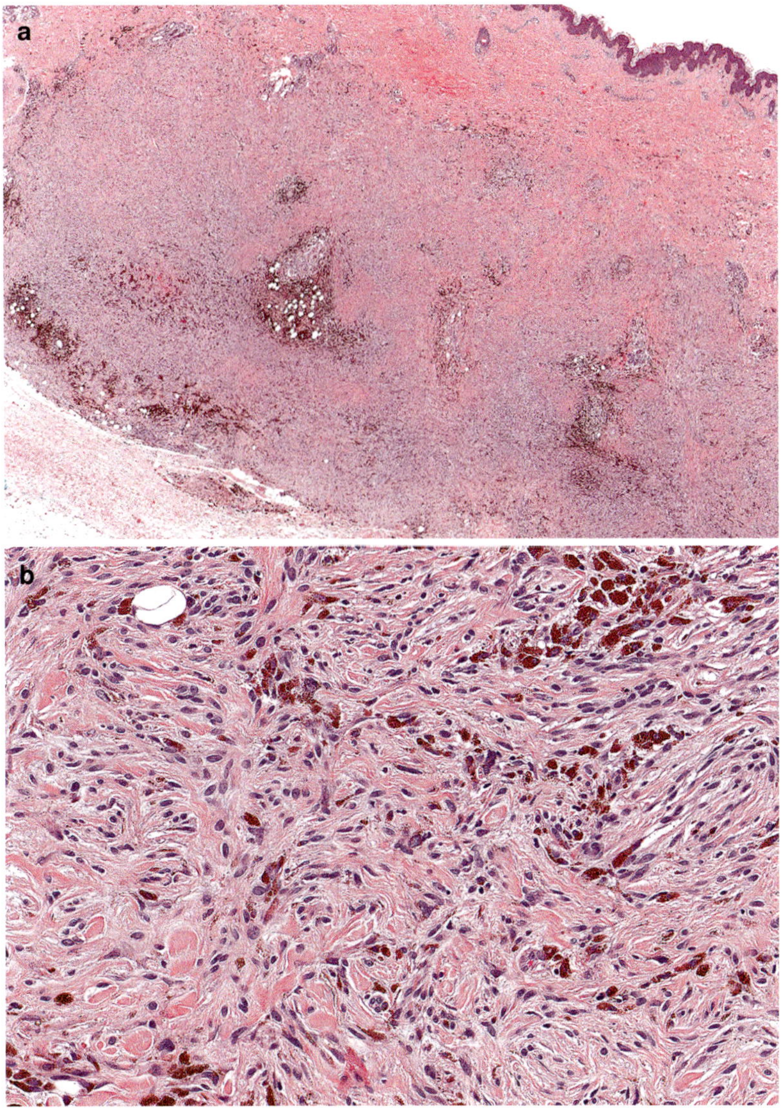

Fig. 3.12 Cellular blue nevus. (**a**). Circumscribed, pushing border is appreciated at low power. (**b**). The tumor is composed of pigmented dendritic melanocytes as well as spindled to ovoid melanocytes with eosinophilic cytoplasm

cellular blue nevi. Although both tumors have the same immunophenotype, clear cell sarcoma has rearrangement of *EWSR1*. FISH to detect this genetic abnormality allows distinction.

Massive Localized Lymphedema

Clinical Features

Massive localized lymphedema (MLL) is a form of secondary lymphedema that occurs in morbidly obese, middle-age adults due to chronic obstruction of lymphatic drainage by excessive adipose tissue. It most often presents as a large, superficial, sometimes pedunculated fatty mass with predilection for the medial thigh, but the arms and legs, abdominal wall, anogenital region, and scrotum can also be affected. MLL is benign but may cause significant clinical and surgical morbidity and rarely may give rise to lymphedema-associated cutaneous angiosarcoma. From the pathologic standpoint, MLL most closely mimics atypical lipomatous tumor/well-differentiated liposarcoma.

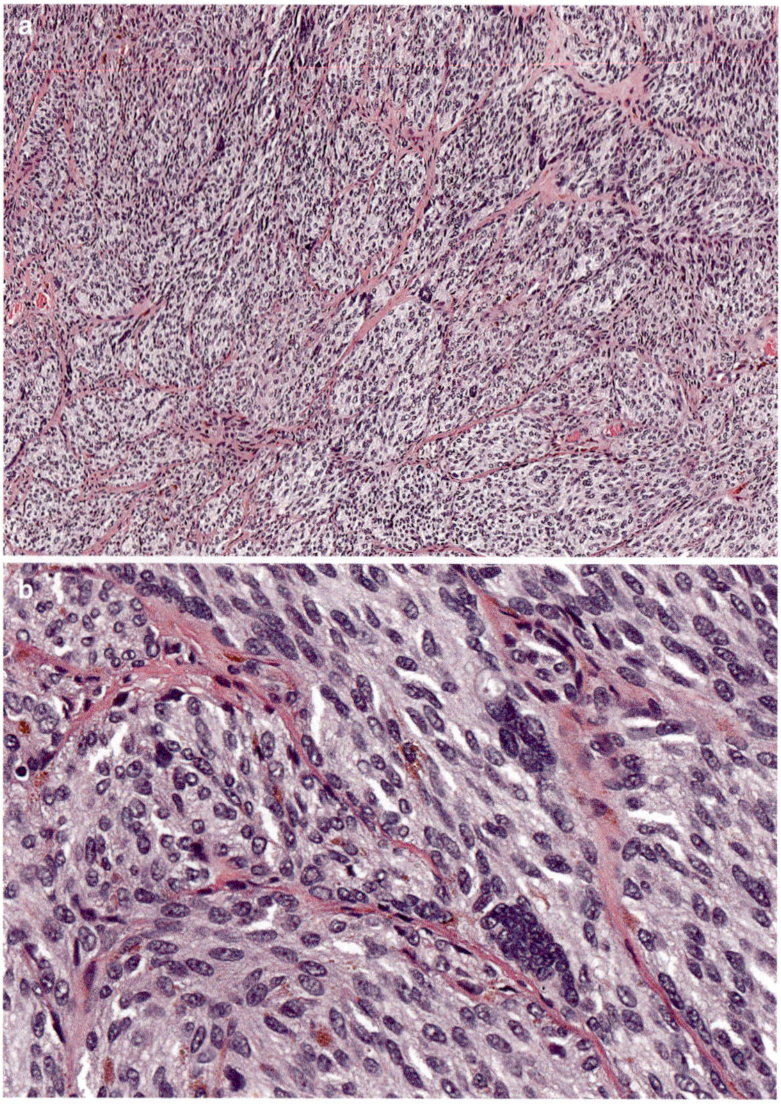

Fig. 3.13 Cellular blue nevus. (**a**). Hypopigmented blue nevus with nests of pale melanocytes and occasional multinucleated cells. (**b**). Higher-power image demonstrating bland nuclear features of hypopigmented blue nevus

Table 3.5 Key pathologic features: cellular blue nevus

Pushing border
Biphasic tumor composed of pigmented dendritic cells and spindled to oval melanocytes with clear to lightly eosinophilic cytoplasm
Bland nuclear features
Positive for S100 protein, SOX10, and melanocyte-specific markers
Lacks *EWSR1* gene rearrangement

Pathologic Features

MLL is usually rather large (mean size, 50 cm) fatty mass covered by thickened nodular skin with peau d'orange-like appearance. Microscopically, the lesion is composed of coarsely lobulated adipose tissue encased by expanded connective tissue bands. The overlying dermis shows edema and varying degrees of fibrosis (Fig. 3.14a, b). A characteristic feature is proliferation of small- to medium-sized lymphatic vessels that may be accompanied by lymphoid aggregates and lymphoid follicles. Reactive-type proliferative capillary network may also develop within fatty lobules, and some long-standing cases demonstrate dystrophic calcifications or heterologous ossification (Fig. 3.15a, b). The fibrous septa contain atypical

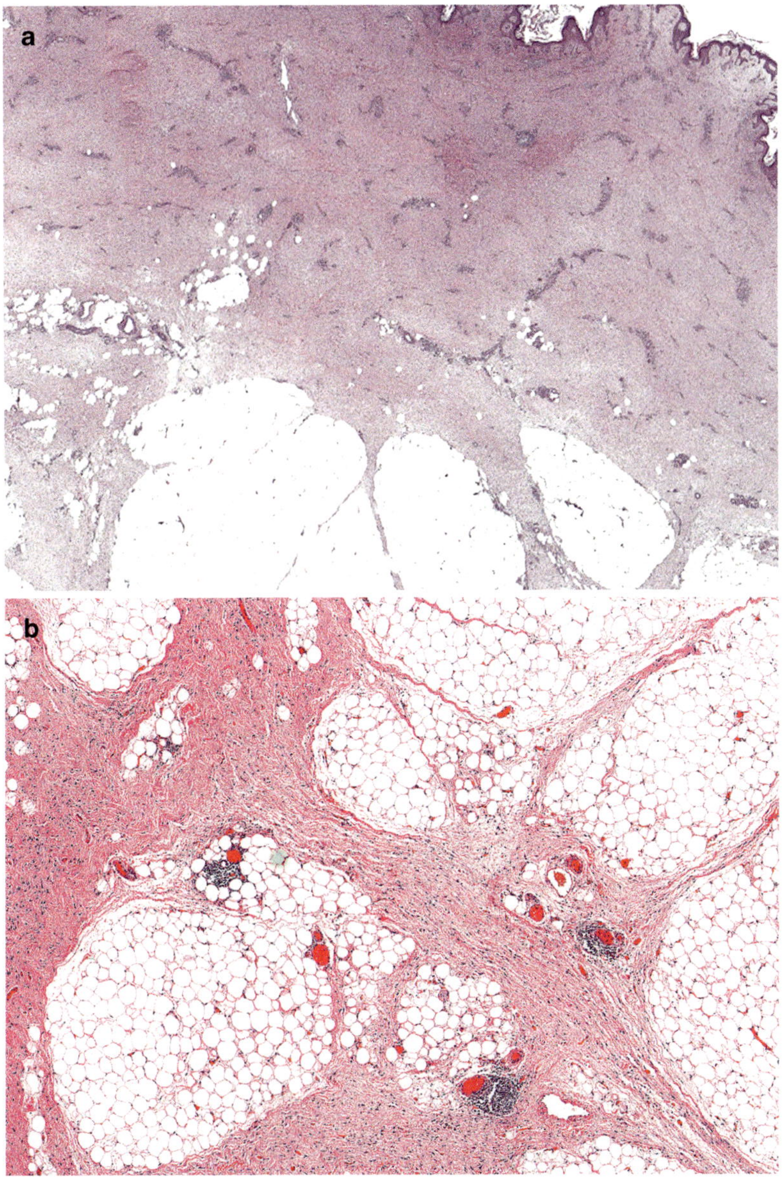

Fig. 3.14 Massive localized lymphedema. (**a**). Lobulated adipose tissue encased by expanded connective tissue bands and overlying dermal fibrosis with angioproliferative changes and thickened nodular skin. (**b**). Fatty mass composed of coarsely lobulated adipose tissue encased by expanded connective tissue bands

hyperchromatic spindle to stellate fibroblasts that closely mimic those seen in atypical lipomatous tumor/well-differentiated liposarcoma, but true lipoblasts are usually not seen (Fig. 3.16a, b). Key pathologic features of massive localized lymphedema are presented in Table 3.6.

Differential Diagnosis

The principal diagnostic mimic is atypical lipomatous tumor/well-differentiated liposarcoma (ALT/WDL). The following histologic clues are very helpful to distinguish MLL from the latter. MLL is superficial in location and nearly always involves the dermis, whereas most ALTs/WDLs are deep-seated, soft tissue or intramuscular tumors that are usually well demarcated from the surrounding tissue, even when superficial. At scanning magnification, MLL shows preservation of lobular fatty architecture, which is completely distorted in ALT/WDL. Dermal edema and a reactive-type capillary proliferation are not prominent in ALT/WDL. FISH testing for *MDM2*

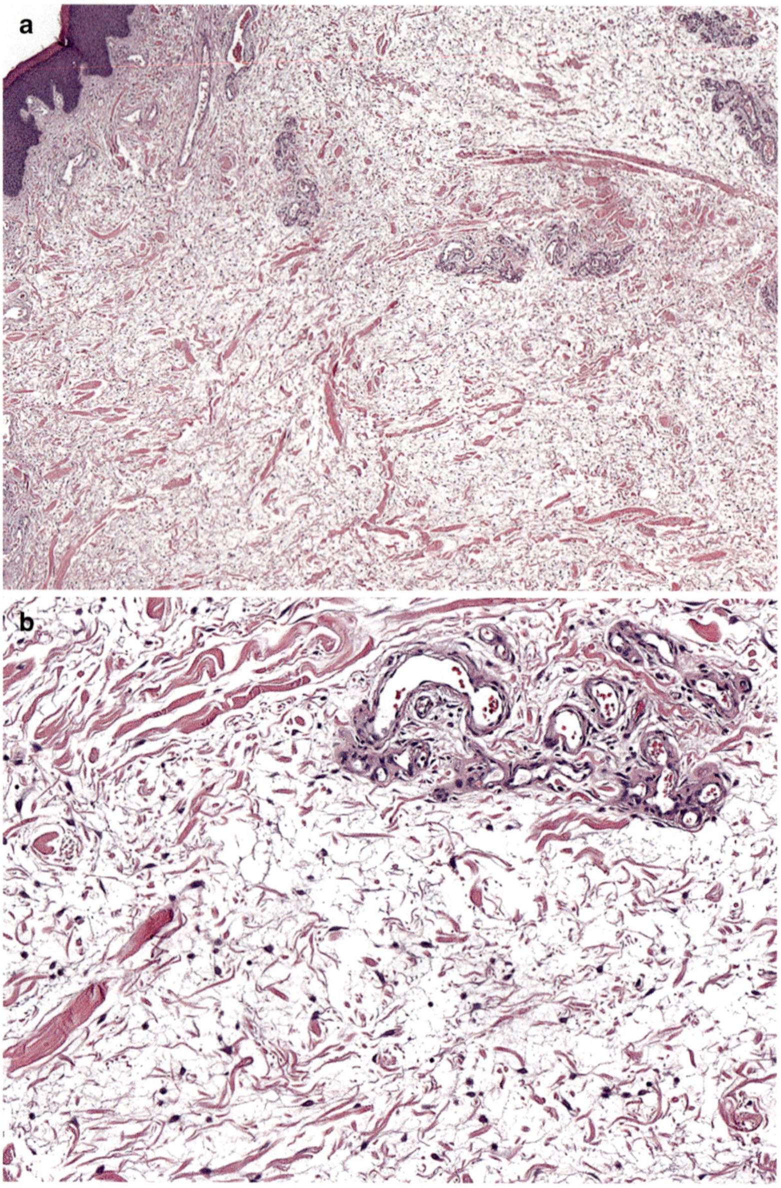

Fig. 3.15 Massive localized lymphedema. (**a**). The stroma is edematous and shows proliferation of small lymphatics and reactive capillaries accompanied by scattered lymphocytes. (**b**). Reactive-type capillaries, a useful diagnostic feature

gene amplification, which is positive in ALT/WDL, can be useful in difficult cases.

Silicone Granuloma

Clinical Features

Silicone is a biomaterial that has been used extensively in reconstructive surgery (breast augmentation) and in cosmetic surgery as an injectable dermal filler. While silicone is a biologically inert material, it may elicit a florid mass-like tissue reaction termed "silicone granuloma" and can rarely cause more significant adverse autoimmune/inflammatory reactions or lymphoma. Silicone granulomas are increasing in frequency due to the popularity of dermal fillers and can be found in the subcutaneous tissue of the face, buttocks, as well as in the breast subcutaneous tissue around ruptured breast implant. The significance of silicone granuloma, aside from cosmetic

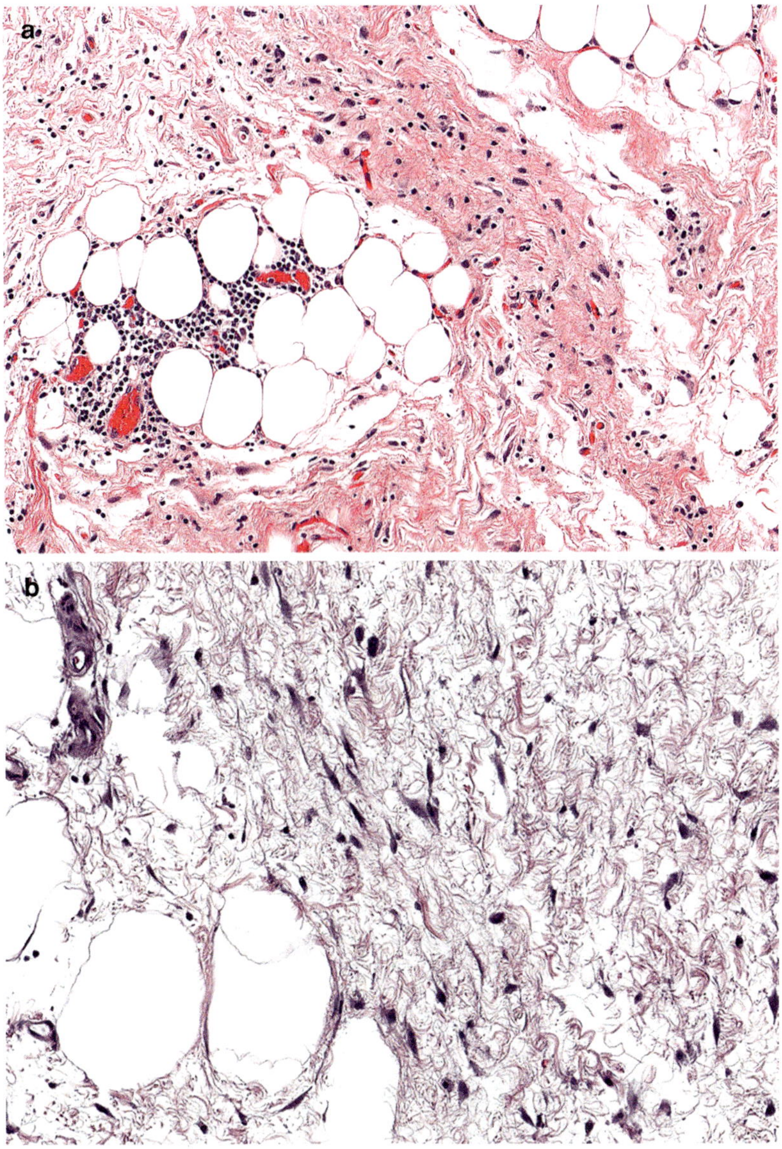

Fig. 3.16 Massive localized lymphedema. (**a** and **b**). Atypical hyperchromatic spindle to stellate fibroblasts mimicking those seen in atypical lipomatous tumor/well-differentiated liposarcoma. True lipoblasts are not seen

Table 3.6 Key pathologic features: massive localized lymphedema

Large, fatty mass, usually from medial thigh
Coarsely lobulated adipose tissue encased by expanded connective tissue bands
Dermal edema, fibrosis, chronic inflammation
Lymphatic and reactive capillary vascular proliferation
Atypical hyperchromatic spindle to stellate fibroblasts that closely mimic those seen in atypical lipomatous tumor/well-differentiated liposarcoma

deformity, is that the granulomatous reaction can mimic liposarcoma.

Pathologic Features

Silicone granuloma represents a collection of vacuolated histiocytes of varying sizes containing silicone material, usually walled off by a fibrous capsule. Mild chronic inflammation may be present. The multivacuolated histiocytes closely resemble lipoblasts and for this reason can mimic liposarcoma (Fig. 3.17a, b). Key pathologic features of silicone granuloma are presented in Table 3.7.

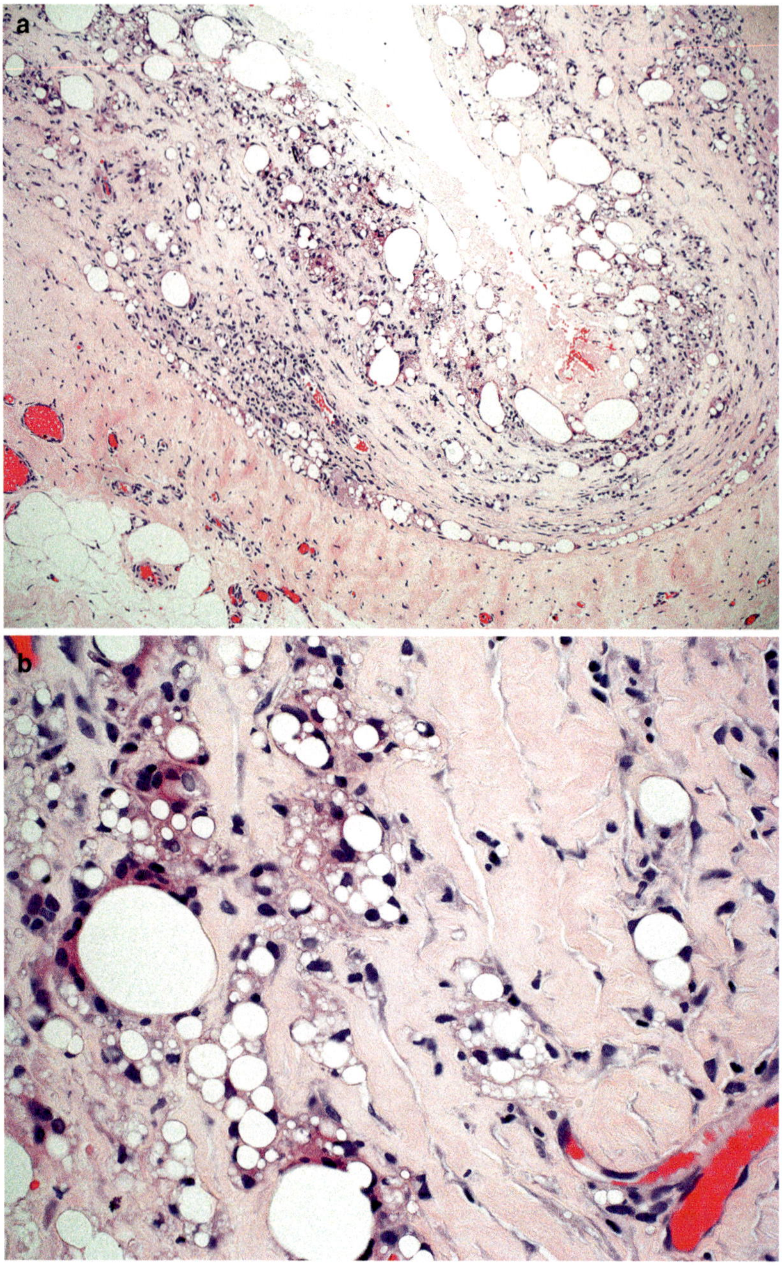

Fig. 3.17 Silicone granuloma. (**a**). Vacuolated histiocytes of varying size containing silicone material walled off by a fibrous capsule. (**b**). The multivacuolated histiocytes closely resemble lipoblasts

Table 3.7 Key pathologic features: silicone granuloma

Collection of vacuolated histiocytes in a fibrous background
Chronic inflammatory reaction
Vacuolated histiocytes resemble true lipoblasts
Lack of cytologic atypia or atypical mitotic figures
Negative for *MDM2* gene amplification
Histiocytes positive for CD68 and CD163

Differential Diagnosis

Silicone granuloma can be mistaken for both atypical lipomatous tumor/well-differentiated liposarcoma (ALT/WDL) and pleomorphic liposarcoma. Atypical hyperchromatic stromal cells, the hallmark of ALT/WDL, are usually not identified in silicone granulomas. Difficult cases may be resolved by immunohistochemistry or FISH testing for *MDM2* gene amplification. Pleomorphic liposarcomas are high-grade pleomorphic sarcomas containing numerous pleomorphic lipoblasts, and should be readily distinguished from silicone granuloma, which lacks significant cytologic atypia or atypical mitotic figures. An immunohistochemical stain for CD68 or CD163 can highlight the histiocytes in silicone granuloma and help distinguish them from lipoblasts seen in liposarcoma.

Mycobacterial Spindle Cell Pseudotumor

Clinical Features

Mycobacterial spindle cell pseudotumor is a rare reactive tumor-like condition caused by mycobacteria, most often *M. avium-intracellulare* followed by *M. tuberculosis*, in immunocompromised patients. Affected sites include primarily lymph nodes and the skin but may involve other sites like the lungs, spleen, nasal cavity, and central nervous system. While classically associated with acquired immunodeficiency syndrome (HIV/AIDS), mycobacterial spindle cell pseudotumor occurs in a variety of immunodeficiency states, including those related to organ transplantation, or induced by immune modulators like tumor necrosis factor inhibitors, and may rarely affect infants after bacille Calmette-Guerin vaccination. The most effective treatment strategy is antimycobacterial therapy; surgical intervention is of limited utility.

Pathologic Features

Mycobacterial spindle cell pseudotumor is composed of a sheets or vague fascicles of spindle cells admixed with inflammatory cells including lymphocytes and plasma cells (Fig. 3.18a, b). The cells have oval nuclei with open chromatin and small nucleoli consistent with fibroblastic/myofibroblastic differentiation, and pale amphophilic cytoplasm, which sometimes appears granular, imparting a more histiocytoid appearance (Fig. 3.19). Cytoplasmic granules seen in this entity represent clumps of acid-fast bacilli that can be detected by acid-fast stains (Fig. 3.20a). Mild cytologic atypia and normal mitotic figures are common, but significant nuclear pleomor-

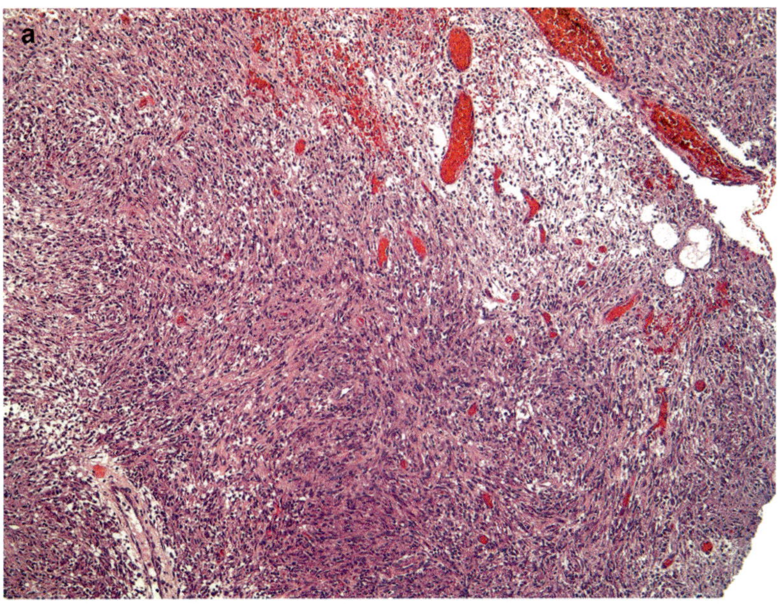

Fig. 3.18 Mycobacterial spindle cell pseudotumor. (**a**). Well-circumscribed unencapsulated cellular mass. (**b**). Fascicles and sheets of spindle cells admixed with inflammatory cells including lymphocytes and plasma cells. (Image courtesy of Dr. Wayne Grayson, Ampath National Laboratories, Johannesburg, South Africa)

Fig. 3.18 (continued)

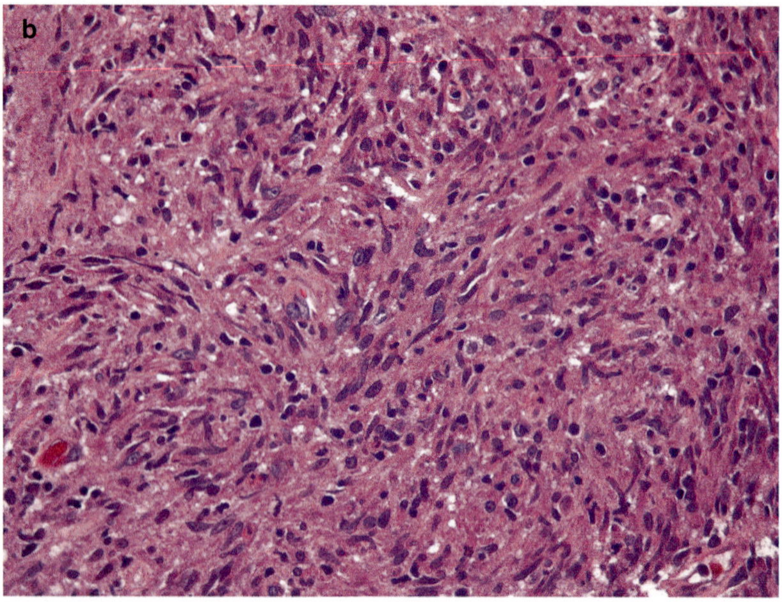

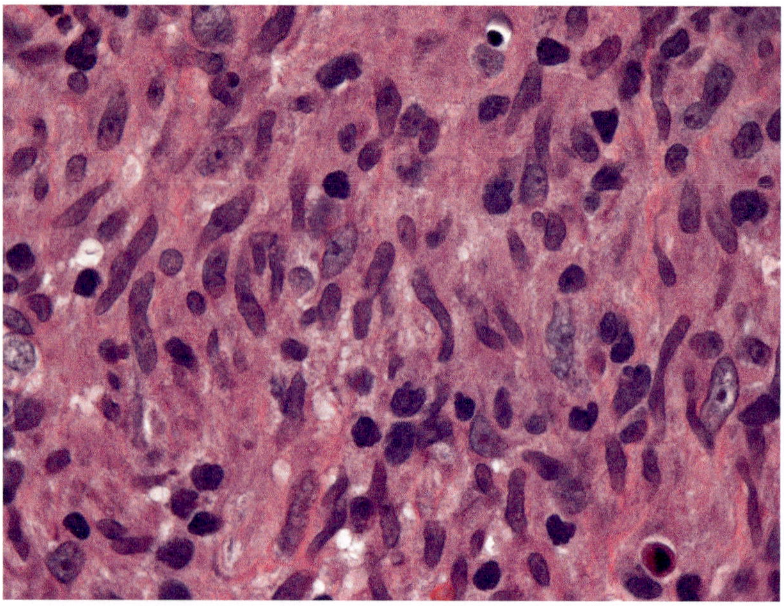

Fig. 3.19 Mycobacterial spindle cell pseudotumor. The cells show oval nuclei with open chromatin and small nucleoli and pale granular cytoplasm imparting a histiocytoid appearance. (Image courtesy of Dr. Wayne Grayson, Ampath National Laboratories, Johannesburg, South Africa)

phism and atypical mitotic figures are not characteristic. By immunohistochemistry, the cells are positive for CD68 (Fig. 3.20b) and may variably co-express SMA, desmin, muscle-specific actin, and CD34, in keeping with fibroblastic/myofibroblastic differentiation. Key pathologic features of mycobacterial spindle cell pseudotumor are presented in Table 3.8.

Differential Diagnosis

Mycobacterial spindle cell pseudotumor is an important mimic of inflammatory myofibroblastic tumor (IMT), spindle cell sarcomas, nodular Kaposi sarcoma, and benign fibrous histiocytoma. Because of the dramatic differences in treatment, we often apply special staining for acid-fast bacilli for fibro-

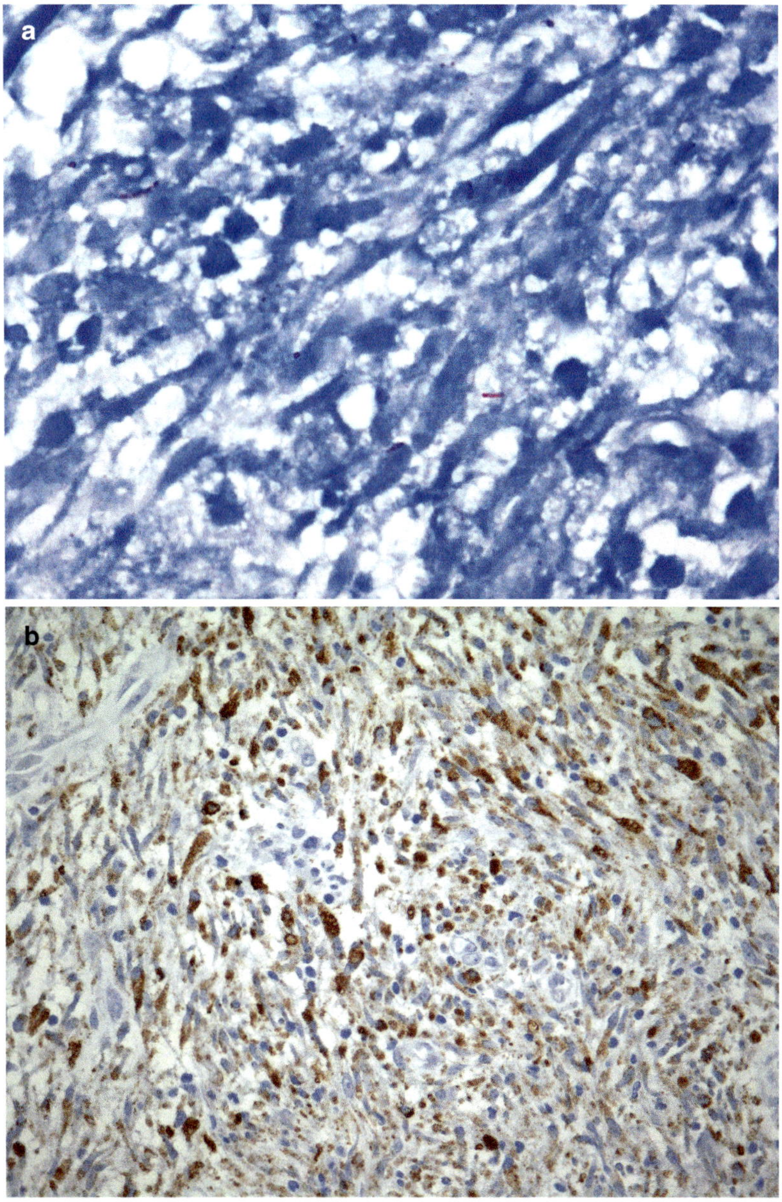

Fig. 3.20 Mycobacterial spindle cell pseudotumor. (**a**). Ziehl-Neelsen stain demonstrates intracytoplasmic acid-fast bacilli. (**b**). The lesional cells are positive for histiocytic marker CD68. (Image courtesy of Dr. Wayne Grayson, Ampath National Laboratories, Johannesburg, South Africa)

Table 3.8 Key pathologic features: mycobacterial spindle cell pseudotumor

HIV/AIDS, solid organ transplant, and other immunocompromised states
Sheets or fascicles of spindle cells admixed with inflammatory cells including lymphocytes and plasma cells
Oval nuclei and pale granular cytoplasm containing clumps of acid-fast bacilli
The mycobacterial organisms can be detected by acid-fast stain

blastic or fibrohistiocytic lesions with an inflammatory component, especially if the clinical context is suggestive. Inflammatory myofibroblastic tumor can be distinguished based on identification of ALK protein expression or *ALK* gene rearrangements. The most helpful features to distinguish mycobacterial spindle cell pseudotumor from pleomorphic spindle cell sarcomas include significant cytologic atypia, pleomorphism, and atypical mitotic figures in the latter. Benign fibrous histiocytomas, especially deep benign fibrous histiocytoma, may be indistinguishable morphologically and immunophenotypically from mycobacterial spindle cell pseudotumor and might require a high index of clinical suspicion and confirmatory staining for acid-fast bacilli. Nodular Kaposi sarcoma (discussed in Chap. 7) expresses vascular markers like CD31 and ERG and is positive for HHV-8.

Acroangiodermatitis

Clinical Features

Acroangiodermatitis (or acroangiodermatitis of Mali) is a florid nonneoplastic cutaneous capillary vascular proliferation in response to venous stasis and associated red blood cell extravasation. It typically affects the lower limbs of older patients with chronic venous insufficiency, amputation stumps, or following coronary bypass surgery or patients with thrombophilia. A similar cutaneous reaction in the setting of underlying arteriovenous malformation or arteriovenous fistula is termed Stewart-Bluefarb syndrome (discussed in Chap. 7). Clinically, acroangiodermatitis presents as red to brown macules, papules, or plaques that are often symmetrically distributed. Acroangiodermatitis is an important clinical and pathologic mimic of Kaposi sarcoma (it used to be called pseudo-Kaposi sarcoma or kaposiform angiodermatitis) and cutaneous angiosarcoma.

Pathologic Features

Acroangiodermatitis is composed of a florid superficial lobular capillary and venular proliferation in a background of chronic inflammation, edema, extravasated red blood cells, and hemosiderin deposits (Fig. 3.21a, b). The vessels lack endothelial atypia and multilayering. Intervening stroma may show reactive myofibroblasts and SMA-positive pericytes, but a significant spindle cell proliferation is not typical of acroangiodermatitis, and therefore the stroma is relatively hypocellular. Key pathologic features of acroangiodermatitis are presented in Table 3.9.

Differential Diagnosis

The most important differential diagnosis is patch stage of Kaposi sarcoma. In contrast to the latter, acroangiodermatitis lacks a significant spindle cell component and the perivascular growth or “promontory sign” seen in Kaposi sarcoma. In difficult cases, immunostaining for HHV8 might be needed to rule out Kaposi sarcoma. In contrast to cutaneous angiosarcoma, acroangiodermatitis maintains a relatively symmetric, lobular architecture at scanning magnification and lacks a dissecting growth pattern, endothelial multilayering, and significant nuclear atypia. In contrast to Kaposi sarcoma and angiosarcoma, the lesional capillaries in acroangiodermatitis are diffusely invested by SMA-positive pericytes.

Bizarre Parosteal Osteochondromatous Proliferation (BPOP, Nora Lesion)

Clinical Features

Until recently, bizarre parosteal osteochondromatous proliferation was considered to represent a reactive lesion of the periosteum, along with florid reactive periostitis (fibro-osseous pseudotumor of digits). Based on the recent demonstration of clonality in this lesion, BPOP is now considered to be a true osteocartilaginous neoplasm. Nonetheless, it is discussed here as this lesion mimics malignant neoplasms like extraosseous osteosarcoma and chondrosarcoma. Florid reactive periostitis (fibro-osseous pseudotumor of digits) is discussed in Chap. 4. BPOP presents as a firm, painless, calcified soft tissue lesion adjacent to the surface of short tubular bones, usually the proximal phalanx of hand in young adult patients. Toes and long bones are less commonly affected. There may be preceding history of trauma. The underlying bone is usually intact. BPOP is usually treated by simple excision but has a propensity for nondestructive local recurrence in approximately 50% of cases.

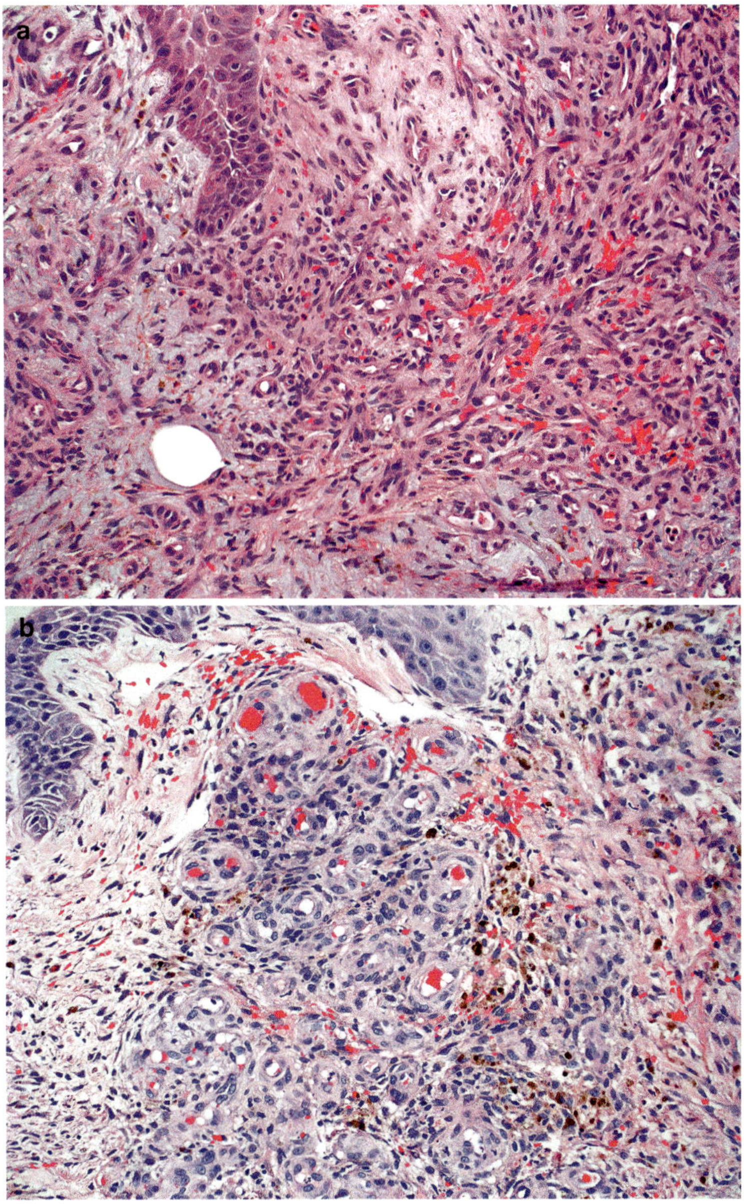

Fig. 3.21 Acroangiodermatitis. (**a**). Florid superficial lobular capillary proliferation in a background of edema and red blood cell extravasation. (**b**). Another example with prominent hemosiderin deposits. The vessels lack significant atypia, endothelial multilayering, or dissecting growth pattern

Table 3.9 Key pathologic features: acroangiodermatitis

Dermal lobular capillary and venular proliferation in a background of edema and chronic inflammation
Extravasated red blood cells and hemosiderin deposits
Negative for cytologic atypia or endothelial multilayering, lacks dissecting growth pattern
Capillaries are invested by SMA-positive pericytes
Negative for HHV-8

Pathologic Features

Histologically, BPOP shows a haphazard admixture of cellular fasciitis-like spindle cell areas and cellular hyaline cartilage transitioning into variably mature woven bone via endochondral ossification (Fig. 3.22). These components (spindle cells, hyaline cartilage, and woven bone) are present in variable amounts in different lesions. Some examples have a well-formed cartilaginous cap at the periphery. The chondrocytes in BPOP are crowded and relatively enlarged and may show mild cytologic atypia and binucleation raising suspicion for chondrosarcoma (Fig. 3.22). Many cases contain characteristic intensely basophilic calcifications like those seen in aneurysmal bone cyst, so-called blue bone. The spindle cell component has the appearance of reactive fibroblasts/myofibroblasts and can directly transition to woven bone. The spindle cells can be mitotically active but lack significant nuclear atypia and atypical mitotic figures (Fig. 3.23). Several

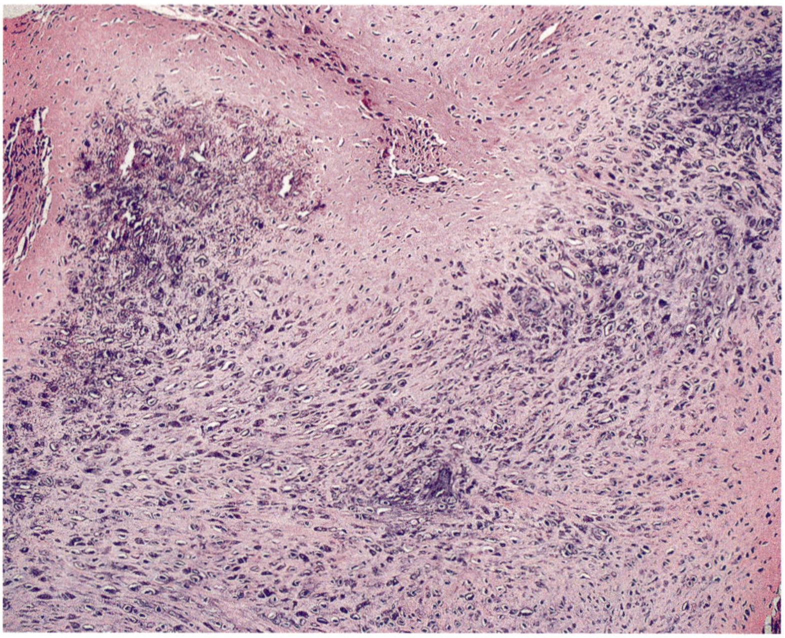

Fig. 3.22 Bizarre parosteal osteochondromatous proliferation (Nora lesion). The lesion consists of cellular hyaline cartilage transitioning into mature woven bone via endochondral ossification, and spindle cell areas. The chondrocytes are crowded and mildly atypical mimicking low-grade chondrosarcoma

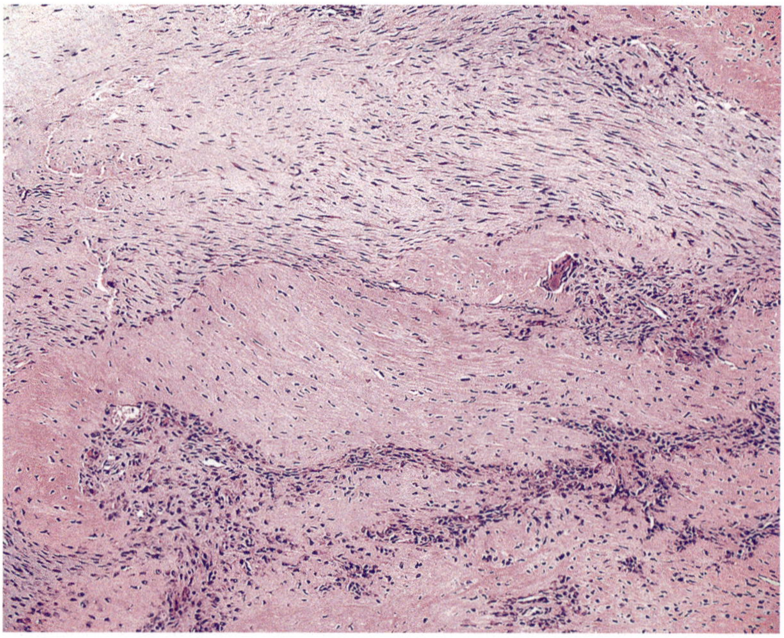

Fig. 3.23 Bizarre parosteal osteochondromatous proliferation (Nora lesion). The spindle cells have the appearance of reactive myofibroblasts without significant nuclear atypia, and are associated with immature woven bone. Osteoclast-type giant cells may be present

Table 3.10 Key pathologic features: bizarre parosteal osteochondromatous proliferation

Soft tissue nodule adjacent to the periosteum of short tubular bones, usually hands
Haphazard admixture of fasciitis-like spindle cell component, cellular hyaline cartilage, and mature woven bone usually formed via endochondral ossification
Basophilic calcifications ("blue bone")
Chondrocytes show crowding and relatively prominent nuclear atypia
Stromal fibroblasts and osteoblasts show no atypia or atypical mitotic figures

recent studies demonstrated a reciprocal translocation t(1;17)(q32;q21) and inversions of chromosome 7, supporting the neoplastic nature of this lesion. Key pathologic features of bizarre parosteal osteochondromatous proliferation are presented in Table 3.10.

Differential Diagnosis

Because of the nuclear atypia, BPOP can be mistaken for extraosseous osteosarcoma or chondrosarcoma. Recognition of the zonal pattern of osseous maturation via endochondral ossification, reactive-appearing woven bone, and lack of cytologic atypia and atypical mitotic figures in the spindle cell component aid in this distinction. From a clinical standpoint, juxtacortical osteosarcoma or chondrosarcoma in the small tubular bones of hands and feet would be very unusual. Of the benign cartilaginous lesions, BPOP can be mistaken for soft tissue chondroma. Soft tissue chondroma is composed of lobules of cytologically banal hyaline cartilage, and while it may have endochondral ossification, it lacks the fasciitis-like spindle cell component seen in BPOP. BPOP is also more cytologically atypical than soft tissue chondroma. BPOP with a well-formed cartilaginous cap may resemble phalangeal osteochondroma but the latter, by definition, shows continuity with the underlying cortical bone and medullary cavity and lacks cytologic atypia seen in BPOP. Clinically, phalangeal osteochondromas are exceptionally rare outside of the hereditary multiple exostoses disorder.

Crystal-Storing Histiocytosis

Clinical Features

Crystal-storing histiocytosis (CSH) is a rare condition characterized by intra-lysosomal accumulation of immunoglobulin crystals in histiocytes. This condition is almost always related to a significant underlying hematolymphoid neoplasm associated with monoclonal immunoglobulins including multiple myeloma/MGUS and lymphoplasmacytic lymphoma. Rarely, it may be associated with autoimmune and connective tissue disorders, chronic infections, drug reactions, hereditary cystinosis, as well as other conditions. Crystal-storing histiocytosis can be localized or generalized and affects a wide variety of sites including the orbit, oral cavity, lung, bone marrow, lymph nodes, spleen, skin, soft tissues, and brain. The typical presentation is that of an asymptomatic mass or swelling, which is discovered incidentally, although some patients present with symptoms related to the affected visceral organ.

Pathologic Features

At scanning magnification CSH represents ill-defined nodules or masses surrounded by inflammatory aggregates (Fig. 3.24). The nodules are composed of sheets of epithelioid to spindled histiocytes with indistinct cell membranes and intensely eosinophilic granular cytoplasm distended by needle-like or rounded refractile immunoglobulin crystals (Fig. 3.25a, b). The background neoplastic lymphoid or plasma cell infiltrate is often obscured by lesional histiocytes. There is no significant cytologic atypia or mitotic activity. The crystals are variably positive on a PAS stain. Immunoglobulins may be highlighted by phosphotungstic acid hematoxylin (PTAH), mass spectrometry, or immunohistochemistry. The immunoprofile of the CSH deposits is represented by all classes of immunoglobulins and can be polyclonal. The lesional histiocytes are positive for CD68 and negative for CD1a, S100, cytokeratins, and muscle markers. Electron microscopy demonstrates membrane-bound dense rhabdoid or rectangular crystals. Key pathologic features of crystal-storing histiocytosis are presented in Table 3.11.

Differential Diagnosis

Awareness of this rare condition is important due to the very significant clinical association with lymphoproliferative disorders. From the standpoint of cutaneous mesenchymal tumors, CSH can be confused with granular cell tumor, xanthogranuloma, deep benign fibrous histiocytoma, mycobacterial spindle cell pseudotumor, Rosai-Dorfman disease, rhabdomyoma, and embryonal rhabdomyosarcoma. Granular cell tumor can be distinguished based on S100 protein, SOX10, and inhibin immunoreactivity, which is negative in CSH, and the former lacks immunoglobulin crystals. Xanthogranulomas and benign fibrous histiocytomas, especially deep benign fibrous histiocytoma, can show significant morphologic overlap, as their constitu-

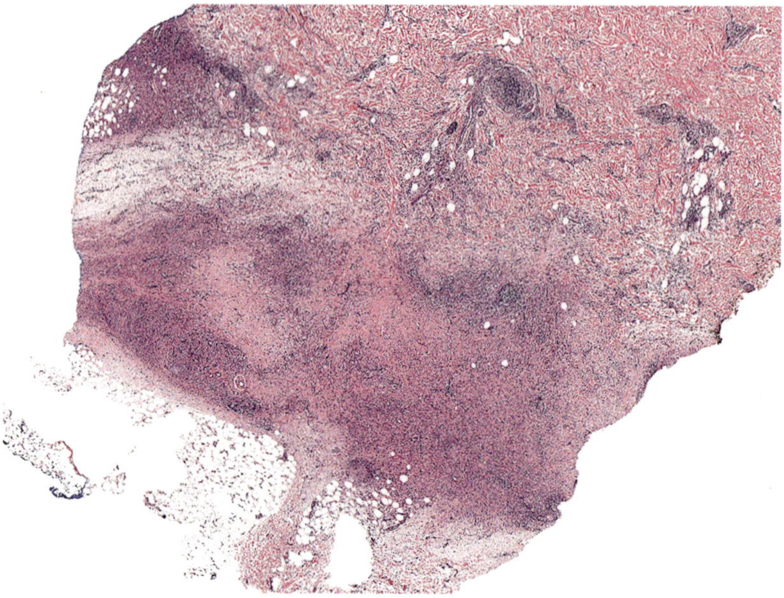

Fig. 3.24 Crystal-storing histiocytosis. An ill-defined nodular infiltrate in the deep dermis and upper subcutis surrounded by inflammatory aggregates

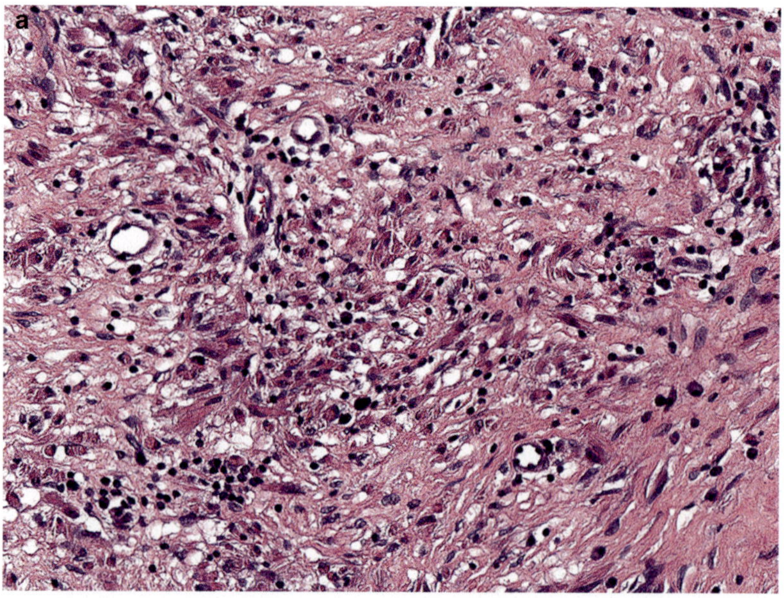

Fig. 3.25 Crystal-storing histiocytosis. (**a**). Sheets of spindle to epithelioid histiocytes with eosinophilic granular cytoplasm admixed with inflammatory cells. (**b**). The cytoplasm contains characteristic, intensely eosinophilic needle-shaped or oval immunoglobulin crystals. The background neoplastic plasma cell infiltrate is obscured by histiocytes in this example

Fig. 3.25 (continued)

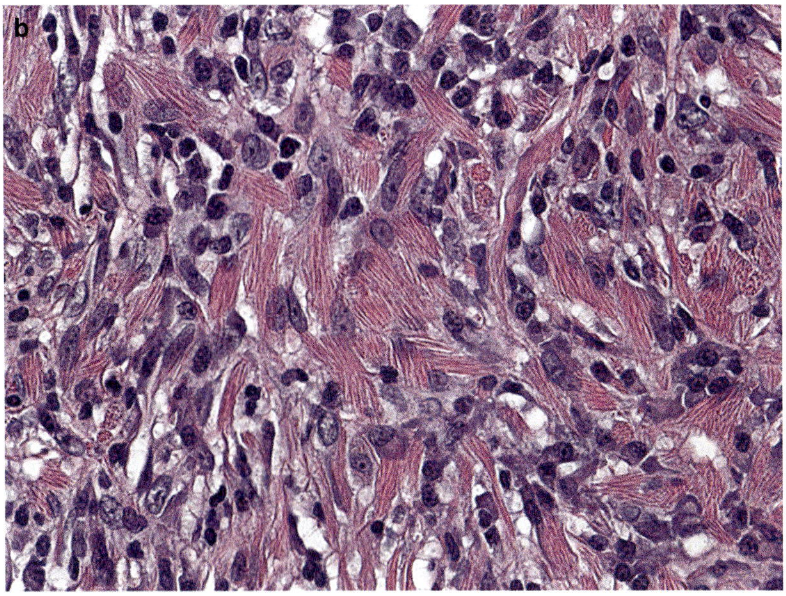

Table 3.11 Key pathologic features: crystal-storing histiocytosis

Sheets of intensely eosinophilic histiocytes distended by numerous needle-like or rounded refractile crystals
Background neoplastic lymphoid or plasma cell infiltrate can be completely obscured by lesional histiocytes
No significant cytologic atypia or mitotic activity
The histiocytes are positive for CD68 and negative for S100 and CD1a
Immunoglobulins of all classes can be identified by PTAH stain, immunohistochemistry, or mass spectrometry

ent histiocytic cells are often palely eosinophilic and granular in appearance. However, these lesions lack intensely eosinophilic refractile crystals. Mycobacterial spindle cell pseudotumor can be excluded based on the clinical history and results of the acid-fast staining. The histiocytes in Rosai-Dorfman disease are more palely eosinophilic and lack distinctive granules and typically show intact lymphocytes within lesional histiocytes (emperipolesis); the histiocytes in Rosai-Dorfman disease are also positive for S100 protein. The eosinophilic refractile crystals within histiocytes may impart a resemblance to the "strap cells" seen in rhabdomyoma and embryonal rhabdomyosarcoma, but in contradistinction to CSH, the latter are positive for skeletal muscle markers, such as desmin, myogenin, and MyoD1.

Erythema Elevatum Diutinum

Clinical Features

Erythema elevatum diutinum (EED) is a localized vasculitis that usually presents in middle-aged adults, as papules and nodules on the extensor surfaces of joints (hands/fingers, wrists, elbows, knees, ankles, feet). The lesions vary from red to violaceous to yellow tinged. Occasional cases present as large masses that clinically mimic neoplasms. EED may be associated with paraproteinemia, hematologic malignancies, inflammatory bowel disease, and autoimmune disease (e.g., rheumatoid arthritis). Lesions may be particularly large in the setting of HIV infection.

Pathologic Features

Early lesions of EED resemble conventional leukocytoclastic vasculitis, often in association with a dense interstitial neutrophilic infiltrate. As the disease progresses, there is a superimposed fibroblastic proliferation within a hyalinized stroma that forms a mass-like lesion (Fig. 3.26a). The fibroblasts often have a storiform pattern and have plump oval-to-spindled nuclei with open chromatin and a distinct nucleolus (Fig. 3.26b). Mitotic figures may be seen, but atypical mitotic figures are absent. Residual leukocytoclasis is typically present, but overt vasculitis is often absent in later stage lesions (Fig. 3.27). Key pathologic features of erythema elevatum diutinum are presented in Table 3.12.

Differential Diagnosis

Late lesions of EED are often mistaken for soft tissue tumors, especially nodular fasciitis, storiform collagenoma/sclerotic fibroma, and sometimes myofibroblastic sarcoma. A clinical presentation of multiple lesions would not be typical of these soft tissue neoplasms. The presence of leukocytoclastic debris and interstitial neutrophils should prompt consideration of EED, as this is not seen in the soft tissue tumors in the differential diagnosis.

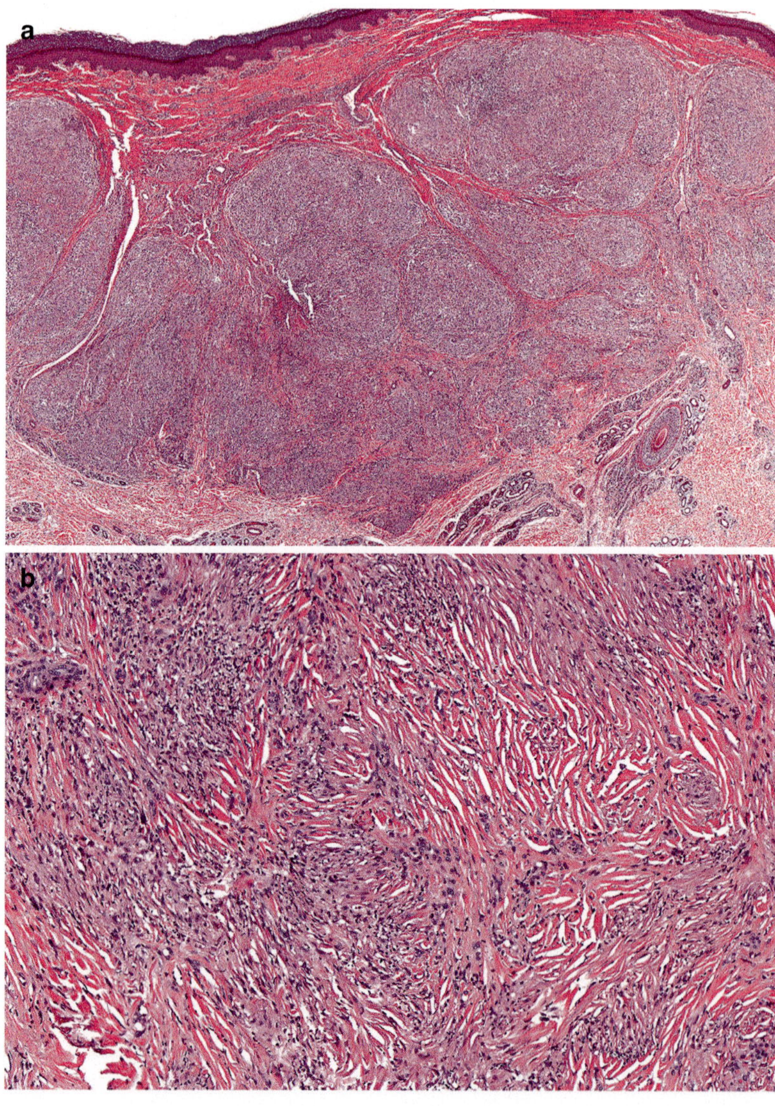

Fig. 3.26 Erythema elevatum diutinum (**a**). Low-power image demonstrating a nodular dermal proliferation of fibroblasts admixed with neutrophils and leukocytoclastic debris. (**b**). The fibroblasts have a storiform pattern and are associated with hyalinized collagen

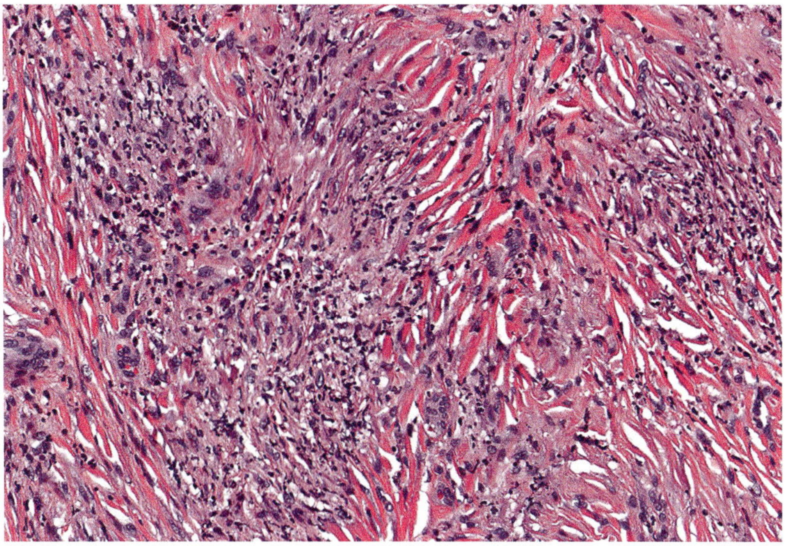

Fig. 3.27 Erythema elevatum diutinum. The fibroblastic proliferation is associated with leukocytoclastic debris but overt leukocytoclastic vasculitis is not seen

Table 3.12 Key pathologic features: erythema elevatum diutinum

Multiple papules and nodules on extensor surfaces of joint
Early lesions: leukocytoclastic vasculitis
Late lesions: storiform proliferation of fibroblasts with hyalinized collagen and leukocytoclastic debris

Metastatic Clear Cell Renal Cell Carcinoma

Clinical Features

Cutaneous metastatic carcinomas with clear cell, eosinophilic, or granular cell cytoplasm may mimic cutaneous perivascular epithelioid cell tumor (PEComa), alveolar soft part sarcoma, granular cell tumor, and clear cell fibrous histiocytoma. While these metastatic carcinomas may originate from a wide variety of visceral sites, including the lung, liver, adrenal, and gynecologic tract, clear cell (renal cell) carcinoma is by far and away the most common and is the focus of this section. Renal cell carcinoma is one of the most common tumors to present with cutaneous metastasis in the setting of an occult primary. The clinical presentation is that of dermal reddish or violaceous nodule, with predilection for head and neck area, especially the scalp.

Pathologic Features

Clear cell renal cell carcinoma is composed of nests or cords of tumor cells with abundant clear cytoplasm and a prominent capillary vasculature. Intratumoral areas of hemorrhage are often present giving the metastatic nodule a violaceous appearance (Fig. 3.28a). Clear cell RCC with eosinophilic features as well as specialized subtypes of RCC like translocation-associated RCC, hereditary leiomyomatosis-associated RCC, and acquired cystic kidney disease-associated RCC can show palely eosinophilic granular cytoplasm (Fig. 3.28b). RCCs with rhabdoid features (a marker of aggressive behavior) demonstrate large cells with eccentric nuclei and eosinophilic perinuclear inclusion (Fig. 3.29). By immunohistochemistry, most metastatic clear cell renal cell carcinomas are positive for cytokeratins, especially CAM5.2, EMA, PAX8 (as are gynecologic tumors), CAIX, CD10, and renal cell carcinoma antigen.

Differential Diagnosis

The differential diagnosis primarily includes PEComa and, to a lesser extent, alveolar soft part sarcoma and more rare neoplasms like clear cell

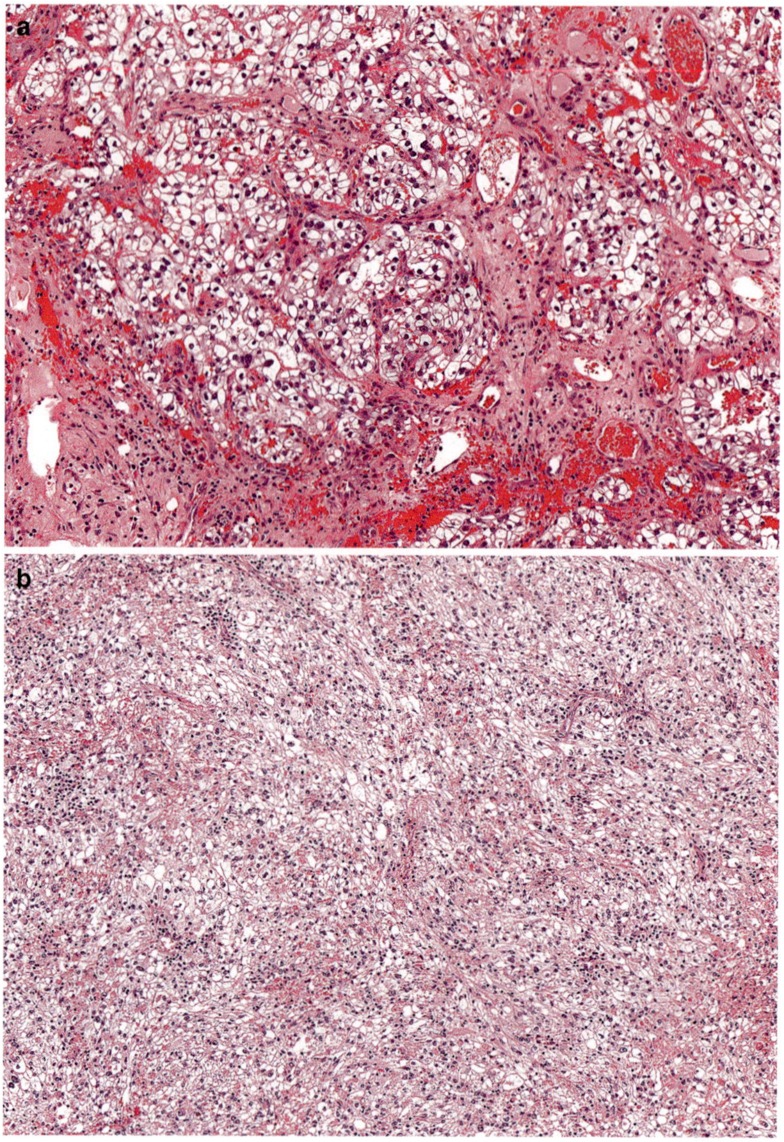

Fig. 3.28 Clear cell renal cell carcinoma (RCC) metastatic to the skin. (**a**). Classic clear cell RCC composed of nests of epithelioid cells with clear cytoplasm separated by prominent capillary vasculature. Stromal hemorrhage is common. (**b**). Eosinophilic clear cell RCC showing nested architecture, eosinophilic granular cytoplasm, and rich vascular pattern. These features can mimic cutaneous PEComa

fibrous histiocytoma or clear cell granular cell tumor. This differential diagnosis is also discussed in detail in Chap. 12. Most of the time, the distinction can be accomplished by application of cytokeratin, EMA, PAX8, CAIX, and other RCC markers which are negative in all of the above entities. An exception is younger patients with Xp11-associated pediatric renal cell carcinomas. These carcinomas tend to lack expression of cytokeratins and EMA and may express TFE3 instead, as would be expected in alveolar soft part sarcoma and a subset of PEComas. Clear cell fibrous histiocytoma shows overlying epidermal hyperplasia, a conventional short spindle cell component with irregular nuclei, and lacks prominent capillary vasculature and any cytokeratin expression. Clear cell granular cell tumor can be distinguished based on a syncytial growth pattern, the absence of nucleoli and prominent capillary vasculature, and expression of S100, SOX10, and inhibin.

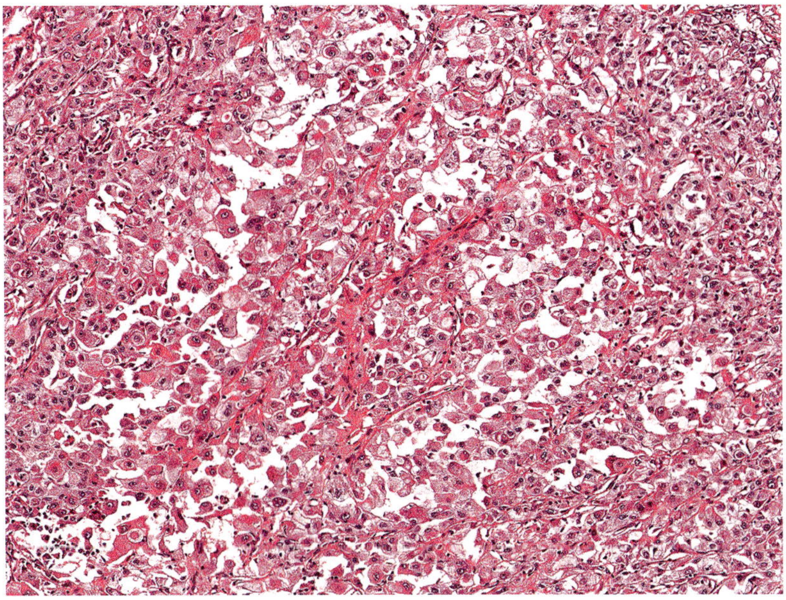

Fig. 3.29 Clear cell carcinoma with rhabdoid features showing large epithelioid cells with eccentric nuclei and eosinophilic inclusion resembling cutaneous PEComa and alveolar soft part sarcoma

Selected References

1. Agaimy A, Specht K, Stoehr R, Lorey T, Märkl B, Niedobitek G, Straub M, Hager T, Reis AC, Schilling B, Schneider-Stock R, Hartmann A, Mentzel T. Metastatic malignant melanoma with complete loss of differentiation markers (undifferentiated/dedifferentiated melanoma): analysis of 14 patients emphasizing phenotypic plasticity and the value of molecular testing as surrogate diagnostic marker. Am J Surg Pathol. 2016;40(2):181–91.
2. Broehm CJ, M'Lady G, Bocklage T, Wenceslao S, Chafey D. Bizarre parosteal osteochondromatous proliferation: a new cytogenetic subgroup characterized by inversion of chromosome 7. Cancer Genet. 2013;206(11):402–5.
3. Campbell K, Kumarapeli AR, Gokden N, Cox RM, Hutchins L, Gardner JM. Metastatic melanoma with dedifferentiation and extensive rhabdomyosarcomatous heterologous component. J Cutan Pathol. 2018;45(5):360–4.
4. Cassarino DS, Derienzo DP, Barr RJ. Cutaneous squamous cell carcinoma: a comprehensive clinicopathologic classification. Part one J Cutan Pathol. 2006a;33(3):191–206.
5. Cassarino DS, Derienzo DP, Barr RJ. Cutaneous squamous cell carcinoma: a comprehensive clinicopathologic classification. Part two J Cutan Pathol. 2006b;33(4):261–79.
6. Dogan S, Barnes L, Cruz-Vetrano WP. Crystal-storing histiocytosis: report of a case, review of the literature (80 cases) and a proposed classification. Head Neck Pathol. 2012;6(1):111–20.
7. Elsensohn A, Shiu J, Grove N, Hosking AM, Barr R, de Feraudy S. Distinguishing Neurofibroma from desmoplastic melanoma: the value of p53. Am J Surg Pathol. 2018;42(3):372–5.
8. Erstine EM, Tetzlaff MT, Ko JS, Prieto VG, Cheah AL, Billings SD. Living on the edge: diagnosing Sarcomatoid melanoma using histopathologic cues at the edge of a dedifferentiated tumor: a report of 2 cases and review of the literature. Am J Dermatopathol. 2017;39(8):593.
9. Fang H, Chiu A, Reichard KK. Crystal-storing Histiocytosis in bone marrow: a Clinicopathologic study of eight cases and review of the literature. Am J Clin Pathol. 2018;149(2):148–63.
10. Kanagal-Shamanna R, Xu-Monette ZY, Miranda RN, Dogan A, Zou D, Luthra R, Weber DM, O'Malley DP, Jorgensen JL, Khoury JD, Bueso-Ramos CE, Orlowski RZ, Medeiros LJ, Young KH. Crystal-storing histiocytosis: a clinicopathological study of 13 cases. Histopathology. 2016;68(4):482–91.
11. Kryvenko ON, Jorda M, Argani P, Epstein JI. Diagnostic approach to eosinophilic renal neoplasms. Arch Pathol Lab Med. 2014;138(11):1531–41.
12. Kurt H, Arnold CA, Payne JE, Miller MJ, Skoracki RJ, Iwenofu OH. Massive localized lymphedema: a clinicopathologic study of 46 patients with an enrichment for multiplicity. Mod Pathol. 2016;29(1):75–82.
13. Llamas-Velasco M, Stengel B, Pérez-González YC, Mentzel T. Late-stage Erythema Elevatum Diutinum Mimicking a fibroblastic tumor: a potential pitfall. Am J Dermatopathol. 2018;40(6):442–4.
14. Manduch M, Oliveira AM, Nascimento AG, Folpe AL. Massive localized lymphoedema: a clinicopathological study of 22 cases and review of the literature. J Clin Pathol. 2009;62(9):808–11.

15. Mc Menamin ME, Goh SG, Poblet E, Gostelow BE, Robson A, Calonje E. Sarcomatoid basal cell carcinoma--predilection for osteosarcomatous differentiation: a series of 11 cases. Am J Surg Pathol. 2006;30(10):1299–308.
16. McCarthy SW, Scolyer RA, Palmer AA. Desmoplastic melanoma: a diagnostic trap for the unwary. Pathology. 2004;36(5):445–51.
17. Meneses MF, Unni KK, Swee RG. Bizarre parosteal osteochondromatous proliferation of bone (Nora's lesion). Am J Surg Pathol. 1993 Jul;17(7):691–7.
18. Momen SE, Jorizzo J, Al-Niaimi F. Erythema elevatum diutinum: a review of presentation and treatment. J Eur Acad Dermatol Venereol. 2014;28(12):1594–602.
19. Nilsson M, Domanski HA, Mertens F, Mandahl N. Molecular cytogenetic characterization of recurrent translocation breakpoints in bizarre parosteal osteochondromatous proliferation (Nora's lesion). Hum Pathol. 2004;35(9):1063–9.
20. Sfeir MM, Schuetz A, Van Besien K, Borczuk AC, Soave R, Jenkins SG, Walsh TJ, Small CB. Mycobacterial spindle cell pseudotumour: epidemiology and clinical outcomes. J Clin Pathol. 2018;71:626–30.
21. Shi KY, Vandergriff T. Late-stage nodular erythema elevatum diutinum mimicking sclerotic fibroma. J Cutan Pathol. 2018;45(1):94–6.
22. Shon W, Ida CM, Boland-Froemming JM, Rose PS, Folpe A. Cutaneous angiosarcoma arising in massive localized lymphedema of the morbidly obese: a report of five cases and review of the literature. J Cutan Pathol. 2011;38(7):560–4.
23. Tran TA, Muller S, Chaudahri PJ, Carlson JA. Cutaneous carcinosarcoma: adnexal vs. epidermal types define high- and low-risk tumors. Results of a meta-analysis. J Cutan Pathol. 2005;32(1):2–11.
24. Wang LL, Thomas WW, Friedman O. Granuloma formation secondary to silicone injection for soft-tissue augmentation in facial cosmetics: Mechanisms and literature review. Ear Nose Throat J. 2018;97(1–2):E46–51.
25. Weissinger SE, Keil P, Silvers DN, Klaus BM, Möller P, Horst BA, Lennerz JK. A diagnostic algorithm to distinguish desmoplastic from spindle cell melanoma. Mod Pathol. 2014;27(4):524–34.
26. Yeh I, Evan G, Jokinen CH. Cutaneous mycobacterial spindle cell pseudotumor: a potential mimic of soft tissue neoplasms. Am J Dermatopathol. 2011;33(6):e66–9.
27. Zembowicz A. Blue nevi and related tumors. Clin Lab Med. 2017;37(3):401–15.

Benign Fibrous, Fibrohistiocytic, and Myofibroblastic Lesions

4

Rajiv M. Patel, Reena Singh, Aaron M. Udager, and Steven D. Billings

Abstract

This chapter covers a large number of benign entities grouped together for convenience under the broad categories of fibrous, fibrohistiocytic, and myofibroblastic lesions. Fibrous lesions generally demonstrate a conspicuous increase in collagen production and varying numbers of fibroblastic spindle cells. "Fibrohistiocytic," a somewhat enigmatic term, is a general descriptor for tumors containing a combination of spindle cells of putative fibroblastic, myofibroblastic, and/or primitive mesenchymal cell origin and histiocytes (bone marrow-derived tissue macrophages and dendritic cells). Myofibroblastic lesions are composed of spindle cells with combined features of smooth muscle cells and fibroblasts.

R. M. Patel (✉) · A. M. Udager
Department of Pathology, University of Michigan Medical School, Ann Arbor, MI, USA
e-mail: rajivpat@umich.edu

R. Singh
Department of Pathology, Oregon Health and Science University School of Medicine, Portland, OR, USA

S. D. Billings
Department of Pathology, Cleveland Clinic, Cleveland, OH, USA

Keloid

Clinical Features

Keloid is a benign fibrous tumor resulting from an abnormal wound-healing response to cutaneous infection and/or injury in susceptible patients, particularly those of African descent. It often occurs in younger patients, demonstrates a strong familial predisposition, and may be solitary or multifocal. Keloid typically presents as a well-demarcated nodular cutaneous mass, which may have an erythematous appearance. Common sites include the head and neck, especially earlobes, and upper torso, particularly the presternal region. Keloids are benign but frequently recur. Surgery combined with intralesional corticosteroids and cryotherapy is considered first-line treatment.

Pathologic Features

Keloid is a hypocellular dermal-based fibroproliferative lesion comprised of prominent thick, glassy bundles of collagen fibers and admixed bland fibroblasts that extend beyond the point of cutaneous injury (Fig. 4.1). Early lesions show variable numbers of small vessels, while older lesions may contain areas of calcification and/or osseous metaplasia. By immunohistochemistry, the spindled cells are usually at least focally positive for SMA, usually exhibiting a membranous (tram-track) staining pattern typical of myofibro-

S. D. Billings et al. (eds.), *Soft Tissue Tumors of the Skin*,
https://doi.org/10.1007/978-1-4939-8812-9_4

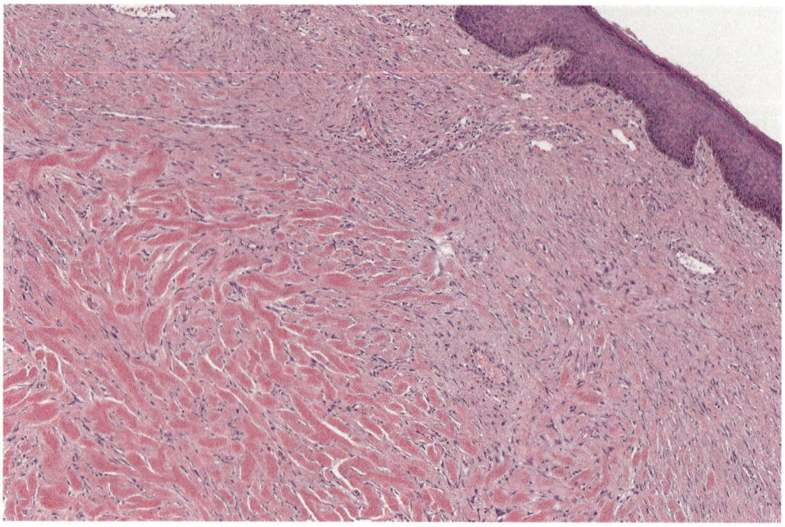

Fig. 4.1 Keloid. A hypocellular dermal-based fibroproliferative lesion composed of prominent, thick glassy eosinophilic collagen bundles admixed with bland fibroblasts

Table 4.1 Key pathologic features: keloid

Hypocellular fibroproliferative lesion
Prominent thick, glassy bundles of collagen admixed with bland fibroblasts
Focal SMA positivity

blasts. HtrA1, a serine protease, may promote keloid development by accelerating cell proliferation and remodeling of keloid-specific extracellular matrix or cell surface molecules (Table 4.1).

Differential Diagnosis

The main differential diagnosis for keloid is hypertrophic scar, although objectively it could be argued that keloid is essentially a form of hypertrophic scar. In contrast to keloid, hypertrophic scars generally are limited to the site of cutaneous injury, contain spindle cells oriented parallel to the overlying epidermis superficially, and do not show prominent thick, glassy bundles of collagen fibers. Older lesions of nodular fasciitis and dermatofibromas may sometimes contain keloidal collagen fibers, but unlike the hypocellular keloid, have cellular areas more typical of those entities.

Fibrous Papule (Angiofibroma)

Clinical Features

Fibrous papule is a member of the broad and diffuse group of superficial angiofibromata that includes the so-called acral angiofibromas (including acral fibrokeratomas, such as acquired digital fibrokeratoma, subungual and periungual Koenen tumors of tuberous sclerosis complex [TSC], and acquired "garlic clove" periungual fibroma), facial angiofibromas of TSC ("adenoma sebaceum"), and pearly penile papules. Only fibrous papule and digital fibrokeratoma (next section) will be discussed at length, as they are the most commonly encountered entities within this group and their key histopathologic features can, to a large degree, be extrapolated to the other lesions with some minor differences. In addition to TSC, angiofibromata have been associated with other syndromes including multiple endocrine neoplasia (MEN) type 1, Birt-Hogg-Dubé syndrome, and Hornstein-Knickenberg syndrome, a phenotypic variant of Birt-Hogg-Dubé syndrome. All are benign lesions cured by simple excision or locally destructive techniques like cryo- or laser therapy. Systemic therapies involving mTOR inhibitors have shown some utility in treating lesions associated with TSC.

Fibrous papules (FP) are small dome-shaped papules, which usually present on the nose and face of adults. Clinically, a melanocytic lesion, wart, or basal cell carcinoma are usually suspected. A subset of FP is seen in association with tuberous sclerosis, or uncommonly in Birt-Hogg-Dubé syndrome, although most appear to be sporadic.

Pathologic Features

All superficial angiofibromata share certain histopathologic features, including a dome-shaped or papillomatous silhouette, the presence of numerous blood vessels, varying amounts of hyalinized collagen, and spindled-to-stellate-to-multinucleated "fibroblastic" cells.

Classic examples of FP demonstrate a paucicellular proliferation of stellate-shaped fibroblasts within a dense fibrous stroma containing small ectatic vessels (Fig. 4.2a). Occasionally, multinucleated cells may be seen (Fig. 4.2b). A variety of histopathologic subtypes, including hypercellular, clear cell, pigmented, pleomorphic, granular cell, inflammatory, and epithelioid variants, have been described. Hypercellular FP shows a dense infiltrate of round-to-ovoid fibroblasts with a nevoid appearance. Clear cell FP contains a proliferation of round cells with foamy cytoplasm resembling foamy macrophages or epithelial cells with clear cell change (Fig. 4.2c and d). The granular cell variant is similar to the clear cell variant, but with much coarser intracytoplasmic granules (Fig. 4.2e). Pleomorphic FP contains stellate fibroblasts with bizarre pleomorphism similar to those seen in pleomorphic fibroma, discussed below (Fig. 4.2f). Pigmented FP differs only by the presence of melanophages within the lesion (Fig. 4.2g). Inflammatory FP has the addition of a brisk inflammatory infiltrate (Fig. 4.2h). Epithelioid fibrous papule contains epithelioid cells with abundant eosinophilic cytoplasm (Fig. 4.2i). The spindled and stellate cells seen in all variants are positive for FXIIIa and negative for S100 protein. CD34 positivity has been rarely reported. Other nonspecific markers such as CD68 and lysozyme may be positive as well. Clinical and histopathologic features are usually sufficient to make the diagnosis, and immunostains are rarely required, except to rule out entities in the differential diagnosis (Table 4.2).

Differential Diagnosis

Hypercellular FP must be differentiated from a melanocytic lesion with melanocytic markers. Clear cell FP often resembles foamy macrophages, which are diffusely positive for CD163, or epithelial neoplasms such as clear cell squamous cell carcinoma and perhaps metastatic renal cell carcinoma, for which keratins and PAX-8 are useful. Pleomorphic FP should be differentiated from atypical fibroxanthoma and pleomorphic dermal sarcoma, both of which have higher cellularity, greater nuclear atypia, and mitotic activity. Pigmented FP typically demonstrate melanocytic hyperplasia and melanophages, similar to a melanocytic lesion, but the latter are positive for melanocytic markers such as S100 protein, Melan-A, and MITF. Depending on the density of the inflammatory infiltrate seen in an inflammatory FP, one might consider a hematolymphoid neoplasm. However, the infiltrate in FP is polymorphous with small and large lymphocytes, plasma cells, tissue macrophages, and scattered eosinophils and neutrophils. Additionally, the identification of the classic fibrous stroma and ectatic vessels seen in all FP variants, as well as the clinical features, helps to differentiate them from histologic mimics.

Acquired Digital Fibrokeratoma

Clinical Features

Acquired digital fibrokeratoma, also known as acral fibrokeratoma, is a benign entity most commonly located on fingers or toes, and less often on palms or soles. The clinical presentation is that of a solitary elongated or pedunculated

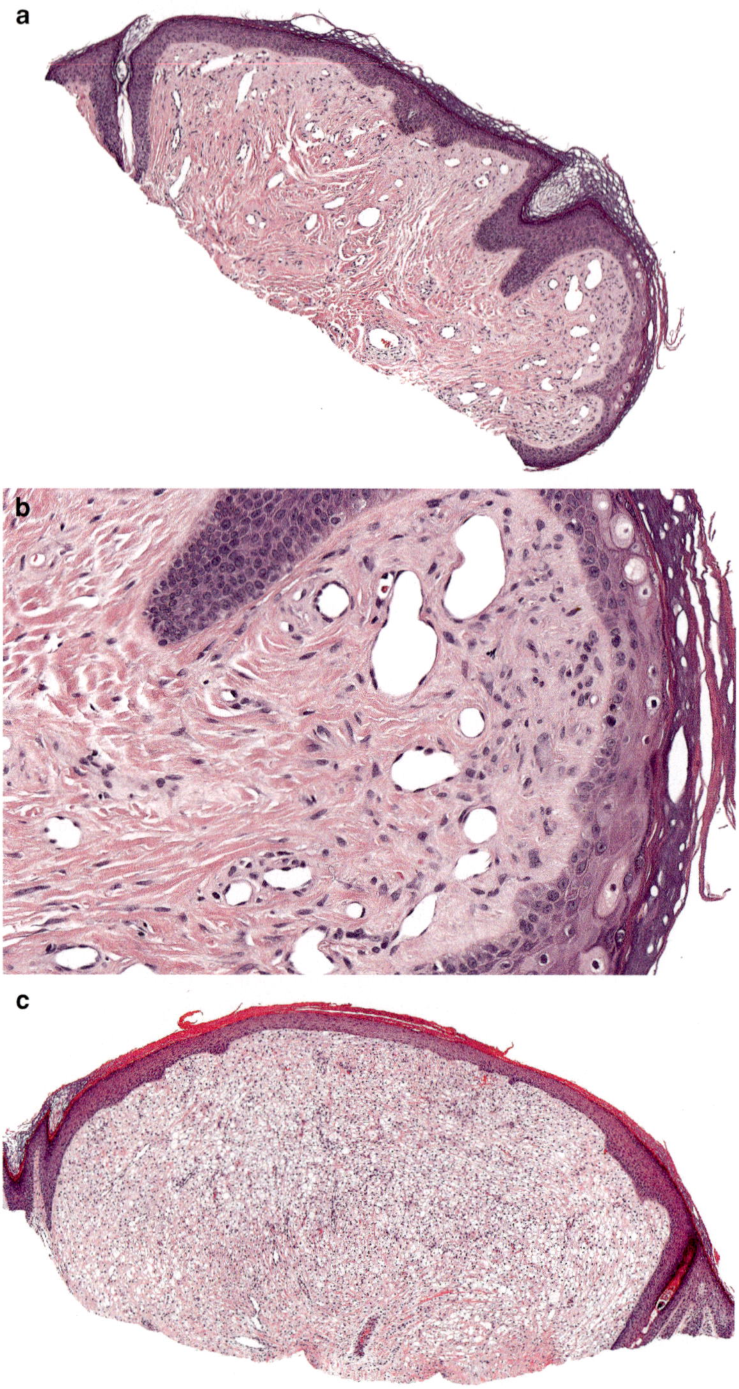

Fig. 4.2 Superficial angiofibroma. (**a**) Fibrous papule with a dome-shaped, paucicellular proliferation of stellate-shaped fibroblasts within a dense fibrous stroma. (**b**) Occasionally, multinucleated cells may be seen. (**c**, **d**) Clear cell fibrous papule containing a proliferation of round cells with foamy clear cytoplasm resembling foamy macrophages or epithelial cells with clear cell change. (**e**) Granular cell fibrous papule is similar to the clear cell variant but contains much coarser granules. (**f**) Pleomorphic fibrous papule contains stellate fibroblasts with bizarre pleomorphism. (**g**) Pigmented fibrous papule containing melanophages. This example is also pleomorphic. (**h**) Inflammatory fibrous papule has similar features to classic fibrous papule with the addition of a brisk inflammatory infiltrate. (**i**) Epithelioid fibrous papule contains epithelioid cells with abundant eosinophilic cytoplasm. (Images **e**–**i** courtesy of Dr. Doug Fullen, University of Michigan)

Fig. 4.2 (continued)

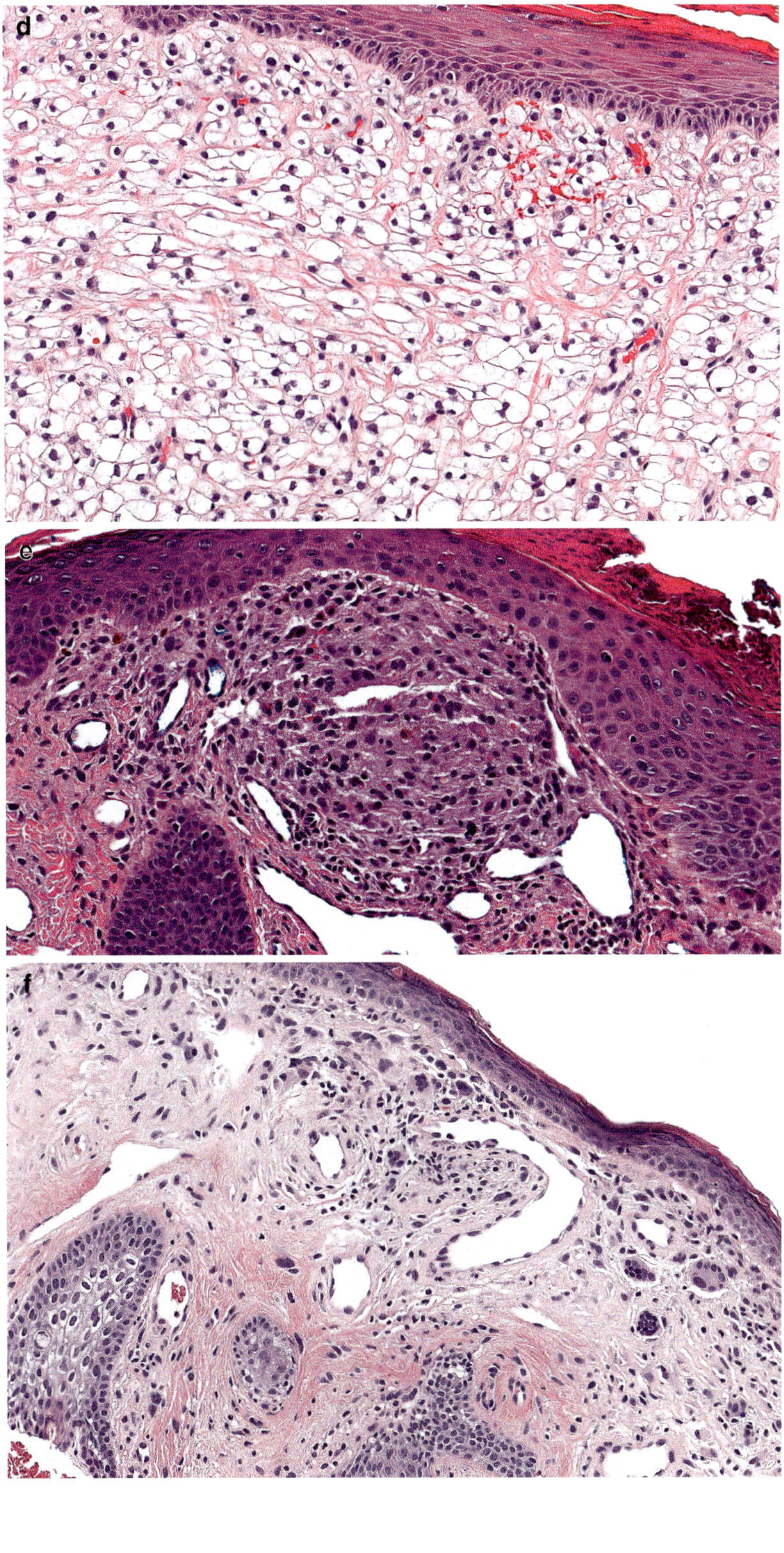

Fig. 4.2 (continued)

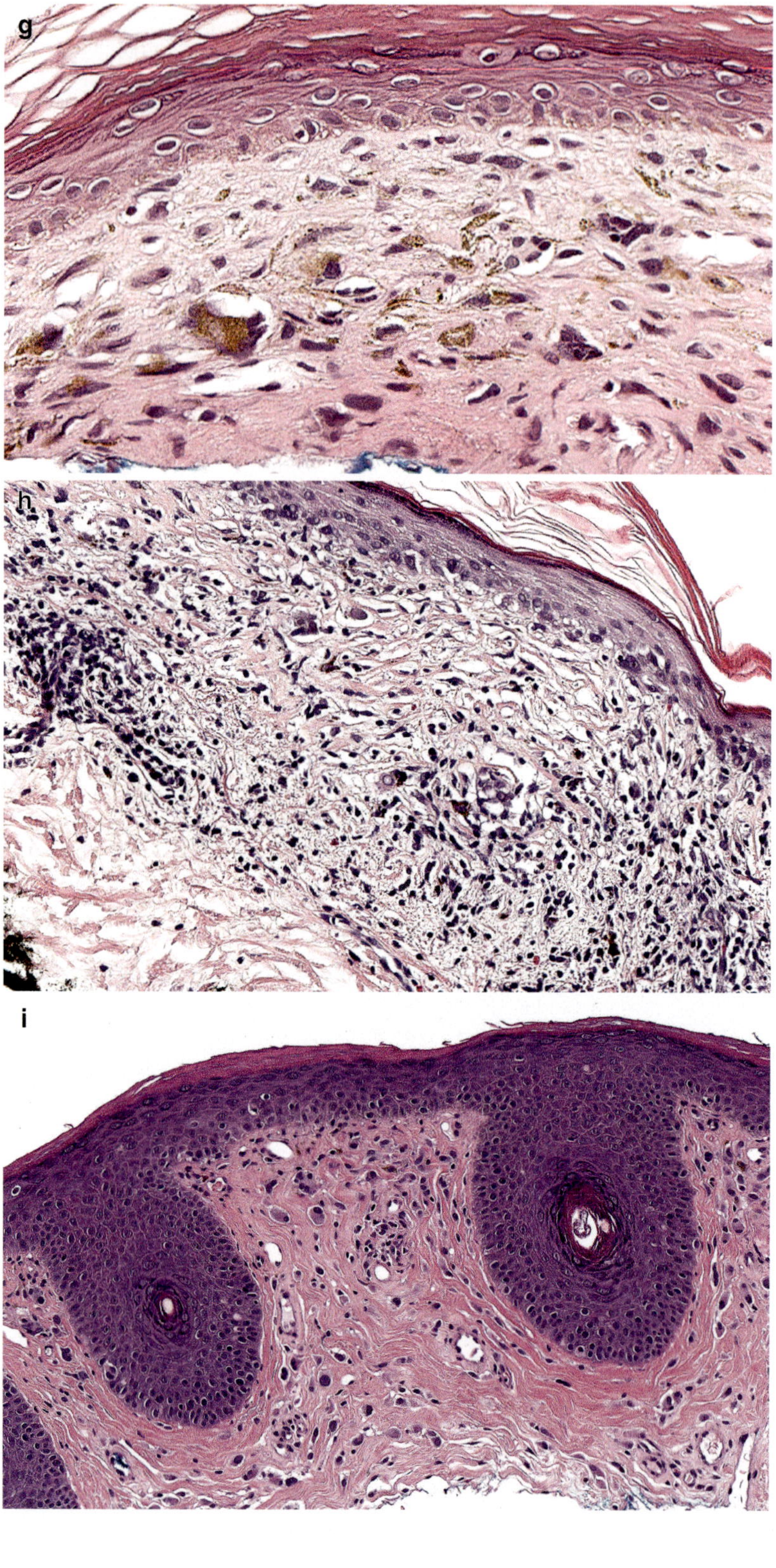

Table 4.2 Key histopathologic features: fibrous papule (angiofibroma)

Paucicellular proliferation of stellate-shaped fibroblasts within a dense fibrous stroma
Ectatic vessels
Occasionally multinucleated cells
Variants: hypercellular, clear cell, pigmented, pleomorphic, epithelioid, granular cell, and inflammatory
Stellate cells positive for FXIIIa, variable for CD68 and lysozyme, negative for S100 protein
CD34 positivity rare

growth with a collarette at the base. Dermoscopic evaluation can enhance visualization of the collarette and reveal a peripheral erythematous region with globular vessels, if this is not evident on initial clinical inspection. Generally, the lesions are small (5 mm or less), but they may become quite elongated, and giant variants have been described. A history of trauma is often present, but development during immunosuppressive therapy has also been noted. Treatment options include excision or laser ablation at the base of the lesion.

Pathologic Features

Histopathology reveals hyperkeratosis and acanthosis overlying thickened collagen bundles arranged along the vertical axis of the lesion. Interstitial fibroblasts are noted to course between collagen, and a characteristic pseudo-nail is often present (Fig. 4.3a and b). Different variants have been described, but all demonstrate the characteristic vertical orientation of collagen bundles. The origin of the lesion may be from dermal connective tissue or from the proximal nail fold and surrounding connective tissue, similar to periungual fibromas (Koenen tumor and "garlic clove" periungual fibroma) (Table 4.3).

Differential Diagnosis

The differential diagnosis includes cellular digital fibroma and superficial acral fibromyxoma, though both of these entities are more cellular and do not have a pseudo-nail. A supernumerary digit similarly appears on fingers or toes, classically on the fifth digit, but is identified by the presence of nerve bundles at its base.

Angiofibroma of Soft Tissue

Clinical Features

Angiofibroma of soft tissue is a distinct, recently described, benign soft tissue tumor with female predominance that typically occurs in middle-aged adults. Tumors usually present as a slowly enlarging painless superficial or deep soft tissue mass in the extremities. This lesion only rarely recurs after surgical excision.

Pathologic Features

Angiofibroma of soft tissue is circumscribed but unencapsulated. The tumors are variably cellular and predominantly comprised of bland-appearing spindle cells with scant pale to amphophilic cytoplasm, hyperchromatic tapered nuclei, and inconspicuous nucleoli. Tumor cells are arranged haphazardly within a variable fibromyxoid stroma with numerous admixed small thin-walled vessels (Fig. 4.4a and b). Scattered tumor cells may express EMA (50% of cases) and CD34, and SMA may be seen in a subset of cases. These tumors are typically negative for S100 protein, desmin, and pan-cytokeratin. Angiofibroma of soft tissue has a t(5;8)(q15;q13) resulting in an *AHRR-NCOA2* fusion (Table 4.4).

Differential Diagnosis

The differential diagnosis for angiofibroma of soft tissue is broad and includes benign, intermediate, and malignant soft tissue tumors, including myxoid dermatofibrosarcoma protuberans, solitary fibrous tumor, myxofibrosarcoma, myxoid liposarcoma, cellular angiofibroma, and low-grade fibromyxoid sarcoma. Myxoid dermatofibrosarcoma protuberans (DFSP) arises in the

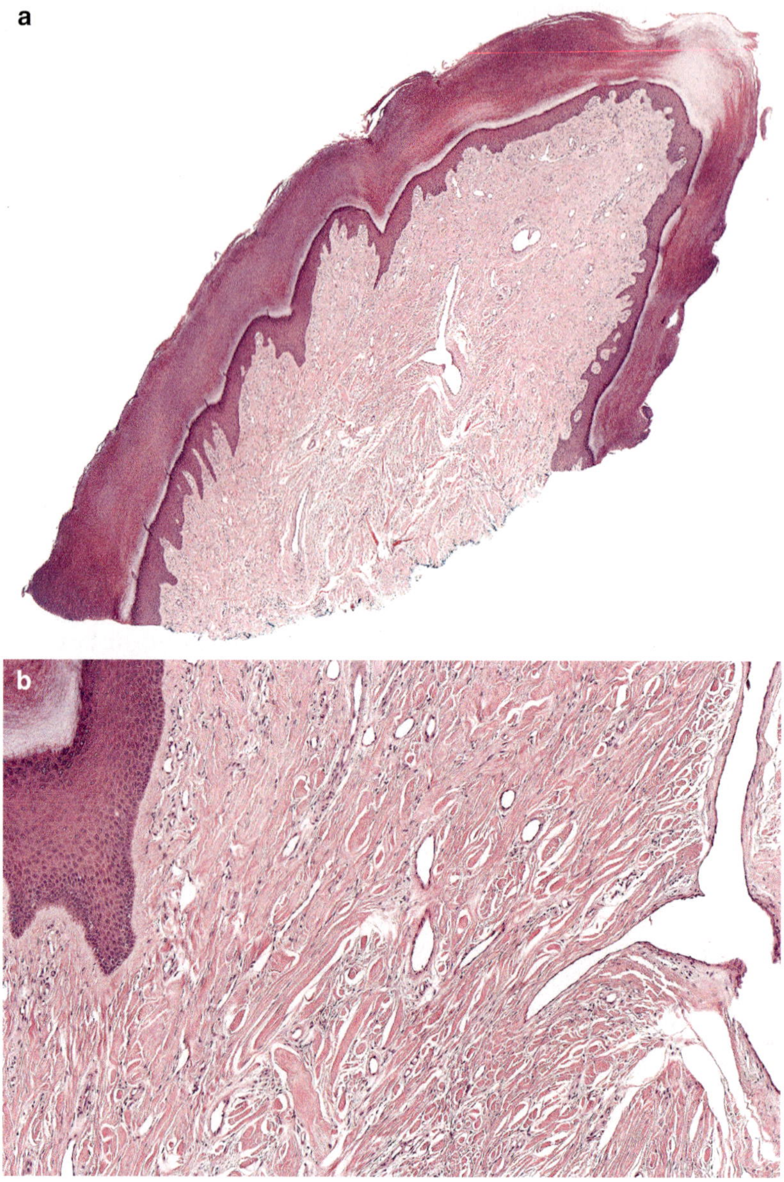

Fig. 4.3 Acquired digital fibrokeratoma. (**a**) Hyperkeratosis and acanthosis overlying vertically oriented collagen bundles. (**b**) Interstitial fibroblasts are present between collagen bundles

dermis, demonstrates fat infiltration, and often shows focal areas of conventional dermatofibrosarcoma protuberans. Solitary fibrous tumor has branching staghorn vessels and is immunoreactive for CD34 and STAT6. Myxofibrosarcoma is infiltrative and has more nuclear atypia and mitotic activity, and widely spaced curvilinear vessels, rather than abundant plexiform vessels. Myxoid liposarcoma has a delicate plexiform vasculature, less uniform cellularity, lipoblasts, and *DDIT3* rearrangement. Low-grade fibromyxoid sarcoma shows alternating fibrous and myxoid zones and is positive for MUC4. Cellular angiofibroma is more similar in name than clinicopathologic features. Unlike soft tissue

Table 4.3 Key pathologic features: acquired digital fibrokeratoma

Epidermal hyperkeratosis and acanthosis
Fibrovascular stroma
Thickened vertically oriented collagen bundles
Characteristic pseudo-nail is often present

angiofibroma, cellular angiofibroma arises most often in the genital region; contains thicker, more hyalinized blood vessels; and has abnormalities of 13q resulting in loss of RB1 expression by immunohistochemistry.

Pleomorphic Fibroma of the Skin

Clinical Features

First described by Kamino et al. in 1989, pleomorphic fibroma (PF) is a solitary, polypoid cutaneous lesion that most commonly arises in the extremities of adults. These lesions are asymptomatic, slow growing, and measure from a few millimeters up to 1.6 cm in greatest dimension. Patients are usually in their third to sixth decades of life, and there is a slight female predominance. Rare subungual cases have been described. These lesions behave in a benign fashion with only rare local recurrences reported. PF are cured by simple excision.

Pathologic Features

Histopathologically, lesions are small, dome-shaped or polypoid, centered in the dermis, densely fibrotic, and sparsely to moderately cellular (Fig. 4.5a). Constituent cells are stellate in shape and have large, pleomorphic, hyperchro-

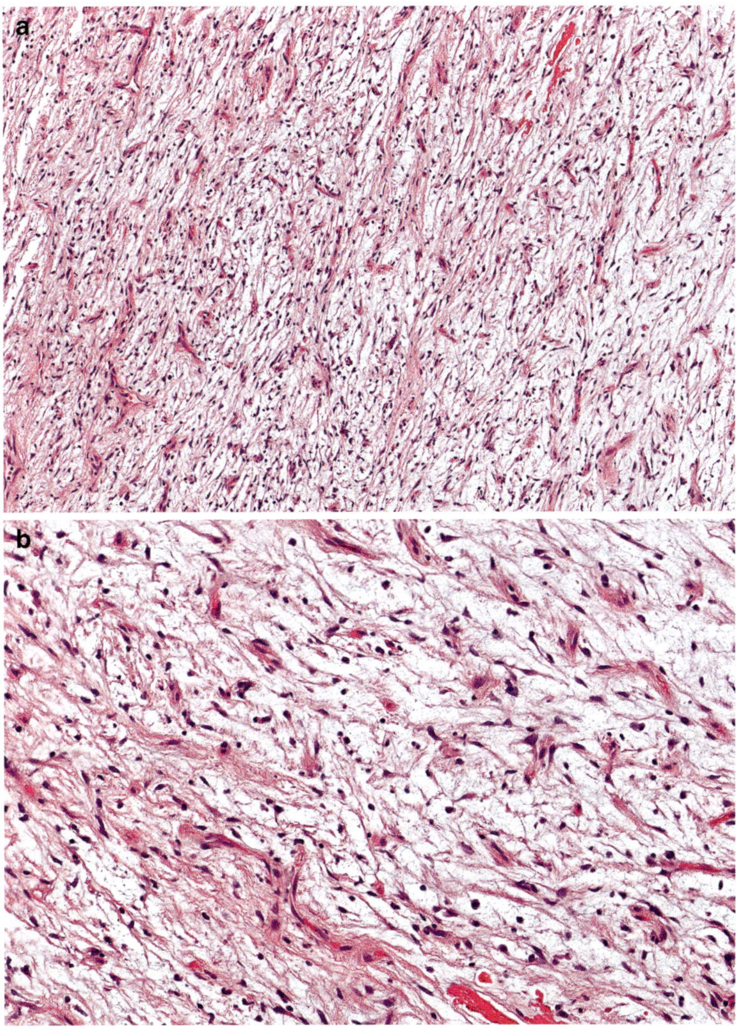

Fig. 4.4 Angiofibroma of soft tissue. (**a**) Bland-appearing spindle cells haphazardly arranged within a variable fibromyxoid stroma in association with small, thin-walled vessels. (**b**) A higher power view. (**c**) A transition zone between myxoid and more fibrous areas

Fig. 4.4 (continued)

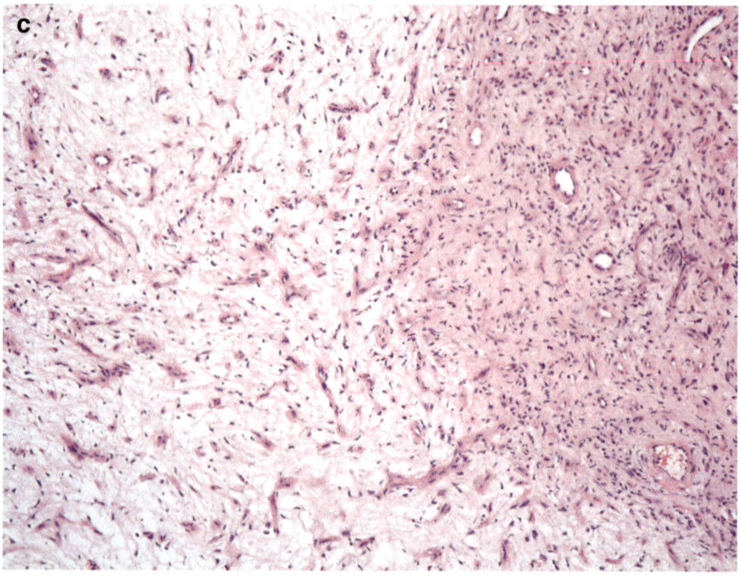

Table 4.4 Key pathologic features: soft tissue angiofibroma

Proliferation of bland, uniform spindle cells
Numerous branching thin-walled blood vessels
Variably myxoid to collagenous stroma
t(5;8) resulting in *AHRR-NCOA2* gene fusion

matic nuclei. Multinucleated cells may be seen (Fig. 4.5b and c). Mitotic figures, including atypical forms, are rarely encountered. A myxoid variant with abundant interstitial mucin has also been reported. The pleomorphic cells are positive for vimentin and CD34, while desmin and S100 protein are negative. Reported immunoreactivity for Factor XIIIa has been variable, with some cases showing positivity in pleomorphic cells, and others demonstrating negativity or only patchy positivity. A recent study demonstrated loss of *RB1* on chromosome 13q in pleomorphic fibromas and loss of RB1 protein expression by immunohistochemistry. These findings indicate that PF shares the same genetic abnormalities as spindle cell/pleomorphic lipoma and other mesenchymal tumors with 13q loss (Table 4.5).

Differential Diagnosis

Atypical fibrous histiocytoma is usually more cellular, has greater levels of nuclear atypia and pleomorphism, and demonstrates other typical features of a dermatofibroma, such as peripheral collagen trapping. Some pleomorphic fibromas have scattered adipocytes leading to consideration of an atypical lipomatous tumor in the differential. These lesions are very rare in the skin and usually spread into the dermis from a deeper-seated lesion. The adipocytic foci in PF lack evidence of cytologic atypia and likely represent entrapped fat cells. In addition, although rare cases of MDM2-positive PFs have been reported, FISH is negative for *MDM2* amplification. Also, atypical lipomatous tumor/well-differentiated liposarcoma does not demonstrate RB1 loss. Atypical fibroxanthoma and pleomorphic dermal sarcoma are usually much more cellular, show significantly more cytologic atypia, and have greater mitotic activity.

Gardner-Associated Fibroma

Clinical Features

Gardner-associated fibroma (GAF) is a benign fibrous soft tissue tumor that is associated with familial adenomatous polyposis (FAP) and desmoid-type fibromatosis. It has a predilection for children and adolescents. Approximately 78% of these lesions appear in the first decade of life (mean age, 5 years). There is a slight male predominance, and lesions are typically solitary, arising in the back and paraspinal region. GAF serve as a sentinel lesion, helping to identify FAP patients who are at a high risk for developing desmoid fibromatoses.

Pathologic Features

GAF is a hypocellular proliferation composed of haphazardly arranged, thickened collagen fibers punctuated by occasional, bland fibroblastic spindle cells, small blood vessels, and mast cells (Fig. 4.6). Nerves, muscle, and adipose tissue are often entrapped at the periphery. The traumatic neuroma-like proliferation of nerve twigs of nuchal-type fibromas is not seen in GAF. By immunohistochemistry most lesions express CD34 and have nuclear immunoreactivity for beta-catenin (approximately 64% of cases in the largest study). The latter finding indicates dysregulation of the Wnt pathway either through *APC* or *CTNNB1* mutations (Table 4.6).

Differential Diagnosis

GAF are benign lesions, which may recur when incompletely excised. As noted previously, these lesions are associated with desmoid tumors but can be separated from them by the latter's increased cellularity arranged in long, intersecting fascicles. The main differential diagnosis is with nuchal-type fibroma. These typically arise in the cervical region of middle-aged adults,

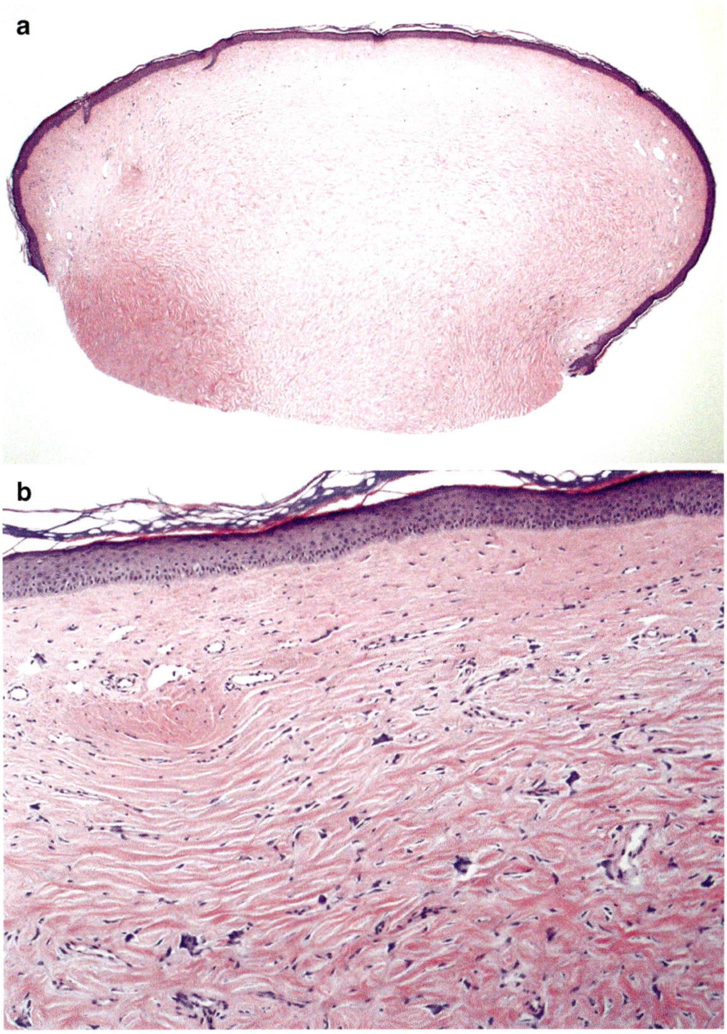

Fig. 4.5 Pleomorphic fibroma. (**a**) A polypoid lesions composed of a densely fibrotic stroma. (**b**, **c**) Constituent cells are stellate with large pleomorphic and hyperchromatic nuclei and are not uncommonly multinucleated. (Images courtesy of Dr. Karen Fritchie, Mayo Clinic)

Fig. 4.5 (continued)

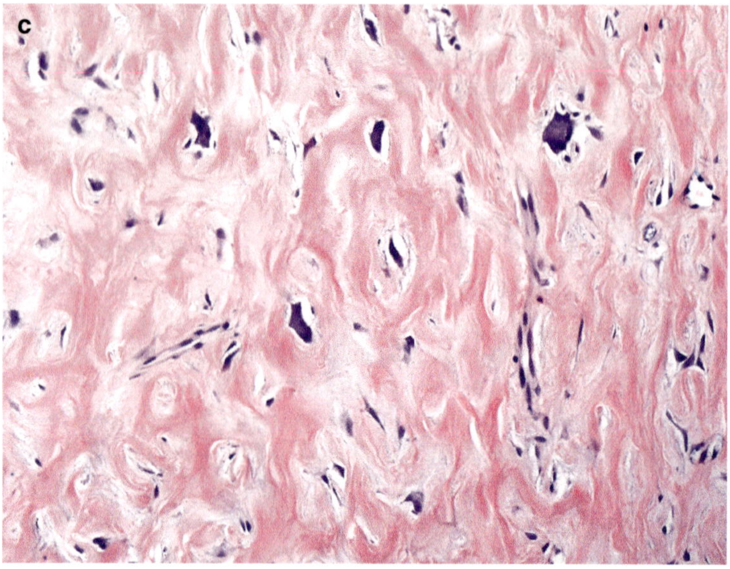

Fig. 4.6 Gardner-associated fibroma. A hypocellular proliferation of haphazardly arranged thickened collagen fibers punctuated by scattered bland fibroblastic spindle cells, occasional small blood vessels, and scattered mast cells

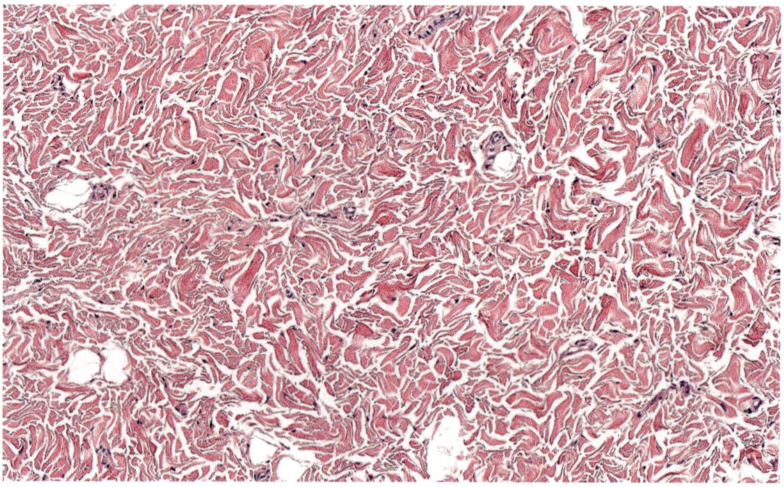

Table 4.5 Key pathologic features: pleomorphic fibroma of the skin

Small, well-circumscribed, dome-shaped, or polypoid lesion
Sparsely to moderately cellular with fibrotic collagen
Stellate cells with large hyperchromatic nuclei
Multinucleated cells may be seen
Pleomorphic cells positive for vimentin and CD34, FXIIIa variable
Desmin and S100 protein negative
Rb1 loss in pleomorphic cells

Table 4.6 Key pathologic features: Gardner-associated fibroma (GAF)

Associated with desmoid and FAP (Gardner syndrome)
Disorganized, thickened collagen bundles and scattered bland spindled fibroblastic cells
Adipose tissue, nerve tissue, and skeletal muscle may be entrapped at the periphery
No traumatic neuroma-like areas
Positive for CD34 and nuclear beta-catenin in 64% of cases

although other sites may also be involved (sacral region, extremities, buttocks). Nuchal-type fibromas are typically solitary lesions that are nearly histologically identical to GAF, but are more likely to have an increased number of entrapped nerve twigs.

Nuchal Fibroma

Clinical Features

Nuchal-type fibroma (NTF) is a rare fibrocollagenous lesion that arises in the posterior neck of middle-aged adults with a slight male predominance. NTF is strongly associated with diabetes mellitus (up to 44% of patients). Other sites of involvement have been reported, and up to 30% of cases include the chest, back, face, and extremities. Earlier cases of NTF were reported in association with Gardner syndrome. However, the clinicopathologic features of NTF are felt to be distinct from Gardner-associated fibroma (see above). NTF are benign lesions that may locally recur after incomplete excision.

Pathologic Features

NTF is typically a solitary, encapsulated, subcutaneous mass composed of a paucicellular proliferation of dense, haphazardly arranged bundles of collagen and scattered fibroblast cells, which entrap lobules of adipose tissue (Fig. 4.7a). Entrapment of adnexal structures and nerve bundles is seen, and there is often a traumatic neuroma-like proliferation of small nerve twigs at the periphery of the lesion (Fig. 4.7b). Constituent spindle cells are positive for CD34 and negative for actin and desmin. Beta-catenin is typically negative. A rare *APC* gene missense mutation and a very rare *MUTYH* gene polymorphism have been reported in one case of extra nuchal-type fibroma (Table 4.7).

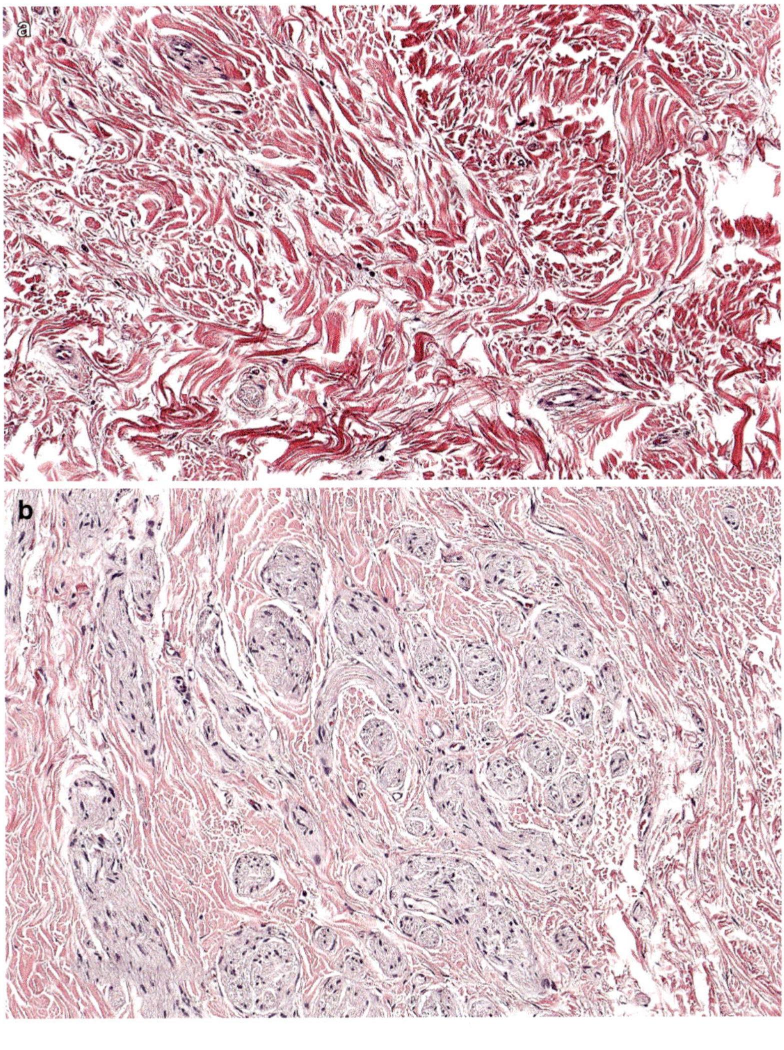

Fig. 4.7 Nuchal-type fibroma. (**a**) A paucicellular proliferation of dense, haphazardly arranged bundles of collagen admixed with scattered fibroblast-like cells and entrapped lobules of adipose tissue. Note the similarity to Gardner-associated fibroma. (**b**) Traumatic neuroma-like area in nuchal-type fibroma

Table 4.7 Key pathologic features: nuchal-type fibroma

Poorly circumscribed mass, 1–8 cm in maximum dimension
Hypocellular with dense hyalinized collagen and fibroblastic cells
Entrapped lobules of adipose tissue
Traumatic neuroma-like changes
Nuclear beta-catenin positivity rare
Negative for S100, SMA, desmin, and EMA

Differential Diagnosis

NTF may be confused with other fibrocollagenous proliferations that contain focal areas of adipose tissue. Gardner-associated fibroma is the most histopathologically similar lesion. Gardner-associated fibroma usually arises in much younger patients, shows a predilection for males, is less likely to present as multiple lesions, and is associated with FAP. Gardner-associated fibromas are more often associated with nuclear beta-catenin positivity. Fibromatoses are more cellular and are less likely to arise in the subcutis. Finally, elastofibroma is a deeper soft tissue lesion associated with abnormal, fragmented elastic fibers and typically presents in the scapular region.

Calcifying Aponeurotic Fibroma

Clinical Features

Calcifying aponeurotic fibroma is a benign, locally infiltrative fibroblastic soft tissue tumor with a slight male predominance, which typically occurs in children and rarely adults. Lesions usually present as a slowly enlarging, painless superficial soft tissue mass of the hands or feet, most commonly the palm or fingers. They may rarely be found along aponeuroses, tendons, and/or fascia at other sites, including the thigh, knee, arm, and elbow. Radiographic imaging may demonstrate intratumoral mineralization. Although calcifying aponeurotic fibroma has a good clinical course, local recurrence after incomplete surgical excision is common (50% of cases). Metastasis and fibrosarcomatous transformation have been reported in exceptionally rare cases. Calcifying aponeurotic fibroma-like lesions has been reported in a family with Albright's hereditary osteodystrophy.

Pathologic Features

The tumors are unencapsulated and poorly circumscribed, dermal masses that often extend into adjacent subcutaneous fat and skeletal muscle (Fig. 4.8a). Microscopically, tumors show variable cellularity and are comprised predominantly of bland-appearing fibroblastic spindle cells with scant eosinophilic cytoplasm, enlarged and slightly irregular hyperchromatic nuclei, and indistinct nucleoli. Tumor cells are arranged in a variety of patterns, including small whorls and short fascicles, within a collagenous stroma. The central portion of the tumor typically contains areas of calcification that are surrounded by epithelioid to chondroid tumor cells (Fig. 4.8b). Some cases may contain multinucleated cells and foci of bland cartilage. The spindle cells show variable SMA, muscle-specific actin, desmin, and CD68 staining, but are negative for S100 protein, beta-catenin, and CD34 expression; cartilaginous foci may express S100 protein. Rare cases may stain with CD34, progesterone receptor, CD57, and EMA. Calcifying aponeurotic fibroma has recurrent *FN1-EGF* fusions (Table 4.8).

Differential Diagnosis

The differential diagnosis for calcifying aponeurotic fibroma includes calcifying fibrous pseudotumor, fibro-osseous pseudotumor of digits, soft tissue chondroma, superficial fibromatosis, and infantile fibromatosis (lipofibromatosis). Although calcifying fibrous pseudotumor, fibro-osseous pseudotumor of digits, and calcifying aponeurotic tumor may have overlapping clinical and morphologic features, specific findings may be helpful for diagnosis (see below). In general, the presence of central cartilage formation with

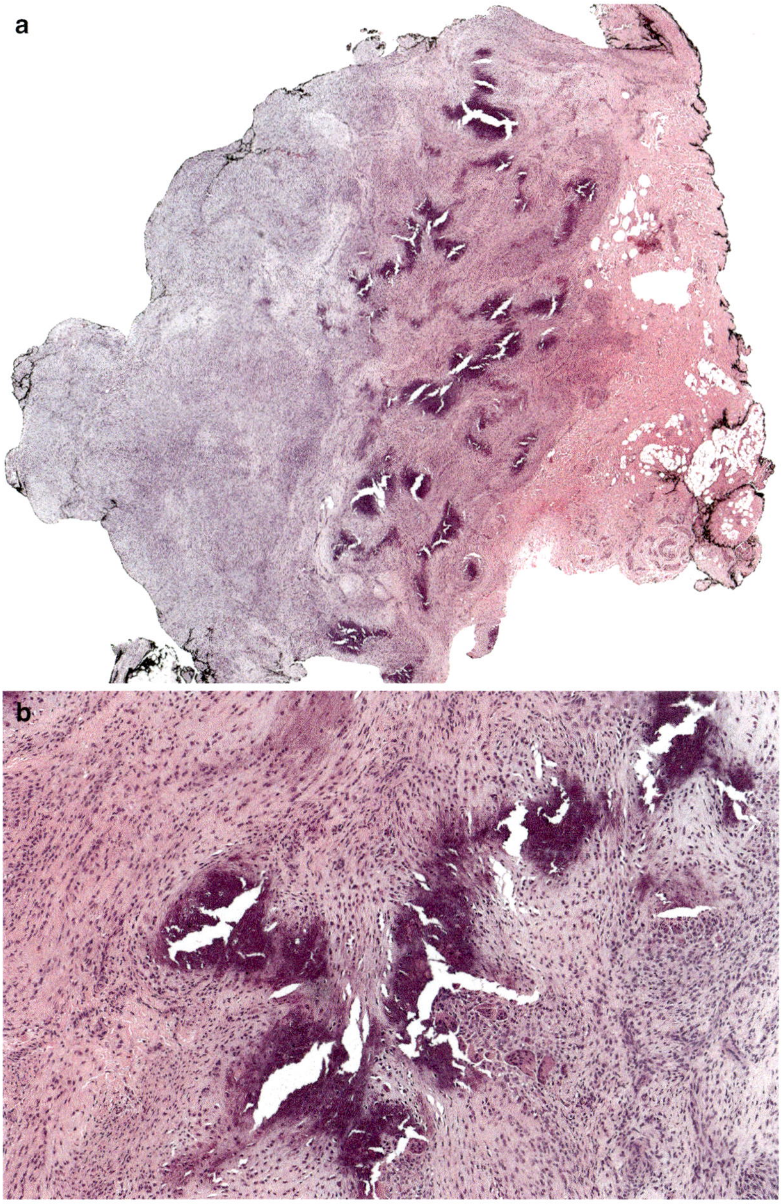

Fig. 4.8 Calcifying aponeurotic fibroma. (**a**) A poorly circumscribed, superficial soft tissue mass extending into adjacent subcutaneous fat and skeletal muscle. (**b**) Bland fibroblastic spindle cells present in whorls and fascicles in a collagenous stroma in association with a central calcified zone surrounded by a radial array of epithelioid to chondroid tumor cells

Table 4.8 Key pathologic features: calcifying aponeurotic fibroma

Spindled-to-ovoid cells arrayed in parallel fascicles
Epithelioid/chondroid cells surrounding calcified zones
Foci of cartilage and multinucleated cells may be seen in some cases
Spindle cells show variable SMA, muscle-specific actin, desmin, and CD68 positivity, negative for S100 protein, beta-catenin, and CD34
Recurrent *FN1-EGF* fusions

calcification favors a diagnosis of calcifying aponeurotic fibroma. Conversely, fibromatosis is more cellular, only rarely shows calcifications, and is not associated with a cartilaginous component. While soft tissue chondromas are benign cartilaginous soft tissue tumors that may show calcification, the presence of an associated spindle cell component favors calcifying aponeurotic fibroma. Unlike calcifying aponeurotic fibroma, infantile fibromatosis (lipofibromatosis) shows fascicles of spindle-to-ovoid cells in a myxoid background infiltrating atrophic skeletal muscle and lipocytes. It has no cartilaginous areas and does not calcify.

Elastofibroma

Clinical Features

Elastofibroma is a benign soft tissue pseudotumor with a strong female predominance that typically presents in elderly adults. A familial predisposition for elastofibroma is seen in up to one third of cases. It usually presents as a slowly growing painless deep soft tissue mass in the upper back near the scapula and may frequently be present bilaterally. There is often a prior history of repetitive trauma, such as intense manual labor. Tumors do not recur after surgical excision.

Pathologic Features

Elastofibromas are unencapsulated, poorly circumscribed hypocellular lesions comprised of bland-appearing fibroblastic spindle cells within dense collagen that contain bundles of degenerated elastic fibers. The elastic fibers have a characteristic serrated and beaded appearance, which can be highlighted with an elastic stain (Fig. 4.9a and b). Admixed lobules of mature adipose tissue may impart a pseudoinfiltrative appearance. The spindle cells are variably positive for CD34 and negative for SMA, desmin, and S100 protein. A variety of chromosomal abnormalities have been reported in elastofibroma including alterations to chromosome 1, t(8;12)(q22;q24.3), copy gains of Xq and t(2;19), and (X;1) rearrangements (Table 4.9).

Differential Diagnosis

The diagnosis of elastofibroma is rarely problematic. Desmoplastic fibroblastoma is perhaps the closest mimic, but the stellate cells of this entity and the lack of altered elastic fibers allow distinction. An elastic stain will confirm the diagnosis of elastofibroma in problematic cases.

Desmoplastic Fibroblastoma (Collagenous Fibroma)

Clinical Features

Desmoplastic fibroblastoma (DFB)/collagenous fibroma is a slow-growing firm mobile mass that rarely causes pain and typically arises in the deep subcutaneous tissue, fascia, or skeletal muscle in adults. It was probably reported as a variant of a fibroma, or other benign mesenchymal tumor in the literature, before the seminal description by Harry Evans in 1995. Patients are usually in the fifth to seventh decades of life, with lesions only rarely being reported in children and adolescents. Males are affected at least twice as commonly as females. Common sites of involvement include the upper and lower extremities, and lesions rarely arise in the head and neck region.

Pathologic Features

Most DFB are well-circumscribed, paucicellular, and composed of distinct, stellate, and bipolar spindle cells, which are widely spaced within a myxocollagenous stroma and demonstrate little to no atypia or mitotic activity (Fig. 4.10a and b). Immunohistochemistry is rarely helpful in making the diagnosis, with at most focal immunoreactivity for SMA and muscle specific actin. Stains for CD34, desmin, and S100 protein are negative. Rare cytokeratin positive cells may be seen. Recently, it has been reported that DFB is positive for FOSL1, a member of the FOS family encoding leucine zipper proteins, by immunohistochemistry, distinguishing this lesion from fibroma of tendon sheath, a morphologic mimic. Genetic abnormalities involving 11q12 are reportedly common in DFB. Though abnormalities involving 11q have also been reported in fibroma of tendon sheath, it is uncertain whether this finding is indicative of a close link between the two lesions (Table 4.10).

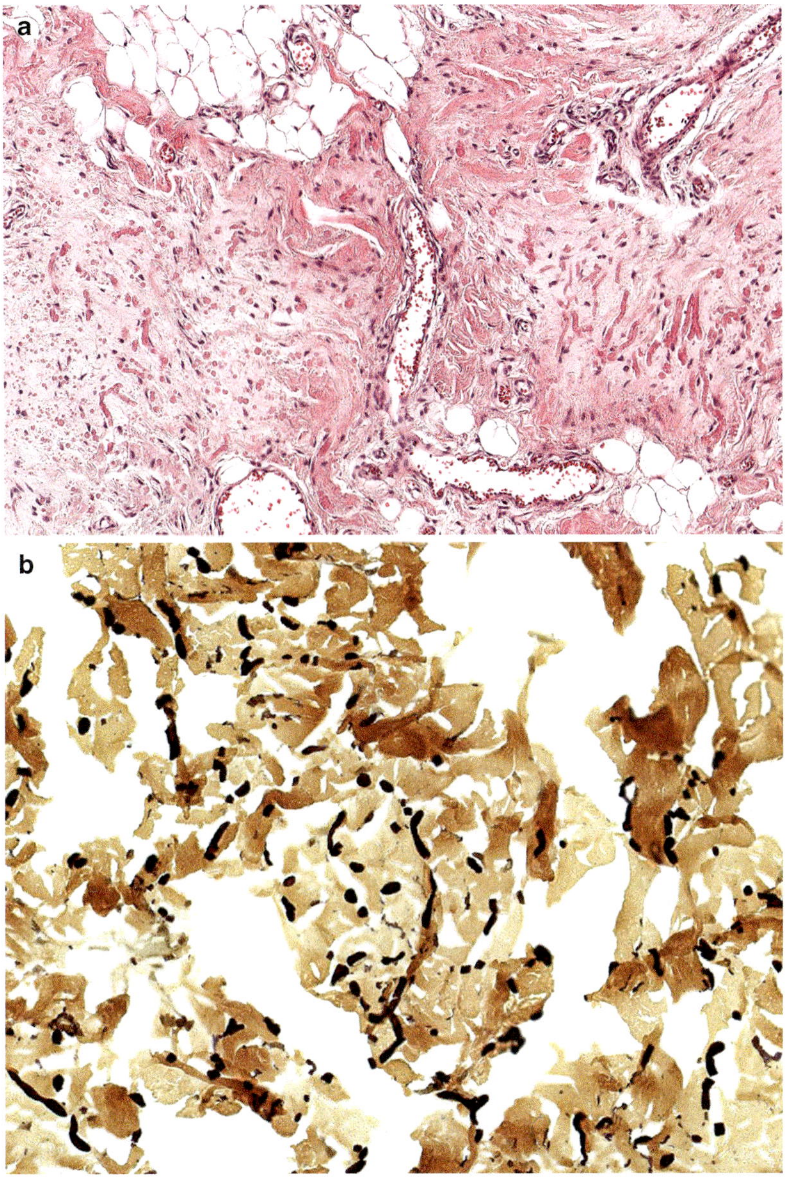

Fig. 4.9 Elastofibroma. (**a**) Bland-appearing fibroblastic spindle cells within dense collagen containing bundles of degenerated elastic fibers with a characteristic serrated and beaded appearance. (**b**) Elastic stain highlighting fibers in black

Table 4.9 Key pathologic features: elastofibroma

Fibroblasts, collagen, and degenerating elastic fibers
Elastic fibers with serrated or beaded appearance
Elastic fibers stain with elastic stain, fibroblasts variably CD34-positive

Differential Diagnosis

A variety of benign and low-grade malignant mesenchymal tumors are in the differential diagnoses. The differential of elastofibroma is discussed above. Fibromatoses are more cellular and have a distinct fascicular growth pattern, infiltrate surrounding tissues, and may have scattered perivascular lymphocytes. Low-grade fibromyxoid sarcoma is more cellular, demonstrates distinct abrupt transition between hypercellular myxoid areas and more hypocellular fibrotic areas, and is positive for MUC4. Calcifying fibrous pseudotumor affects young adults and children and typically contains psam-

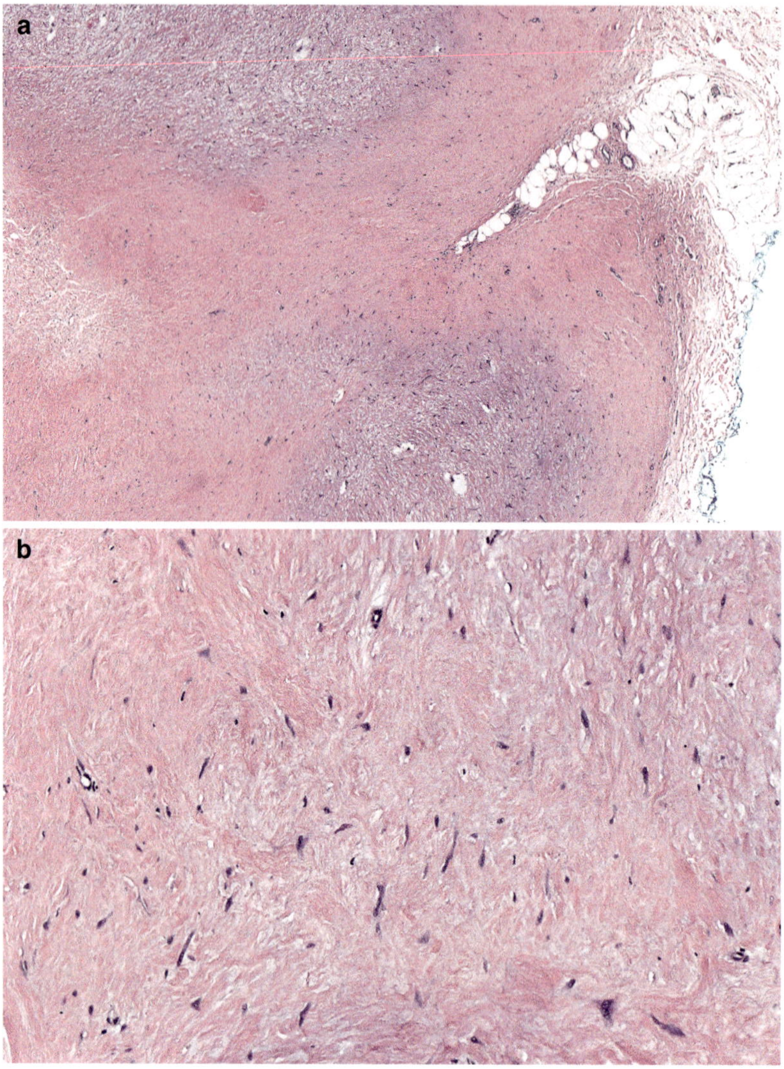

Fig. 4.10 Desmoplastic fibroblastoma (collagenous fibroma). (**a**) Well-circumscribed, paucicellular lesion composed of distinct, widely spaced, stellate to bipolar spindle cells. (**b**) Higher-power view of stellate cells in a dense myxocollagenous to collagenous stroma

Table 4.10 Key pathologic features: desmoplastic fibroblastoma (collagenous fibroma)

Abundant hypovascular myxocollagenous or collagenous stroma
Low to moderately cellular proliferation of uniformly distributed bipolar-to-stellate cells with small nucleoli
No significant atypia; mitoses uncommon
Positive for FOSL1 and focally positive for SMA and muscle specific actin; negative for S100, CD34, desmin, and EMA. Rare keratin-positive cells may sometimes be seen
t(2;11)(q31;q12) reportedly common

momatous calcifications and a lymphoplasmacytic infiltrate. Hypocellular or myxoid variants of neurofibroma may resemble DFB, but there is usually a characteristic combination of fine collagen fibers with bland spindle cells with wavy buckled nuclei and scattered mast cells. Neurofibromas are also strongly and diffuse positive for S100 protein unlike DFB. Older lesions of nodular fasciitis may become hyalinized and somewhat more paucicellular. However, typical cellular areas of nodular fasciitis with a tissue culture-like growth pattern, myxoid degeneration, and extravasated erythrocytes are usually present to allow distinction.

Sclerotic Fibroma (Storiform Collagenoma)

Clinical Features

Sclerotic fibroma (SF) is a distinctive benign cutaneous fibrous lesion that typically presents as a slow-growing, firm, skin-colored to hyperpigmented solitary nodule. It may arise in any part of the body, but the head and neck region and arms are commonly affected. Adults are typically affected with no gender preference. Multiple lesions are a marker of Cowden syndrome (a member of PTEN hamartoma tumor syndrome, which also includes Bannayan-Riley-Ruvalcaba syndrome, PTEN-related Proteus syndrome, and Proteus-like syndrome). These lesions may also be sporadic. Simple excision is curative.

Pathologic Features

SF is a well-demarcated, hypocellular dermal nodule made up of sclerotic collagen with extensive clefting artifact and containing a storiform proliferation of bland spindle cells (Fig. 4.11a). The storiform pattern is so extensive as to impart a "plywood-like" pattern, which has led some to describe these as plywood fibromas (Fig. 4.11b). Cases with bizarre multinucleated giant cells, myxoid change, and high cellularity have also been described. By immunohistochemistry the spindle cells express Factor XIIIa and SMA, and to a lesser extent CD34 (Table 4.11).

Differential Diagnosis

The differential diagnoses include sclerotic neurofibroma and dermatofibroma and hypocellular fibroma of tendon sheath. Unlike SF, neurofibroma is composed of S100 protein-positive spindle cells with wavy, buckled nuclei in association with collagen bundles and mast cells. Dermatofibroma may be distinguished from SF by the presence of features typical of the former including secondary elements (e.g., hemosiderin and foam-laden cells, Touton-type giant cells, etc.), peripheral collagen trapping, and epidermal hyperplasia. Fibroma of tendon sheath has clefting artifact similar to SF, but the former does not arise in the dermis, is usually intimately associated with tendon sheaths, has characteristic slit-like vessels, and resembles burnt-out nodular fasciitis at least focally.

Fibrous Hamartoma of Infancy

Clinical Features

Fibrous hamartoma of infancy (FHI) is a rare soft tissue lesion, which typically affects infants and young children. Classically, lesions involve the axilla, back, or upper arm, but unusual locations including the scrotum, chest wall, thigh, breast, forearm, abdominal wall, buttock, cheek, scalp, hip, and orbit have been reported. There is a strong male predominance, and the mean patient age is 15 months. Approximately 20% of cases may arise congenitally. These lesions are benign, with only local recurrences (15% of cases) reported and no metastases.

Pathologic Features

Histopathologically, these lesions display a classic triphasic morphology: fibrous bands composed of bland spindle-shaped fibroblasts and myofibroblasts in fascicles separated by collagen; more cellular, immature, round to spindled cells in a myxoid matrix; and variable amounts of mature adipose tissue (Fig. 4.12a–d). A recent large study from the Mayo Clinic reported cases with a resemblance to giant cell fibroblastoma and two tumors with sarcomatous features. The one sarcomatous case with follow-up showed the patient to be alive and well after radical resection 4 years after presentation. Fibroblastic cells are SMA-positive, but mesenchymal cells are nega-

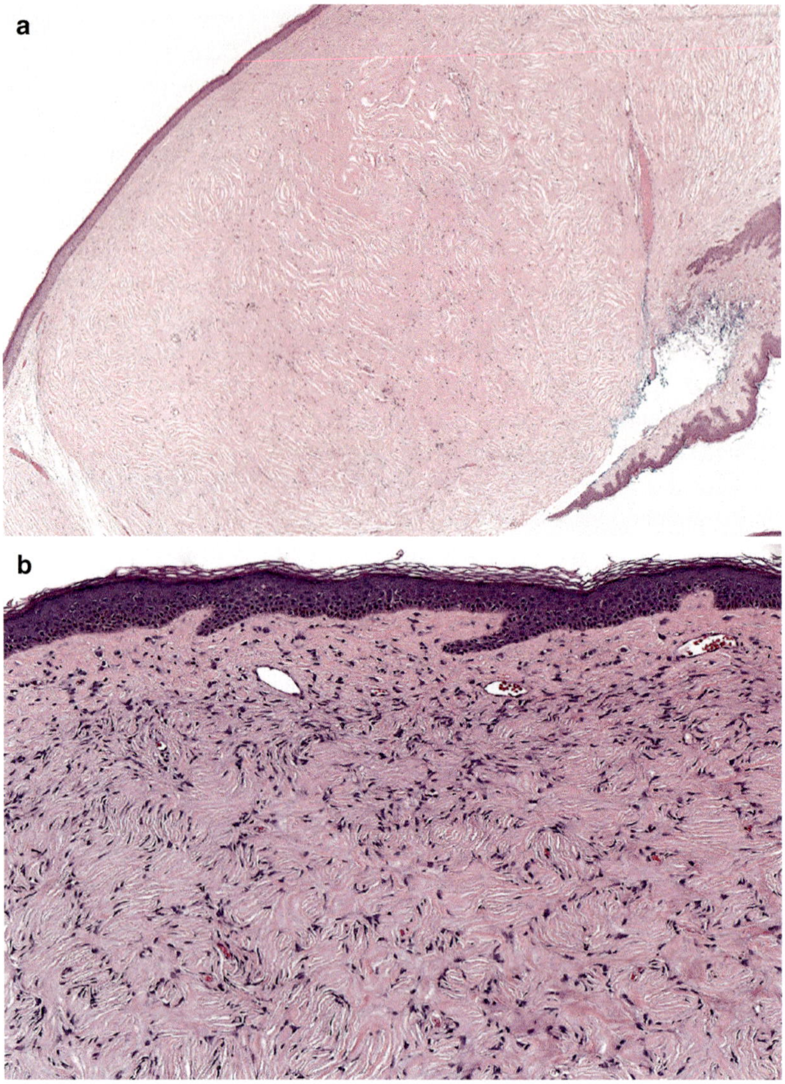

Fig. 4.11 Sclerotic fibroma (storiform collagenoma). (**a**) A well-demarcated hypocellular dermal nodule made up of a storiform proliferation of bland spindle cells embedded in sclerotic collagen with extensive clefting artifact. (**b**) The pattern of the stroma imparts a "plywood-like" pattern

Table 4.11 Key pathologic features: sclerotic fibroma

Polypoid, well-circumscribed lesion with abundant collagen
"Plywood-like" clefting artifact
Bland spindle cells in prominent storiform growth pattern
Myxoid change, multinucleated giant cells, and high cellularity may be seen
FXIIIa, SMA, and CD34 (variable)-positive; desmin, cytokeratin, and S100 protein are negative
Lesions associated with Cowden syndrome have loss of *PTEN* (10q23.3)

tive. The fibroadipose tissue is positive for S100, and sclerotic zones are CD34-positive. Little is known about the genetic events which cause this lesion. Small numbers of cases have been reported to show cytogenetic abnormalities, including complex karyotypes involving gains and losses of multiple chromosomes, a complex t(6; 12;8) (q25;q24.3;q13) and a reciprocal t(2;3) (q31;q21). The latter findings suggest that these lesions are neoplasms rather than hamartomas (Table 4.12).

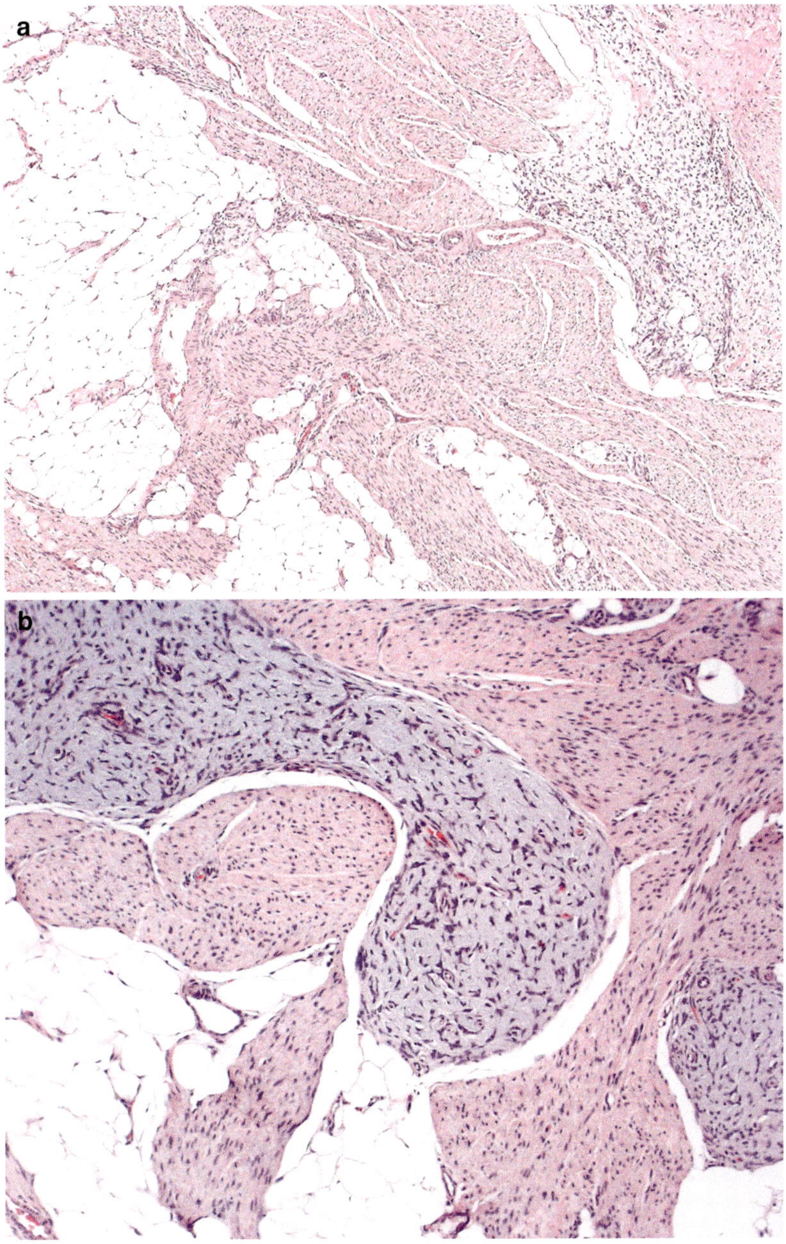

Fig. 4.12 Fibrous hamartoma of infancy. (**a**) Triphasic morphology consisting of fibrous bands composed of bland spindle cells, primitive spindled-to-ovoid mesenchymal cells, and variable amounts of mature adipose tissue. (**b**) High-power view of the three components of fibrous hamartoma: fibrous bands containing bland spindle cells, primitive mesenchymal cells, and adipose tissue. (**c**) High-power view of spindled-to-ovoid primitive mesenchymal cells. (**d**) An example of fibrous hamartoma with more adipose tissue

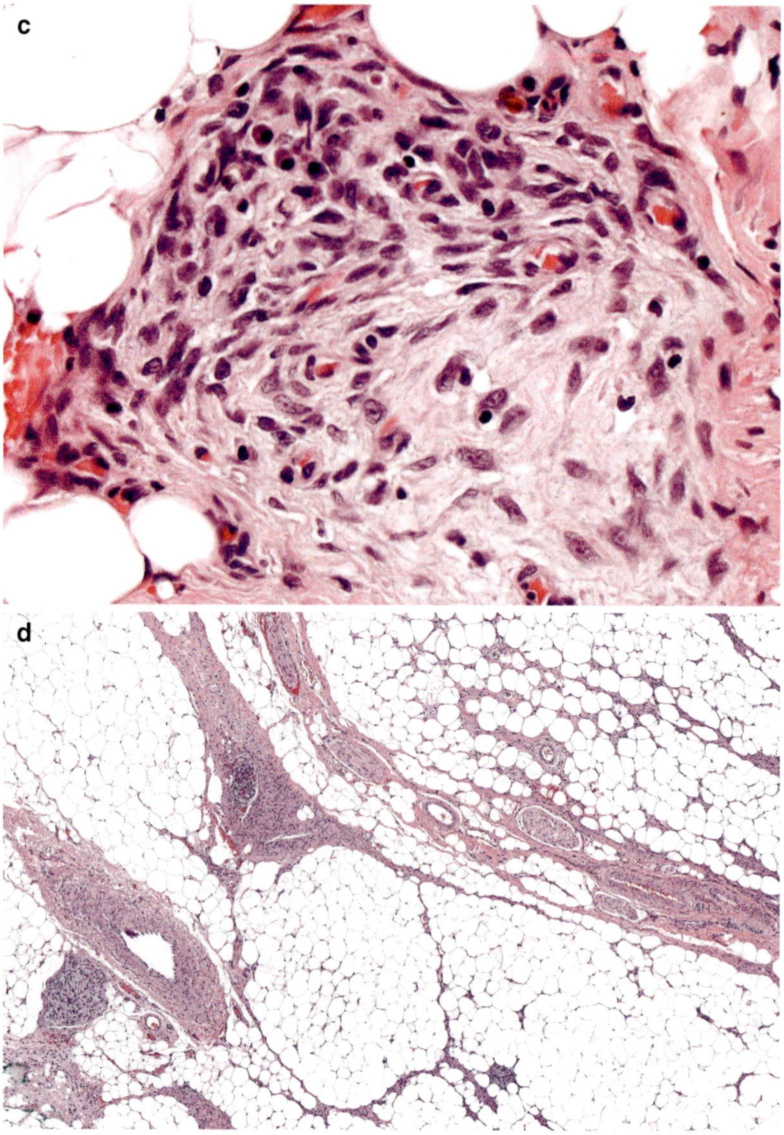

Fig. 4.12 (continued)

Table 4.12 Key histopathologic features: fibrous hamartoma of infancy

Classic triphasic morphology:
Bland fibroblastic myofibroblastic cells in fascicles
Myxoid nodules with primitive spindled to stellate cells
Varying amounts of adipose tissue

Differential Diagnosis

The differential is broad and includes tumors with varying amounts of adipose tissue, fibrous tissue, and primitive-appearing spindle cells. These lesions include lipofibromatosis, so-called lipofibromatosis-like neural tumor and maturing lipoblastoma. Lipofibromatosis occurs on the distal extremities. "Lipofibromatosis-like neural tumor" has S100 protein-positive spindle cells and *NTRK1* rearrangement. Lipoblastoma tends to be circumscribed and has *PLAG1* rearrangements. The predominantly fibroblastic lesions in the differential include fibromatosis, myofibroma, and calcifying aponeurotic fibroma. Fibromatosis lacks the triphasic appearance, and many cases have nuclear beta-catenin localization. Myofibroma has a biphasic appearance with dark- and light-staining areas. Calcifying aponeurotic fibroma has zones of calcification surrounded by epithelioid to chondroid cells. Those rare cases with sarcomatous areas need to be distinguished from infantile fibrosarcoma and spindle cell rhabdomyosarcoma by documenting the absence of *ETV6* rearrangement and myogenin or MyoD1 expression, respectively.

Infantile Digital Fibroma (Inclusion Body Fibromatosis)

Clinical Features

Infantile digital fibroma/fibromatosis (IDF) is a benign myofibroblastic proliferation described in 1965 by Reye, also known as Reye's tumor or inclusion body fibromatosis. IDF occurs as small (<2 cm), dome-shaped, non-tender, single, or multiple nodules on the fingers and, less commonly, toes. The lesion favors the dorsal or lateral aspect of the distal digit, with the second to fifth digits most commonly affected. Involvement of the thumb or great toe is exceptional. Nearly all lesions present before the age of 3 years with most presenting within the first year of life.

Although there is a high rate of recurrence following surgery (up to 74%), IDF carries an excellent prognosis. Interestingly, many lesions will spontaneously regress given adequate time. Therefore, in the absence of rapid growth or functional impairment, some authors suggest expectant management. Additionally, intralesional corticosteroids may be helpful in the treatment of IDF.

Pathologic Features

On histopathology, IDF is a poorly circumscribed, uniform proliferation of bland fibroblasts within a dense collagenous stroma. This dermal-based proliferation surrounds adnexal structures and extends into the deep dermis and subcutis (Fig. 4.13a and b). On closer inspection, characteristic small round eosinophilic inclusions of variable size (3–15 microns) are present within the cytoplasm of fibroblasts, separated from the nucleus by a thin clear zone (Fig. 4.13c).

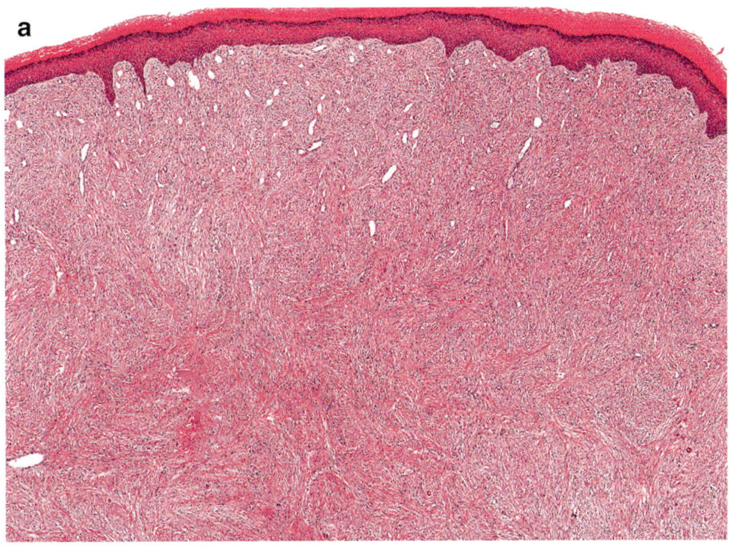

Fig. 4.13 Infantile digital fibroma (inclusion body fibromatosis). (**a**, **b**) A poorly circumscribed, uniform proliferation of bland fibroblasts within a dense collagenous stroma. (**c**) Characteristic small round eosinophilic inclusions of variable size (3–15 microns) are present within the cytoplasm of fibroblasts, separated from the nucleus by a thin clear zone. (**d**) Inclusions are highlighted on a trichrome special stain

Fig. 4.13 (continued)

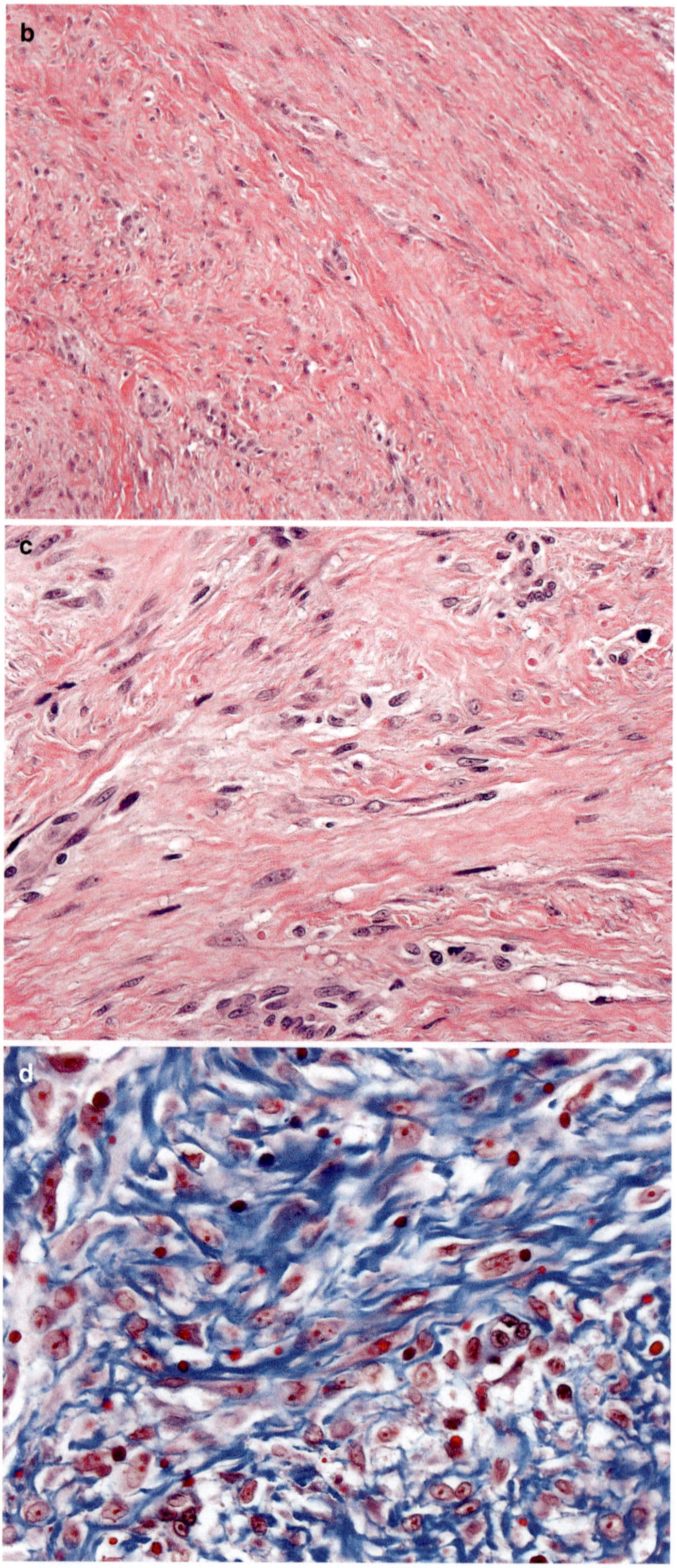

Table 4.13 Key pathologic features: infantile digital fibroma

Poorly circumscribed, uniform proliferation of bland fibroblastic cells in dense collagenous stroma
Lesional cells have round eosinophilic intracytoplasmic inclusions (3–15 microns)

Inclusions may be numerous or rare, in which case trichrome staining may be helpful in highlighting them (Fig. 4.13d). On ultrastructural and immunohistochemical examination, these inclusions have been shown to be densely packed actin microfilaments (Table 4.13).

Differential Diagnosis

The differential diagnosis includes palmoplantar fibromatosis, which lacks the characteristic eosinophilic inclusions. Benign digital fibromas (superficial acral fibromyxoma or cellular digital fibroma) may also be considered, but these lesions are typically seen in older patients and demonstrate diffuse CD34 immunoreactivity.

Plaque-Like CD34-Positive Dermal Fibroma

Clinical Features

Plaque-like CD34-positive dermal fibroma is a benign dermal spindle cell neoplasm first described by Rodriguez-Jurado and colleagues in 2004 as "medallion-like dermal dendrocyte hamartoma." Lesions are acquired or congenital, well-demarcated, slightly pigmented, indurated annular plaques that can affect any age group and arise at any anatomic site, with a slight female predominance. Clinical diagnoses typically included dermatofibroma, atrophic and plaque-like DFSP, and cutis laxa. There has been controversy regarding whether this is a neoplastic or hamartomatous lesion, or neither. However, recent work suggests that this is a neoplastic fibroblastic proliferation. This lesion is completely benign and cured by simple excision. Recurrence and malignant transformation have not been reported.

Pathologic Features

Lesions are composed of a band-like proliferation of bland, spindled fibroblasts in the mid to upper dermis. A grenz zone may be present, and extension into the subcutis is rare (Fig. 4.14a). Spindle cells in the superficial dermis are arrayed perpendicular to the epidermis, while deeper constituent cells take on a more storiform growth pattern. In areas, spindle cells are concentrically arrayed around the numerous capillaries. There is a paucity of elastic fibers, which may occasionally be entirely absent. Atypia is not appreciated, and mitoses are inconspicuous. A hypocellular variant of plaque-like CD34-positive dermal fibroma has been described. By immunohistochemistry the spindle cells are strongly and diffusely positive for CD34 and fascin (Fig. 4.14b). Immunoreactivity for SMA and FXIIIa is inconsistent at best (Table 4.14).

Differential Diagnosis

The differential diagnoses of plaque-like CD34-positive dermal fibroma include plaque-like and atrophic dermatofibrosarcoma protuberans, fibroblastic connective tissue nevus, diffuse neurofibroma, and dermatomyofibroma. Plaque-like and atrophic variants of dermatofibrosarcoma protuberans demonstrate clinical features similar to plaque-like CD34-positive dermal fibroma. The former entities are usually less well circumscribed both clinically and histopathologically, while the latter has a distinctly band-like, well-delineated proliferation within the papillary and upper reticular dermis. The perpendicular arrangement of superficial tumor cells alternating with parallel arrangement of deeper tumor cells of CD34-positive dermal fibroma is not seen in dermatofibrosarcoma protuberans. In difficult cases molecular studies for the *COL1A1-PDGFB* gene fusion allow for distinction between dermatofibrosarcoma protuberans and plaque-like CD34-positive dermal fibroma.

Fibroblastic connective tissue nevus also has a plaque-like clinical appearance and presents on the trunk of young adults and children but is composed

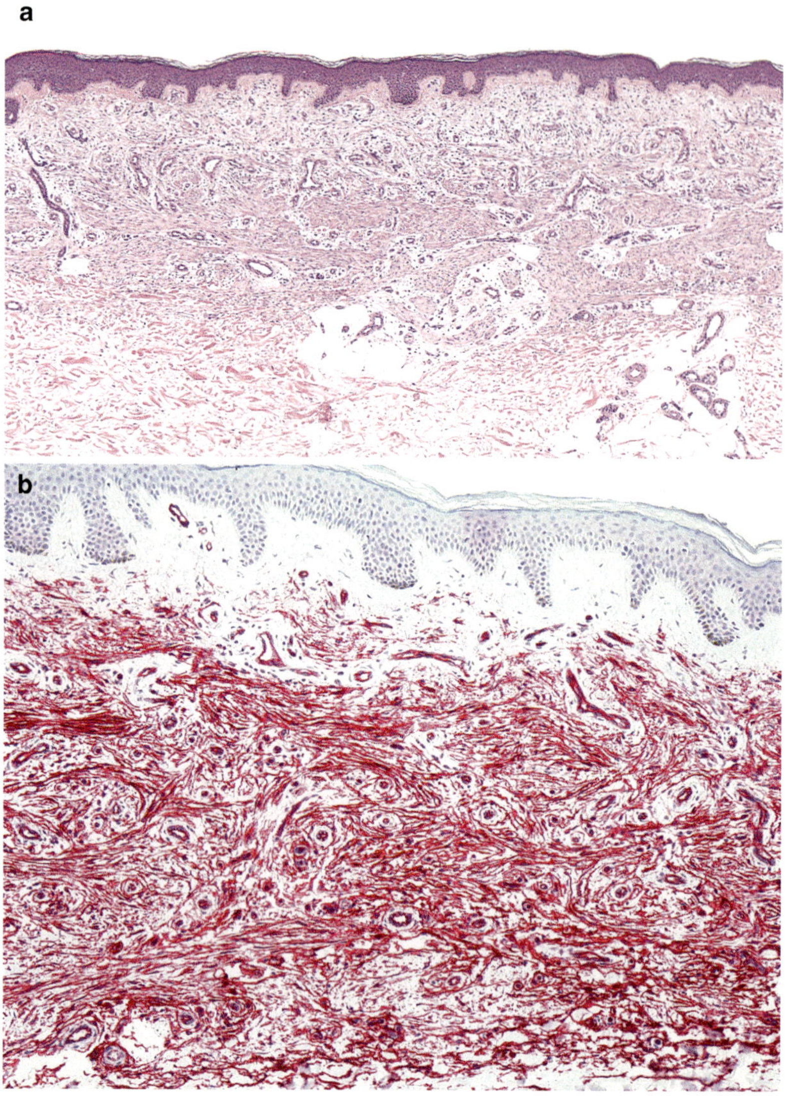

Fig. 4.14 Plaque-like CD34+ dermal fibroma. (**a**) A band-like proliferation of bland spindled fibroblastic cells in the mid to upper dermis beneath a grenz zone. Spindle cells in the superficial dermis are arrayed perpendicular to the epidermis (shown here), while deeper constituent cells take on a more storiform growth pattern. (**b**) CD34 immunostain is diffusely positive in the spindle cells. (Images courtesy of Dr. Thomas Mentzel, Dermatopathology Bodensee, Friedrichshafen, Germany)

Table 4.14 Key pathologic features: plaque-like CD34-positive dermal fibroma

Well-circumscribed spindle cell proliferation in papillary and reticular dermis with grenz zone
Cells oriented perpendicularly in superficial portions and parallel in deeper portion with respect to the epidermis
Diminished or absent elastic fibers
Scattered capillary vessels throughout
Rare mitotic figures and no atypia

of short fascicles of spindle cells present in a haphazard pattern involving the full thickness of the reticular dermis. Adnexal structures, vessels, and nerves may be entrapped, and there is often mature adipose tissue in the reticular dermis. The epidermis overlying the lesion is typically hyperplastic, unlike the epidermis in plaque-like CD34-positive dermal fibroma. Diffuse neurofibromas typically have more haphazardly arranged spindle cells in association with dermal collagen bundles and mast cells. Constituent cells have wavy and buckled, dark nuclei. Neurofibromas are positive for S100 protein. Unlike plaque-like CD34-positive dermal fibroma, dermatomyofibroma contains horizontally arranged, densely packed bundles and fascicles of bland spindle cells and is CD34-negative.

Dermatomyofibroma

Clinical Features

Dermatomyofibroma is an uncommon benign soft tissue tumor with a slight female predominance that typically occurs in young to middle-aged adults. Tumors usually present as slowly growing, painless cutaneous nodules or plaques involving the head and neck, thorax, or abdomen. These tumors only very rarely recur after surgical excision, even when incompletely excised. Rarely dermatomyofibroma may arise in children and be quite large or multicentric.

Pathologic Features

Microscopically, tumors are relatively hypocellular and comprised of bland-appearing fibroblastic/myofibroblastic spindle cells arranged in fascicles parallel to the epidermis within a collagenous stroma. Tumors are usually confined to the dermis but may rarely show focal involvement of the superficial subcutaneous fat (Fig. 4.15a). No significant cytologic atypia, mitotic activity, or necrosis is present (Fig. 4.15b). Tumor cells in early lesions express SMA, but older lesions are negative for this marker, as well as S100 protein, desmin, and CD34. Elastic stains often demonstrates increased numbers of fibers (Table 4.15).

Differential Diagnosis

The primary differential diagnosis is with fibroblastic connective tissue nevus, but other entities in the differential include fibrous histiocytoma, leiomyoma, dermatofibrosarcoma protuberans,

a

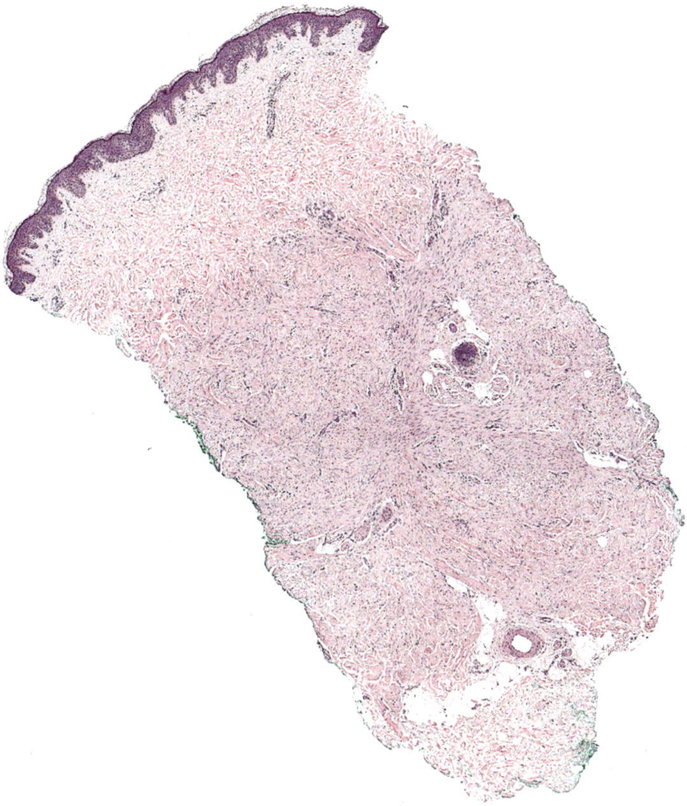

Fig. 4.15 Dermatomyofibroma. (**a**) A dermal-based, fibroblastic/myofibroblastic spindle cell proliferation arranged in horizontal fascicles (parallel to the epidermis) within a collagenous stroma. (**b**) The bland fibroblastic and myofibroblastic cells are devoid of atypia, mitoses, and necrosis

Fig. 4.15 (continued)

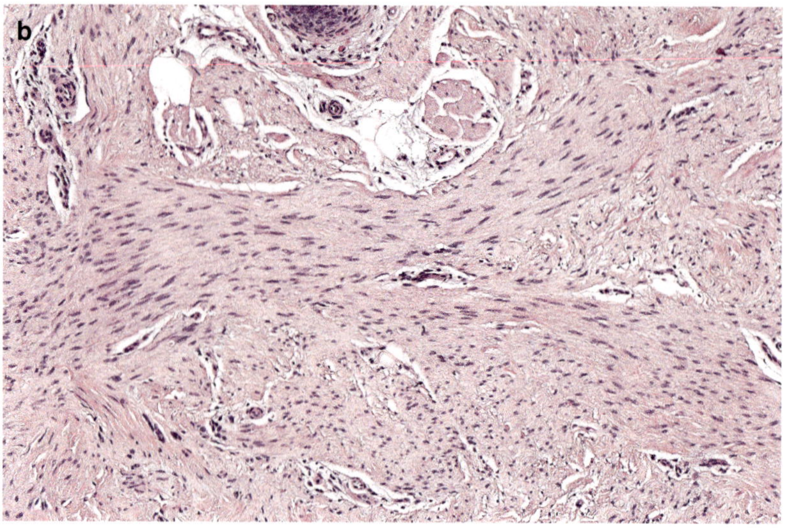

Table 4.15 Key pathologic features: dermatomyofibroma

Hypocellular lesion of bland-appearing fibroblastic/myofibroblastic spindle cells in fascicles parallel to the epidermis
Collagenous stroma
Rarely and only focally involves the subcutis
No atypia, mitoses, or necrosis
Only early lesions positive for SMA

fibrous hamartoma of infancy, superficial fibromatosis, and hypertrophic scar. Fibroblastic connective tissue nevus has shorter fascicles of spindle cells, often in association with collections of adipocytes in the reticular dermis, epidermal papillomatous hyperplasia, and usually CD34 expression. In some cases, the distinction can be very difficult but is of little consequence. Benign fibrous histiocytoma lacks the parallel fascicular pattern and demonstrates collagen trapping. Leiomyoma has an intersecting fascicular pattern of spindle cells with abundant eosinophilic cytoplasm, blunt-ended nuclei with perinuclear vacuoles, and SMA positivity. Dermatofibrosarcoma protuberans has a tight storiform proliferation of spindle cells and broad "honeycomb" infiltration of the subcutis. Unlike dermatomyofibroma, fibrous hamartoma arises in infants and young children and demonstrates triphasic histomorphology with immature mesenchymal spindle cells and bands of fibrocollagenous tissue and adipose tissue. Superficial fibromatoses are multinodular and hypercellular and lack the parallel arrangement of spindle cells. Hypertrophic scars have effacement of the rete pegs in the overlying epidermis, more conspicuous vertically oriented blood vessels, and may contain keloidal collagen.

Fibroblastic Connective Tissue Nevus

Clinical Features

Fibroblastic connective tissue nevus (FCTN) most commonly presents in children but can affect a wide age range, including middle-aged adults. Women are affected about twice as commonly as men. Lesions typically present as a plaque involving the trunk, extremities, or head and neck. Agminate and congenital cases have been reported. FCTN is a benign lesion without risk of recurrence or metastasis, even in cases with positive margins.

Pathologic Features

The overlying epidermis is papillomatous in the majority of cases (Fig. 4.16a). FCTN is poorly circumscribed and comprised of short intersecting fascicles of bland fibroblastic/myofibroblastic spindle cells present primarily in the reticular

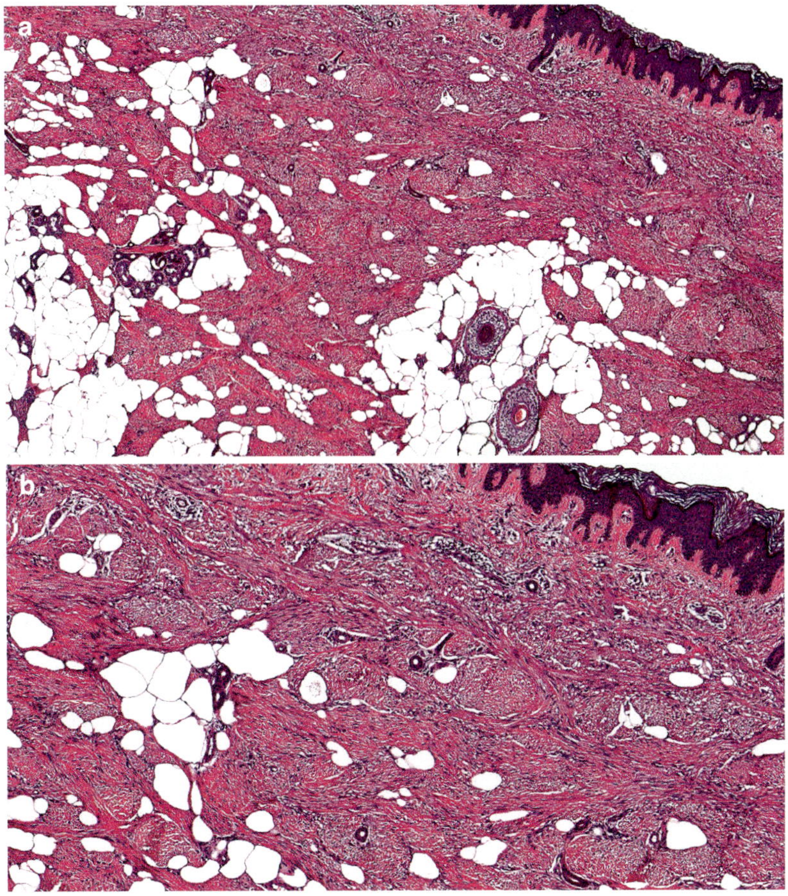

Fig. 4.16 Fibroblastic connective tissue nevus. (**a**) Papillomatous epidermis with underlying poorly circumscribed reticular dermal spindle cell proliferation that infiltrates into the subcutis. (**b**) The spindle cell proliferation is composed of short intersecting fascicles of bland fibroblastic/myofibroblastic cells present primarily in the reticular dermis. Note also collections of adipocytes within the reticular dermis

Table 4.16 Key pathologic features: fibroblastic connective tissue nevus

Poorly circumscribed lesion of short fascicles of bland fibroblastic/myofibroblastic spindle cells in the reticular dermis
Adipocytes within the reticular dermis
Frequent extension into the subcutis
No significant mitotic activity or cytologic atypia
CD34-positive, focal SMA immunoreactivity in half of cases, and negative for S100 protein and desmin

dermis with frequent extension into the subcutis (Fig. 4.16b). Collections of adipocytes within the reticular dermis are also present in the majority of cases. Mitotic activity and cytologic atypia are typically absent. By immunohistochemistry, most are CD34-positive and roughly half show some expression of SMA, while S100 and desmin are negative (Table 4.16).

Differential Diagnosis

FCTN has a broad differential diagnosis, the most important of which includes dermatomyofibroma, plaque-like CD34-positive dermal fibroma, pilar leiomyoma, dermatofibrosarcoma protuberans, and lipofibromatosis. The differentiating features of dermatomyofibroma are addressed above. Plaque-like CD34-positive dermal fibroma has a similar clinical presentation but typically has an atrophic rather than papillomatous epidermis. Also, the spindle cell proliferation of plaque-like CD34-positive dermal fibroma is usually restricted to the papillary and superficial reticular dermis, with vertical orientation of the spindle cells in the papillary dermis. Unlike in FCTN, collections of adipocytes in the reticular dermis are not a feature. Pilar leiomyoma is distinguished from FCTN by its dermal proliferation of intersecting fascicles of spindle cells with abundant eosinophilic cytoplasm and cigar-shaped nuclei with perinuclear vacuoles. There is diffuse expression for SMA and variable desmin positivity. Dermatofibrosarcoma protuberans is composed of a tighter, more storiform proliferation of mildly atypical CD34-positive spindle cells involving the entire dermis and extending into the subcutis with a "honeycomb" pattern of infiltration. Lipofibromatosis has similar clinical features to FCTN but demonstrates biphasic histology consisting of spindle cells arranged in fascicles and with abundant adipose tissue infiltrating through skeletal muscle.

Superficial Fibromatoses

Clinical Features

Fibromatoses are a large group of benign, though sometimes locally aggressive, soft tissue tumors that occur across a wide age spectrum. In general, fibromatoses are subdivided into superficial (fascial) and deep types. Superficial fibromatoses usually occur in older adults without gender predilection and present as a slowly enlarging, multinodular soft tissue mass of the hands, feet, or penis. Palmar and plantar fibromatoses are also known as Dupuytren contracture and Ledderhose disease, respectively, while penile fibromatosis is also known as Peyronie disease. They have an autosomal dominant inheritance pattern with incomplete penetrance. While superficial fibromatoses have a benign clinical course, local recurrences after surgical excision are common, and other nonsurgical approaches may show variable efficacy. In contrast to superficial fibromatoses, deep fibromatoses (also known as desmoid-type fibromatoses) usually occur in younger adults and present as a slow-growing deep soft tissue mass in the extremities or trunk or intra-abdominally. In addition, a subset of patients with intra-abdominal deep fibromatoses may have familial adenomatous polyposis (FAP) syndrome and, thus, manifest other syndromic features, including intestinal polyposis, osteomas, and Gardner-associated fibromas (Gardner syndrome). In general, deep fibromatoses may show a more aggressive clinical course, with frequent local recurrences after surgical excision and occasional deaths despite multimodal therapeutic approaches (i.e., systemic chemotherapy, radiation therapy, etc.). There is an increasing trend for avoiding surgery unless medically necessary.

Pathologic Features

Superficial fibromatoses are multinodular, unencapsulated, but relatively circumscribed tumors (Fig. 4.17a). Deep fibromatoses are often poorly circumscribed and demonstrate prominent local infiltration of adjacent soft tissue and/or visceral organs. Microscopically, fibromatoses are variably cellular and comprised predominantly of bland-appearing fibroblasts/myofibroblasts with scant eosinophilic to amphophilic cytoplasm, tapered vesicular nuclei that have undulating nuclear membranes, and inconspicuous nucleoli. Tumor cells are arranged in long, intersecting fascicles within a collagenous stroma containing thin-walled curvilinear vessels with frequent associated mild perivascular lymphocytic inflammation and edema (Fig. 4.17b). Plantar fibromatoses, particularly those in younger patients, may be relatively hypercellular, with focally increased cytologic atypia, scattered multinucleated cells, and/or mitotic activity (Fig. 4.17c and d). In contrast, a subset of superficial fibromatoses, particularly those involving the hands or penis, may be relatively hypocellular with hyalinized stroma (Fig. 4.17e). Tumor cells typically express smooth muscle and/or muscle-specific actin and are negative for S100 protein, CD34, desmin, and pan-cytokeratin expression. Sporadic deep fibromatoses show recurrent somatic activating *CTNNB1* mutations, whereas FAP-associated deep fibromatoses demonstrate inactivating *APC* mutations with somatic loss of heterozygosity; as such, beta-catenin immunostains usually show strong and diffuse nuclear accumulation in deep fibromatoses. Nuclear positivity for beta-catenin is seen in approximately 50% of superficial fibromatoses and is typically focal. Gains of whole

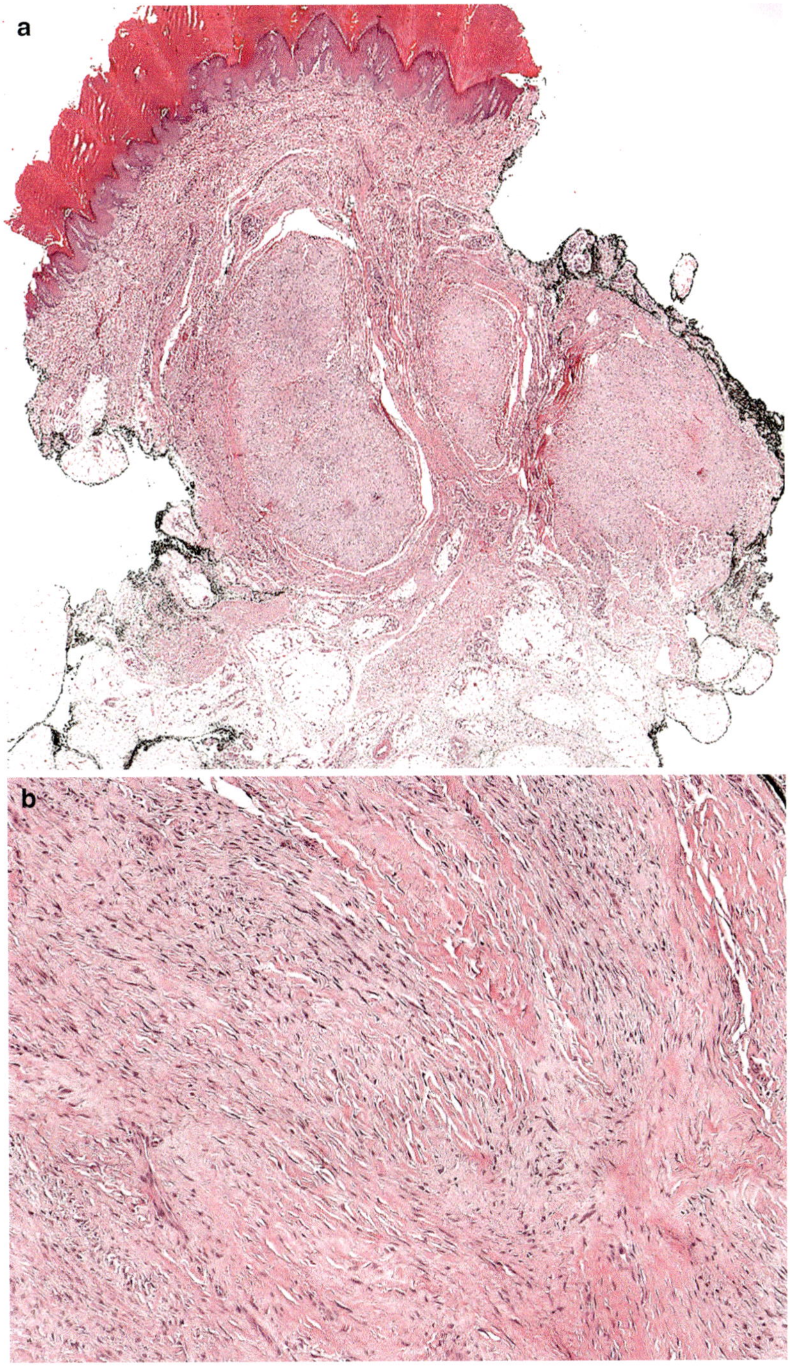

Fig. 4.17 Superficial fibromatoses. (**a**) Tumors are multinodular, unencapsulated, but relatively circumscribed. (**b**) An example of palmar fibromatosis composed of a variably cellular proliferation of bland-appearing fibroblastic spindle cells arranged in long, intersecting fascicles set within a collagenous stroma. (**c**) Some cases, particularly plantar fibromatosis in younger patients, may be somewhat more cellular. Thin-walled vessels with mild perivascular inflammation are noted in both **b** and **c**. (**d**) Multinucleated cells are relatively common in plantar fibromatosis. (**e**) Some cases, particularly those involving the penis, may be hypocellular

Fig. 4.17 (continued)

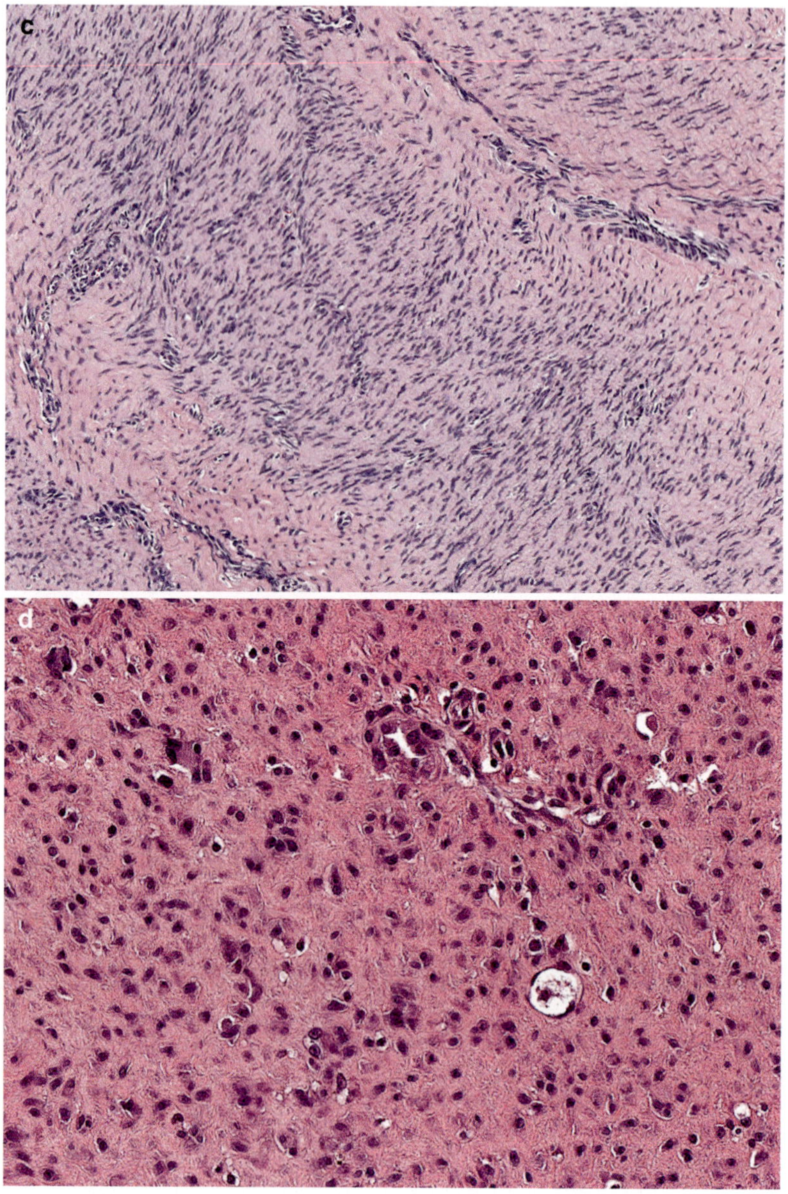

Fig. 4.17 (continued)

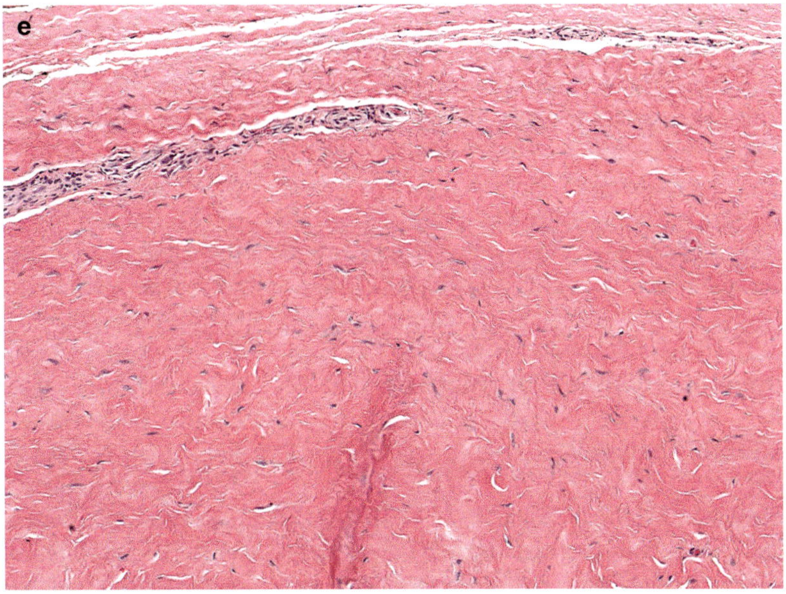

chromosomes 7 and 8 are seen in palmar fibromatoses, and gains of 8 and 14 are present in plantar fibromatoses. Palmar fibromatoses may also demonstrate abnormalities involving 14q11.2 and 7p14.1 (Table 4.17).

Differential Diagnosis

The primary differential diagnosis of superficial fibromatosis is with fibroma of tendon sheath. Fibroma of tendon sheath is typically less cellular and lacks the fascicular growth pattern of fibromatosis. Cellular examples of fibroma of tendon sheath do not have long fascicles, as discussed above. Calcifying aponeurotic fibromas also present in acral surfaces, but have distinct calcified and chondroid areas. Dermatomyofibroma and fibroblastic connective tissue nevus do not typically involve acral sites or the penis and are primarily located in the dermis. Both superficial acral and deep (desmoid) fibromatoses do not typically involve the dermis. Cellular fibrous histiocytoma has a central fascicular growth pattern

Table 4.17 Key pathologic features: superficial fibromatoses

Key pathologic features: superficial fibromatoses
Long fascicles of fibroblasts and myofibroblasts in a collagenous stroma
Focally SMA and muscle-specific actin-positive, nuclear beta-catenin positive in 50% of cases (focal)
Palmar fibromatosis (Dupuytren contracture)
Relatively hypocellular
Gains of whole chromosomes 7 and 8 and abnormalities involving 14q11.2 and 7p14.1
Plantar fibromatosis (Ledderhose disease)
Relatively hypercellular, especially in younger patients
Focal increased cytologic atypia, multinucleated cells, and/or mitoses
Gains of whole chromosomes 8 and 14
Penile fibromatosis (Peyronie disease)
Relatively hypocellular with prominent hyalinized stroma
Key pathologic features: deep fibromatoses
Same histologic features as with superficial fibromatosis
May have variable stromal myxoid change
Somatic cases with activating *CTNNB1* mutations, FAP-associated cases with inactivating *APC* mutations
Nuclear beta-catenin diffusely present in most cases

resembling fibromatosis, but the peripheries show typical features of conventional fibrous histiocytoma, such as storiform growth and peripheral collagen trapping. Synovial sarcoma can present in the peripheral extremities, but unlike fibromatosis is composed of plumper spindle cells with overlapping nuclei, often has a staghorn vasculature, is positive for TLE, is usually focally positive for cytokeratins, and has a t(X;18).

Juvenile Hyaline Fibromatosis

Clinical Features

Juvenile hyaline fibromatosis (JHF), also known as fibromatosis hyalinica multiplex juvenilis and Murray-Puretic-Drescher syndrome, is a rare autosomal recessive genodermatosis with variable penetrance, that is characterized by hyalinizing fibrosis of the skin and internal organs. Approximately 70 cases have been reported to date. Patients typically present in early childhood, usually during the first 2 years of life, with multiple papular skin lesions, gingival hyperplasia, joint contractures, and osteolytic bone lesions. Males are affected slightly more than females. Clinically, skin lesions may resemble an adnexal neoplasm or non-melanoma skin cancer. The systemic variant of JHF is known as infantile systemic hyalinosis (ISH) and has an earlier onset and poor prognosis. Hyaline fibromatosis syndrome (HFS) has been suggested as a unifying descriptor to include patients with either JHF or ISH. Treatment of JHF usually involves multiple resections of cutaneous nodules, due to a high recurrence rate. Radiotherapy is ineffective. Intralesional steroid injection may reduce the size of lesions. In patients with ISH, gingivectomy can help improve nourishment, and penicillamine has been reported to improve joint mobility. Nonetheless, the prognosis for ISH is poor with most patients dying of malnutrition, infection, or intractable diarrhea before the age of 2.

Pathologic Features

Microscopy shows skin lesions to be composed of bland spindle-shaped fibroblastic cells embedded within a PAS/Alcian blue-positive, Congo red-negative, densely hyalinized stroma (Fig. 4.18a and b). Elastic tissue is not present. Early lesions are more cellular than older lesions (Fig. 4.18c). Some cases may contain spherical calcified particles resembling psammoma bodies. By immunohistochemistry spindle cells are negative for SMA, and there is a population of CD68-positive macrophages in between the spindle cells. Loss-of-function mutations in capillary morphogenesis gene 2 (*CMG2/ANTXR2*), a transmembrane surface protein, result in accumulation of collagen IV in the extracellular matrix, which leads to the manifestations of HFS (Table 4.18).

Differential Diagnosis

Due to the deposition of amorphous material, cutaneous lesions of HFS may clinically and histopathologically resemble lipoid proteinosis, amyloidosis, scleromyxedema, or myofibroma. Lipoid proteinosis is a rare autosomal recessive genodermatosis caused by a loss-of-function mutation or reduced expression of the gene encoding extracellular matrix protein 1 (ECM1) on chromosome 1q21. This leads to the deposition of hyaline material within the skin and submucosa, which manifests as the pathognomonic dermatologic finding of this disorder, beaded papules over the lid margins termed "moniliform blepharosis." These features distinguish this disorder from HFS. Amyloidosis demonstrates apple-green birefringence on Congo red staining, which is not seen in HFS. Unlike HFS, scleromyxedema is a chronic fibromucinous disorder characterized by monoclonal gammopathy and generalized papular and sclerodermoid skin lesions, which by histology demonstrate dermal mucin, increased collagen deposition, and a proliferation of fibroblasts. Myofibromas are not hyalinized like

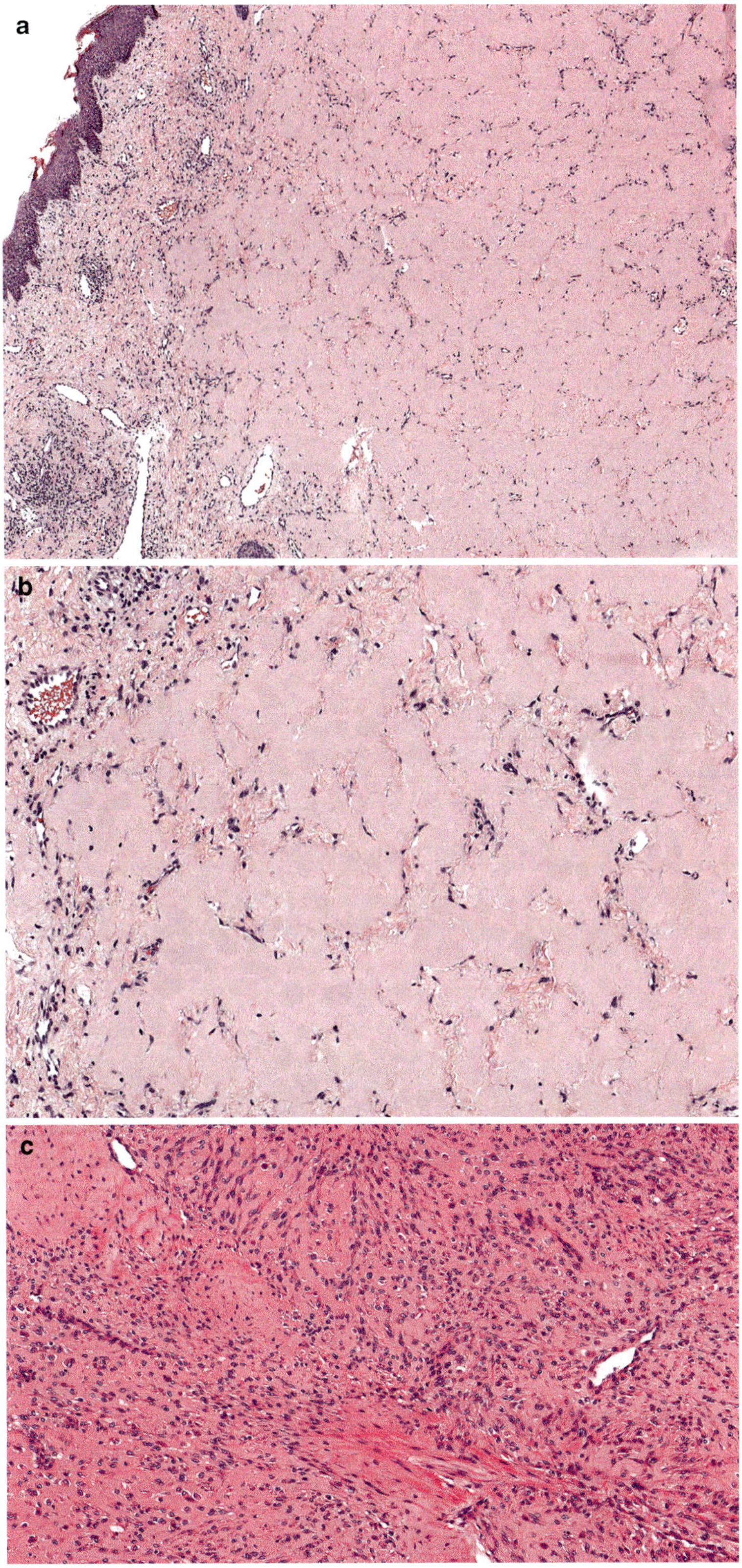

Fig. 4.18 Juvenile hyaline fibromatosis. (**a**, **b**) A skin lesion of juvenile hyaline fibromatosis composed of bland spindle-shaped fibroblastic cells embedded within a densely hyalinized stroma. (**c**) Early lesions of juvenile hyaline fibromatosis are more cellular, as in this case

Table 4.18 Key histopathologic features: juvenile hyaline fibromatosis/infantile systemic hyalinosis/hyaline fibromatosis syndrome

Bland spindle-shaped fibroblastic cells within PAS/Alcian blue-positive, densely hyalinized stroma
Early lesions more cellular than older ones
May contain spherical calcified particles resembling psammoma bodies
Spindle cells negative for SMA
Population of CD68-positive macrophages in between spindle cells
Loss-of-function mutations in capillary morphogenesis gene 2 (*CMG2/ANTXR2*) result in accumulation of collagen IV in the extracellular matrix

lesions of HFS, but instead are composed of a well-circumscribed, paucicellular proliferation of SMA-positive, desmin-negative "myoid" spindle cells in association with a prominent hemangiopericytomatous (staghorn) vasculature.

Infantile Fibromatosis (Lipofibromatosis)

Clinical Features

Two distinct morphological types of fibromatosis occurring in infancy and childhood have been described. The first is extremely rare, essentially identical to adult desmoid fibromatosis, and will not be discussed further. The other variant, also called lipofibromatosis or mesenchymal-type infantile fibromatosis, is an uncommon benign soft tissue tumor with slight male predominance that typically occurs in infants and children, including a small subset of congenital cases. Tumors usually present as a rapidly enlarging deep soft tissue mass in the extremities, thorax, abdomen, or head and neck and may recur locally after incomplete surgical excision. These lesions, however, do not metastasize.

Pathologic Features

Lipofibromatosis is a poorly circumscribed, hypercellular tumor comprised predominantly of bland-appearing round-to-ovoid cells with a moderate amount of eosinophilic cytoplasm, enlarged and slightly irregular nuclei, and inconspicuous nucleoli. Tumor cells are arranged haphazardly or form small bundles and fascicles within a fibromyxoid stroma and show a characteristic diffuse, infiltrative growth into adjacent soft tissue, including adipose tissue and skeletal muscle (Fig. 4.19a). Some of the smaller fat cells (adipocytes) observed in these lesions are likely a result of fatty proliferation due to muscular atrophy secondary to tumor infiltration of skeletal muscle (Fig. 4.19b). Although mitotic activity and cellularity may be focally increased, cytologic atypia is minimal, and necrosis is absent. Tumor cells typically express smooth muscle and/or muscle-specific actin and are negative for S100, CD34, desmin, and pan-cytokeratin. No recurrent genetic abnormalities have been described, but a case with a three-way t(4;9;6) has been reported (Table 4.19).

Differential Diagnosis

The major differential diagnosis for infantile fibromatosis (lipofibromatosis) is with infantile (congenital) fibrosarcoma. Despite the possibility of significant morphologic and immunophenotypic overlap, cellular infantile fibromatosis (lipofibromatosis) can typically be distinguished from infantile (congenital) fibrosarcoma by its lack of a herringbone growth pattern. Additionally, a diffuse infiltrative pattern and variation in cellularity is suggestive of lipofibromatosis, while uniform hypercellularity, marked mitotic activity, and/or necrosis favor a diagnosis of infantile (congenital) fibrosarcoma. In difficult cases, demonstration of the *ETV6-NTRK3* gene fusion of infantile fibrosarcoma rules out lipofibromatosis. Interestingly, a group of superficial soft tissue tumors occurring in children and young adults reminiscent of lipofibromatosis, with variable cytologic atypia and a distinct immunophenotype of S100 protein and CD34 positivity suggestive of neural differentiation and recurrent gene fusions involving the *NTRK1* gene, has been recently reported. The relationship, if any, of these to lipofibromatosis remains to be determined. Lipofibromatosis demonstrates infiltrative growth into adipose tissue mimicking the growth

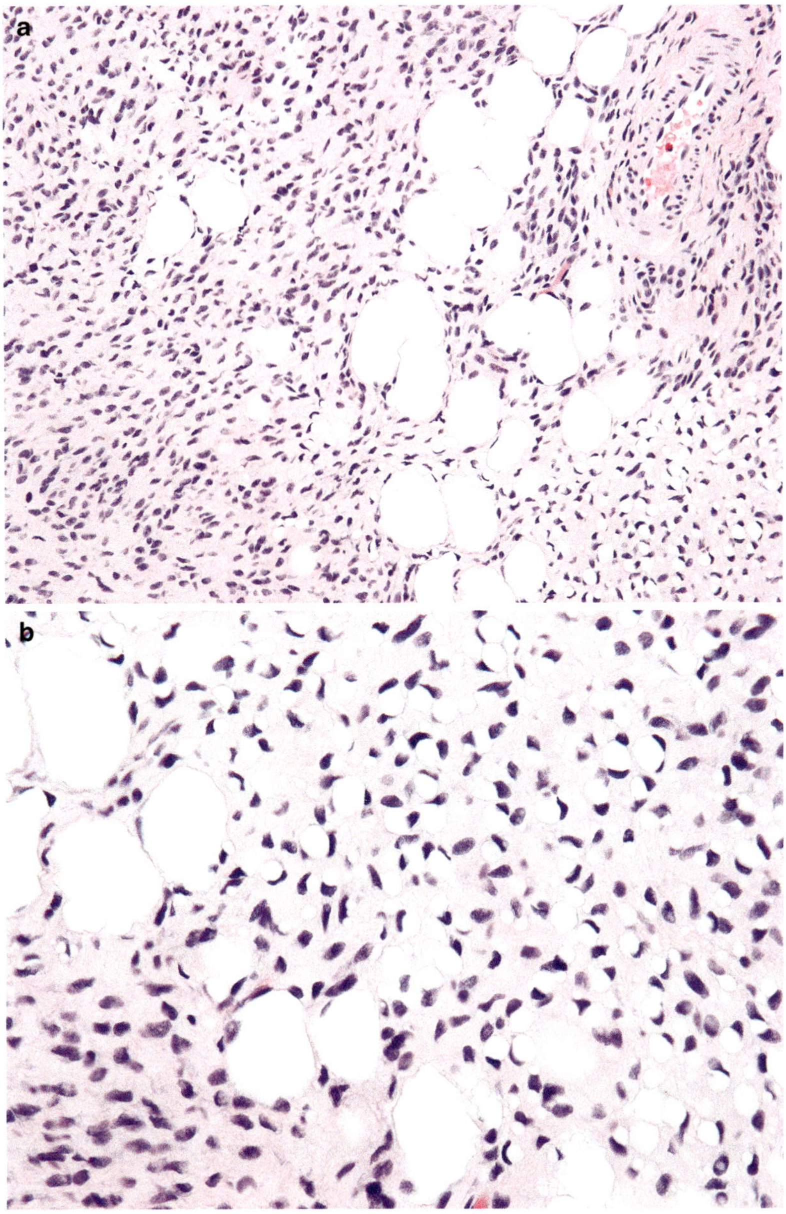

Fig. 4.19 Infantile fibromatosis (lipofibromatosis). (**a**) A poorly circumscribed, hypercellular tumor comprised of bland-appearing round-to-ovoid cells arranged haphazardly or forming small bundles and fascicles within a fibromyxoid stroma. (**b**) A case with more prominent small lipocytes. These cells are likely due to fatty proliferation in response to muscular atrophy secondary to tumor infiltration of skeletal muscle. (Images courtesy of Dr. Andrew Folpe, Mayo Clinic)

Table 4.19 Key pathologic features: infantile fibromatosis (lipofibromatosis)

Poorly circumscribed tumor with haphazardly arranged fibroblast-like or primitive mesenchymal cells in a myxoid stroma
Prominent infiltration into skeletal muscle and adipose tissue
Proliferation of lipocytes secondary to skeletal muscle atrophy may be extensive
Mitotically active cellular spindle cell areas with fascicular growth resemble infantile fibrosarcoma
Variable staining for smooth muscle and muscle-specific actin, desmin typically negative

pattern seen in DFSP and diffuse neurofibroma. DFSP has a predominantly storiform growth pattern, is diffusely CD34-positive, and has a *COL1A1-PDGFRB* fusion, features not seen in lipofibromatosis. The infiltration of adipose tissue by lipofibromatosis may also lead to consideration of a lipogenic tumor such as myxoid liposarcoma or lipoblastoma. Myxoid liposarcoma is vanishingly rare in infants and children, has a distinctive "chicken-wire" vascular pattern, and has *DDIT3* translocation, which can be demonstrated by FISH. Lipoblastoma is more myxoid with a prominent lobular growth pattern and uniformity in the size of adipocytes, unlike lipofibromatosis.

Benign Fibrous Histiocytoma (Dermatofibroma)

Clinical Features

Benign fibrous histiocytoma (dermatofibroma) encompasses a family of benign tumors with overlapping clinical and histologic features. They are usually ≥1 cm in diameter, but may reach up to 10 cm in size, and involve the extremities of young-to-middle-aged adults (but may occur at any age). They often present as a superficial, slow-growing papulonodular lesion with variably increased pigmentation. Conventional fibrous histiocytoma/dermatofibroma is more common in younger women and has a propensity to arise on the legs. Other variants have a largely equal sex distribution. Occasional lesions may arise in the arms, trunk, and distal extremities. Involvement of the head and neck and face is uncommon, except for the cellular variant. Rare cases may be multiple and distributed widely or agminated and arise in the deep dermis or subcutis and can be quite large. In general, these tumors demonstrate indolent behavior with a low risk of local recurrence. Certain histologic types (those involving the face, cellular, aneurysmal/hemosiderotic, deep, and atypical variants) are associated with an increased risk of local recurrence (up to 20% in some series). Exceptionally, metastases and even death from disease have been reported and, similar to the increased risk for local recurrence, are also associated with the aforementioned histologic subtypes. It should be stressed that metastasis and death are so rare that all of the members of this group are still best regarded as benign entities, with some risk for local nondestructive recurrence. Simple excision is curative in most cases. In general, we recommend conservative re-excision of the subtypes at increased risk for recurrence with due consideration for cosmetically sensitive locations.

Pathologic Features

All members of this group share certain histopathologic features, including relative circumscription, origin in the reticular dermis, and frequent overlying epidermal hyperplasia with increased basilar pigmentation (Fig. 4.20a). Occasional cases will show follicular or sebaceous induction in the overlying epidermis (Fig. 4.20b). Cases in the deeper dermis or subcutis usually lack overlying epidermal change and are larger. At the periphery of the tumor, the constituent spindle cells will interdigitate with peripheral collagen fibers of the reticular dermis, so-called collagen trapping (Fig. 4.20c). For larger or more deeply situated tumors, involve-

Fig. 4.20 Benign fibrous histiocytoma (dermatofibroma). (**a**) Circumscribed dermal proliferation with epidermal hyperplasia. (**b**) Occasional cases may show follicular or sebaceous induction. (**c**) Peripheral collagen trapping. (**d**) Extension into subcutaneous fat with fat necrosis and inflammation. (**e**) Conventional benign fibrous histiocytoma with spindle cells in vaguely storiform arrangement (bottom) and siderophages, histiocytes, Touton-like giant cells, and scattered small lymphocytes (top). (**f**) The lipidized (ankle-type) variant tends to be hypocellular with foamy histiocytes in a hyalinized background. (**g**) The cellular variant has intersecting fascicles of tumor cells with little to no secondary elements and may demonstrate necrosis in up to 10% of cases. Cytologic atypia and atypical mitoses will be absent, assuaging the concern for malignancy. (**h**) Aneurysmal and/or hemosiderotic variant with hemorrhagic pseudovascular spaces and siderophages. (**i**) Atypical fibrous histiocytoma demonstrating admixed hyperchromatic, pleomorphic, and multinucleated cells. Other features of conventional dermatofibroma such as collagen trapping (seen here) allow distinction from atypical fibroxanthoma/pleomorphic dermal sarcoma and undifferentiated pleomorphic sarcomas. (**j**) Deep benign fibrous histiocytoma demonstrating a prominent staghorn (hemangiopericytomatous) vasculature. (**k**) Granular cell variant containing plump spindled-to-ovoid cells with abundant eosinophilic granular cytoplasm. (**l**) A rare myxoid example of benign fibrous histiocytoma. (**m**) Keloidal variant of benign fibrous histiocytoma. (Image courtesy of Dr. Thomas Brenn, University of Calgary). (**n**) CD34 is generally negative, but can be positive at the periphery of benign fibrous histiocytomas

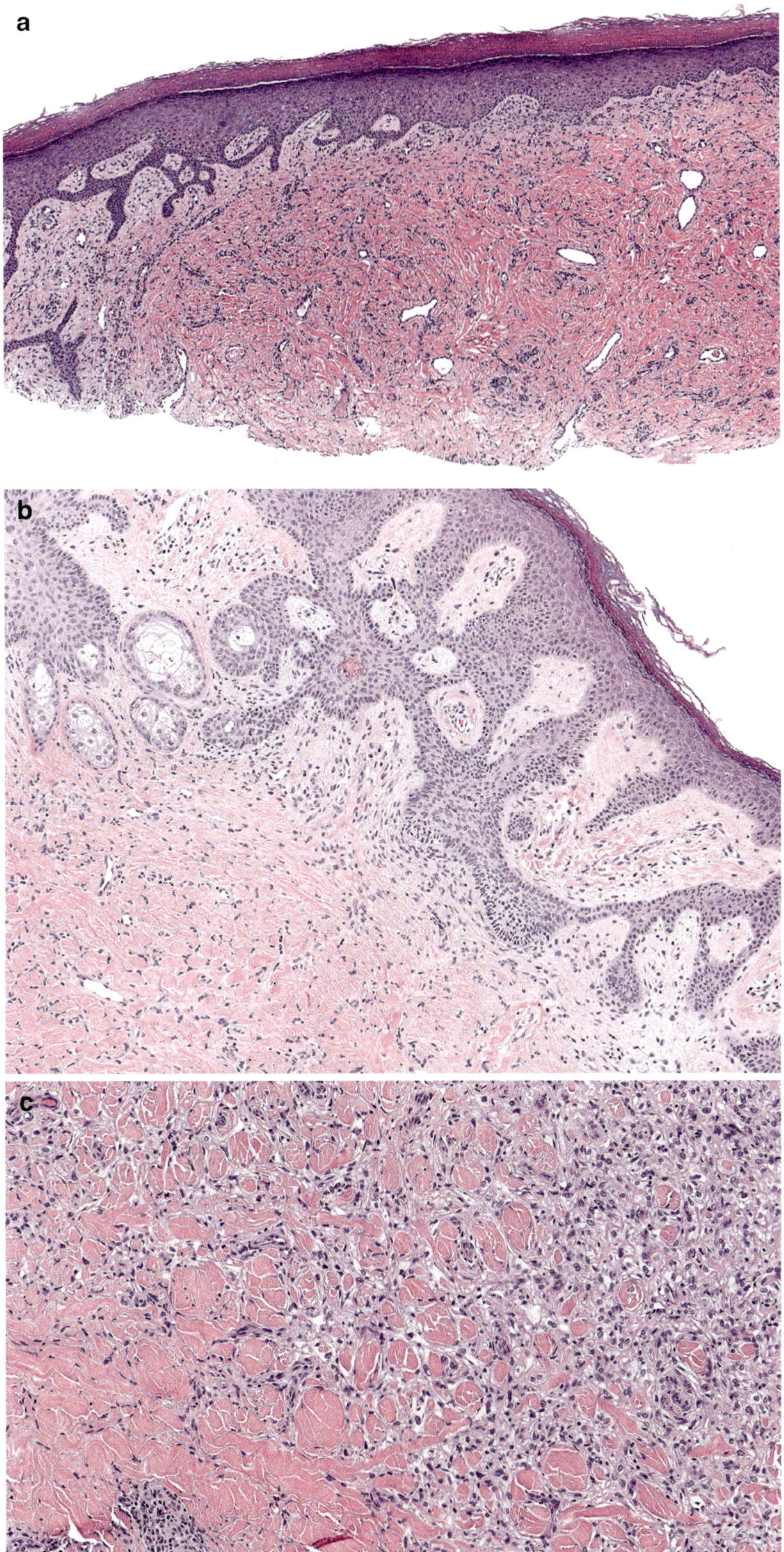

Fig. 4.20 (continued)

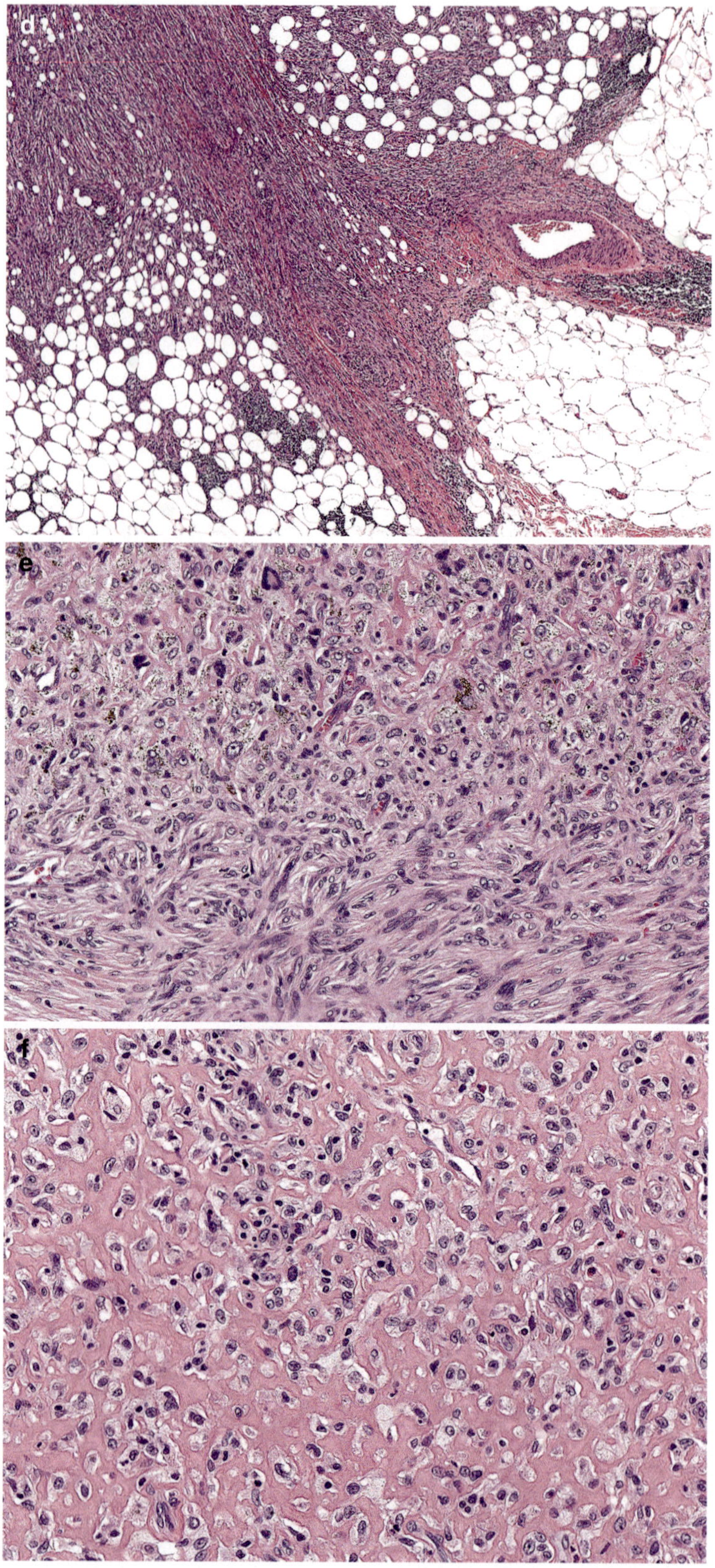

Fig. 4.20 (continued)

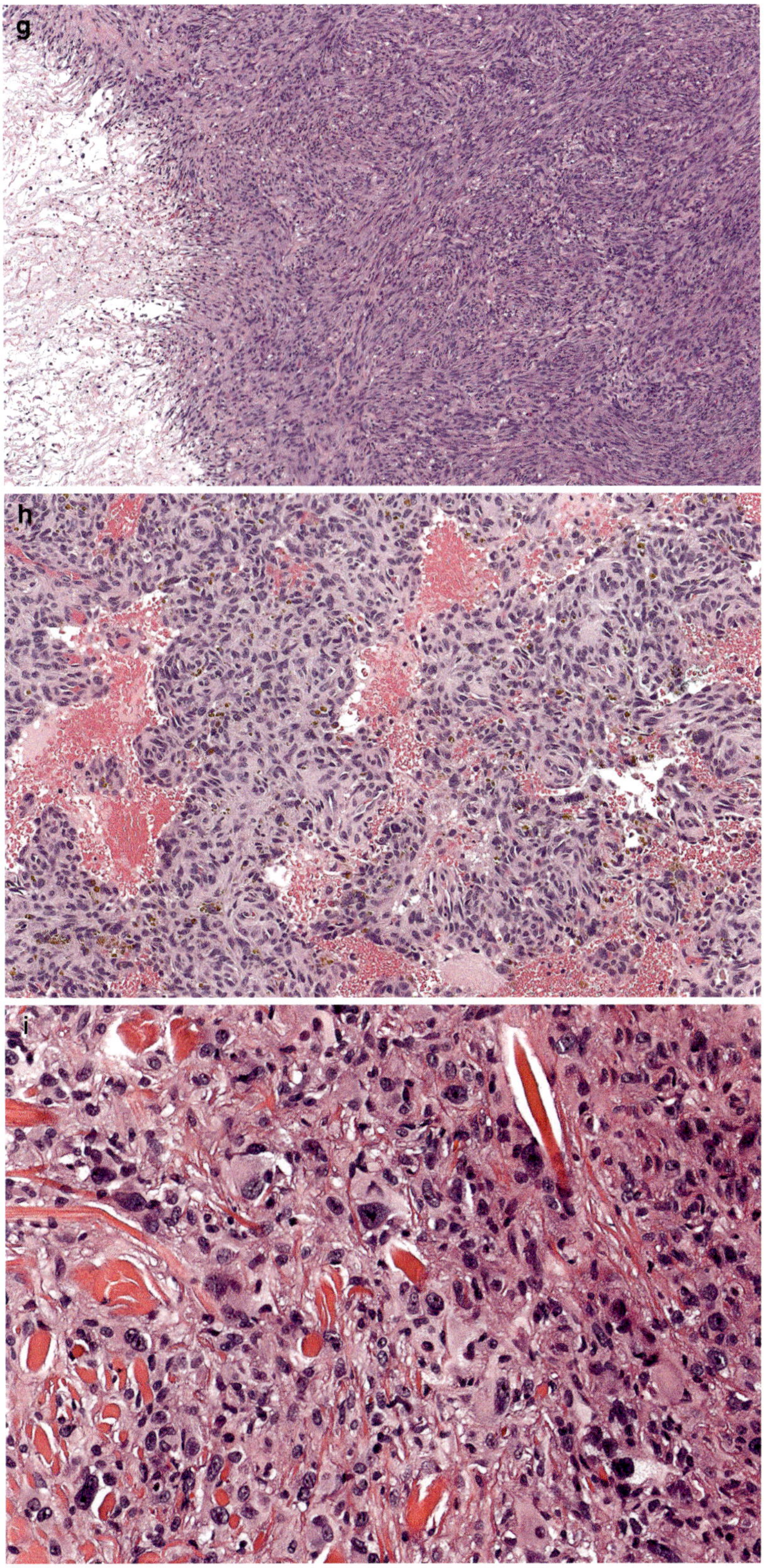

Fig. 4.20 (continued)

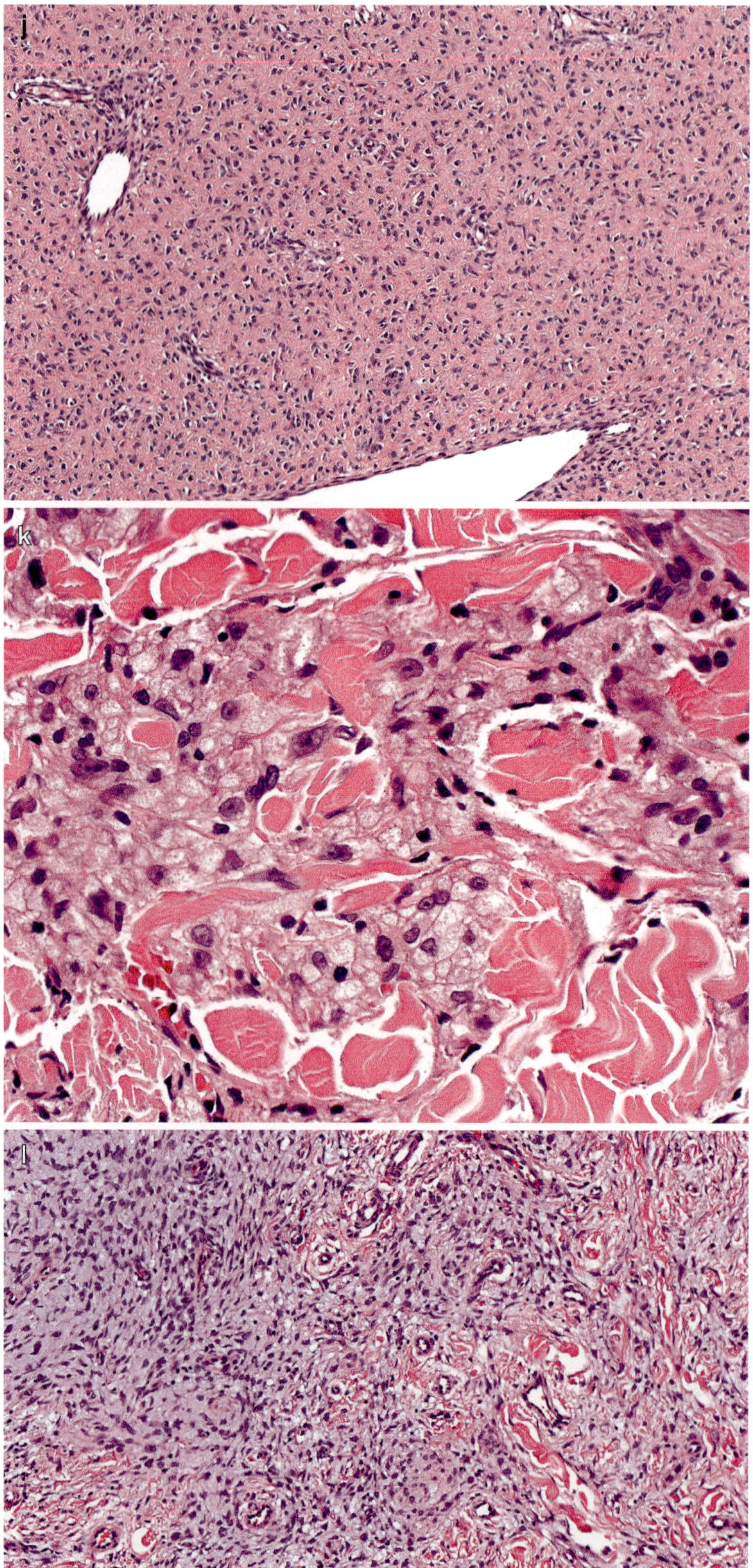

Fig. 4.20 (continued)

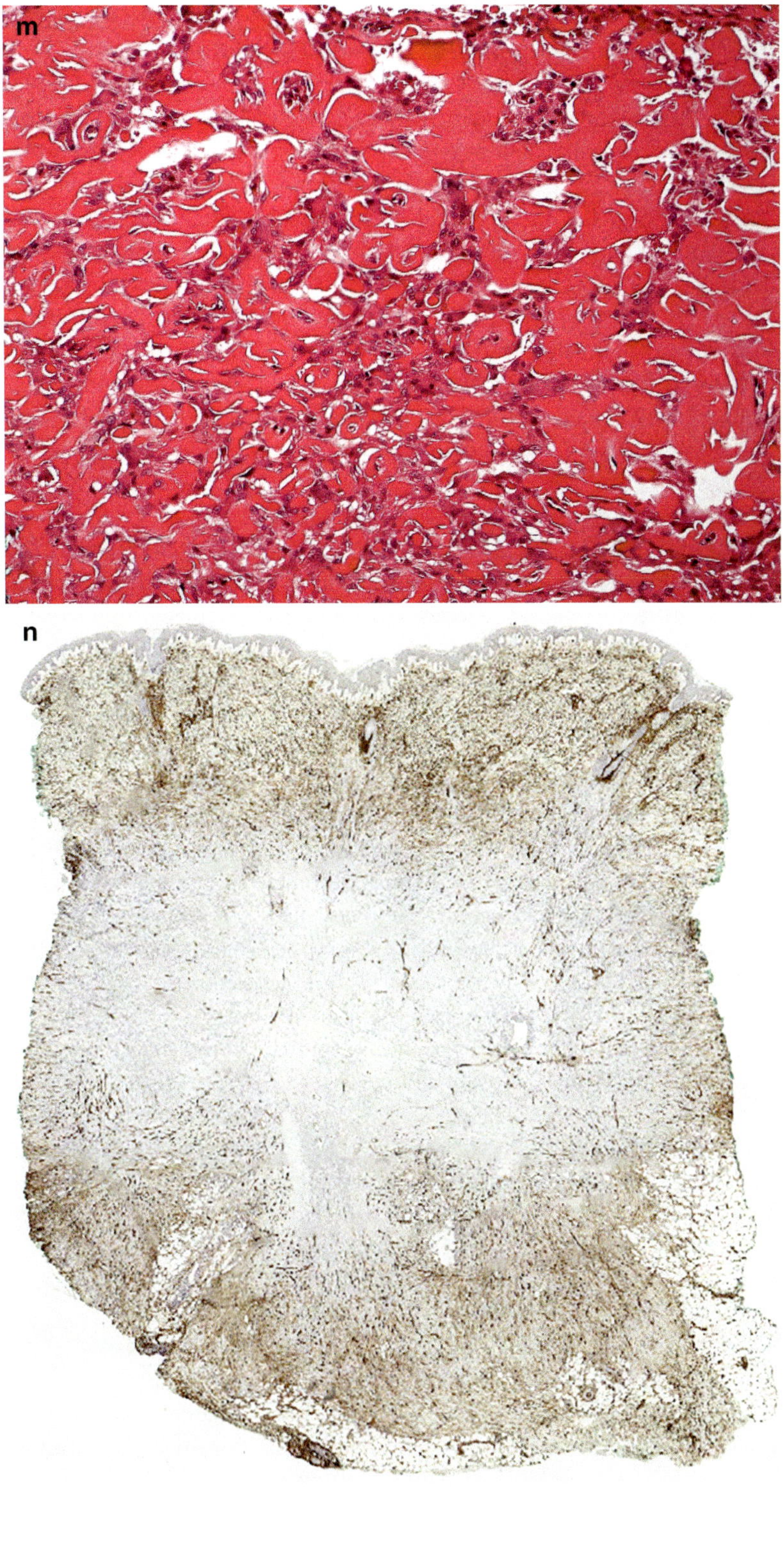

ment of the subcutis is common. Infiltration into the subcutis occurs in a limited, relatively circumscribed fashion along expanded fibrous septa. This infiltration is often associated with foci of fat necrosis and a lymphohistiocytic infiltrate (Fig. 4.20d). There are numerous histologic variants of DF. The distinguishing features of the most important subtypes are described below.

Conventional Benign Fibrous Histiocytoma/Dermatofibroma

Conventional benign fibrous histiocytoma/dermatofibroma is classically a polymorphous tumor composed of an admixture of bland, lightly eosinophilic spindle cells in a focally storiform growth pattern, fibroblasts, histiocytes, siderophages, multinucleated cells (including Touton-type giant cells), and scattered lymphocytes (Fig. 4.20e). The cellularity is variable. Burned-out cases may show fibrosis and relatively low cellularity.

Lipidized (Ankle-Type) Fibrous Histiocytoma

Lipidized (ankle-type) fibrous histiocytoma is very similar to a conventional dermatofibroma with the notable addition of numerous foamy histiocytes and background hyalinizing fibrosis (Fig. 4.20f). These lesions often tend to be somewhat hypocellular and are seen most commonly on the distal lower extremity, hence the alternative designation as "ankle-type" dermatofibromas.

Cellular Fibrous Histiocytoma

Cellular fibrous histiocytoma differs from the conventional form by its relative uniform cellularity and predominantly fascicular growth pattern. The tumor is composed of fascicles of uniform spindled cells with little to no secondary elements (i.e., admixed histiocytes and lymphocytes) (Fig. 4.20g). Mitotic activity is common (up to 5–10 mitoses/10 HPFs), but atypical mitotic figures are not seen. Necrosis may be seen in up to 10% of cases. The latter features may raise concern for malignancy. Approximately 20% of this subtype arise on the head and neck and face and account for approximately 80% of head and neck benign fibrous histiocytomas.

Aneurysmal and/or Hemosiderotic Fibrous Histiocytoma

Aneurysmal and/or hemosiderotic fibrous histiocytomas demonstrate varying amounts of intratumoral hemorrhage, typically consisting of large collections of blood in pseudocystic spaces not lined by endothelial cells in association with numerous siderophages (Fig. 4.20h). The background tumor can resemble a conventional benign fibrous histiocytoma, atypical fibrous histiocytoma (see below), or, frequently, cellular fibrous histiocytoma.

Atypical Fibrous Histiocytoma/Dermatofibroma with Monster Cells

Atypical fibrous histiocytoma, also known as dermatofibroma with monster cells, resembles a conventional benign fibrous histiocytoma with admixed hyperchromatic, pleomorphic, and multinucleated cells (Fig. 4.20i). Mitotic figures may be seen, and in contrast to other fibrous histiocytomas, atypical forms may be present. Features of conventional dermatofibroma, such as collagen trapping and secondary elements, are also present allowing distinction from atypical fibroxanthoma/pleomorphic dermal sarcoma and undifferentiated pleomorphic sarcomas.

Deep Fibrous Histiocytoma

Deep fibrous histiocytomas arise in the deep dermis or subcutis, tend to be large, are less fibrous, are more cellular, and often have a prominent staghorn (hemangiopericytomatous) vasculature (Fig. 4.20j). In our experience, this variant and cellular fibrous histiocytoma are most often mistaken for a sarcoma.

Rare Variants

Rarely encountered variants include clear cell, granular cell (Fig. 4.20k), balloon cell, myxoid (Fig. 4.20l), and keloidal dermatofibroma (Fig. 4.20m).

Immunohistochemistry is rarely necessary for the diagnosis of benign fibrous histiocytomas. Classically, they are immunoreactive for FXIIIa and

Table 4.20 Key pathologic features: benign fibrous histiocytoma (dermatofibroma)

Conventional benign fibrous histiocytoma (dermatofibroma)
Varying amounts of epidermal hyperplasia, basal layer hyperpigmentation, and follicular induction
Circumscribed but unencapsulated tumor arising in the reticular dermis
Composed of bland lightly eosinophilic spindle cells present in a focally storiform growth pattern
Secondary elements including Touton-type giant cells, hemosiderin and foam-laden cells, and a lymphohistiocytic infiltrate
Peripheral collagen trapping
FXIIIa positive, variable immunoreactivity for SMA, CD68, and CD10. Negative for CD34, S100 (except in dendritic cells), and desmin
Lipidized fibrous histiocytoma
Tendency to arise in the lower extremity particularly around the ankle
Similar to conventional dermatofibroma with the addition of extensive hyalinizing fibrosis and numerous foamy histiocytes
Cellular fibrous histiocytoma
Cellular proliferation of uniform spindle cells in a fascicular growth pattern
Few if any secondary elements
Increased mitotic activity, but no atypical forms
Focal necrosis in up to 10% of cases
20% arise on the head, neck, or face
May have a peripheral rim of CD34-positive spindle cells
Aneurysmal and/or hemosiderotic fibrous histiocytoma
Varying amounts of intratumoral hemorrhage often contained within pseudocystic spaces
Abundant hemosiderin
Background tumor may be conventional, atypical, or cellular fibrous histiocytoma
Intratumoral hemorrhage may cause rapid clinical change in size and pigmentation raising concern for melanoma
Atypical fibrous histiocytoma/dermatofibroma with monster cells
Resembles conventional benign fibrous histiocytoma with varying numbers of hyperchromatic, pleomorphic, and multinucleated cells
Mitotic figures including atypical forms may be seen
Deep fibrous histiocytoma
Arises in the deep dermis or subcutis
Often large, less fibrous, and more cellular than typical fibrous histiocytoma
May have a prominent staghorn (hemangiopericytomatous) vasculature
Most common variant, in addition to cellular fibrous histiocytoma, to be mistaken for a sarcoma

negative for CD34. It should be mentioned that cellular fibrous histiocytoma is often negative for FXIIIa. It is also common for reactive CD34 cells to be present at the periphery of the tumor (Fig. 4.20n), leading to concern for DFSP. Unlike DFSP, the central portion of the tumor, with rare exceptions, is negative for CD34 in lesional cells. Variable immunoreactivity for SMA, CD68, CD163, and CD10 is common. Immunohistochemical stains for S100 protein are negative, but entrapped dendritic cells are frequently highlighted with this stain. Dermatofibromas are negative for desmin and cytokeratins. It should be stressed that histologic features rather than immunohistochemical stains should be the basis for diagnosis. We rarely order immunohistochemical stains for this group of tumors.

Previously it has been suggested that dermatofibromas represent a reactive process due to the fact that a subset are associated with arthropod bites, trauma, or folliculitis. However, molecular studies have demonstrated clonality, chromosomal copy number gains and losses, and gene fusions involving a number of different loci, including protein kinase C genes, *PRKCB* and *PRKCD*, as well *LAMTOR1*, and genes for CD63 and podoplanin. These genetic findings support the interpretation that this group of tumors represents true neoplasms, rather than reactive proliferations (Table 4.20).

Differential Diagnosis

The primary differential diagnosis for conventional benign fibrous histiocytoma and the cellular variant is dermatofibrosarcoma protuberans. Dermatofibrosarcoma protuberans (DFSP) lacks the overlying epidermal changes, has little to no collagen trapping, and usually demonstrates diffuse infiltration into the subcutaneous fat in the absence of fat necrosis and inflammation. DFSP is more monomorphic than conventional benign fibrous histiocytoma and has a tighter storiform growth pattern and more slender, hyperchromatic nuclei than are seen in cellular fibrous histiocytoma. DFSP is diffusely positive for CD34 with only focal immunoreactivity for FXIIa and has a *COL1A1-PDGFRB* fusion.

Hypocellular examples of conventional benign fibrous histiocytoma can be confused with sclerotic blue nevus, neurofibroma, and sclerosing perineurioma. In sclerotic blue nevi, the pigmented cells contain melanin rather than hemosiderin. Neurofibromas produce their own more delicate "shredded carrot" collagen, whereas the spindle cells of benign fibrous histiocytomas intercalate between pre-existing reticular dermal collagen bundles. Both blue nevus and neurofibroma lack the secondary elements of conventional benign fibrous histiocytoma and are positive for S100 protein and SOX10. Sclerosing perineurioma arises almost exclusively in the digits, an unusual site for fibrous histiocytomas, and is positive for EMA and GLUT-1. Occasional cases of interstitial granuloma annulare can superficially resemble benign fibrous histiocytoma. Evidence of collagen alterations and interstitial mucin helps in the distinction.

Aneurysmal fibrous histiocytoma may be confused with angiomatoid fibrous histiocytoma, though this is largely due to similarity in nomenclature, rather than any shared histopathologic features. Angiomatoid fibrous histiocytoma has a fibrous pseudocapsule with a peripheral lymphoid cuff, features not seen in aneurysmal fibrous histiocytoma. Angiomatoid fibrous histiocytoma is discussed in more detail in the next chapter.

Lipidized forms of benign fibrous histiocytoma should be distinguished from xanthogranuloma and xanthoma. The latter two lesions are more uniformly composed of histiocytes and lack overlying epidermal change and collagen trapping. Xanthogranuloma often has admixed eosinophils, which are not typically present in benign fibrous histiocytoma.

Atypical fibrous histiocytoma needs to be distinguished from atypical fibroxanthoma/pleomorphic dermal sarcoma, undifferentiated pleomorphic sarcoma, and pleomorphic fibroma. The tumors comprising the spectrum of atypical fibroxanthoma/pleomorphic dermal sarcoma can largely be excluded on clinical grounds, as the vast majority arise in sun-damaged skin of the head and neck. Undifferentiated pleomorphic sarcoma is larger and more deeply seated, has an infiltrative growth pattern and a more diffuse atypia, and is more mitotically active. Pleomorphic fibroma discussed above is often polypoid, consists of scattered pleomorphic cells without a distinctive growth pattern, is positive for CD34, and shows loss of RB1. None of these tumors have the background features of conventional fibrous histiocytoma present in all cases of atypical fibrous histiocytoma.

Multinucleate Cell Angiohistiocytoma

Clinical Features

Multinucleate cell angiohistiocytoma (MCAH) is a peculiar vascular and fibrohistiocytic lesion first described by Smith and Wilson Jones in 1985. While some regard it as an entity sui generis, others believe it to be a variant of fibrous histiocytoma (dermatofibroma) or angiofibroma (most notably fibrous papule of the face). As initially described, lesions are grouped, non-regressing asymptomatic, red-to-violaceous papules that develop over weeks to months on the face or acral sites of elderly women. Papules may coalesce or take on annular or linear configurations. Other variations from the initial clinical description include isolated papules arising at a variety of anatomic sites, coexisting epidermal proliferations or atrophy, fibrosis, and extensive angiomatous changes; a case with generalized distribution has also been reported. The clinical differential diagnosis includes lichen planus, cutaneous lymphoid hyperplasia, Kaposi sarcoma, acroangiodermatitis (pseudo-Kaposi sarcoma), insect bites, granuloma annulare, and sarcoidosis. MCAH is a benign lesion with an indolent, but sometimes progressive, course. Spontaneous resolution has been reported, which some argue is supportive of a reactive rather than neoplastic process. Treatment is not necessary, but excision, cryotherapy, and lasers may be used to eradicate pruritic or cosmetically unacceptable lesions.

Pathologic Features

By histology MCAH are characterized by bizarre multinucleated cells with scalloped, angulated cytoplasm seen in association with a proliferation of dilated capillary dermal vessels, scattered lymphohistiocytic infiltrate, dense collagen in the upper dermis, and an increased number of interstitial mononuclear cells (Fig. 4.21a and b). Varying amounts of background fibrosis, epidermal hyperplasia, and mast cells may also be seen. By immunohistochemistry, mononuclear cells are positive for vimentin, FXIIIa, CD68, and lysozyme, but negative for S100 protein and CD1a. Multinucleated cells are positive for vimentin, and variably so for CD68, but negative for other monocyte/macrophage markers. Estrogen receptor (ER) positivity has been reported in interstitial and perivascular spindle cells and occasionally multinucleated cells. The etiology and pathogenesis of MCAH are largely unknown. The female predominance and ER positivity suggests the possibility of a hormonal

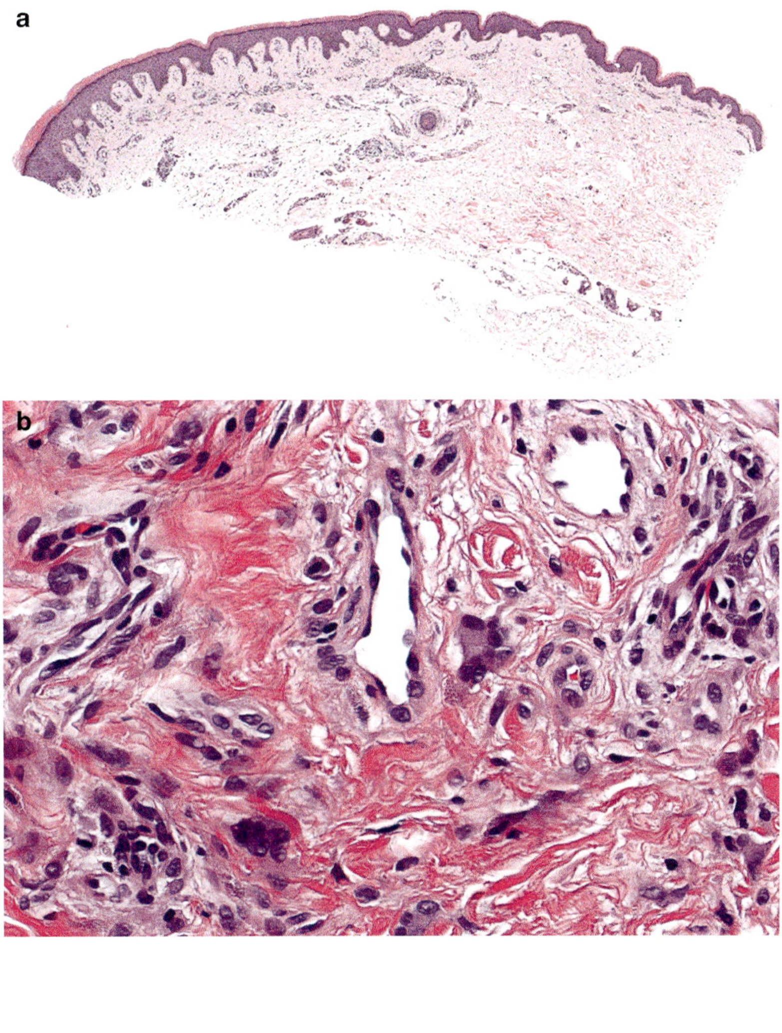

Fig. 4.21 Multinucleate cell angiohistiocytoma. (**a**) Dilated capillary dermal vessels. (**b**) Bizarre multinucleated cells with scalloped, angulated cytoplasm near dilated vessels

Table 4.21 Key pathologic features: multinucleated cell angiohistiocytoma

Bizarre multinucleated cells with scalloped, angulated cytoplasm
Proliferation of dilated capillary dermal vessels
Scattered lymphohistiocytic infiltrate
Dense collagen in the upper dermis
Increased interstitial mononuclear cells
Varying fibrosis, epidermal hyperplasia, and mast cells
Mononuclear cells positive for vimentin, Factor XIIIa, CD68, ER, and lysozyme and negative for S100 and CD1a
Multinucleated cells positive for vimentin, variably so for ER and CD68, but negative for other monocyte/macrophage markers

influence. IL-4 from mast cell degranulation has been postulated to play a role in the morphogenesis of the multinucleate cells. MCAH is a benign lesion with an indolent, but sometimes progressive, course (Table 4.21).

Differential Diagnosis

The histologic differential diagnosis of MCAH includes fibrous histiocytoma (dermatofibroma, particularly the atrophic vascular variant), angiofibroma (especially fibrous papule), Kaposi sarcoma and pseudo-Kaposi sarcoma (acroangiodermatitis), and microvenular hemangioma. Unlike dermatofibroma, MCAH typically arises in crops on the face and acral sites. Dermatofibromas more commonly have epidermal hyperplasia, collagen trapping, basal layer hyperpigmentation, a denser population of FXIIIa-positive dendrocytes, and more of a storiform growth pattern. Fibrous papule has an increased number of dilated capillaries and occasional multinucleated cells, but collagen bundles are perifollicular in distribution, or more vertically oriented and multinucleated cells are much fewer in number compared to MCAH. Kaposi sarcoma does not contain multinucleated cells and is HHV-8-positive. Pseudo-Kaposi sarcoma (acroangiodermatitis) tends to affect the lower extremities and has tortuous, thick-walled vessels and abundant hemosiderin deposition, unlike MCAH. Microvenular hemangioma consists of compressed venules lined by a prominent endothelium with surrounding pericyte layer and lacks multinucleated cells.

Epithelioid Fibrous Histiocytoma

Clinical Features

Epithelioid fibrous histiocytoma (EFH), also known as epithelioid histiocytoma, is now considered a distinct entity separate from the family of benign fibrous histiocytomas discussed above. Clinically, EFH usually presents on the extremities of young to middle-aged adults, as an erythematous, polypoid lesion. It is benign and cured by simple excision.

Pathologic Features

EFH is a well-circumscribed but unencapsulated tumor composed of uniform epithelioid to polygonal cells arranged in a sheetlike growth pattern (Fig. 4.22a). A dilated, sometimes branching, capillary vasculature is often seen at the periphery of the tumor. The individual tumor cells have enlarged, uniform nuclei with fine chromatin and a small nucleolus, and relatively abundant eosinophilic cytoplasm (Fig. 4.22b). Scattered mitotic figures may be seen, but cytologic atypia is minimal to absent. In contradistinction to dermatofibromas, collagen trapping is not a conspicuous feature. An epidermal collarette is often present in EFH. By immunohistochemistry, EFH is diffusely positive for FXIIIa. Recently, it has been documented that almost all EFH have rearrangements involving *ALK* and that close to 90% are positive for ALK by immunohistochemistry, which correlates with *ALK* gene rearrangement (Fig. 4.22c). EFH are often positive for EMA and are negative for cytokeratins and S100 protein (Table 4.22).

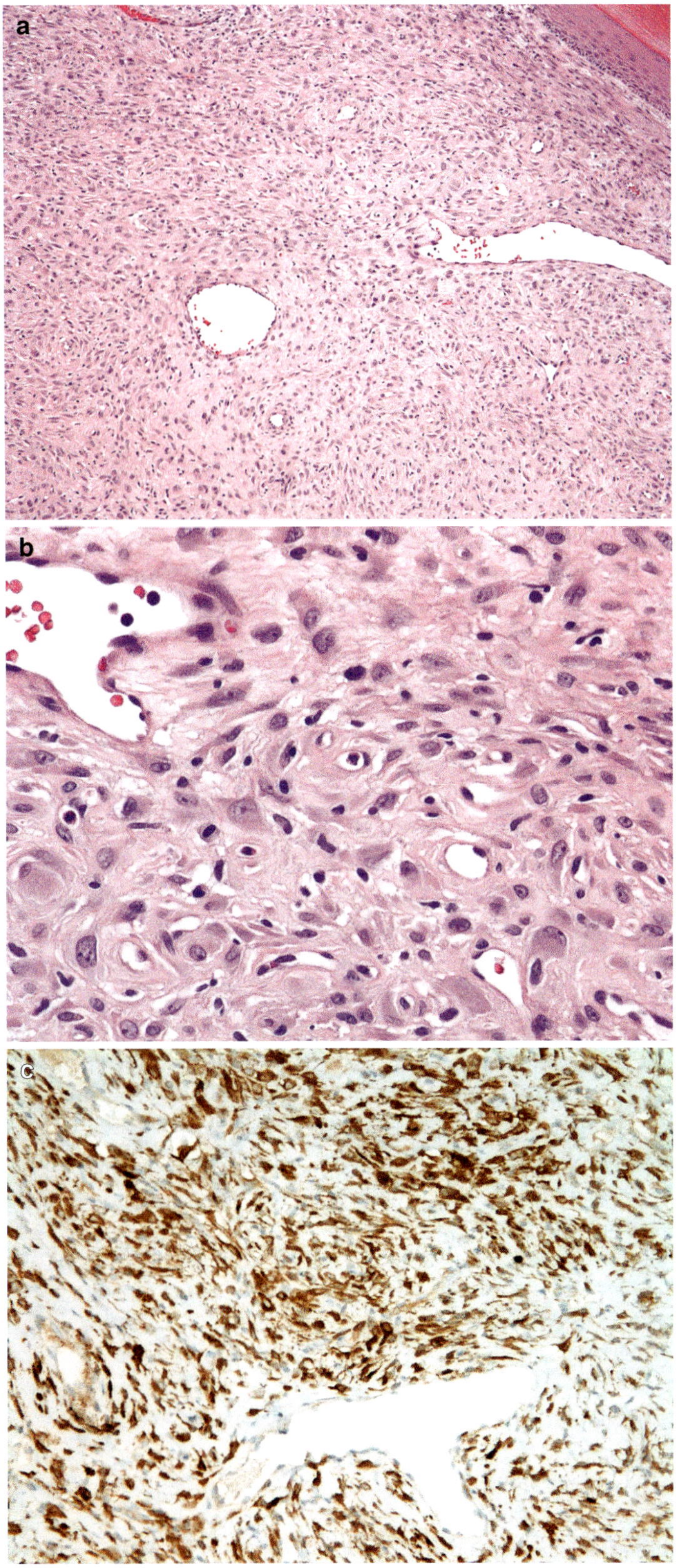

Fig. 4.22 Epithelioid fibrous histiocytoma. (**a**) Sheetlike growth of uniform epithelioid cells. Dilated vessels are seen at the periphery. (**b**) Individual tumor cells have enlarged, uniform nuclei with fine chromatin and a small nucleolus, and an abundant amount of eosinophilic cytoplasm. (**c**) ALK positivity in epithelioid fibrous histiocytoma

Table 4.22 Key pathologic features: epithelioid fibrous histiocytoma

Well-circumscribed dermal proliferation of uniform epithelioid to polygonal cells with abundant eosinophilic cytoplasm arranged in a sheetlike growth pattern
Epidermal collarette
Dilated capillary vasculature
Scattered mitotic figures but limited cytologic atypia
ALK rearrangements with close to 90% are positivity for ALK by IHC
Positive for FXIIIa and often EMA, negative for cytokeratins and S100

Differential Diagnosis

Perhaps the most difficult differential diagnosis is with cutaneous syncytial myoepithelioma (CSM). Both have similar cytomorphologic features. However, CSM is positive for EMA and typically variably positive for S100 protein, cytokeratins, and SOX10, but negative for ALK. CSM also demonstrates *EWSR1* rearrangement by FISH, which is not seen in EFH. Cellular neurothekeomas (CNTK) are more spindled and nested, lack a polypoid silhouette, and are positive for NKI-C3, PGP9.5, and CD10, unlike EFH. Neither CSM nor CNTK are immunoreactive for ALK by immunohistochemistry. Spitz nevi enter the differential diagnosis due to shared epithelioid cytomorphology, but are also immunoreactive for melanocytic markers, such as S100 protein, Melan-A, MiTF, and SOX10. Of note, a subset of Spitz nevi are also positive for ALK. Conventional DF may enter the differential, but are distinguished by the presence of secondary elements (Touton-type giant cells, hemosiderin, foam cells), peripheral collagen trapping, and lack of immunoreactivity for ALK and EMA.

Juvenile (Solitary) Xanthogranuloma

Clinical Features

Solitary (juvenile) xanthogranuloma (JXG) is a benign soft tissue tumor belonging to the broad group of non-Langerhans cell histiocytoses that occurs without gender predilection most frequently in children, including a significant portion of congenital lesions. JXG typically present as a solitary, slow-growing cutaneous papule or nodule of the head and neck, chest, abdomen, or extremities, although a subset of multifocal tumors in children (<5% of cases) will involve the eye, deep soft tissues, or visceral organs (i.e., liver, lung, etc.). JXG near the eye in children should prompt ophthalmologic referral to rule out eye and ocular adnexal involvement. Juvenile myelomonocytic leukemia (JMML), as well as germline mutations in *NF1* and *NF2*, has been reported in children with JXG. Tumors that present in children frequently grow and then spontaneously regress, leaving only hyperpigmented skin, while tumors that present in adulthood may persist as a mass lesion. Xanthogranuloma is a benign lesion, with infrequent local recurrence after surgical excision. Extraordinarily rare cases of death have been reported in patients with multifocal, systemic disease. Symptomatic patients with multisystem disease can successfully be treated with LCH-based regimens that include both corticosteroids and vinca alkaloids.

Pathologic Features

JXG are unencapsulated, but circumscribed, hypercellular tumors comprised predominantly of bland-appearing histiocytes with abundant pale cytoplasm and enlarged, slightly irregular vesicular nuclei with conspicuous nucleoli. Tumor cells are arranged in diffuse nodular sheets within the dermis and frequently closely abut the overlying flattened epidermis (Fig. 4.23a). In most cases, varying numbers of giant cells, including Touton and osteoclast-type giant cells, are distributed evenly throughout the tumor, and a conspicuous mixed acute and chronic inflammatory infiltrate with lymphocytes, eosinophils, and plasma cells is present (Fig. 4.23b). It should be noted that early tumors and visceral forms may lack Touton-type giant cells and an inflammatory infiltrate. In some tumors, there is prominent intracytoplasmic lipid accumulation, and regressed tumors may show

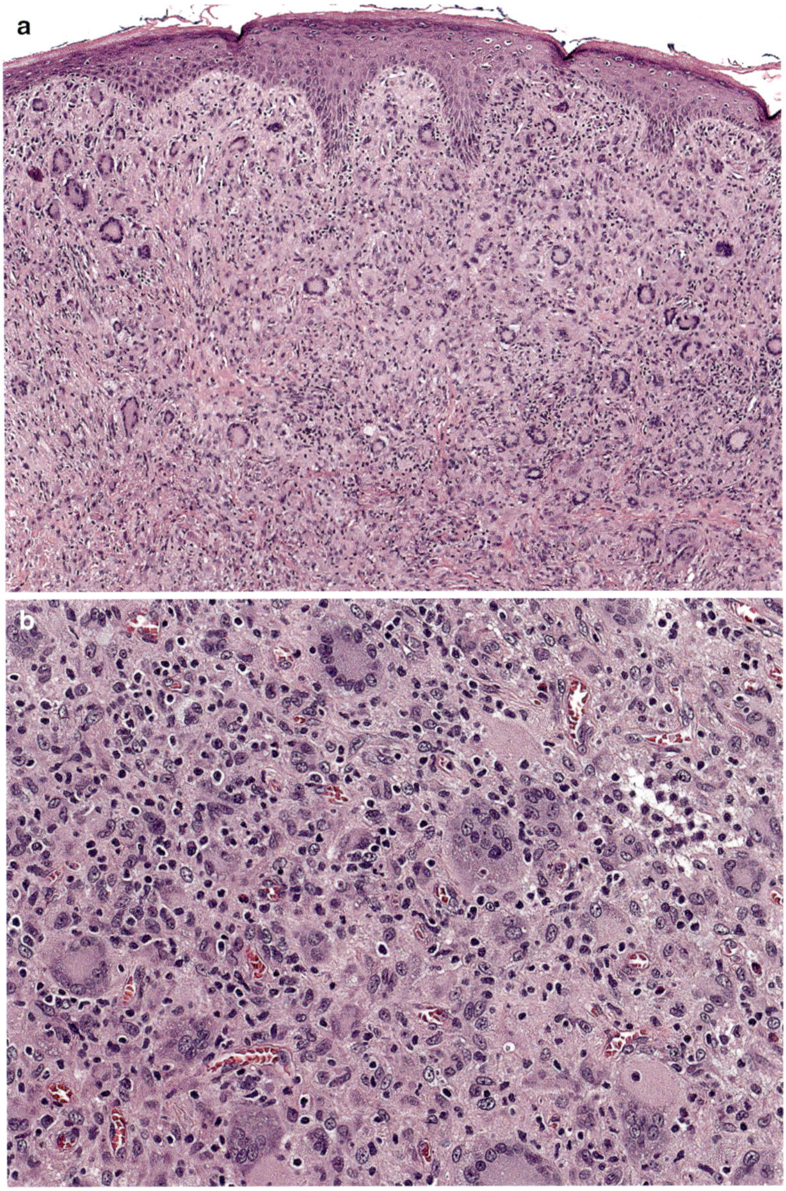

Fig. 4.23 Juvenile (solitary) xanthogranuloma. (**a**) The tumor cells are arranged in diffuse nodular sheets within the dermis abutting the epidermis. (**b**) Touton- and osteoclast-type giant cells are distributed evenly with admixed inflammatory cells

fibrosis with a storiform growth pattern. Tumor cells express CD68, CD163, and FXIIIa but are negative for S100 protein and CD1a expression.

Molecular studies have provided evidence of clonality in juvenile xanthogranuloma, in support of a neoplastic process. Recently, mutations involving *NRAS*, *KRAS*, *ARAF*, or *MAP2K1* were found in 7 out of 12 systemic juvenile xanthogranuloma cases, suggesting a role for MAPK signaling in JXG. Two cases of mixed Langerhans cell histiocytosis/juvenile xanthogranuloma have been reported to have V600E mutations, and a *RNF11-BRAF* fusion was identified in one case of systemic juvenile xanthogranuloma. A *PIK3CD* mutation in serial biopsies from a single patient suggests that the PI3K pathway may also be involved in juvenile xanthogranuloma progression. Finally, copy number alterations or copy neutral loss of heterozygosity including trisomy 5 and 17 and loss of heterozygosity in 5q have been reported in two lesions from a case of diffuse JXG. The same study found only two

Table 4.23 Key pathologic features: solitary (juvenile) xanthogranuloma

Circumscribed hypercellular tumor composed of bland histiocytes with abundant pale cytoplasm
Variable numbers of giant cells, particularly of the Touton-type
Mixed acute and chronic inflammation with lymphocytes, eosinophils, and plasma cells
Early and visceral lesions may lack Touton-type giant cells and inflammation
Older lesions may show more spindle cells, a storiform growth pattern, and fibrosis
Positive for CD68, CD163, and Factor XIIIa, negative for S100 and CD1a

cases of solitary JXG with molecular abnormalities, one showing gains on 1q and 11q and the other loss in 3p (Table 4.23).

Differential Diagnosis

The differential diagnosis for solitary (juvenile) xanthogranuloma includes xanthoma, benign fibrous histiocytoma, and solitary reticulohistiocytoma. Although some xanthoma subtypes may show multinucleated osteoclast-type giant cells, Touton-type giant cells are typically absent. Benign fibrous histiocytomas may have Touton-type giant cells, but typically are more polymorphous and have collagen trapping and frequently epidermal hyperplasia. Solitary reticulohistiocytoma has ground-glass histiocytes, lacks Touton giant cells, and is negative for Factor XIIIa expression.

Solitary Reticulohistiocytoma/ Multicentric Reticulohistiocytosis

Clinical Features

Solitary reticulohistiocytoma is a rare benign soft tissue tumor with slight male predominance that typically occurs in younger adults. Tumors usually present as a solitary slowly enlarging cutaneous soft tissue mass in the chest, abdomen, extremities, or head and neck and do not recur after surgical excision.

Multicentric reticulohistiocytosis is a multifocal counterpart to solitary reticulohistiocytoma. It usually presents in middle-aged adults with a slight female predominance. Lesions present as multiple slowly enlarging soft tissue masses in the skin, mucosa, soft tissue, and/or joints. A subset of cases may be associated with a rheumatologic disorder or underlying malignancy, such as carcinoma of the breast, lung, colon, ovary, or cervix, as well as sarcoma and lymphoma. Multicentric reticulohistiocytosis often shows a variable clinical course, with periods of relative improvement and worsening of disease. Some patients develop significant arthritis with deforming arthropathy. In patients with a malignancy or rheumatologic disorder, treatment of the underlying condition may improve the clinical symptoms associated with multicentric reticulohistiocytosis.

Pathologic Features

Microscopically, tumors are circumscribed, unencapsulated tumors comprised predominantly of large epithelioid histiocytes with abundant pale to eosinophilic cytoplasm, enlarged and irregular vesicular nuclei, prominent nucleoli, and frequent multinucleation (Fig. 4.24). Tumor cells are arranged in diffuse nodular sheets within the dermis, with prominent admixed collagen bundles; a conspicuous chronic inflammatory infiltrate is often present as well. Although focally increased cytologic atypia and mitotic activity may be noted, necrosis is not identified. Tumor cells express CD68 and CD163, but are negative for Factor XIIIa, S100, and CD1a expression. The pathologic findings in multicentric reticulohistiocytosis are identical to those of the solitary form (Table 4.24).

Differential Diagnosis

The differential diagnosis of solitary reticulohistiocytoma includes Langerhans cell histiocytosis, Rosai-Dorfman disease, epithelioid fibrous histiocytoma, and benign fibrous histiocytoma. In

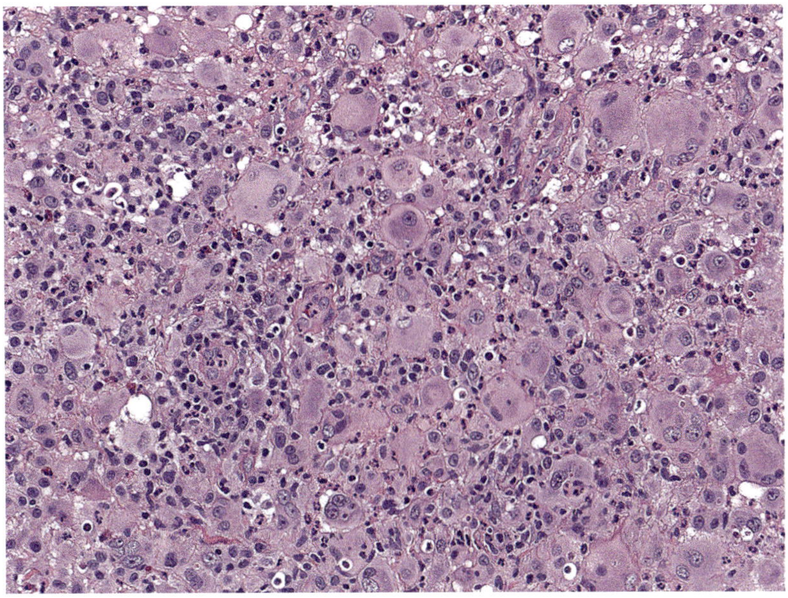

Fig. 4.24 Solitary reticulohistiocytoma/multicentric reticulohistiocytosis. Large epithelioid histiocytes with abundant pale to eosinophilic cytoplasm, enlarged and irregular vesicular nuclei, prominent nucleoli, and frequent multinucleation. Note the associated inflammatory infiltrate

Table 4.24 Key pathologic features: solitary reticulohistiocytoma/multicentric reticulohistiocytosis

Circumscribed but unencapsulated proliferation of deeply eosinophilic (ground-glass) epithelioid cells among scattered inflammation
Multinucleation and spindling of cells common
Only mild atypia and occasional mitoses
Positive for CD68 and CD163, variable immunoreactivity for lysozyme, negative for S100 protein

contrast to reticulohistiocytoma, Langerhans cell histiocytosis and Rosai-Dorfman disease both express S100 protein and, in the case of Langerhans cell histiocytosis, CD1a. Epithelioid fibrous histiocytoma is positive for ALK and often has a more conspicuous capillary vasculature. Benign fibrous histiocytoma is more polymorphous and has peripheral collagen trapping.

The differential diagnosis for multicentric reticulohistiocytosis is similar to that discussed above for solitary reticulohistiocytoma; however, given its unique clinical associations (including the possibility of concurrent malignancy or rheumatologic disease) and variable, but often progressive clinical course, it is important to distinguish multicentric reticulohistiocytosis from solitary reticulohistiocytoma on clinical findings.

Xanthomas

Clinical Features

Xanthoma is a benign soft tissue lesion that occurs due to accumulation of excess serum lipids, most frequently in patients with hyperlipoproteinemias. These lesions typically present as a slowly growing cutaneous soft tissue mass, but may occur in tendons, synovium, deep soft tissue, and/or bone. There are five types of xanthoma: eruptive, tuberous, plane, xanthelasma, and tendinous. Eruptive xanthomas typically occur in patients with types I, III, or V hyperlipoproteinemia, are small and multiple, and show predilection for the buttocks. Eruptive xanthomas can also occur as a reaction to tattoos. Tuberous xanthomas usually arise in patients with types IIa or III hyperlipoproteinemia, are large with plaque-like growth, and demonstrate predilection for the buttocks,

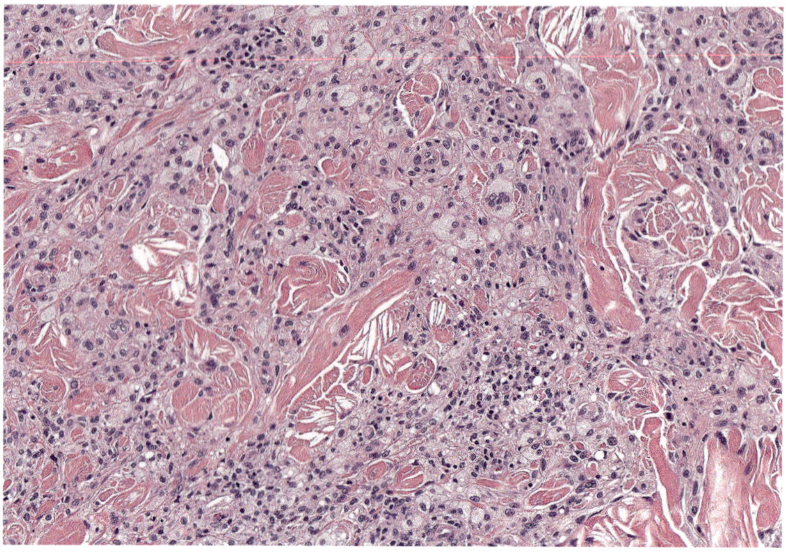

Fig. 4.25 Xanthoma. Relatively hypercellular lesion composed predominantly of lipid-laden ("foamy") histiocytes with moderate pale to amphophilic cytoplasm, small pyknotic nuclei, and inconspicuous nucleoli, arranged in diffuse nodular sheets within the dermis

knees, elbows, and fingers. Plane xanthomas are typically found in the palmar creases of patients with primary biliary cirrhosis III, but may also be present in normolipemic patients with an underlying hematolymphoid malignancy. Xanthelasmas arise on the eyelids of patients with types IIa or III hyperlipoproteinemia. Finally, tendinous xanthomas occur in patients with type IIa hyperlipoproteinemia or cerebrotendinous xanthomatosis. Because xanthomas represent a reactive accumulation of lipid-laden histiocytes often due to excess serum lipids, they may regress with systemic medical therapy; surgical excision is generally not necessary.

Pathologic Features

Grossly, xanthomas are unencapsulated, but well-circumscribed skin and/or soft tissue lesions. Microscopically, xanthomas are relatively hypercellular and composed predominantly of lipid-laden ("foamy") histiocytes with moderate pale to amphophilic cytoplasm, small pyknotic nuclei, and inconspicuous nucleoli, arranged in diffuse nodular sheets within the dermis (Fig. 4.25). In addition to foamy histiocytes, eruptive xanthomas show numerous admixed non-foamy histiocytes and chronic inflammatory cells, while tuberous and tendinous xanthomas frequently contain cholesterol clefts with multinucleated giant cells and fibrosis (Table 4.25).

Table 4.25 Key pathologic features: xanthoma

Foamy macrophages admixed with inflammatory cells
Cholesterol clefts flanked by multinucleated giant cells
Varying fibrosis, most conspicuous in long-standing lesions
Eruptive xanthoma has larger proportion of non-foamy macrophages
Sheets of xanthoma cells and less fibrosis in plane xanthoma and xanthelasma

Differential Diagnosis

While the diagnosis of xanthoma is often straightforward, some xanthoma subtypes may show morphologic overlap with other benign or intermediate malignant soft tissue tumors, including benign fibrous histiocytoma, solitary (juvenile) xanthogranuloma, tenosynovial giant cell tumor, and giant cell tumor of soft tissue. Peripheral collagen-trapping and the presence of non-foamy histiocytes favor a diagnosis of benign fibrous histiocytoma, while the presence of Touton-type multinucleated giant cells is consistent with solitary (juvenile) xanthogranuloma. Finally, tenosynovial giant cell tumor and giant cell tumor of soft tissue both show a prominent population of epithelioid histiocyte-like mononuclear cells, which are not typically seen in xanthomas.

Tenosynovial Giant Cell Tumor

Clinical Features

Tenosynovial giant cell tumor (TSGCT) is a benign soft tissue tumor with slight female predominance that typically occurs in middle-aged patients. Tumors usually present as a slowly enlarging soft tissue mass along tendons of the hands and feet or associated with large joints, including the knee, ankle, and wrist. There are two types of tenosynovial giant cell tumor: localized and diffuse. The localized type (also known as giant cell tumor of tendon sheath) most commonly involves the digits of the hands and has a relatively low, but significant risk of local recurrence after surgical excision. In contrast to the localized type, the diffuse type (also known as extra-articular pigmented villonodular synovitis) is relatively uncommon, occurs in a younger age group, and is characterized by extra-articular soft tissue involvement with predilection for the knee; diffuse type tumors show a significant local recurrence rate after surgical excision and may be associated with malignant transformation and subsequent metastasis. Radiotherapy alone or in combination with surgical excision may decrease the likelihood of recurrence of diffuse-type tenosynovial giant cell tumor. Clinical trials of agents such as imatinib mesylate that target the CSF1 receptor are ongoing.

Pathologic Features

All tenosynovial giant cell tumors show common morphologic features; however, there are characteristic gross and microscopic differences between the localized and diffuse types. Grossly, most localized type tenosynovial giant cell tumors are small, encapsulated, circumscribed solid masses with firm tan cut surfaces. In contrast, diffuse type tumors tend to be larger, unencapsulated, and poorly circumscribed; in addition, they may have a conspicuous pigmented "rust-brown" appearance and typically show prominent villonodular growth (for obvious reasons, such tumors have also been called "pigmented villonodular synovitis"). Microscopically, both types of tenosynovial giant cell tumor are typically hypercellular and composed of varying amounts of three cell types: epithelioid mononuclear cells, multinucleated giant cells, and foamy histiocytes (Fig. 4.26a). It should be noted that occasional cases have very few multinucleated giant cells (giant cell-poor TSGCT). In addition, the diffuse type of TSGCT usually shows conspicuous villonodular architecture and intratumoral hemosiderin accumulation/deposition (Fig. 4.26b). Mitoses up to 3/10 high-power fields may be seen in greater than 10% of cases, but this does not portend a more aggressive clinical course. Rare malignant diffuse-type TSGCTs (malignant pigmented villonodular synovitis) show significant cytologic atypia, mitotic activity, and foci of necrosis (Fig. 4.26c). The epithelioid mononuclear cells of TSGCT express clusterin and are often positive for MiTF (a significant pitfall), but are negative for CD163, though entrapped histiocytes are CD163-positive. TSGCT also can contain desmin-positive dendritic cells, which may be mistaken for evidence of rhabdomyosarcoma. Tenosynovial giant cell tumors harbor characteristic *CSF1* gene fusions, most commonly a *COL6A3-CSF1* gene fusion resulting from t(1;2) genomic rearrangements (Table 4.26).

Differential Diagnosis

The differential diagnosis for TSGCT includes fibroma of tendon sheath, xanthoma, benign fibrous histiocytoma, and giant cell tumor of soft tissue. Although they share some clinical features, fibroma of tendon sheath does not show the characteristic foamy histiocytes or multinucleated osteoclast-type giant cells of tenosynovial giant cell tumor. Similarly, the presence of a distinct population of epithelioid histiocyte-like mononuclear cells argues against xanthoma and benign fibrous histiocytoma. Finally, while

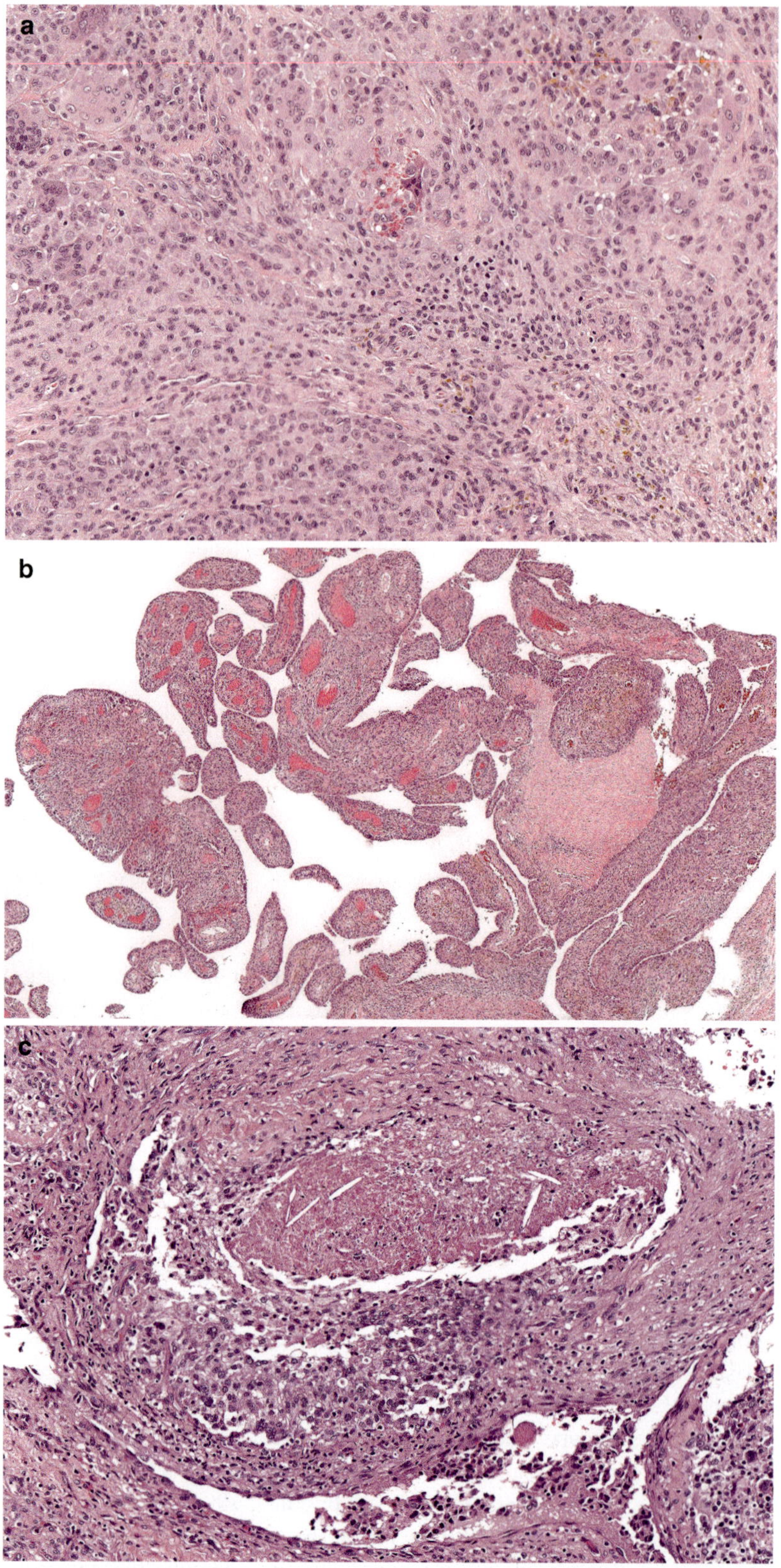

Fig. 4.26 Tenosynovial giant cell tumor. (**a**) Hypercellular lesion comprised of varying amounts of three cell types: epithelioid mononuclear cells, multinucleated giant cells, and foamy histiocytes. (**b**) Diffuse type of tenosynovial giant cell tumors usually shows conspicuous villonodular architecture and intratumoral hemosiderin accumulation/deposition. (**c**) Malignant tenosynovial giants cell tumor with necrosis

Table 4.26 Key pathologic features: tenosynovial giant cell tumor

Tenosynovial giant cell tumor – localized type
Small, well-circumscribed lobulated mass often associated with tendon sheath
Moderately cellular tumor composed of sheets of polygonal-to-round cells
Hypocellular collagenized zones
Scattered multinucleated giant cells
Varying proportions of foam cells, hemosiderin, giant cells, mononuclear cells, and collagen
Rare cartilaginous and osseous metaplasia
Tenosynovial giant cell tumor – diffuse type
Poorly circumscribed, extensively destructive mass associated with large joints
Pronounced cellularity with expansive sheets of round-to-polygonal cells punctuated by pseudoglandular spaces
Less numerous giant cells
Other features similar to localized type tenosynovial giant cell tumor
Malignant diffuse-type tenosynovial giant cell tumor (malignant pigmented villonodular synovitis)
As per diffuse-type tenosynovial giant cell tumor with the addition of significant cytologic atypia and mitotic activity and foci of necrosis

TSGCT and giant cell tumor of soft tissue show significant morphologic overlap, clinical features (including anatomic site) should assist in this differential diagnosis; in addition, in contrast to tenosynovial giant cell tumor, giant cell tumor of soft tissue often shows a multinodular growth pattern with prominent intervening fibrous septa.

Superficial Acral Fibromyxoma (Digital Fibromyxoma) and Cellular Digital Fibroma

Clinical Features

Superficial acral fibromyxoma (SAF) is a benign soft tissue tumor with a male predominance that typically occurs in middle-aged adults. Tumors nearly always present as a slowly growing soft tissue mass on the finger or toe, most commonly associated with the nail bed. Cellular digital fibroma (CDF) likely represents a variant of SAF. It tends to be smaller, but otherwise has the same clinical presentation. SAF may also be related to the acral fibrokeratomas, which some consider a subset of acral angiofibromata (see above). Superficial acral fibromyxoma is benign, but may recur locally (~20%), likely the result of the difficulty of achieving negative margins in acral locations. Conservative, but complete excision is recommended.

Pathologic Features

SAF is unencapsulated and relatively circumscribed and almost always arises adjacent to the nail bed (Fig. 4.27a). It is somewhat hypocellular and comprised predominantly of small bland-appearing spindle cells with scant eosinophilic cytoplasm and hyperchromatic tapered nuclei with inconspicuous nucleoli. Tumor cells are evenly distributed within a variably fibrous and myxoid stroma containing frequent admixed small vessels (Fig. 4.27b). Multinucleated stromal cells and associated mast cells may be present. Cytologic atypia and mitotic activity is minimal, and necrosis is not identified. CDF is more cellular and composed of shorter fascicles of bland spindled cells (Fig. 4.27c). SAF and CDF consistently express CD34. SAF may show some immunoreactivity for EMA, SMA, CD10, and nestin and shows frequent loss of RB1 expression. The tumor cells are negative for desmin, S100 protein, MUC4, STAT6, GFAP, and pan-cytokeratin (Table 4.27).

Differential Diagnosis

The differential diagnosis for SAF includes cutaneous myxoma, neurofibroma, dermatofibrosarcoma protuberans, sclerosing perineurioma, and low-grade fibromyxoid sarcoma. SAF is a more cellular lesion than cutaneous myxoma and the stroma contains more collagen. In contrast to neurofibroma, the tumor cells of SAF are not comma-shaped, and the vasculature is more conspicuous. SAF is also negative for S100 protein. Dermatofibrosarcoma protuberans is more cellular than SAF. CDF is more likely to be confused with dermatofibrosarcoma protuberans in that it

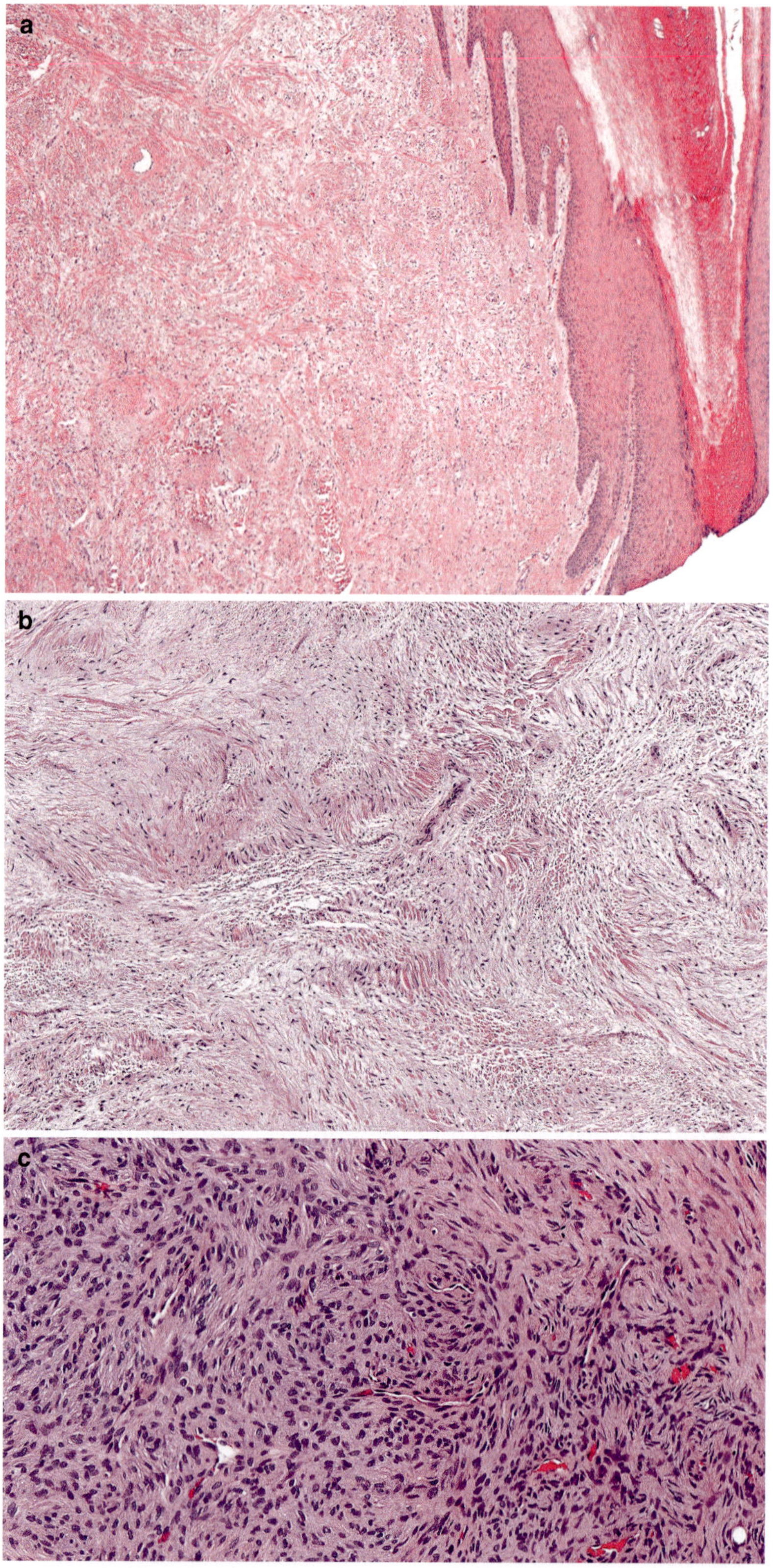

Fig. 4.27 Superficial acral fibromyxoma (digital fibromyxoma) and cellular digital fibroma. (**a**) Superficial acral fibromyxoma is an unencapsulated but circumscribed hypocellular lesion that nearly always arises adjacent to the nail bed. (**b**) The bland spindle cells are set within a fibrous and myxoid stroma containing small vessels. (**c**) Cellular digital fibroma is more cellular with short fascicles of bland spindled cells

Table 4.27 Key pathologic features: superficial acral fibromyxoma (digital fibromyxoma) and cellular digital fibroma

Hypocellular proliferation of bland spindle cells
Variable fibrous-to-myxoid stroma containing small vessels
Multinucleated stromal and mast cells may be present
CDF is likely a more cellular variant of SAFM composed of shorter fascicles of bland spindled cells
SAF and CDF consistently express CD34. SAF shows variable staining with EMA, SMA, CD10, and nestin and has frequent loss of RB1 expression. Both are negative for desmin, S100, MUC4, STAT6, GFAP, and pan-cytokeratin

is more cellular than SAF, but it can be distinguished by its circumscription and lack of a storiform growth pattern. Dermatofibrosarcoma protuberans demonstrates a *COL1A1-PDGFRB* fusion, while SAF and CDF do not. Sclerosing perineurioma has a cord-like growth pattern and lacks myxoid stroma and a conspicuous vasculature. Low-grade fibromyxoid sarcoma typically has abrupt transitions from cellular fibrous to hypocellular myxoid zones and is positive for MUC4.

Cutaneous Myxoma/Superficial Angiomyxoma

Clinical Features

Cutaneous myxomas are benign paucicellular multilobular, papulonodular, or polypoid lesions commonly occurring in adults (median age of 45.5 years). Lesions arise on the trunk, head and neck, or lower limbs most often; there is no sexual predisposition. Multiple lesions are associated with Carney complex, but multiple lesions have been described in the absence of this syndrome. Cutaneous myxomas are benign, but may recur in up to 38% of cases when incompletely excised.

Pathologic Features

Lesions are typically poorly circumscribed, but a multilobular silhouette is often present (Fig. 4.28a). Lobules are composed of an abundant myxoid stroma containing stellate to bipolar fibroblastic cells in association with mucin pools, a sparse mixed inflammatory infiltrate characteristically containing scattered neutrophils, and numerous small blood vessels. Lesions with an extensive vasculature are often designated as superficial angiomyxomas (Fig. 4.28b). There is little to no cytologic atypia or mitotic activity encountered. Isolated epithelial elements including epidermal inclusion cysts, strands of squamous or basaloid epithelium, and adnexal induction may be seen, particularly in the setting of Carney complex (Fig. 4.28c).

By immunohistochemistry constituent cells may be variably positive for SMA, typically in a tram-track myofibroblastic pattern of immunoreactivity. Cytokeratins, S100 protein, FXIIIa, desmin, and CD68 stains are negative. Some studies have found focal CD34 positivity. Patients presenting with multiple lesions in the setting of Carney complex have a mutation in the *PRKAR1A* gene, which encodes one of the four subunits of protein kinase A (Table 4.28).

Differential Diagnosis

Cutaneous myxomas can be confused with other myxoid lesions, which may arise in the skin and superficial soft tissues including myxofibrosarcoma, aggressive angiomyxoma, dermal nerve sheath myxoma, trichodiscoma/fibrofolliculoma, and focal cutaneous mucinoses. Myxofibrosarcoma is typically a larger lesion originating in the deeper soft tissues and secondarily extending into the skin with significant cytologic atypia and pleomorphism, and a characteristic arcuate vasculature with prominent tumor cell condensation. Imaging studies will also reveal a larger deep-seated mass. Cutaneous angiomyxomas involving the genital region should be distinguished from aggressive angiomyxoma, which is typically a more deeply seated, large mass within pelvic soft tissues that is extensively infiltrative and has a characteristic vasculature composed of small capillaries and thick-walled vessels with distinct perivascular

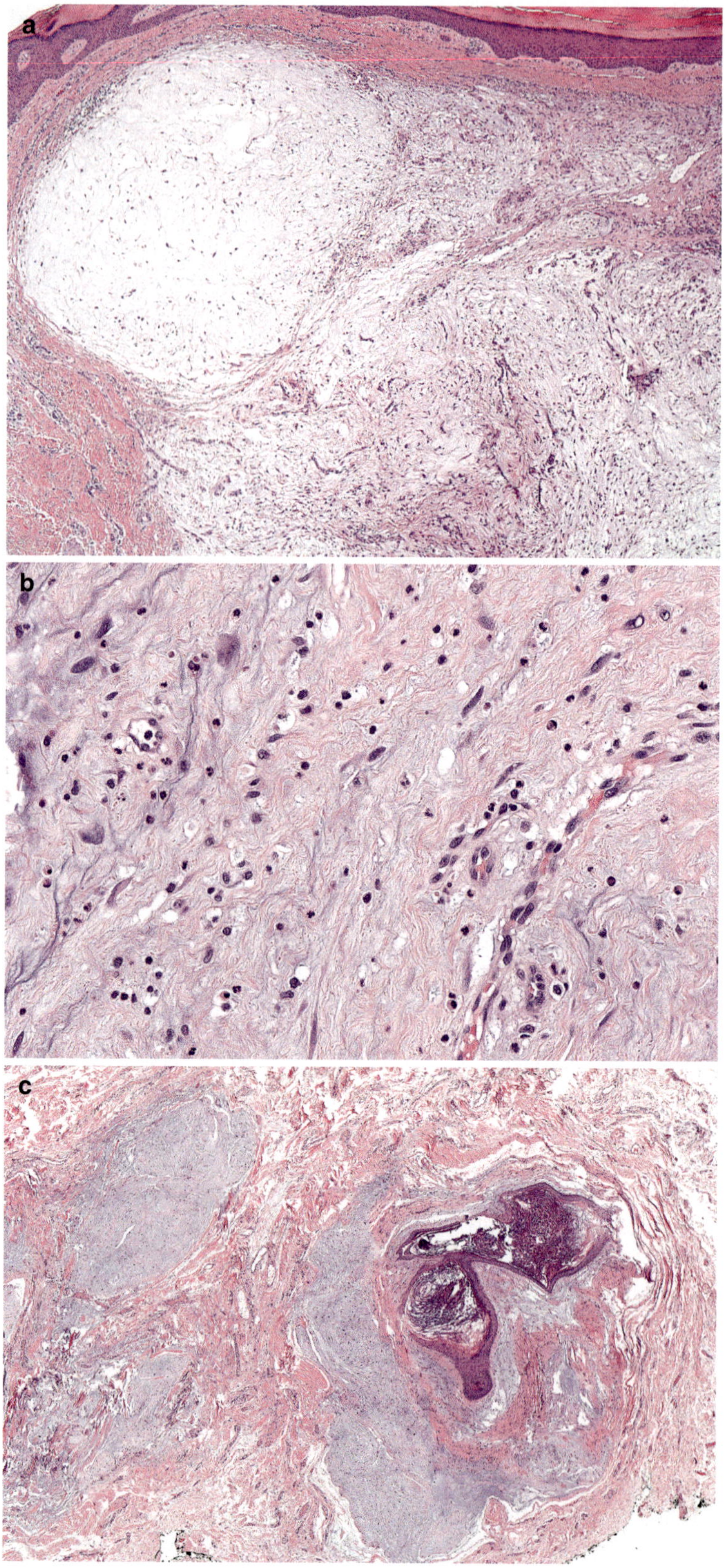

Fig. 4.28 Cutaneous myxoma/superficial angiomyxoma. (**a**) Cutaneous myxoma. A myxoid dermal tumor with a multilobular architecture. (**b**) Superficial angiomyxoma with prominent vessels and neutrophils. (**c**) Isolated epithelial elements, including epidermal inclusion cysts, may be seen

Table 4.28 Key pathologic features: cutaneous myxoma/superficial angiomyxoma

Poorly circumscribed myxoid nodules with lobular silhouette
Stellate to bipolar fibroblastic cells and muciphages
Sparse mixed inflammatory infiltrate characteristically containing neutrophils
Varying cellularity
Numerous small blood vessels (when prominent designated as superficial or cutaneous angiomyxoma)
Positive for SMA (tram-track myofibroblastic pattern), variable CD34 immunoreactivity
Negative for S100 protein, FXIIIa, and desmin

hyalinization. Dermal nerve sheath myxoma typically arises in the extremities, particularly the fingers, and has more spindled to epithelioid Schwann cells present in nests, cords and syncytial aggregates; these cells are positive for S100 protein, GFAP, neuron-specific enolase, p75, and CD57, all of which are negative in cutaneous myxomas. Myxoid variants of trichodiscoma/fibrofolliculoma may also enter the differential diagnosis of cutaneous myxoma. Trichodiscoma/fibrofolliculoma is predominantly a fibrous tumor associated with hair follicles. These lesions likely arise from perifollicular mesenchymal spindle cells and present in the head and neck region.

Cellular Neurothekeoma

Clinical Features

Cellular neurothekeoma (CNTK) is a benign soft tissue tumor with a female predominance that typically occurs in younger adults. Tumors usually present as a slowly enlarging cutaneous soft tissue mass of the head and neck or extremities and only rarely recur after surgical excision.

Pathologic Features

Cellular neurothekeoma is a circumscribed tumor arising in the dermis. It is typically composed of discrete nests or fascicles of epithelioid to spindled cells often delineated by fibrous septa (Fig. 4.29a and b). The tumor cells have oval nuclei with fine chromatin, small nucleoli, and relatively abundant eosinophilic cytoplasm. In some cases, hemorrhage and osteoclast-type giant cells are present in tumor nests. Focal nuclear atypia is relatively common and is sometimes prominent (atypical cellular neurothekeoma) (Fig. 4.29c). Constituent spindle cells are embedded in a collagenous stroma, but focal myxoid change is relatively common. Predominately myxoid variants (Fig. 4.29d) have been described as well as variants with prominent hyalinized stroma (desmoplastic cellular neurothekeoma) (Fig. 4.29e). Tumors may also be more cellular with solid sheets and fascicles of tumor cells. Perineural invasion and lymphovascular invasion have also been described in atypical cellular neurothekeoma, but none of these features seem to impact clinical behavior. Tumor cells express NKI-C3, CD10, and PGP9.5, though none of these markers are terribly specific and thus need to be interpreted in light of the histologic features. Variable expression of MiTF (60–80%) and SMA is seen (10–50%). The tumor cells are negative for SOX10, S100 protein, CD34, desmin, and pan-cytokeratin expression.

Originally considered a nerve sheath tumor due to morphologic similarity to dermal nerve sheath myxoma (myxoid neurothekeoma), cellular neurothekeoma is now considered a fibrohistiocytic tumor. No definitive ultrastructural or immunophenotypic evidence of nerve sheath differentiation has been reported. Genetic analysis of cellular neurothekeoma has demonstrated overlap with benign fibrous histiocytomas (Table 4.29).

Differential Diagnosis

The differential diagnosis for neurothekeoma includes dermal nerve sheath myxoma, plexiform fibrohistiocytic tumor, benign fibrous histiocytoma, and melanocytic tumors. Dermal nerve sheath myxoma has distinct fibrous septations,

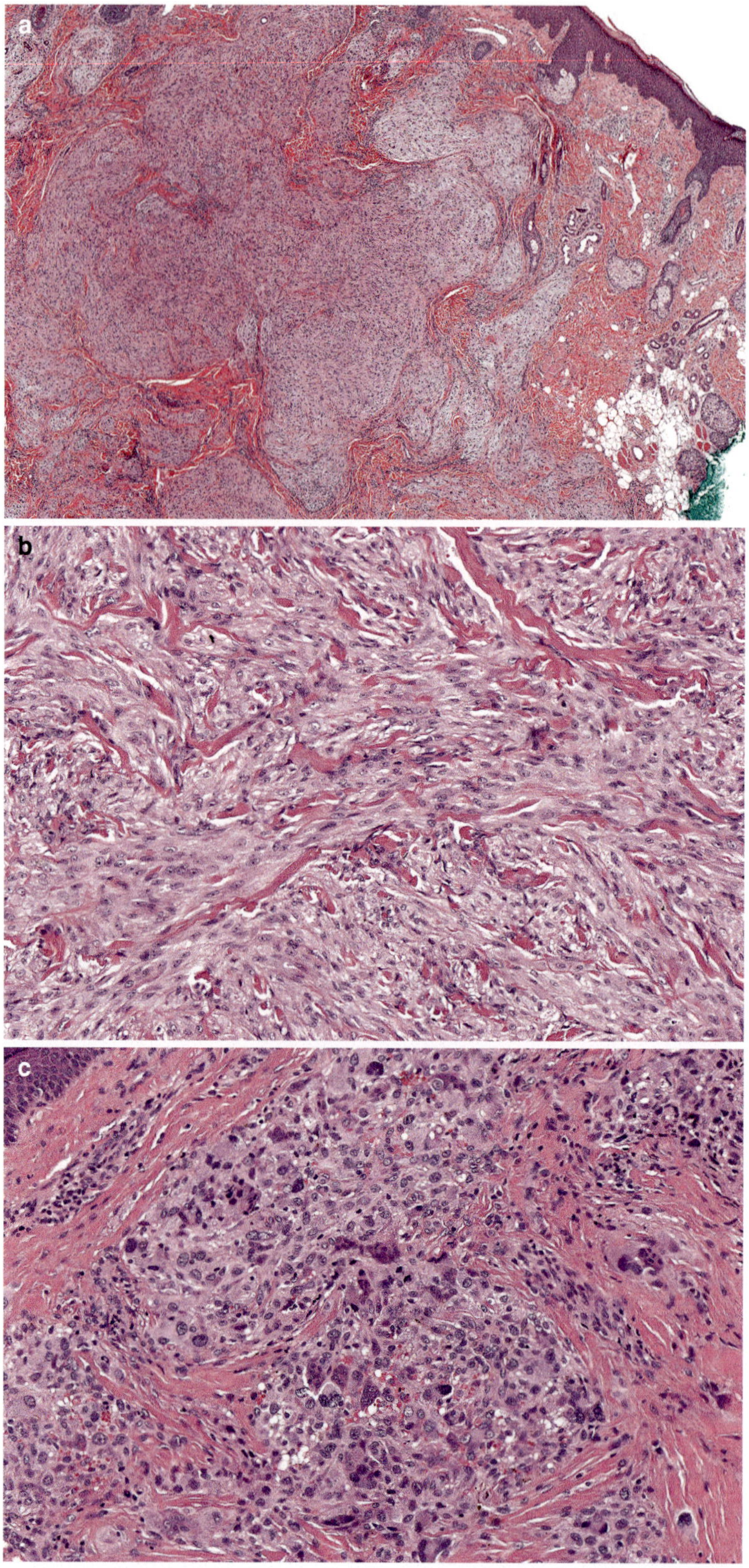

Fig. 4.29 Cellular neurothekeoma. (**a**) Circumscribed tumor in dermis comprised of nests of bland spindle cells delineated by fibrous septa. (**b**) Tumor cells may be epithelioid to spindled. (**c**) Atypical cellular neurothekeoma with significant cellular atypia and pleomorphism. This case also has admixed osteoclast-like giant cells. (**d**) Myxoid variant cellular neurothekeoma. (**e**) Desmoplastic cellular neurothekeoma with cords of tumor cells embedded in a dense collagenous stroma

Fig. 4.29 (continued)

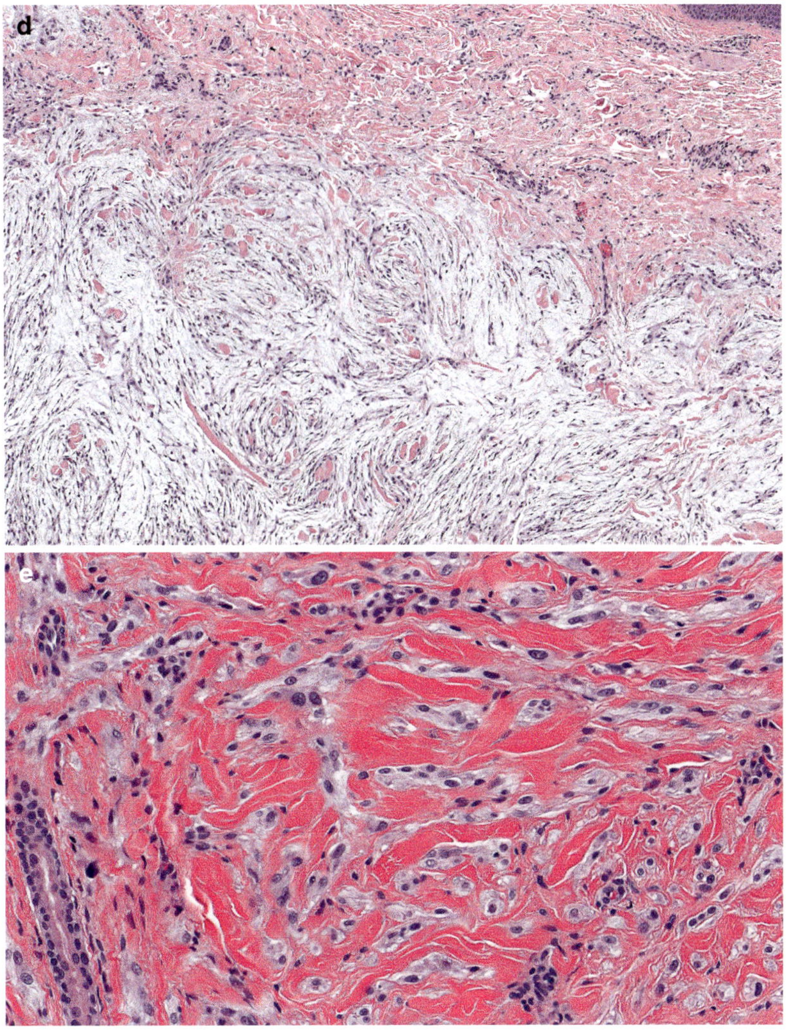

Table 4.29 Key pathologic features: cellular neurothekeoma

Circumscribed dermal tumor
Discrete nests or fascicles of spindled to epithelioid cells often delineated by fibrous septa
Collagenous to focally myxoid stroma
Cases with atypical features including large size (>5 cm), infiltrative growth, high mitotic rate, high cellularity, cytologic atypia, and perineural and lymphovascular invasion have the same prognosis as typical CNTK
NKI-C3, CD10, and PGP9.5 positive. Variable expression of CD68, MiTF (60–68%), and SMA (10–50%). Negative for SOX10, S100 protein, CD34, desmin, pan-cytokeratin, and EMA

more myxoid stroma, and a predominantly spindled morphology and is consistently positive for S100 protein. The tumor nodules of cellular neurothekeoma can bear a striking resemblance to the histiocytoid nodules of plexiform fibrohistiocytic tumor, but the latter has an infiltrative growth pattern and is usually biphasic with histiocytoid nodules and fascicles of spindled cells. Benign fibrous histiocytoma has peripheral collagen trapping and epidermal hyperplasia and does not have a nested growth pattern. Melanocytic tumors are consistently positive for S100 protein and SOX10.

Nodular Fasciitis

Clinical Features

Nodular fasciitis most often occurs in younger patients and affects men and women equally. It typically presents as a solitary, small, rapidly growing mass of the upper extremity, trunk/chest wall, or head and neck region. A history of antecedent trauma is noted in approximately 50% of patients. Nodular fasciitis of the scalp and underlying skull (i.e., cranial fasciitis) typically occurs in young infants and may be associated with birth trauma in a subset of cases. Intradermal, ossifying, and intravascular variants have also been described. Nodular fasciitis is a benign neoplasm with a low risk of recurrence that often spontaneously regresses. Tumors from the head and neck have a higher risk of recurrence compared with cases arising in other locations.

Pathologic Features

Nodular fasciitis is unencapsulated and variably circumscribed. Most cases arise in the subcutis, but as noted above, cases arising in the dermis and within vessels have been reported (Fig. 4.30a). Dermal cases tend to be relatively circumscribed, but nodular fasciitis arising in the subcutis may extend along subcutaneous septa (Fig. 4.30b). Typically, nodular fasciitis is composed of irregular fascicles of bland, lightly eosinophilic spindle cells with a swirling, so-called tissue culture growth pattern (Fig. 4.30c). Constituent tumor cells have elongated delicate cytoplasmic processes and vesicular nuclei with small nucleoli (Fig. 4.30d). Mitotic figures are frequent, but atypical forms are not seen. The background stroma is frequently myxoid with extravasated erythrocytes and areas of cystic breakdown often being present (Fig. 4.30e). These stromal features are important clues to the diagnosis. Older cases may show hyalinization, and some cases will develop keloidal collagen fibers (Fig. 4.30f). Intravascular forms demonstrated vessels expanded by a proliferation of myofibroblasts similar to conventional nodular fasciitis. Intravascular forms often have numerous osteoclast-type giant cells (Fig. 4.30g). Constituent spindle cells demonstrate a "myofibroblastic" immunophenotype and pattern of staining, namely, membranous (tram-track) accentuation of immunoreactivity with immunohistochemical stains to actins (e.g., SMA, caldesmon, and calponin) (Fig. 4.30h). Previously thought to be a reactive process, nodular fasciitis is now known to be a true neoplasm. Over 90% of cases have a translocation involving *USP6*, the same gene involved in aneurysmal bone cysts (Table 4.30).

Differential Diagnosis

Due to its high cellularity and mitotic activity and sometimes prominent areas of myxoid change, nodular fasciitis can be mistaken for myxofibrosarcoma. Myxofibrosarcoma has a greater number of atypical hyperchromatic cells, more prominent myxoid stroma, and usually a distinctive curvilinear vasculature with surrounding tumor cell condensation. Cases of nodular fasciitis arising in the dermis can be mistaken for cellular fibrous histiocytoma and dermatofibrosarcoma protuberans. Cellular fibrous histiocytoma has features of conventional benign fibrous histiocytoma, such as peripheral collagen trapping, and lacks the myxoid stroma and cystic degeneration of nodular fasciitis. Dermatofibrosarcoma protuberans has a tighter more storiform growth pattern, contains spindled cells with slender hyperchromatic nuclei, and infiltrates the fat in a diffuse "honeycomb" pattern, rather than following subcutaneous septa. Immunohistochemical stains play little role in the differential diagnosis, as stains such as SMA and CD34 can be positive at least focally in fasciitis and all the lesions considered in the differential diagnosis. In partial samples or difficult cases, FISH to detect *USP6* rearrangement can confirm the diagnosis.

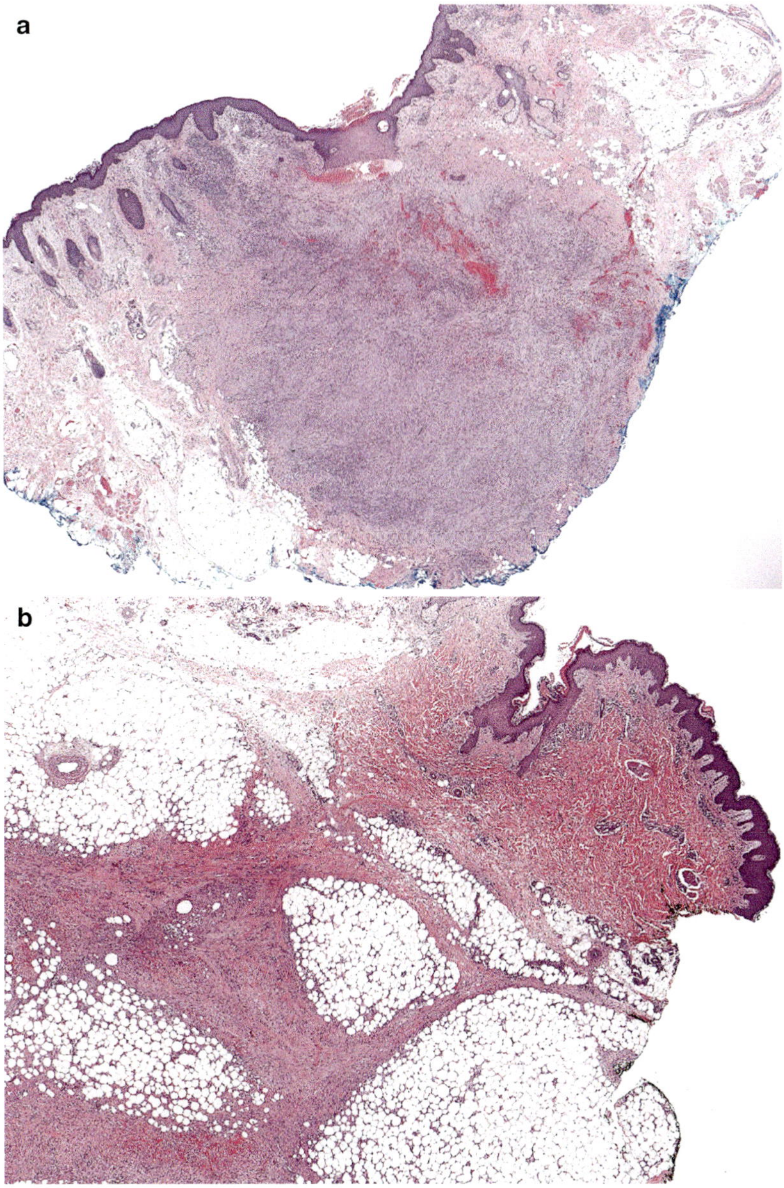

Fig. 4.30 Nodular fasciitis. (**a**) Nodular fasciitis arising in the dermis, showing an unencapsulated but circumscribed proliferation of myofibroblastic spindle cells. (**b**) Cases arising in subcutis tend to extend along fibrous septa. (**c**) Irregular fascicles of lightly eosinophilic spindle cells with a "tissue culture" growth pattern. (**d**) Tumor cells have elongated delicate cytoplasmic processes and vesicular nuclei with small nucleoli. (**e**) Extravasated erythrocytes and myxoid degeneration are helpful diagnostic features. (**f**) An example of nodular fasciitis with keloidal collagen. (**g**) An example of intravascular fasciitis. Note the osteoclast-type giant cells. (**h**) SMA tram-track pattern of immunoreactivity in nodular fasciitis

Fig. 4.30 (continued)

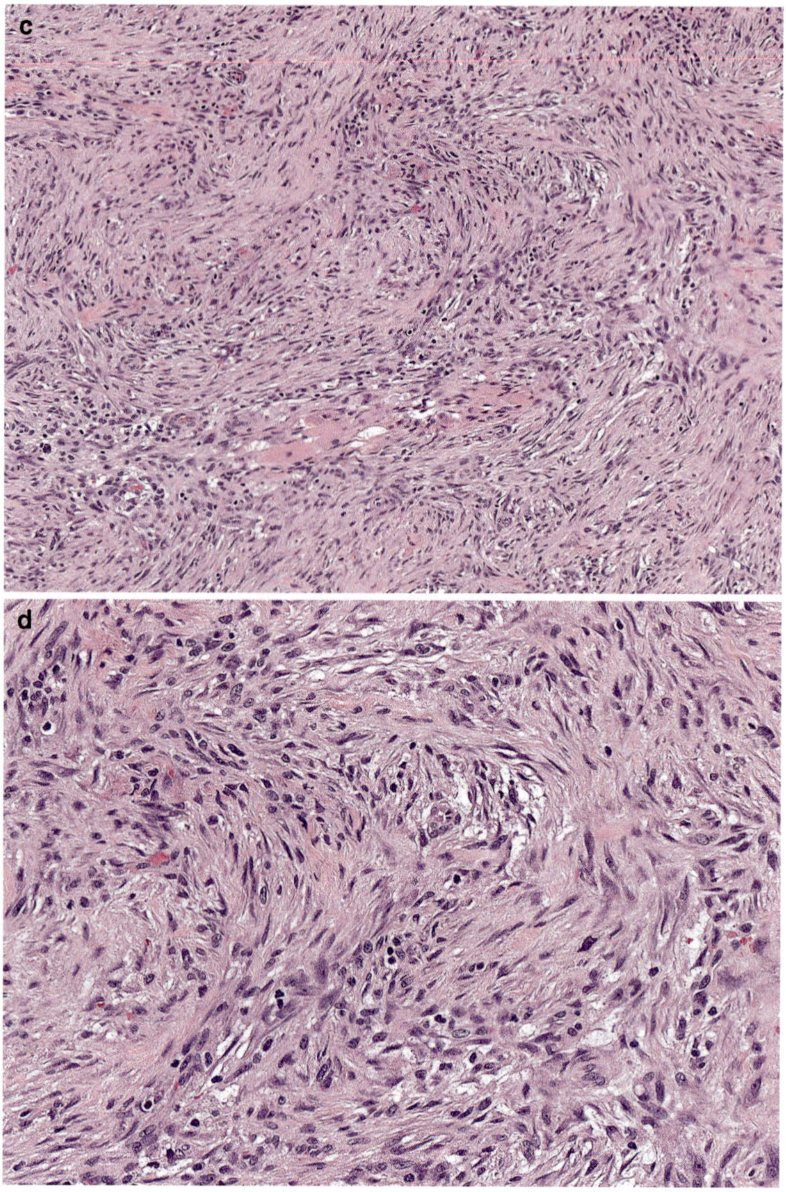

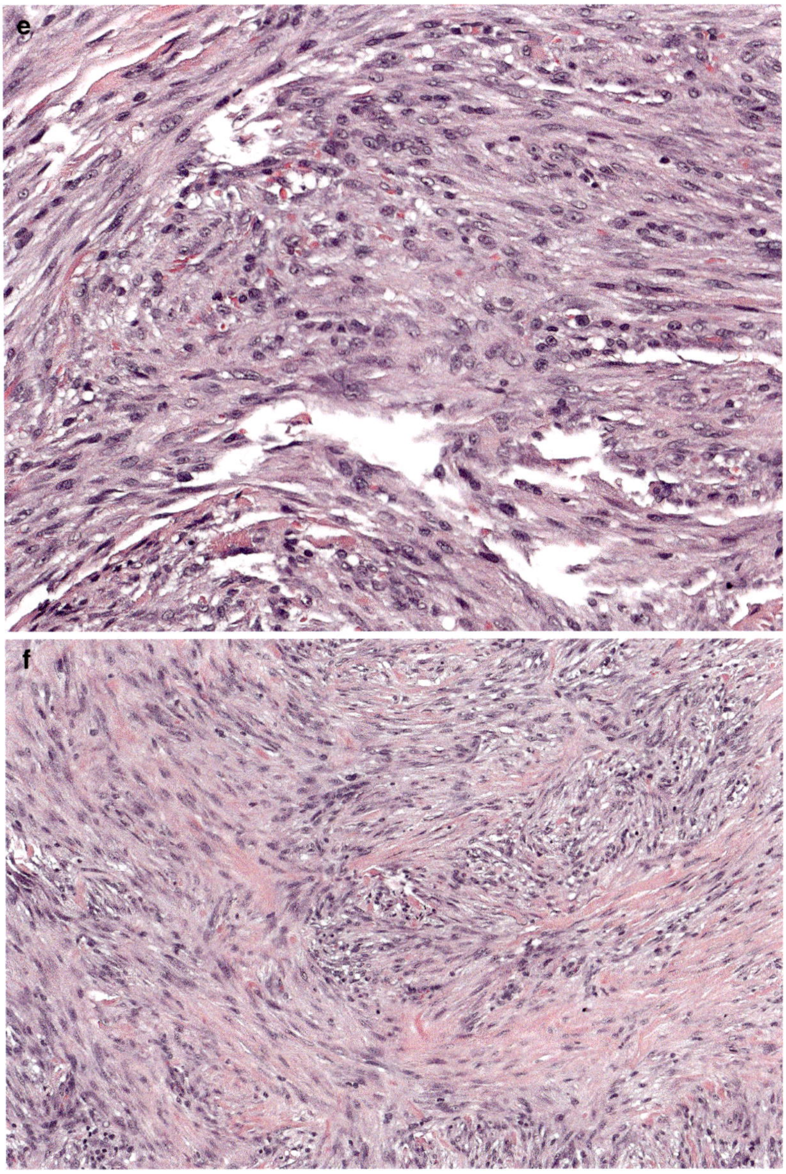

Fig. 4.30 (continued)

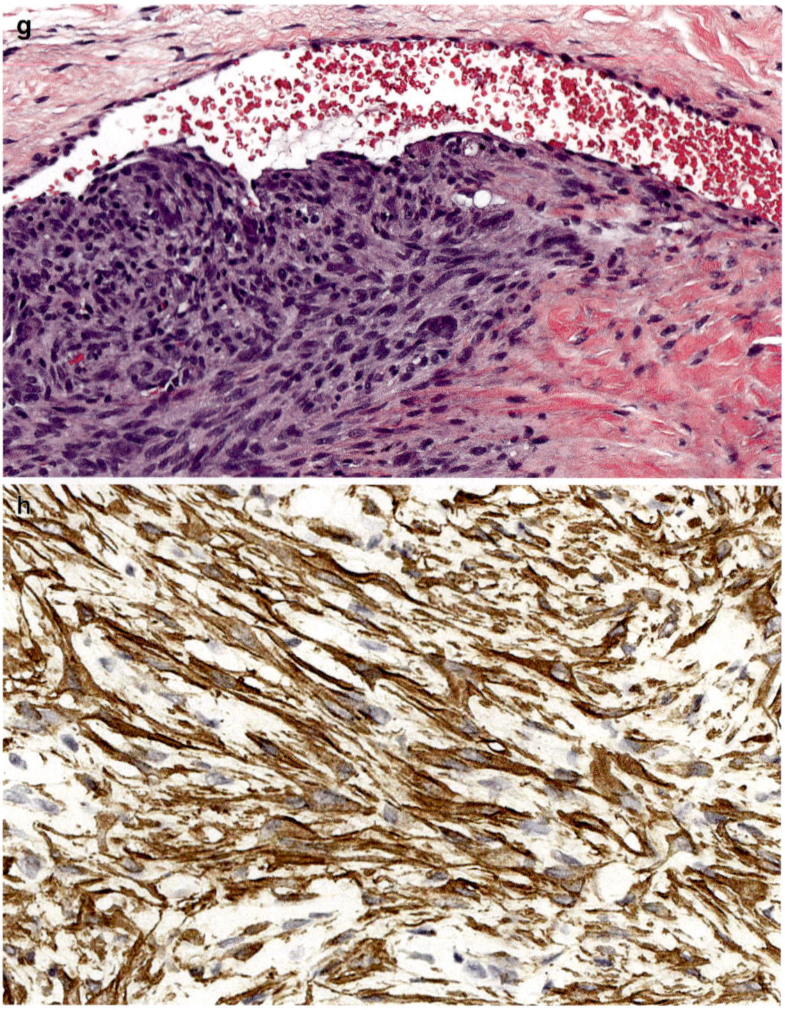

Fig. 4.30 (continued)

Table 4.30 Key pathologic features: nodular fasciitis

Irregular fascicles of bland lightly eosinophilic spindled cells with a "tissue culture" growth pattern
Mitotically active but no atypical mitoses
Variably myxoid stroma with extravasated erythrocytes and areas of cystic breakdown
Hyalinized stroma with keloid-like collagen in older lesions
Osteoclast-type giant cells may be seen, particularly in intravascular variant
Spindle cells usually positive for actins (SMA, caldesmon, calponin) often in a "tram-track" myofibroblastic pattern
USP6 gene rearrangement

Proliferative Fasciitis

Clinical Features

Proliferative fasciitis, first described by Chung and Enzinger in 1975, has significant clinical overlap with nodular fasciitis including a similar anatomic distribution and association with trauma, but usually presents in a slightly older patient population, with occasional cases presenting in children. Lesions occur in the subcutis of the extremities, trunk, or rarely the head and neck and are usually less than 5 cm in maximum dimension. Lesions present as firm, but mobile subcutaneous nodules, which may be painful. A history of rapid growth is typical.

Pathologic Features

Most cases of proliferative fasciitis have overlapping features with nodular fasciitis, with a tissue culture-like pattern of spindled cells, myxoid stroma, and extravasation of erythrocytes. The defining histologic feature of proliferative fasciitis is the presence of ganglion-like myofibroblasts interspersed among the spindled cells. These cells have enlarged eccentrically placed nuclei with prominent nucleoli and relatively abundant eosinophilic cytoplasm (Fig. 4.31a and b). Interestingly, pediatric cases may demonstrate a more diffuse, sheetlike growth pattern of ganglion-like myofibroblasts, sometimes with focal areas of necrosis (Fig. 4.31c). Proliferative fasciitis is usually immunoreactive for SMA ("tram-track") and sometimes focally for desmin. Rearrangement of *USP6* has not been identified to date (Table 4.31).

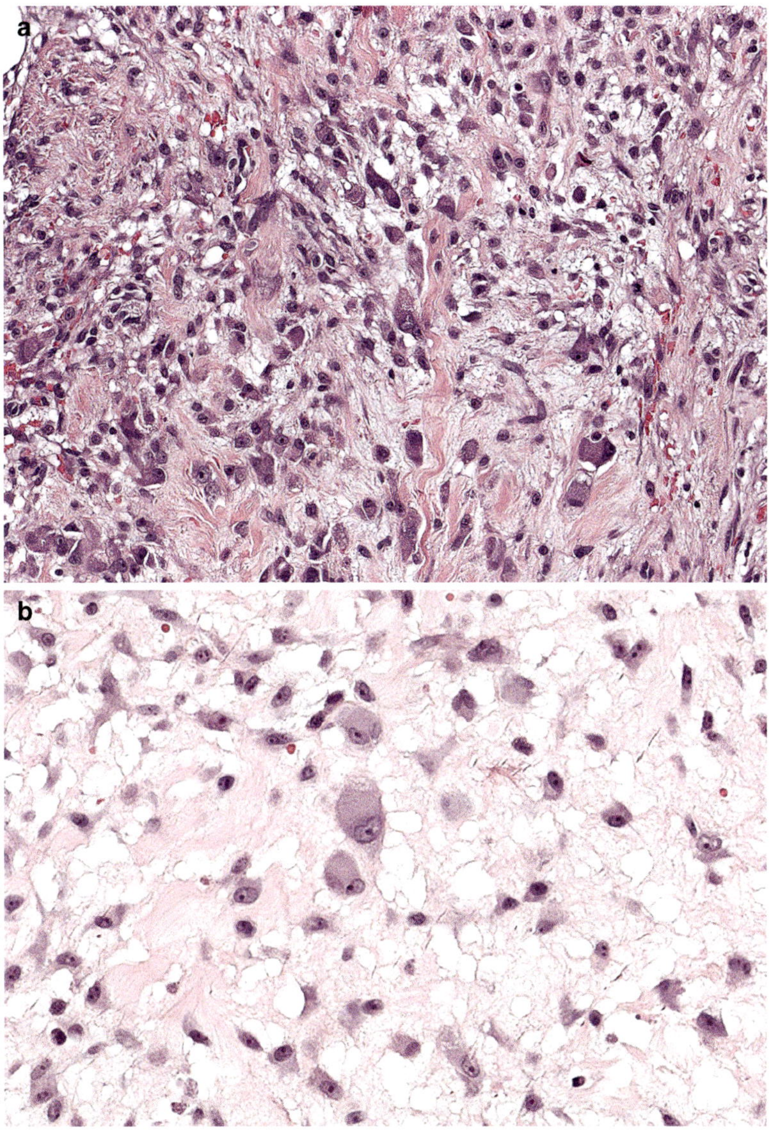

Fig. 4.31 Proliferative fasciitis. (**a**) Overlapping histologic features with nodular fasciitis including spindled myofibroblastic cells and tissue culture-like architecture. Note scattered ganglion-like myofibroblasts. (**b**) High-power view of ganglion-like cells, the defining feature of proliferative fasciitis. (**c**) Pediatric cases may have a diffuse, sheetlike growth of ganglion-like myofibroblasts. Necrosis may also be focally present

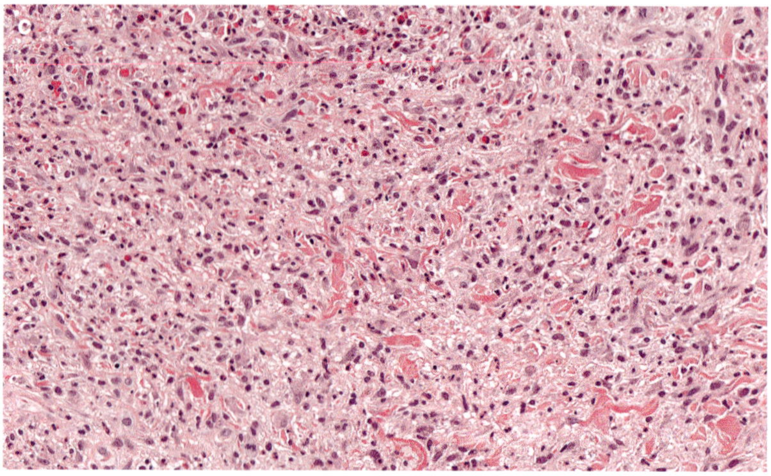

Fig. 4.31 (continued)

Table 4.31 Key pathologic features: proliferative fasciitis

Overlapping features with nodular fasciitis, including tissue culture-like pattern of spindled cells, myxoid stroma, and extravasation of erythrocytes
Interspersed ganglion-like myofibroblasts are a defining feature
Pediatric cases may have sheetlike growth of ganglion-like cells and foci of necrosis

Differential Diagnosis

The differential of proliferative fasciitis overlaps with the differential diagnosis of nodular fasciitis, as discussed above. The same comments are applicable to proliferative fasciitis. In cases with numerous ganglion-like myofibroblasts, the differential diagnosis can include metastatic melanoma, anaplastic large cell lymphoma, myxoinflammatory fibroblastic sarcoma, epithelioid sarcoma, and, in pediatric cases, rhabdomyosarcoma. With the exception of myxoinflammatory fibroblastic sarcoma, all of the entities in the differential diagnosis can be sorted out with a carefully selected panel of immunohistochemical stains, including S100 protein (melanoma), CD30 (anaplastic large cell lymphoma), epithelioid sarcoma (AE1/3 and INI1), and myogenin (rhabdomyosarcoma). The degree of cytologic atypia and extent of the associated inflammatory infiltrate seen in myxoinflammatory fibroblastic sarcoma exceeds that typically seen in proliferative fasciitis.

Ischemic Fasciitis

Clinical Features

Ischemic fasciitis (also known as decubital ischemic fasciitis or atypical decubital fibroplasia) usually occurs at sites of intermittent pressure-induced ischemia, most commonly in soft tissue overlying bony prominences (e.g., sacrum, hip, shoulder, elbow). It is usually seen in elderly and debilitated patients, but presentation in younger patients is increasingly recognized, especially in cases involving the elbows.

Pathologic Features

Ischemic fasciitis involves the subcutis and demonstrates a characteristic zonal pattern, with central fibrinoid necrosis, adjacent loose myxoid stroma, and a surrounding proliferation of myofibroblastic cells similar to those of nodular fasciitis with admixed ganglion-like myofibroblasts (Fig. 4.32a). A reactive, thin-walled vascular proliferation is also commonly present surrounding the zone of fibrinoid necrosis (Fig. 4.32b). A subset of the reactive myofibroblasts can demonstrate significant hyperchromasia and pleomorphism (Fig. 4.32c), leading to a misdiagnosis of a pleomorphic sarcoma. Similar to other forms of nodular fasciitis, immunoreactivity for SMA is common. Rearrangement of *USP6* is not

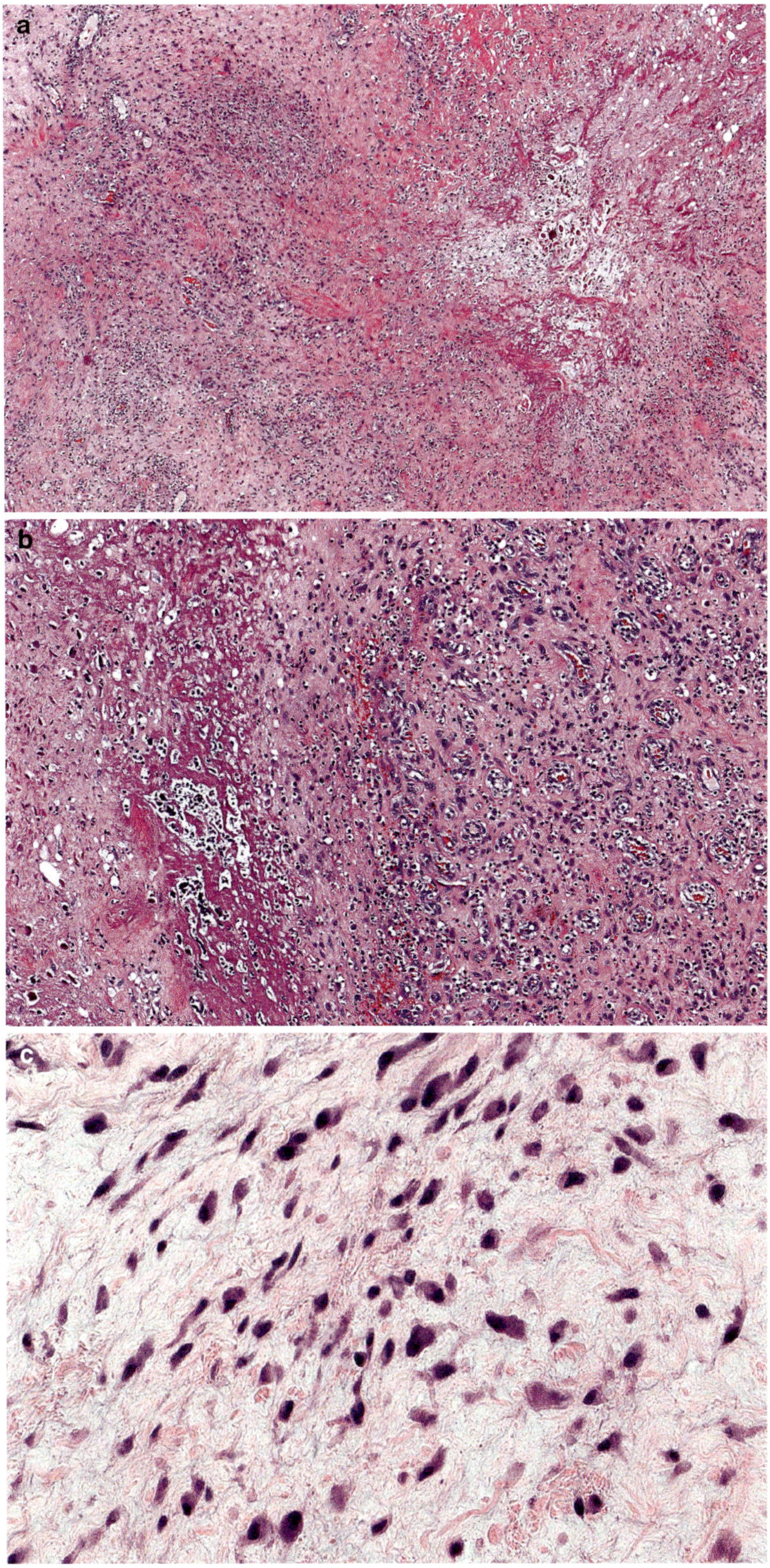

Fig. 4.32 Ischemic fasciitis. (**a**) A reactive spindle cell proliferation with a zonal pattern including a central zone of fibrinoid necrosis surrounded by reactive myofibroblasts. (**b**) Reactive thin-walled vascular proliferation around a zone of fibrinoid necrosis. (**c**) Myofibroblasts with significant hyperchromasia and pleomorphism may be mistaken for evidence of a sarcoma

Table 4.32 Key pathologic features: ischemic fasciitis

Characteristic zonal histology
Central fibrinoid necrosis, adjacent loose myxoid stroma surrounded by a proliferation of myofibroblastic spindle cells
Scattered admixed atypical ganglion-like myofibroblasts

a feature. However, recently novel t(1;2)(p36.1;q23) and t(7;19)(q32;q13.3) chromosomal translocations have been identified in a single case of ischemic fasciitis, suggesting a possible clonal pathogenetic link. The clinical significance of these findings remains to be determined (Table 4.32).

Differential Diagnosis

Ischemic fasciitis is most frequently confused with myxofibrosarcoma and undifferentiated pleomorphic sarcoma. Both of these entities have greater nuclear atypia and lack the distinct zonation of ischemic fasciitis. Immunohistochemistry plays no role in resolving the differential diagnosis.

Fibroma of Tendon Sheath

Clinical Features

Fibroma of tendon sheath (FTS) is a myofibroblastic proliferation related to nodular fasciitis, which arises in tenosynovial soft tissues. Most FTS arise in the upper extremities, with the first three fingers being the most frequent sites of involvement. FTS in the knee, elbow, and wrist have been rarely reported. Affected patients are typically in the second through fifth decades of life. FTS is a benign lesion, which may locally recur in approximately 20–25% of cases, but does not metastasize.

Pathologic Features

Lesions are slow-growing, small (≤3 cm), firm, well-circumscribed nodules typically attached, or directly adjacent, to tendon sheaths. Cleft-like spaces are often seen at the periphery (Fig. 4.33a). Most FTS are hypocellular and contain myofibroblastic spindle cells with elongated, tapered nuclei with indistinct eosinophilic cytoplasmic processes embedded in an eosinophilic hyalinized stroma (Fig. 4.33b). Most lesions have a low mitotic rate and lack significant cytologic atypia. A pleomorphic variant has been described in which a significant level of nuclear hyperchromasia and pleomorphism contrasts with the generally low mitotic activity seen in these lesions as a whole; a degenerative phenomenon has been suggested to reconcile these disparate features (Fig. 4.33c). In newly eruptive lesions, the hyalinized areas alternate with foci more typical of nodular fasciitis, including foci with extensive myxoid change and tissue culture-like architecture, as well as extravasated red cells (Fig. 4.33d). Older lesions are more fibrotic and paucicellular (Fig. 4.33e). In some lesions the tumor has zones of increased cellularity and a more fascicular growth pattern (cellular fibroma of tendon sheath) (Fig. 4.33f). Some lesions contain multinucleated osteoclast-type giant cells, but other secondary elements such as hemosiderin and foam cells are not noted. Similar to nodular fasciitis and related lesions, constituent cells express smooth muscle markers in a reactive tram-track pattern (SMA, caldesmon, and calponin), but are negative for desmin. *USP6* rearrangements have been reported in cellular fibroma of tendon sheath, but not other variants. These lesions are benign but may recur after incomplete excision (Table 4.33).

Differential Diagnosis

Hypocellular collagenized lesions are usually very characteristic and rarely confused with other entities. More cellular variants can resemble classic nodular fasciitis or a cellular fibrous histiocytoma (dermatofibroma). Tenosynovial giant cell tumor has a similar anatomic distribution, but these lesions tend to have more rounded cells, as opposed to the spindled cells seen in FTS. Unlike FTS, osteoclast-type giant cells and other secondary elements, such as xanthoma cells and hemosiderin-laden macrophages, are common in

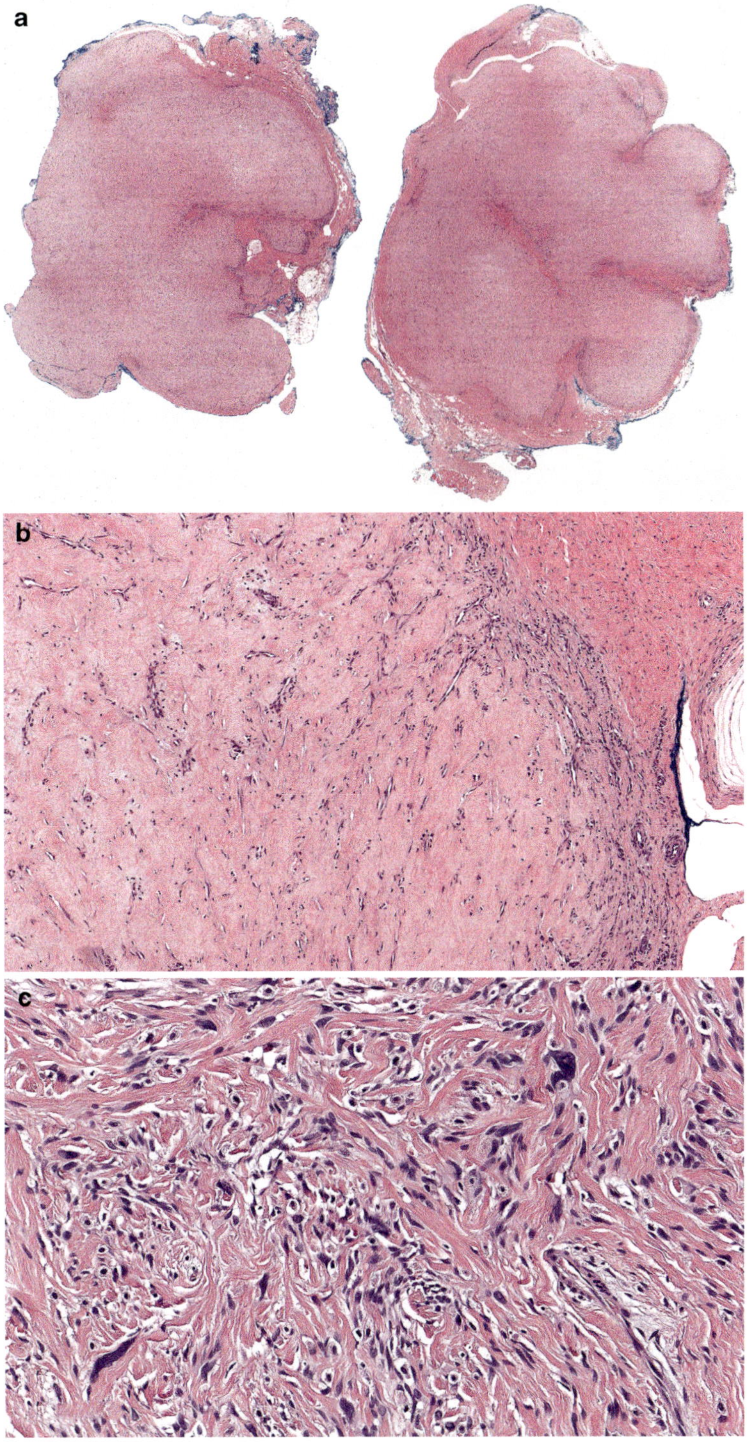

Fig. 4.33 Fibroma of tendon sheath. (**a**) Low-power view illustrating the multinodular architecture of fibroma of tendon sheath. (**b**) A hypocellular lesion composed of myofibroblastic spindle cells with elongated, tapered nuclei with indistinct eosinophilic cytoplasmic processes embedded in a hyalinized stroma. (**c**) Pleomorphic fibroma of tendon sheath is likely due to a degenerative phenomenon resulting in nuclear hyperchromasia and pleomorphism. (**d**) Extensive myxoid change and tissue culture-like architecture, as well as extravasated red cells in a newly eruptive lesion. (**e**) Extensive fibrosis typical of an older lesion. (**f**) Cellular fibroma of tendon sheath showing zones of increased cellularity

Fig. 4.33 (continued)

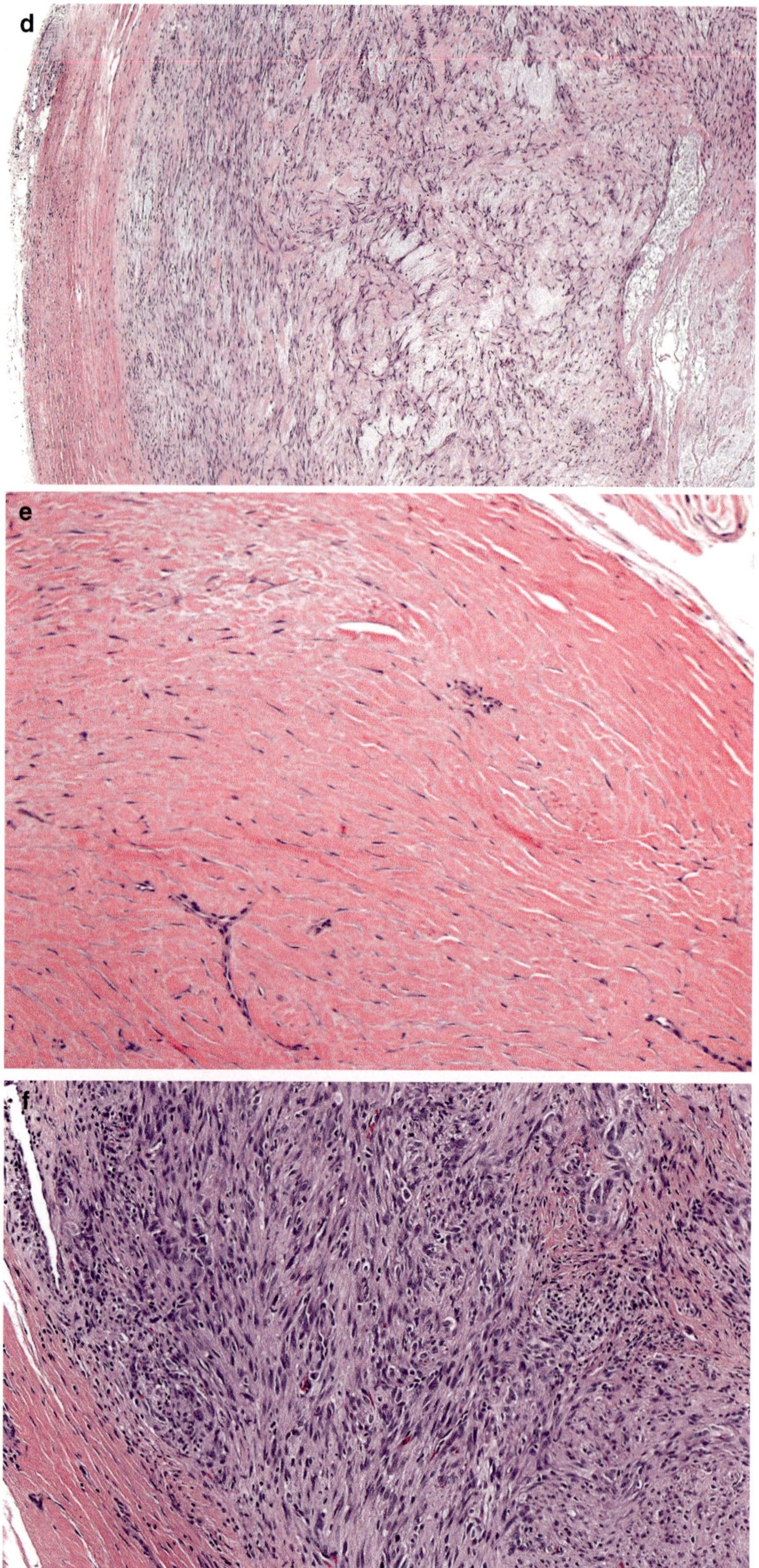

Table 4.33 Key pathologic features: fibroma of tendon sheath

Bland spindle cells in a heavily collagenized matrix surrounding slit-like vessels
Increased cellularity and nuclear atypia in cellular and pleomorphic variants, respectively
Tram-track immunoreactivity for actins but not desmin
Translocations involving the long t(2:11) (q31–32; q12), a finding shared with giant cell tumor of tendon sheath, but showing different break points
USP6 gene rearrangements seen in a subset of cellular fibromas of tendon sheath, but not other variants

tenosynovial giant cell tumor. Finally, pleomorphic variants of FTS can be confused with pleomorphic sarcomas, which in general demonstrate greater mitotic activity, cellularity, and pleomorphism.

Calcifying Fibrous Pseudotumor

Clinical Features

Calcifying fibrous pseudotumor is a rare benign soft tissue pseudotumor with slight female predominance that typically occurs in children and young adults. Tumors usually present as slowly growing painless soft tissue masses in the extremities, thorax, abdomen, or head and neck, although tumors can occur at essentially any site in the body, including visceral sites, such as the gastrointestinal tract. It shares several clinical and morphologic features with IgG4-related sclerosing diseases, although this link remains unsubstantiated. Radiographic imaging may demonstrate a soft tissue mass with intralesional mineralization. Tumors demonstrate indolent clinical behavior, with only rare local recurrences after surgical excision.

Pathologic Features

Grossly, tumors are unencapsulated, but circumscribed solid superficial or deep soft tissue masses. Microscopically, tumors are relatively circumscribed, hypocellular, and comprised of bland-appearing fibroblastic spindle cells within densely collagenous stroma. Variable mixed chronic inflammatory cells, including lymphocytes and plasma cells, are present, and characteristic focal to diffuse dystrophic and/or psammomatous calcifications are noted (Fig. 4.34a). Spindle cells show variable SMA, muscle-specific actin, desmin, CD34, and FXIIIa staining but are negative for S100 protein, pancytokeratin, and ALK expression. The presence of IgG4-positive plasma cells in these tumors, particularly those arising in the GI tract, has raised the possibility that they represent a variant in the spectrum of IgG4-related sclerosing diseases. A recent study identified novel deleterious mutations in *ZN717*, *FRG1*, and *CDC27* genes as well as significant copy number losses on eight chromosomes with a large loss common to all samples on chromosome 6. These mutations deleteriously altered coding domains in a manner predicted to be damaging to protein function, suggesting a role in CFTP tumorigenesis (Table 4.34).

Differential Diagnosis

The differential diagnosis for calcifying fibrous pseudotumor includes burned-out nodular fasciitis, fibromatosis, inflammatory myofibroblastic tumor, fibro-osseous pseudotumor of digits, and calcifying aponeurotic fibroma. In general, late-stage nodular fasciitis still has more cellular areas than calcifying fibrous pseudotumor and does not typically show prominent calcifications. Fibromatosis generally demonstrates prominent fascicular growth and only rarely shows calcifications. Inflammatory myofibroblastic tumor (IMT) is an important differential diagnostic consideration, as it can show significant morphologic overlap with calcifying fibrous pseudotumor, although in general, inflammatory myofibroblastic tumors are more cellular and show a more prominent inflammatory infiltrate; documentation of an *ALK* gene rearrangement or ALK protein expression argues against the diagnosis of calcifying fibrous pseudotumor and in favor of IMT. Finally, depending on the clinical features, fibro-osseous pseudotumor of digits and/or calci-

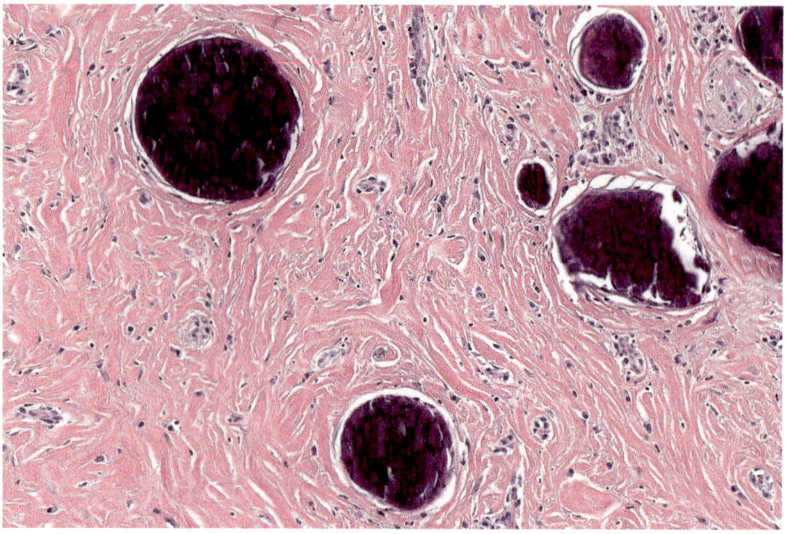

Fig. 4.34 Calcifying fibrous pseudotumor. Calcified deposits and fibroblastic cells within a fibrous stroma in a case of calcifying fibrous pseudotumor

Table 4.34 Key pathologic features: calcifying fibrous pseudotumor

Well-circumscribed mass composed of hyalinized fibrosclerotic tissue
Variable inflammatory infiltrate composed of lymphocytes and plasma cells
Psammomatous calcifications are a characteristic feature
Scattered, bland fibroblastic, and myofibroblastic spindle cells
Spindle cells show variable immunoreactivity for SMA, MSA, CD34, and FXIIIa
IgG4-positive plasma cells present in a subset

fying aponeurotic fibroma may enter the differential diagnosis of calcifying fibrous pseudotumor. The presence of maturing osteoid, osteoblastic rimming, and admixed multinucleated osteoclast-like giant cells, as well as the distinctive clinical presentation, suggests fibro-osseous pseudotumor of digits, while central cartilage formation and calcification favors a diagnosis of calcifying aponeurotic fibroma.

Fibroosseous Pseudotumor of Digits

Clinical Features

Fibro-osseous pseudotumor of digits (FOPT) is a form of heterotopic ossification originally described under the name "florid reactive periostitis of the tubular bones of the hands and feet" in 1981 and renamed FOPT in 1986. It has been likened to myositis ossificans and presents as a small, painful papule on the second or third finger. It is more common in women and young adults and has been associated with repetitive trauma secondary to manual labor. Tumors usually present as enlarging painful and/or swollen soft tissue masses. Radiographic imaging may demonstrate a vague soft tissue mass with disorganized intralesional mineralization, and the tumor may appear to involve the underlying cortical bone (Fig. 4.35a). Tumors show benign clinical behavior without local recurrence after surgical excision.

Pathologic Features

The tumors are unencapsulated but circumscribed solid superficial soft tissue masses. Microscopically, tumors are typically hypercellular and comprised of plump fibroblastic spindle cells with moderate eosinophilic cytoplasm, enlarged and slightly irregular vesicular nuclei, and inconspicuous nucleoli. Tumor cells are arranged haphazardly and in short fascicles within variable fibromyxoid stroma. Admixed foci of osteoid formation with osteoblastic rimming, patchy calcification, and scattered multinucleated osteoclast-like giant cells are present (Fig. 4.35b). Although mitotic activity may be present, there is no significant cytologic atypia

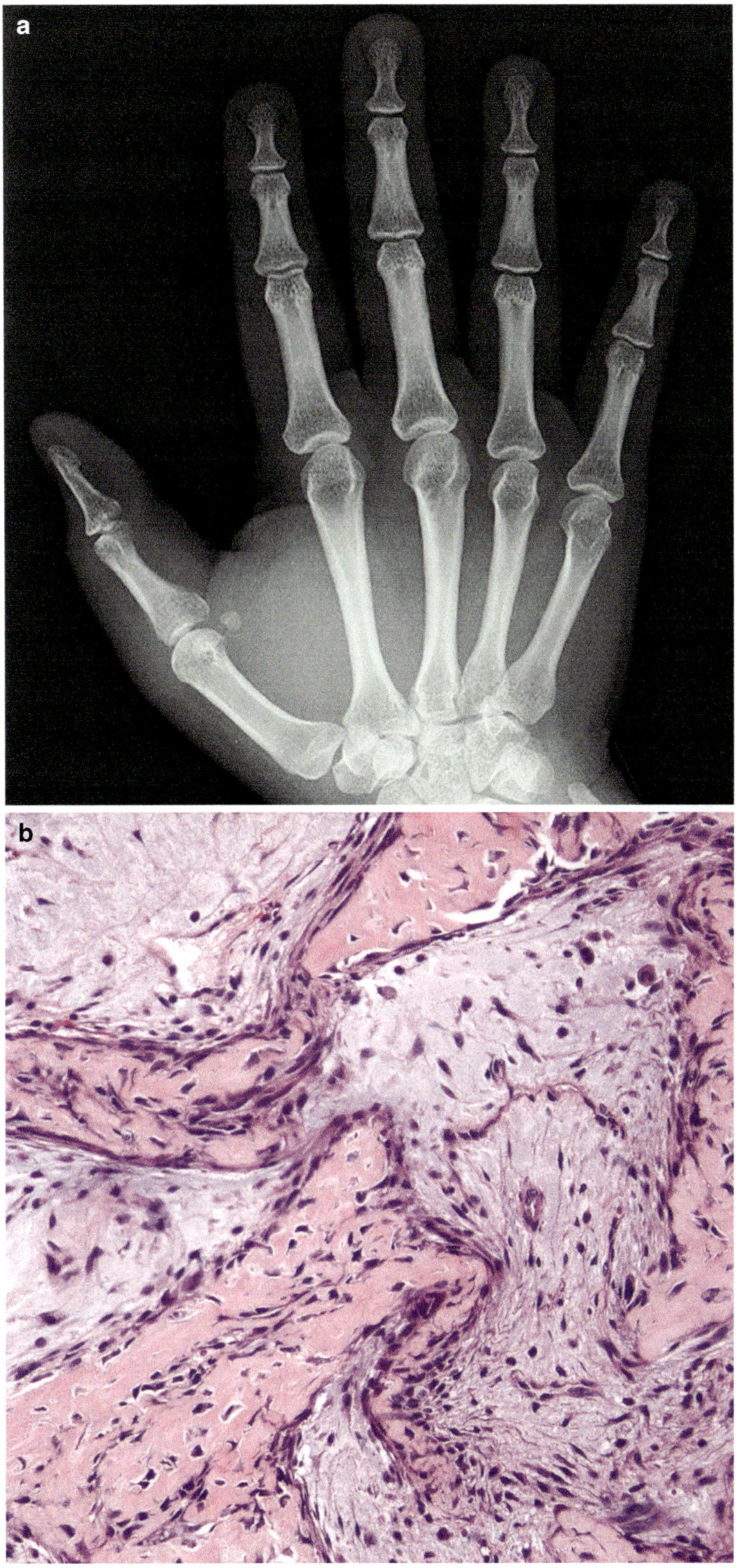

Fig. 4.35 Fibro-osseous tumor of digits. (**a**) Radiograph demonstrating a vague soft tissue mass with disorganized intralesional mineralization between the thumb and index finger. The tumor may appear to involve the underlying cortical bone. (**b**) Plump fibroblasts within a fibromyxoid stroma with osteoid formation. (Images courtesy of Dr. David Lucas, University of Michigan)

Table 4.35 Key pathologic features: fibro-osseous pseudotumor of digits

Digital subcutaneous multinodular lesion extending into fibrous tissues
Cellular proliferation of haphazardly arranged myofibroblastic cells
Foci of osteoid and bone formation with osteoblastic rimming, patchy calcification, and scattered multinucleated osteoclast-like giant cells
Spindle cells express SMA ("tram-track" pattern) but are negative for desmin, S100, CD34, and pan-cytokeratin
Subset demonstrate *USP6* rearrangement

or necrosis. The spindle cells express SMA, but are negative for desmin, S100, CD34, and pancytokeratin expression. In a recent study, four of five cases of FOPT demonstrated *USP6* rearrangements placing these lesions in the group of transient neoplasms including nodular fasciitis and myositis ossificans (Table 4.35).

Differential Diagnosis

The differential diagnosis of fibro-osseous pseudotumor of digits includes subungual exostosis, soft tissue giant cell tumor, giant cell tumor of bone, and theoretically, osteosarcoma. Of these entities, subungual exostosis is the only one with significant clinical overlap involving presentation in the digits. Subungual exostosis is usually less cellular, and radiographs will demonstrate origin from the underlying bone. Presentation of the other entities in the digits is exceptional. Both giant cell tumor of bone and most cases of osteosarcoma arise from bone. Osseous and extraskeletal osteosarcoma typically exhibit a much greater degree of cytologic atypia.

Selected References

1. Aceñero MJ, Vorwald PW, Yamauchi SC. Calcifying fibrous pseudotumor affecting the retroperitoneum: could it be a new entity within the spectrum of IgG-4 sclerosing disease? Virchows Arch. 2010;456(6):719–21.
2. Agaimy A, Michal M, Giedl J, Hadravsky L, Michal M. Superficial acral fibromyxoma: clinicopathological, immunohistochemical, and molecular study of 11 cases highlighting frequent Rb1 loss/deletions. Hum Pathol. 2017;60:192–8. PMID:27825811.
3. Agaram NP, Zhang L, Sung YS, Chen CL, Chung CT, Antonescu CR, Fletcher CD. Recurrent NTRK1 Gene Fusions Define a Novel Subset of Locally Aggressive Lipofibromatosis-like Neural Tumors. Am J Surg Pathol. 2016;40(10):1407–16.
4. Al-Ibraheemi A, Martinez A, Weiss SW, Kozakewich HP, Perez-Atayde AR, Tran H, Parham DM, Sukov WR, Fritchie KJ, Folpe AL. Fibrous hamartoma of infancy: a clinicopathologic study of 145 cases, including 2 with sarcomatous features. Mod Pathol. 2017;30(4):474–85.
5. Allen PW. Nodular fasciitis. Pathology. 1972;4(1): 9–26.
6. Allen PW, Dymock RB, MacCormac LB. Superficial angiomyxomas with and without epithelial components. Report of 30 tumors in 28 patients. Am J Surg Pathol. 1988;12(7):519–30.
7. Al-Zaid T, Wang WL, Lopez-Terrada D, Lev D, Hornick JL, Hafeez-Diwan A, Fletcher CD, Lazar AJ. Pleomorphic fibroma and dermal atypical lipomatous tumor: Are they related? J Cutan Pathol. 2013;40(4):378–84.
8. Amaravati R. Rare malignant transformation of a calcifying aponeurotic fibroma. J Bone Joint Surg Am. 2002;84-A(10):1889, author reply 1889.
9. Balachandran K, Allen PW, MacCormac LB. Nuchal fibroma. A clinicopathological study of nine cases. Am J Surg Pathol. 1995;19(3):313–7. PMID:7872429.
10. Bansal C, Stewart D, Li A, et al. Histologic variants of fibrous papule. J Cutan Pathol. 2005;32:424–8. 15953376.
11. Barnhill RL, Mihm MC Jr. Cellular neurothekeoma. A distinctive variant of neurothekeoma mimicking nevomelanocytic tumors. Am J Surg Pathol. 1990;14:113–20.
12. Beerman H. Lipid diseases as manifested in the skin. Med Clin N Am. 1951;35(2):433–56.
13. Bertoni F, Unni KK, Beabout JW, et al. Malignant giant cell tumor of the tendon sheaths and joints (malignant pigmented villonodular synovitis). Am J Surg Pathol. 1997;21(2):153–63.
14. Boland JM, Folpe AL, Hornick JL, et al. Clusterin is expressed in normal synoviocytes and in tenosynovial giant cell tumors of localized and diffuse types: diagnostic and histogenetic implications. Am J Surg Pathol. 2009;33(8):1225–9.
15. Brazzelli V, Rivetti N, Carugno A, Barruscotti S, Croci GA, Perani G, Borroni G. Eruptive xanthomas after extensive tattooing: a case report and literature review. G Ital Dermatol Venereol. 2015;150(6):770–1.Wilkes LL. Tendon xanthoma in type IV hyperlipoproteinemia. South Med J [Case Reports]. 1977;70(2):254–5.
16. Briganti A, Salonia A, Deho F, Zanni G, Rokkas K, Rigatti P, et al. Peyronie's disease: a review. Curr Opin Urol. 2003;13(5):417–22.
17. Bürgi J, Kunz B, Abrami L, Deuquet J, Piersigilli A, Scholl-Bürgi S, Lausch E, Unger S, Superti-Furga A,

Bonaldo P, et al. CMG2/ANTXR2 regulates extracellular collagen VI which accumulates in hyaline fibromatosis syndrome. Nat Commun. 2017;8:15861. https://doi.org/10.1038/ncomms15861.
18. Busam KJ, Mentzel T, Colpaert C, Barnhill RL, Fletcher CD. Atypical or worrisome features in cellular neurothekeoma: a study of 10 cases. Am J Surg Pathol. 1998;22:1067–72.
19. Calonje E, Mentzel T, Fletcher CD, Path MRC. Cellular benign fibrous histiocytoma. Clinicopathologic analysis of 74 cases of a distinctive variant of cutaneous fibrous histiocytoma with frequent recurrence. Am J Surg Pathol. 1994;18(7):668–76.
20. Calonje E, Guerin D, McCormick D, Fletcher CD. Superficial angiomyxoma: clinicopathologic analysis of a series of distinctive but poorly recognized cutaneous tumors with tendency for recurrence. Am J Surg Pathol. 1999;23(8):910–7.
21. Carter JM, Wang X, Dong J, Westendorf J, Choux MM, Oliveira AM. USP6 genetic arrangements in cellular fibroma of tendon sheath. Mod Pathol. 2016;29(8):865–9.
22. Cassier PA, Gelderblom H, Stacchiotti S, Thomas D, Maki RG, Kroep JR, van der Graaf WT, Italiano A, Seddon B, Dômont J, Bompas E, Wagner AJ, Blay JY. Efficacy of imatinib mesylate for the treatment of locally advanced and/or metastatic tenosynovial giant cell tumor/pigmented villonodular synovitis. Cancer. 2012;118(6):1649–55.
23. Chaudhry IH, Kazakov DV, Michal M, Mentzel T, Luzar B, Calonje E. Fibro-osseous pseudotumor of the digit: a clinicopathological study of 17 cases. J Cutan Pathol. 2010;37(3):323–9.
24. Chung EB, Enzinger FM. Proliferative fasciitis. Cancer. 1975;36(4):1450–8.
25. Chung EB, Enzinger FM. Fibroma of tendon sheath. Cancer. 1979;44(5):1945–54.
26. Coffin CM, Hornick JL, Zhou H, Fletcher CDM. Gardner fibroma: A clinical, pathologic, and immunohistochemical analysis of 45 patients with 57 fibromas. Am J Surg Pathol. 2007;31(3):410–6.
27. Cohen BA, Hood A. Xanthogranuloma: report on clinical and histologic findings in 64 patients. Pediatr Dermatol. 1989;6(4):262–6.
28. Cullen D, Díaz Recuero JL, Cullen R, Rodríguez Peralto JL, Kutzner H, Requena L. Superficial acral fibromyxoma: report of 13 cases with new immunohistochemical findings. Am J Dermatopathol. 2017;39(1):14–22. PMID:28045748.
29. Darling TN, Skarulis MC, Steinberg SM, et al. Multiple facial angiofibromas and collagenomas in patients with multiple endocrine neoplasia type 1. Arch Dermatol. 1997;133:853–7.
30. de Feraudy S, Fletcher CDM. Intradermal nodular fasciitis: a rare lesion analyzed in a series of 24 cases. Am J Surg Pathol. 2010;34(9):1377–81.
31. de Feraudy S, Fletcher CD. Fibroblastic connective tissue nevus: a rare cutaneous lesion analyzed in a series of 25 cases. Am J Surg Pathol. 2012;36:1509.
32. de Silva MV, Reid R. Myositis ossificans and fibroosseous pseudotumor of digits: a clinicopathologic review of 64 cases with emphasis on diagnostic pitfalls. Int J Surg Pathol. 2003;11:187–95.
33. De Wever I, Dal Cin P, Fletcher CD, Mandahl N, Mertens F, Mitelman F, et al. Cytogenetic, clinical, and morphologic correlations in 78 cases of fibromatosis: a report from the CHAMP Study Group. Chromosomes and Morphology. Mod Pathol. 2000;13(10):1080–5. PMID:11048801.
34. Dehner LP. Juvenile xanthogranulomas in the first two decades of life: a clinicopathologic study of 174 cases with cutaneous and extracutaneous manifestations. Am J Surg Pathol. 2003;27(5):579–93.
35. Denadai R, Bertola DR, Stelini RF, et al. Additional thoughts about juvenile hyaline fibromatosis and infantile systemic hyalinosis. Adv Anat Pathol. 2012;19(3):191–2; author reply 192.
36. Downey C, Requena L, Bagué S, Sánchez Martínez MÁ, Lloreta J, Baselga E. Agminated fibroblastic connective tissue nevus: a new clinical presentation. Pediatr Dermatol. 2016;33(4):e240–3.
37. Doyle LA, Fletcher CD. Metastasizing "benign" cutaneous fibrous histiocytoma: a clinicopathologic analysis of 16 cases. Am J Surg Pathol. 2013;37(4):484–95.
38. Doyle LA, Marino-Enriquez A, Fletcher CDM, Hornick JL. ALK rearrangement and overexpression in epithelioid fibrous histiocytoma. Mod Pathol. 2015;28:904–12.
39. Dupree WB, Enzinger FM. Fibro-osseous pseudotumor of the digits. Cancer. 1986;58:2103–9.
40. Edgar MA, Lauer SR, Bridge JA, et al. Soft tissue angiofibroma: report of 2 cases of a recently described tumor. Hum Pathol. 2013;44(3):438–41.
41. Erickson-Johnson MR, Chou MM, Evers BR, et al. Nodular fasciitis: a novel model of transient neoplasia induced by MYH9-USP6 gene fusion. Lab Investig. 2011;91(10):1427–33.
42. Estela JR, Rico MT, Pérez A, Unamuno B, Garcías J, Cubells L, et al. Dermatofibroma of the face: a clinicopathologic study of 20 cases. Actas Dermosifiliogr. 2014;105(2):172–7. PMID: 24275565.
43. Evans HL. Desmoplastic fibroblastoma. A report of 7 cases. Am J Surg Pathol. 1995;19:1077–81.
44. Evans HL. Multinucleated giant cells in plantar fibromatosis. Am J Surg Pathol. 2002; 26(2):244–248. PMID:11812947.
45. Fanti PA, Dika E, Piraccini BM, Infusino SD, Baraldi C, Misciali C. Superficial acral fibromyxoma: a clinicopathological and immunohistochemical analysis of 12 cases of a distinctive soft tissue tumor with a predilection for the fingers and toes. G Ital Dermatol Venereol. 2011;146(4):283–7.
46. Fetsch JF, Miettinen M. Calcifying aponeurotic fibroma: a clinicopathologic study of 22 cases arising in uncommon sites. Hum Pathol. 1998;29(12):1504–10. PMID:9865839.
47. Fetsch JF, Miettinen M, Laskin WB, et al. A clinicopathologic study of 45 pediatric soft tissue tumors

with an admixture of adipose tissue and fibroblastic elements, and a proposal for classification as lipofibromatosis. Am J Surg Pathol. 2000;24(11):1491–500.
48. Fetsch JF, Laskin WB, Miettinen M. Superficial acral fibromyxoma: a clinicopathologic and immunohistochemical analysis of 37 cases of a distinctive soft tissue tumor with a predilection for the fingers and toes. Hum Pathol. 2001;32(7):704–14.
49. Fetsch JF, Laskin WB, Miettinen M. Palmar-plantar fibromatosis in children and preadolescents: a clinicopathologic study of 56 cases with newly recognized demographics and extended follow-up information. Am J Surg Pathol. 2005;29(8):1095–105.
50. Fetsch JF, Laskin WB, Hallman JR, Lupton GP, Miettinen M. Neurothekeoma: an analysis of 178 tumors with detailed immunohistochemical data and long-term patient follow-up information. Am J Surg Pathol. 2007;31:1103–14.
51. Fletcher CD, Powell G, van Noorden S, et al. Fibrous hamartoma of infancy: a histochemical and immunohistochemical study. Histopathology. 1988;12:65–74.
52. Flucke U, Shepard SJ, Bekers EM, Tirabasco R, van Diest PJ, Creytens D, van Gorp JM. Fibro-osseous pseudotumor of digits- Expanding the spectrum of clonal transient neoplasms harboring *USP6* rearrangement. Ann Diagn Pathol. 2018;35:53–5.
53. Folpe AL, Weiss SW, Fletcher CD, et al. Tenosynovial giant cell tumors: evidence for a desmin-positive dendritic cell subpopulation. Mod Pathol. 1998;11(10):939–44.
54. Frew JW. Multinucleate cell angiohistiocytoma: clinicopathological correlation of 142 cases with insights into etiology and pathogenesis. Am J Dermatopathol. 2015;37:222–8.
55. Fullen DR, Lowe L, Su LD. Antibody to S100a6 protein is a sensitive immunohistochemical marker for neurothekeoma. J Cutan Pathol. 2003;30:118–22.
56. Gauchotte G, Bressenot A, Serradori T, et al. Reactive nodular fibrous pseudotumor: a first report of gastric localization and clinicopathologic review. Gastroenterol Clin Biol. 2009;33(12):1076–81.
57. Gleason BC, Fletcher CD. Deep "benign" fibrous histiocytoma: clinicopathologic analysis of 69 cases of a rare tumor indicating occasional metastatic potential. Am J Surg Pathol. 2008;32(3):354–62.
58. Glusac EJ, Barr RJ, Everett MA, et al. Epithelioid cell histiocytoma. A report of 10 cases including a new cellular variant. Am J Surg Pathol. 1994;18(6):583–90.
59. Guitart J, Bergfeld WF, Tuthill RJ. Fibrous papule of the nose with granular cells: Two cases. J Cutan Pathol. 1991;18:284–7.
60. Hall LD, Ferringer T. The best diagnosis is: Eruptive xanthoma. Cutis. 2012;90(1):12, 15–6.
61. Hanft VN, Shea CR, McNutt NS, Pullitzer D, Horenstein MG, Prieto VG. Expression of CD34 in sclerotic ("plywood") fibromas. Am J Dermatopathol. 2000;22(1):17–21.
62. Hepple R, Kreysel HW. Cutaneous angiomyxoma: a benign neoplasm distinct from cutaneous focal mucinosis. J Am Acad Dermatol. 1995;33(2 Pt 2):352–5.
63. Hernández JL, Rodríguez-Parets JO, Valero JM, Muñoz MA, Benito MR, Hernandez JM, Bullón A. High-resolution genome-wide analysis of chromosomal alterations in elastofibroma. Virchows Arch. 2010;456(6):–681, 7.
64. Heymann WR. Infantile digital fibromatosis. J Am Acad Dermatol. 2008;59(1):122–3.
65. Hill KA, Gonzalez-Crussi F, Omeroglu A, et al. Calcifying fibrous pseudotumor involving the neck of a five-week-old infant. Presence of factor XIIIa in the lesional cells. Pathol Res Pract. 2000;196(7):527–31.
66. Hinds B, Ajello-Perez AD, LeBoit PE, McCalmont TH, North JP. Loss of retinoblastoma in pleomorphic fibroma: an immunohistochemical and genomic analysis. J Cutan Pathol. 2017;44(8):665–761.
67. Hollmann TJ, Bovée JV, Fletcher CD. Digital fibromyxoma (superficial acral fibromyxoma): a detailed characterization of 124 cases. Am J Surg Pathol. 2012;36(6):789–98.
68. Hsieh YJ, Lin YC, Wu YH, Su HY, Billings SD, Hood AF. Subungual pleomorphic fibroma. J Cutan Pathol. 2003;30(9):569–71.
69. Iwata J, Fletcher CD. Lipidized fibrous histiocytoma: clinicopathologic analysis of 22 cases. Am J Dermatopathol. 2000;22(2):126–34.
70. Jain A, Maheshwari V, Alam K, et al. Calcifying fibrous pseudotumor of peritoneum. J Postgrad Med. 2007;53(3):189–90.
71. Jang KS, Oh YH, Han HX, et al. Calcifying fibrous pseudotumor of the pleura. Ann Thorac Surg. 2004;78(6):e87–8.
72. Janssen D, Harms D. Juvenile xanthogranuloma in childhood and adolescence: a clinicopathologic study of 129 patients from the Kiel pediatric tumor registry. Am J Surg Pathol. 2005;29(1):21–8.
73. Jiménez-Heffernan JA, Urbano J, Tobio R, et al. Calcifying fibrous pseudotumor: a rare entity related to inflammatory pseudotumor. Acta Cytol. 2000;44(5):932–4.
74. Jin Y, Möller E, Nord KH, et al. Fusion of the AHRR and NCOA2 genes through a recurrent translocation t(5;8)(p15;q13) in soft tissue angiofibroma results in upregulation of aryl hydrocarbon receptor target genes. Genes Chromosomes Cancer. 2012;51(5):510–20.
75. Jumper N, Paus R, Bayat A. Functional histopathology of keloid disease. Histol Histopathol. 2015;30(9):1033–57.
76. Kaddu S, McMenamin ME, Fletcher CD. Atypical fibrous histiocytoma of the skin: clinicopathologic analysis of 59 cases with evidence of infrequent metastasis. Am J Surg Pathol. 2002;26(1):35–46.
77. Kamino H, Jacobson M. Dermatofibroma extending into the subcutaneous tissue. Differential diagnosis

from dermatofibrosarcoma protuberans. Am J Surg Pathol. 1990;14(12):1156–64.

78. Kamino H, Lee JY, Berke A. Pleomorphic fibroma of the skin: a benign neoplasm with cytologic atypia. A clinical pathologic study of 8 cases. Am J Surg Pathol. 1989;13:107–13.
79. Kamino H, Reddy VB, Gero M, Greco MA. Dermatomyofibroma. A benign cutaneous, plaque-like proliferation of fibroblasts and myofibroblasts in young adults. J Cutan Pathol. 1992;19:85.
80. Kan AE, Rogers M. Juvenile hyaline fibromatosis: an expanded clinicopathologic spectrum. Pediatr Dermatol. 1989;6(2):68–75.
81. Kato I, Yoshida A, Ikegami M, Okuma T, Tonooka A, Horiguchi S, Funata N, Kawai A, Goto T, Hishima T, Aoki I, Motoi T. FOS1 immunohistochemistry clarifies distinction between desmoplastic fibroblastoma and fibroma of tendon sheath. Histopathology. 2016;69(6):1012–20.
82. Kayaselçuk F, Demirhan B, Kayaselçuk U, Ozerdem OR, Tuncer I. Vimentin, SMA, desmin, S-100 protein, p53, and estrogen receptor expression in elastofibroma and nodular fasciitis. Ann Diagn Pathol. 2002;6(2):94–9.
83. Kazakov DV, Kyrpychova L, Martinek P, Grossmann P, Steiner P, Vanecek T, Pavlovsky M, Bencik V, Michal M, Michal M. ALK gene fusions in epithelioid fibrous histiocytoma: a study of 14 cases, with new histopathologic findings. Am J Dermatopathol. 2018. https://doi.org/10.1097/DAD.0000000000001085.
84. Keasbey LE. Juvenile aponeurotic fibroma (calcifying fibroma); a distinctive tumor arising in the palms and soles of young children. Cancer. 1953;6(2):338–46.
85. Kitano Y. Juvenile hyalin fibromatosis. Arch Dermatol. 1976;112(1):86–8.
86. Kucher C, McNiff JM. Epithelial fibrous papule-a new variant. J Cutan Pathol. 2007;34:571–5.
87. Kumar E, Patel NR, Demicco EG, Bovee JV, Olivera AM, Lopez-Terrada DH, Billings SD, Lazar AJ, Wang WL. Cutaneous nodular fasciitis with genetic analysis: a case series. J Cutan Pathol. 2016;43(12):1143–9.
88. Kuo TT, Hu S, Chan HL. Keloidal dermatofibroma: report of 10 cases of a new variant. Am J Surg Pathol. 1998;22(5):564–8.
89. Kuo TT, Chen TC, Lee LY. Sclerosing angiomatoid nodular transformation of the spleen (SANT): clinicopathological study of 10 cases with or without abdominal disseminated calcifying fibrous tumors, and the presence of a significant number of IgG4+ plasma cells. Pathol Int. 2009;59(12):844–50.
90. Kutzner H, Mentzel T, Palmedo G, Hantschke M, Rütten A, Paredes BE, Schärer L, Guillen CS, Requena L. Plaque-like CD34 positive dermal fibroma ("medallion-like dermal dendrocyte hamartoma"): clinicopathologic, immunohistochemical, and molecular analysis of 5 cases emphasizing its distinction from superficial, plaque-like dermatofibrosarcoma protuberans. Am J Surg Pathol. 2010;34(2):190–201.
91. Lambert CM, Nuki G. Multicentric reticulohistiocytosis with arthritis and cardiac infiltration: regression following treatment for underlying malignancy. Ann Rheum Dis [Case Reports]. 1992;51(6):815–7.
92. Lamovec J, Bracko M, Voncina D. Pleomorphic fibroma of tendon sheath. Am J Surg Pathol. 1991;15:1202–5.
93. Laskin WB, Miettinen M, Fetsch JF. Infantile digital fibroma/fibromatosis: a clinicopathologic and immunohistochemical study of 69 tumors from 57 patients with long-term follow-up. Am J Surg Pathol. 2009;33(1):1–13.
94. Lauer DH, Enzinger FM. Cranial fasciitis of childhood. Cancer. 1980;45(2):401–6.
95. Lehmer LM, Moore JB, Ragsdale BD. Ischemic fasciitis: enhanced diagnostic resolution through clinical, histopathologic and radiologic correlation in 17 cases. J Cutan Pathol. 2016;43(9):740–8.
96. Liegl B, Fletcher CD. Ischemic fasciitis: analysis of 44 cases indicating an inconsistent association with immobility or debilitation. Am J Surg Pathol. 2008;32(10):1546–52.
97. Linos K, Sedivcová M, Cerna K, Sima R, Kazakov DV, Nazeer T, et al. Extra nuchal-type fibroma associated with elastosis, traumatic neuroma, a rare APC gene missense mutation, and a very rare MUTYH gene polymorphism: a case report and review of the literature. J Cutan Pathol. 2011;38(11):911–8. PMID:21752055.
98. Macchia G, Trombetta D, Möller E, Mertens F, Storlazzi CT, Debeiec-Rychter M, Sciot R, Nord KH. FOSL1 as a candidate target gene for 11q12 rearrangements in desmoplastic fibroblastoma. Lab Investig. 2012;92(5):735–43.
99. Maeda A, Kawabata K, Kusuzaki K. Rapid recurrence of calcifying fibrous pseudotumor (a case report). Anticancer Res. 2002;22(3):1795–7.
100. Magro G, Michal M, Alaggio R, et al. Intradermal proliferative fasciitis in childhood: a potential diagnostic pitfall. J Cutan Pathol. 2011;38(1):59–62.
101. Marcoval J, Moreno A, Bordas X, et al. Diffuse plane xanthoma: clinicopathologic study of 8 cases. J Am Acad Dermatol. 1998;39(3):439–42.
102. Marino-Enriquez A, Fletcher CD. Angiofibroma of soft tissue: clinicopathologic characterization of a distinctive benign fibrovascular neoplasm in a series of 37 cases. Am J Surg Pathol. 2012;36(4):500–8.
103. Marque M, Bessis D, Pedeutour F, Viseux V, Guillot B, Fraitag-Spinner S. Medallion-like dermal dendrocyte hamartoma: the main diagnostic pitfall is congenital atrophic dermatofibrosarcoma. Br J Dermatol. 2009;160(1):190–3.
104. McNiff JM, Subtil A, Cowper SE, Lazova R, Glusac EJ. Cellular digital fibromas: distinctive CD34-positive lesions that may mimic dermatofibrosarcoma protuberans. J Cutan Pathol. 2005;32(6):413–8.

105. Mehrad M, LaFramboise WA, Lyons MA, Trejo Bittar HE, Yousem SA. Whole exome sequencing identifies unique mutations and copy number losses in calcifying fibrous tumor of the pleura: report of three cases and review of the literature. Hum Pathol. 2018. pii: S0046-8177(18)30125-4. https://doi.org/10.1016/j.humpath.2018.04.005. [Epub ahead of print].
106. Meis JM, Enzinger FM. Proliferative fasciitis and myositis of childhood. Am J Surg Pathol. 1992;16(4):364–72.
107. Mentzel T, Kutzner H. Dermatomyofibroma: clinicopathologic and immunohistochemical analysis of 56 cases and reappraisal of a rare and distinct cutaneous neoplasm. Am J Dermatopathol. 2009;31:44.
108. Mentzel T, Kutzner H, Rütten A, Hügel H. Benign fibrous histiocytoma (dermatofibroma) of the face: clinicopathologic and immunohistochemical study of 34 cases associated with an aggressive clinical course. Am J Dermatopathol. 2001;23(5):419–26.
109. Mentzel T, Wiesner T, Cerroni L, Hantschke M, Kutzner H, Rütten A, et al. Malignant dermatofibroma: clinicopathological, immunohistochemical, and molecular analysis of seven cases. Mod Pathol. 2013;26(2):256–67.
110. Metcalf JS, Maize JC, LeBoit PE. Circumscribed storiform collagenoma (sclerosing fibroma). Am J Dermatopathol. 1991;13(2):122–9.
111. Michael M, Fetsch JF, Hes O, Miettinen M. Nuchal-type fibroma: A clinical pathologic study 52 cases. Cancer. 1999;85(1):156–63.
112. Michal M, Mukensnabl P, Chlumska A, et al. Fibrous hamartoma of infancy. A study of eight cases with immunohistochemical and electron microscopical findings. Pathol Res Pract. 1992;188:1049–53.
113. Miettinen M, Fetch JF. Collagenous fibroma (desmoplastic fibroblastoma): A clinicopathologic analysis of 63 cases of a distinctive soft tissue lesion with stellate-shaped fibroblasts. Hum Pathol. 1998;29:676–82.
114. Miettinen M, Fetsch JF. Reticulohistiocytoma (solitary epithelioid histiocytoma): a clinicopathologic and immunohistochemical study of 44 cases. Am J Surg Pathol. 2006;30(4):521–8.
115. Monaghan H, Salter DM, Al-Nafussi A. Giant cell tumour of tendon sheath (localised nodular tenosynovitis): clinicopathological features of 71 cases. J Clin Pathol. 2001;54(5):404–7.
116. Montgomery EA, Meis JM. Nodular fasciitis. Its morphologic spectrum and immunohistochemical profile. Am J Surg Pathol. 1991;15(10):942–8.
117. Montgomery H, Osterberg AE. Xanthomatosis: correlation of clinical histopathologic and chemical studies of cutaneous xanthoma. Arch Dermatol Syph. 1938;37:373.
118. Montgomery E, Lee JH, Abraham SC, Wu TT. Superficial fibromatoses are genetically distinct from deep fibromatoses. Mod Pathol. 2001;14(7):695–701. PMID:11455002.
119. Moosavi CA, Al-Nahar LA, Murphey MD, Fanburg-Smith JC. Fibroosseous pseudotumor of the digit: a clinicopathologic study of 43 new cases. Ann Diagn Pathol. 2008;12(1):21–8.
120. Nagamine N, Nohara Y, Ito E. Elastofibroma in Okinawa. A clinicopathologic study of 170 cases. Cancer. 1982;50(9):1794–805.
121. Nascimento AG. A clinicopathologic and immunohistochemical comparative study of cutaneous and intramuscular forms of juvenile xanthogranuloma. Am J Surg Pathol. 1997;21(6):645–52.
122. Nofal A, Sanad M, Assaf M, et al. Juvenile hyaline fibromatosis and infantile systemic hyalinosis: a unifying term and a proposed grading system. J Am Acad Dermatol. 2009;61(4):695–700.
123. Page RN, King R, Mihm MC Jr, Googe PB. Microphthalmia transcription factor and NKI/C3 expression in cellular neurothekeoma. Mod Pathol. 2004;17:230–4.
124. Patchefsky AS, Enzinger FM. Intravascular fasciitis: a report of 17 cases. Am J Surg Pathol. 1981;5(1):29–36.
125. Paties C, Vassallo G, Taccagni GL. Clear cell dermatofibroma. Am J Surg Pathol. 1997;21(2):250–2.
126. Paxton CN, O'Malley DP, Bellizzi AM, Alkapalan D, Fedoriw Y, Hornick JL, Perkins SL, South ST, Andersen EF. Genetic evaluation of juvenile xanthogranuloma: genomic abnormalities are uncommon in solitary lesions, advanced cases may show more complexity. Mod Pathol. 2017;30(9):1234–40.
127. Pennacchia I, Kutzner H, Kazakov DV, Mentzel T. Fibroblastic connective tissue nevus: clinicopathological and immunohistochemical study of 14 cases. J Cutan Pathol. 2017;44(10):827–34.
128. Pérez LP, Zulaica A, Rodríguez L, Campo MC, Peñaranda JM, Fernández-Redondo V, et al. Multinucleate cell angiohistiocytoma. Report of five cases. J Cutan Pathol. 2006;33:349–52.
129. Perosio PM, Weiss SW. Ischemic fasciitis: a juxta-skeletal fibroblastic proliferation with a predilection for elderly patients. Mod Pathol. 1993;6(1):69–72.
130. Pezhouh MK, Rezaei MK, Shabihkhani M, Ghosh A, Belchis D, Montgomery EA, Voltaggio L. Clinicopathologic study of calcifying fibrous tumor of the gastrointestinal tract: a case series. Hum Pathol. 2017;62:199–205.
131. Pulitzer DR, Martin PC, Reed RJ. Fibroma of tendon sheath. A clinicopathologic study of 32 cases. Am J Surg Pathol. 1989;13(6):472–9.
132. Puls F, Hofvander J, Magnusson L, Nilsson J, Haywood E, Sumathi VP, et al. FN1-EGF gene fusions are recurrent in calcifying aponeurotic fibroma. J Pathol. 2016;238(4):502–7. PMID:26691015.
133. Rao AS, Vigorita VJ. Pigmented villonodular synovitis (giant-cell tumor of the tendon sheath and synovial membrane). A review of eighty-one cases. J Bone Joint Surg Am. 1984;66(1):76–94.
134. Rapini RP, Golitz LE. Sclerotic fibromas of the skin. J Am Acad Dermatol. 1989;20(2 Pt 1):266–271. PMID:2464630.
135. Ravić-Nikolić A, Mladenović V, Mitrović S, Miličić V, Djukić A, Jovović-Dagović B, Savčić G. Generalized

eruptive xanthomas associated with diabetic dyslipidemia. Eur J Dermatol. 2014;24(3):394–5.
136. Requena L, Gutiérrez J, Sánchez Yus E. Multiple sclerotic fibromas of the skin. A cutaneous marker of Cowden's disease. J Cutan Pathol. 1992;19(4):346–351. PMID:1430474.
137. Reye RD. Recurring digital fibrous tumors of childhood. Arch Pathol. 1965;80:228–31.
138. Rosa G, Billings SD. A report of three cases of pediatric proliferative fasciitis. J Cutan Pathol. 2014;41(9):720–3.
139. Rougemont AL, Fetni R, Murthy S, et al. A complex translocation (6;12;8)(q25;q24.3;q13) in a fibrous hamartoma of infancy. Cancer Genet Cytogenet. 2006;171:115–8.
140. Saab ST, McClain CM, Coffin CM. Fibrous hamartoma of infancy: a clinicopathologic analysis of 60 cases. Am J Surg Pathol. 2014;38(3):394–401.
141. Sachak T, Heerema NA, Mayerson J, Payne JE, Parwani A, Iwenofu OH. Novel t(1;2)(p36.1;q23) and t(7;19)(q32;q13.3) chromosomal translocations in ischemic fasciitis: expanding the spectrum of pseudosarcomatous lesions with clonal pathogenetic link. Diagn Pathol. 2018;13(1):18.
142. Schaffer JV, Gohara MA, McNiff JM, et al. Multiple facial angiofibromas: A cutaneous manifestation of Birt–Hogg–Dubé syndrome. J Am Acad Dermatol. 2005;53:S108–11.
143. Sciot R, Samson I, van den Berghe H, van Damme B, Dal CP. Collagenous fibroma (desmoplastic fibroblastoma): Genetic link with fibroma of tendon sheath? Mod Pathol. 1999a;12:565–8.
144. Sciot R, Rosai J, Dal Cin P, et al. Analysis of 35 cases of localized and diffuse tenosynovial giant cell tumor: a report from the Chromosomes and Morphology (CHAMP) study group. Mod Pathol. 1999b;12(6):576–9.
145. Shek TW, Chan AC, Ma L. Extra-nuchal nuchal fibroma. Am J Surg Pathol. 1996;20(7):902–3.
146. Shimizu S, Hashimoto H, Enjoji M. Nodular fasciitis: an analysis of 250 patients. Pathology. 1984;16(2):161–6.
147. Sigel JE, Smith TA, Reith JD, et al. Immunohistochemical analysis of anaplastic lymphoma kinase expression in deep soft tissue calcifying fibrous pseudotumor: evidence of a late sclerosing stage of inflammatory myofibroblastic tumor? Ann Diagn Pathol. 2001;5(1):10–4.
148. Singh Gomez C, Calonje E, Fletcher CD. Epithelioid benign fibrous histiocytoma of skin: clinicopathological analysis of 20 cases of a poorly known variant. Histopathology. 1994;24(2):123–9.
149. Smith NP, Wilson JE. Multinucleate cell angiohistiocytoma: a new entity. Br J Dermatol. 1985; 113:15.
150. Somerhausen NS, Fletcher CD. Diffuse-type giant cell tumor: clinicopathologic and immunohistochemical analysis of 50 cases with extraarticular disease. Am J Surg Pathol. 2000;24(4):479–92.
151. Soyer HP, Kutzner H, Metze D, et al. Clear-cell fibrous papule. J Cutan Pathol. 1996;23:62.
152. Stratton J, Billings SD. Cellular neurothekeoma: analysis of 37 cases emphasizing atypical histologic features. Mod Pathol. 2014;27:701–10.
153. Stuart LN, Hiatt KM, Zohreh Z, Gardner JM, Shalin SC. Plaque-like CD34-positive dermal fibroma/medallion-like dendrocyte hamartoma: an unusual spindle cell neoplasm. J Cutan Pathol. 2014;41:625–9.
154. Tamada S, Ackerman AB. Dermatofibroma with monster cells. Am J Dermatopathol. 1987;9(5):380–7. PMID:2825558.
155. Tardío JC, Butrón M, Martín-Fragueiro LM. Superficial acral fibromyxoma: report of 4 cases with CD10 expression and lipomatous component, two previously under recognized features. Am J Dermatopathol. 2008;30(5):431–5.
156. Tashakori M, Pimentl J, Howitt BE, Sanchez J, Michalowski S, Chitale D, Ormsby AH, Williamson SR. Pleomorphic fibroma of the skin with MDM2 immunoreactivity: A potential diagnostic pitfall. J Cutan Pathol. 2018;45(1):59–62.
157. Techavichit P, Sosothikul D, Chaichana T, Teerapakpinyo C, Thorner PS, Shuangshoti S. BRAF V600E mutation in pediatric intracranial and cranial juvenile xanthogranuloma. Hum Pathol. 2017;69:118–22.
158. Tran P, McLemore M. Atypical cellular neurothekeoma: a potential diagnostic pitfall for benign and malignant spindle cell lesions in skin. J Cutan Pathol. 2018. https://doi.org/10.1111/cup.13274. [Epub ahead of print].
159. Tran TA, Hayner-Buchan A, Jones DM, McRorie D, Carlson JA. Cutaneous balloon cell dermatofibroma (fibrous histiocytoma). Am J Dermatopathol. 2007;29(2):197–200.
160. Ushijima M, Tsuneyoshi M, Enjoji M. Dupuytren type fibromatoses. A clinicopathologic study of 62 cases. Acta Pathol Jpn. 1984;34(5):991–1001. PMID:6507097.
161. Ushijima M, Hashimoto H, Tsuneyoshi M, et al. Giant cell tumor of the tendon sheath (nodular tenosynovitis). A study of 207 cases to compare the large joint group with the common digit group. Cancer. 1986;57(4):875–84.
162. Val-Bernal JF, Mira C. Dermatofibroma with granular cells. J Cutan Pathol. 1996;23(6):562–5. PMID:9001988.
163. Van Dorpe J, Ectors N, Geboes K, et al. Is calcifying fibrous pseudotumor a late sclerosing stage of inflammatory myofibroblastic tumor? Am J Surg Pathol. 1999;23(3):329–35.
164. Vanni R, Fletcher CD, Sciot R, Dal Cin P, De Wever I, Mandahl N, et al. Cytogenetic evidence of clonality in cutaneous benign fibrous histiocytomas: a report of the CHAMP study group. Histopathology. 2000;37(3):212–7. PMID:10971696.
165. Veugelers M, Wilkes D, Burton K, McDermott DA, Song Y, Goldstein MM, et al. Comparative PRKAR1A genotype-phenotype analyses in humans with Carney complex and prkar1a haploinsufficient mice. Proc Natl Acad Sci U S A. 2004;101(39):14222–7.

166. Walther C, Hofvander J, Nilsson J, Magnusson L, Domanski HA, Gisselsson D, et al. Gene fusion detection in formalin-fixed paraffin-embedded benign fibrous histiocytomas using fluorescence in situ hybridization and RNA sequencing. Lab Investig. 2015;95(9):1071–6. PMID:26121314.
167. Wambacher-Gasser B, Zelger B, Zelger BG, Steiner H. Clear cell dermatofibroma. Histopathology. 1997;30(1):64–9. PMID:9023559.
168. Wang GY, Nazarian RM, Zhao L, Hristov AC, Patel RM, Fullen DR, Chan MP. Protein gene product 9.5 (PGP9.5) expression in benign cutaneous mesenchymal, histiocytic, and melanocytic lesions: comparison with cellular neurothekeoma. Pathology. 2017;49(1):44–9.
169. Wehrli BM, Weiss SW, Yandow S, Coffin CM. Gardner associated fibromas (GAF) in young patients: A distinct fibrous lesion that identifies unsuspected Gardner's syndrome and risk for fibromatosis. Am J Surg Pathol. 2001;25(5):645–51.
170. Weinreb I, Shaw AJ, Perez-Ordoñez B, et al. Nodular fasciitis of the head and neck region: a clinicopathologic description in a series of 30 cases. J Cutan Pathol. 2009;36(11):1168–73.
171. West RB, Rubin BP, Miller MA, et al. A landscape effect in tenosynovial giant-cell tumor from activation of CSF1 expression by a translocation in a minority of tumor cells. Proc Natl Acad Sci U S A. 2006;103(3):690–5.
172. Winkelmann RK. Cutaneous syndromes of non-X histiocytosis. A review of the macrophage-histiocyte diseases of the skin. Arch Dermatol. 1981;117(10):667–72.
173. Yamada Y, Yamamoto H, Kohashi K, Ishii T, Iura K, Maekawa A, Bekki H, Otsuka H, Yamashita K, Tanaka H, Hiraki T, Mukai M, Shirakawa A, Shinnou Y, Jinno M, Yanai H, Taguchi K, Maehara Y, Iwamoto Y, Oda Y. Histological spectrum of angiofibroma of soft tissue: histological and genetic analysis of 13 cases. Histopathology. 2016;69(3):459–69.
174. Yamawaki S, Naitoh M, Kubota H, Aya R, Katayama Y, Ishiko T, Tamura T, Yoshikawa K, Enoshiri T, Ikeda M, Suzuki S. Htra1 is specifically up-regulated in active keloid lesions and stimulates keloid development. Int J Mol Sci. 2018;19(5):pii: E1275.
175. Yantiss RK, Nielsen GP, Lauwers GY, et al. Reactive nodular fibrous pseudotumor of the gastrointestinal tract and mesentery: a clinicopathologic study of five cases. Am J Surg Pathol. 2003;27(4):532–40.
176. Zelger B, Cerio R, Soyer HP, et al. Reticulohistiocytoma and multicentric reticulohistiocytosis. Histopathologic and immunophenotypic distinct entities. Am J Dermatopathol [Comparative Study]. 1994;16(6):577–84.
177. Zelger BW, Zelger BG, Steiner H, Ofner D. Aneurysmal and haemangiopericytoma-like fibrous histiocytoma. J Clin Pathol. 1996;49(4):313–8.

Fibrous, Fibrohistiocytic, and Myofibroblastic Tumors of Intermediate Malignancy

5

Reena Singh, Aaron M. Udager, Steven D. Billings, and Rajiv M. Patel

Abstract

Fibrous, fibrohistiocytic, and myofibroblastic tumors of intermediate malignancy comprise a group of lesions that has a relatively high risk of local recurrence, but a limited risk of metastasis. Most of these tumors present in young adults as superficial masses. Members of this group include dermatofibrosarcoma protuberans and its numerous variants, plexiform fibrohistiocytic tumor, angiomatoid fibrous histiocytoma, giant cell tumor of soft tissue, and inflammatory myofibroblastic tumor.

R. Singh
Department of Pathology, Oregon Health and Science University School of Medicine, Portland, OR, USA

A. M. Udager · R. M. Patel (✉)
Department of Pathology, University of Michigan Medical School, Ann Arbor, MI, USA
e-mail: rajivpat@umich.edu

S. D. Billings
Department of Pathology, Cleveland Clinic, Cleveland, OH, USA

Dermatofibrosarcoma Protuberans

Clinical Features

Dermatofibrosarcoma protuberans (DFSP) is the most common dermal sarcoma. It generally affects adults aged 20–50 years, but any age group may be affected. Pediatric cases account for 6% of all DFSP cases. Giant cell fibroblastoma (GCF) is considered a pediatric form of DFSP. GCF typically presents in children less than 10 years of age and is more common in boys. Rare congenital cases and adult cases have been described. Pigmented DFSP, or Bednar tumor, appears to occur more often in dark-skinned patients, but the other DFSP variants lack any racial or ethnic predilection.

The most commonly affected sites are the trunk, proximal extremities, and head and neck in descending frequency. A series of distal extremity and acral cases have also recently been reported. A prolonged period of slow growth correlating with clinically indurated plaques is followed by rapid progression and development of multiple protruding nodules from the precursor plaques. This latter characteristic clinical feature lends the tumor its namesake. Bednar tumor usually has a blue to black appearance depending on the degree of melanin pigmentation present. The atrophic variant of DFSP does not have a protuberant phase, maintaining its clinical appearance as a depressed plaque.

S. D. Billings et al. (eds.), *Soft Tissue Tumors of the Skin*,
https://doi.org/10.1007/978-1-4939-8812-9_5

The rate of local recurrence is 20–50% with incomplete excision, but the risk of metastasis is low (<5%) and usually happens only after multiple recurrences. DFSP with fibrosarcomatous transformation (DFSP-FS) has a higher rate of local recurrence (exceeding 50%) and distant metastasis (10–15%). Clinical outcome is not impacted by the percent of fibrosarcomatous transformation present in a given case. The lungs are the most common site of metastasis, and nodal metastases are rare. Mohs micrographic surgery has lower rates of local recurrence than conventional wide excision; this improved outcome is likely related to the often asymmetric growth of DFSP and the technical limitations of wide excision to achieve tumor-free margins in this setting. For inoperable or metastatic cases, chemotherapy with tyrosine kinase inhibitors, such as imatinib mesylate, has been shown to have clinical benefit in a significant proportion of patients.

Pathologic Features

Conventional DFSP is a poorly circumscribed, low-grade fibroblastic tumor involving the dermis and subcutis (Fig. 5.1a). Rare solitary subcutaneous tumors without dermal involvement can rarely occur (Fig. 5.1b). The overlying epidermis is usually slightly atrophic or near normal in appearance. The tumor cells are arranged in a collagenous stroma in either a storiform pattern (Fig. 5.1c, d) or in short intersecting fascicles that run parallel to the overlying skin. Conventional DFSP has finely collagenous stroma, but there may be foci of extensive hyalinization or myxoid change. As long as the aforementioned stromal changes involve less than 50% of the tumor, it can be designated as conventional DFSP.

The tumor cells have scant cytoplasm and uniform nuclei with little or no pleomorphism and mitotic activity. Extension into the surrounding tissue occurs via tentacles that spread along tissue septa, and infiltration into the subcutis imparts a characteristic honeycomb appearance without appreciable fat necrosis or inflammation (Fig. 5.1e). There may be invasion into deeper structures, including fascia, muscle, periosteum, and bone. Lesions on the scalp are associated with early periosteal involvement. Secondary features, including inflammatory cells, hemosiderin, multinucleated giant cells, and histiocytes, are uncommon. There are numerous histologic variants of DFSP, which are described below.

Diffuse immunoreactivity for CD34 is observed in 80–100% of cases. DFSP is negative for FXIIIa, smooth muscle actin, desmin, S100, and keratins. In general, the aforementioned immunophenotype is common to all variants of DFSP, and any differences will be subsequently noted. Greater than 90% of tumors harbor a recurrent t(17;22)(q22;q13) translocation, resulting in *COL1A1-PDGFB* gene fusion and amplification, yielding constitutive activation of the PDGFB tyrosine kinase receptor. This genetic aberration is present in all histologic DFSP subtypes. FISH remains a more reliable means of detecting the rearrangement over RT-PCR, due to the variable breakpoints for *COL1A1*. The remaining percentage of DFSP (<10%) have variant genetic aberrations.

Pigmented Variant (Bednar Tumor)

Bednar tumor is similar to conventional DFSP, but with the addition of variable amounts of melanin-containing dendritic cells (Fig. 5.2). The entire tumor is positive for CD34, but only the dendritic cells are positive for S100 protein and SOX10 and/or other melanocytic markers, such as Melan-A and HMB45.

Giant Cell Fibroblastoma

GCF is comprised of ovoid fibroblastic cells and pleomorphic multinucleated giant cells in a variably fibrous to myxoid stroma. Pseudovascular spaces lined by moderately atypical tumor cells and/or multinucleated tumor cells are commonly present (Fig. 5.3a–c). Perivascular lymphocytes arranged in an onionskin pattern may be present (Fig. 5.3d). GCF may have areas of conventional or myxoid DFSP. Recurrent lesions may maintain the morphology of GCF, have hybrid features of conventional DFSP, or be completely composed of conventional DFSP.

Myxoid DFSP

A designation of myxoid DFSP is used when myxoid change accounts for more than 50% of the tumor. Myxoid DFSP often has a multinodular growth pattern. The stellate and fusiform spindle cells are uniformly distributed in a random fashion within a myxoid stroma. Scattered thin-walled vessels are especially prominent in this variant (Fig. 5.4a), as are occasional multinucleated cells reminiscent of those seen in GCF. Areas of conventional DFSP and/or GCF aid in the diagnosis and are present in approximately 60% of adequately sampled cases (Fig. 5.4b).

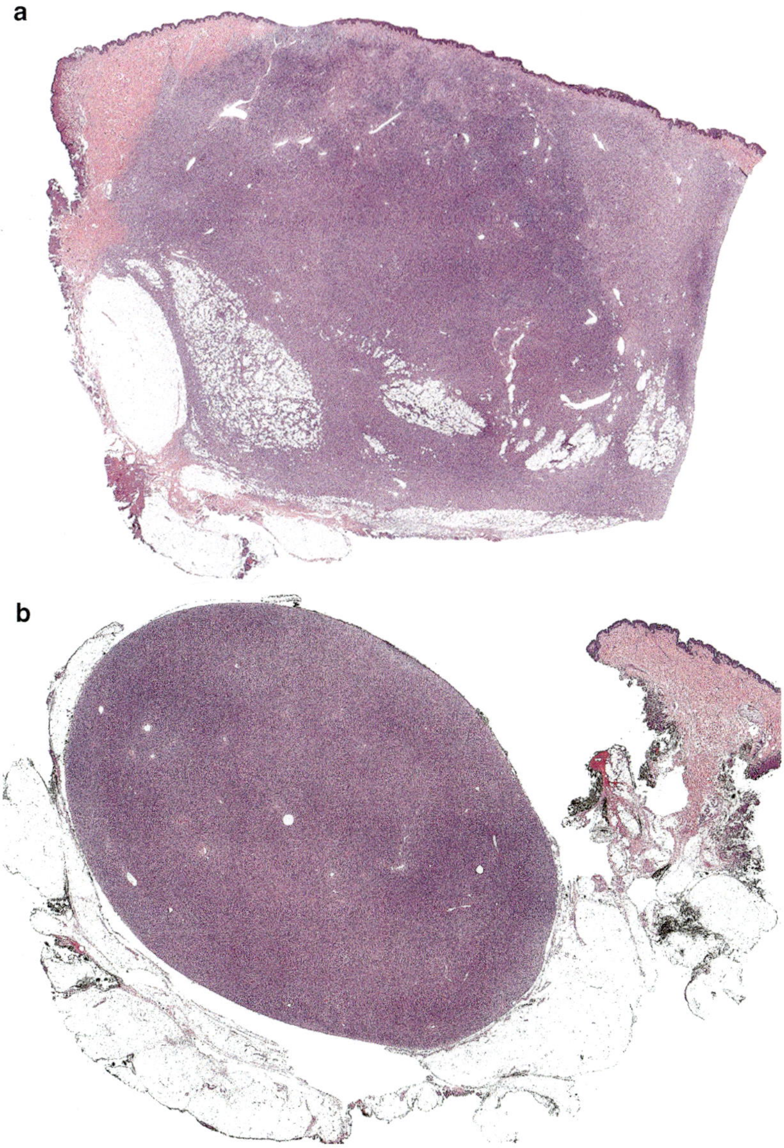

Fig. 5.1 (**a**) Conventional dermatofibrosarcoma protuberans involving dermis and subcutis. (**b**) Rarely cases may be restricted to the subcutis. (**c**) Tumor cells are typically arranged in a storiform pattern. (**d**) Spindled tumor cells with minimal pleomorphism and sparse mitotic activity within a collagenous stroma. (**e**) Honeycomb pattern of infiltration into subcutaneous fat

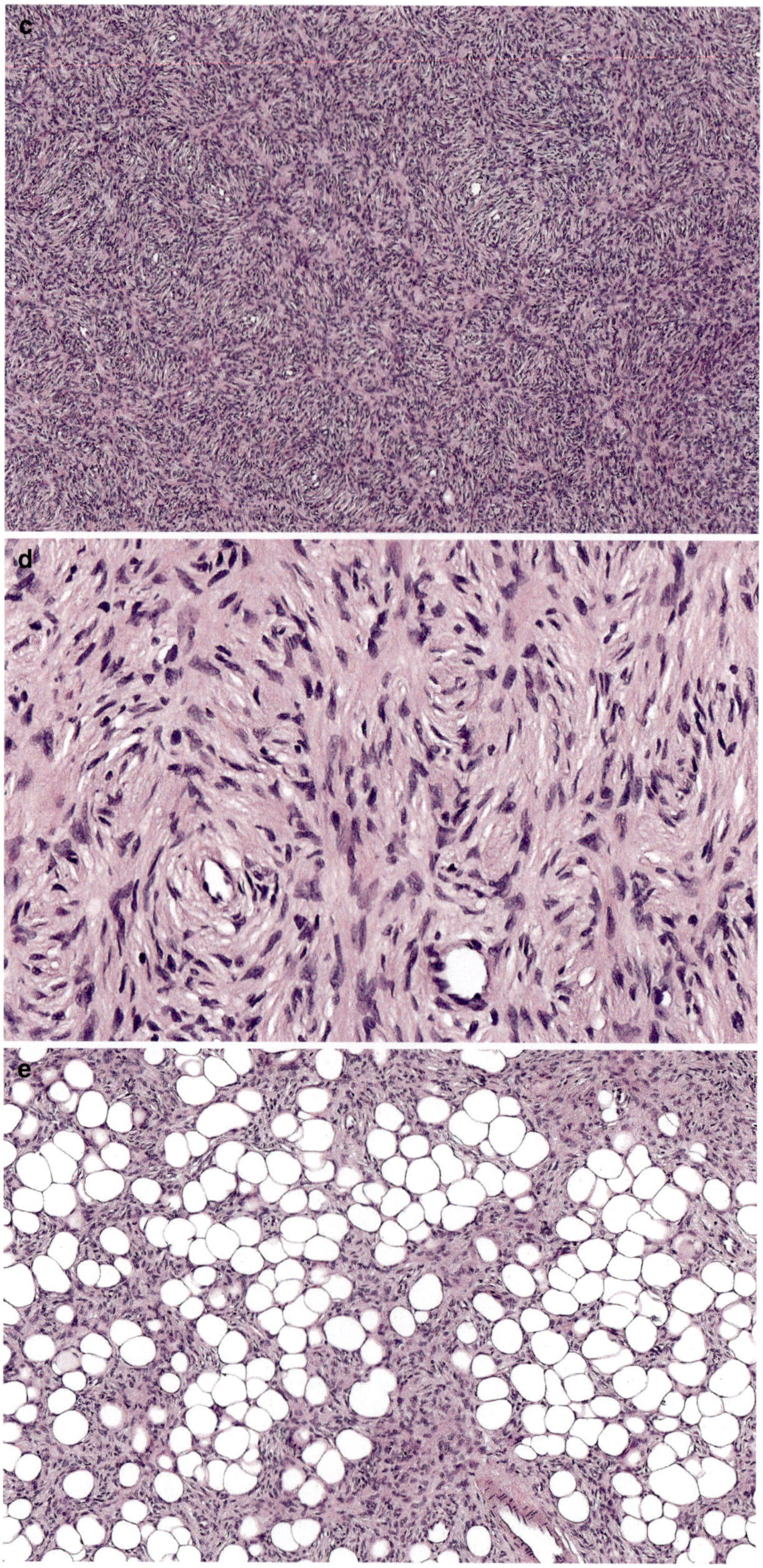

Fig. 5.1 (continued)

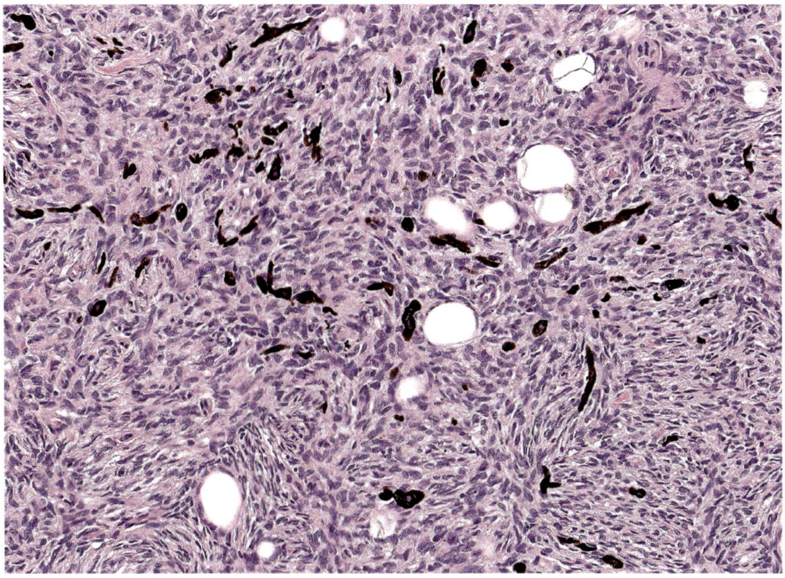

Fig. 5.2 Bednar tumor demonstrating admixed melanin-containing dendritic cells

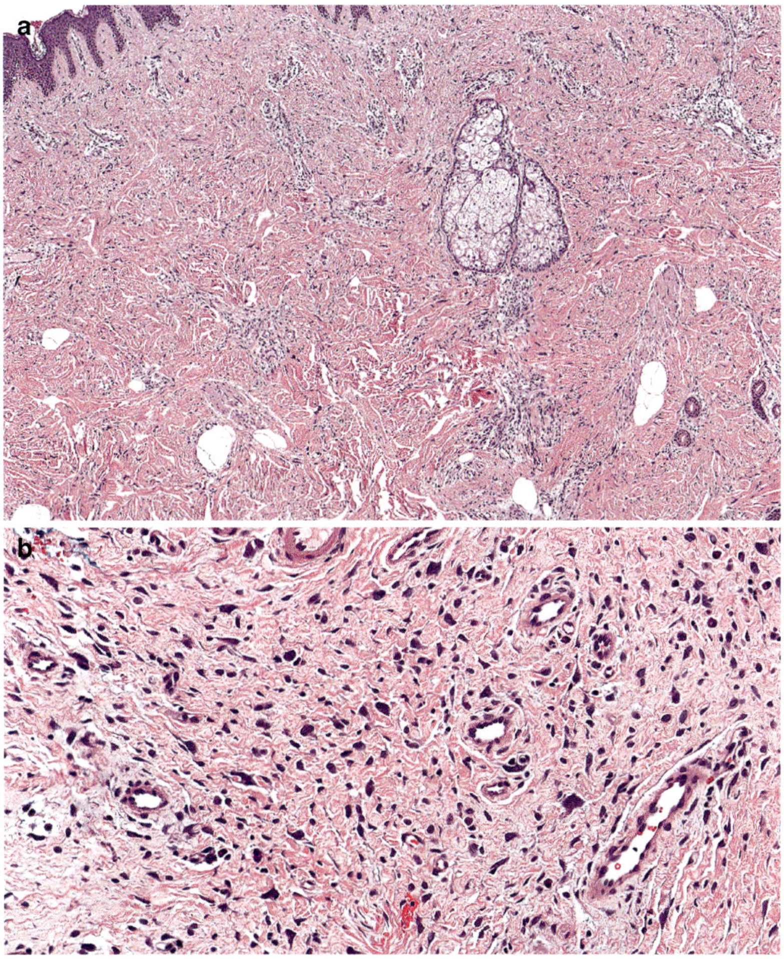

Fig. 5.3 (**a**) Low-power view of giant cell fibroblastoma. (**b**) Higher-power examination of fibroblastic cells and pleomorphic multinucleated giant cells. (**c**) Pseudovascular spaces are lined by atypical tumor cells. (**d**) Perivascular extravasation of lymphocytes in an onionskin pattern

Fig. 5.3 (continued)

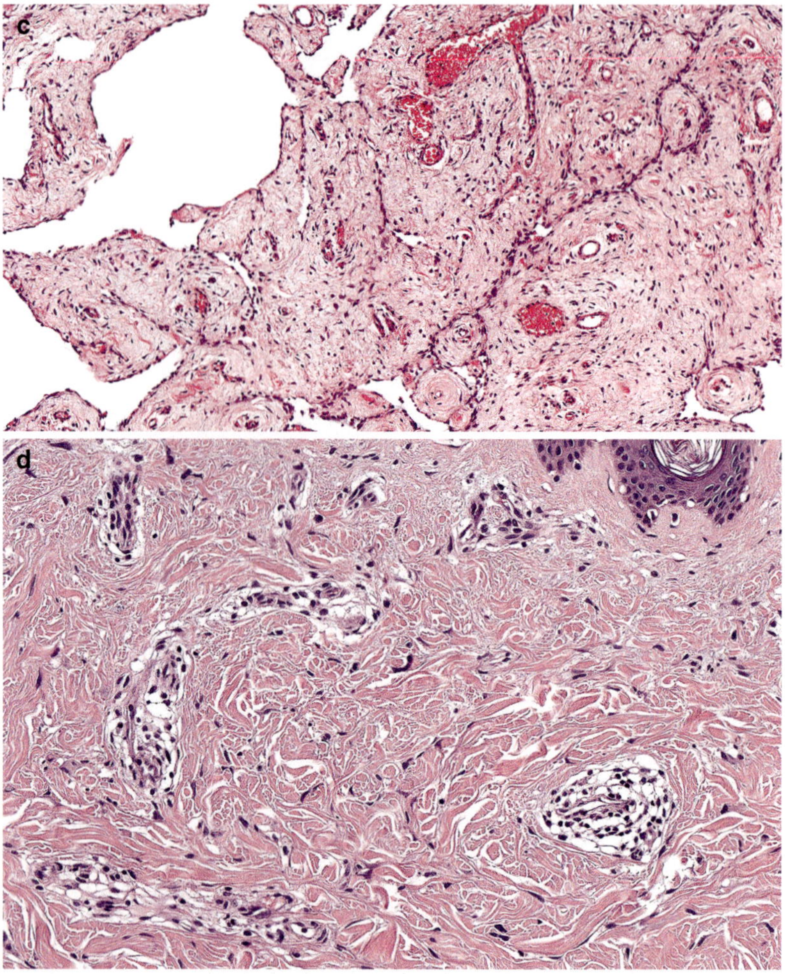

Atrophic Variant

Histologically, the atrophic variant demonstrates greater than 50% thinning of the involved dermis when compared to the surrounding, uninvolved dermis and a parallel arrangement of lesional cells (Fig. 5.5a–c). Both the clinical appearance of a plaque and the aforementioned histologic features are required for the diagnosis of this DFSP variant.

Sclerosing Variant

The sclerosing variant is characterized by paucicellular or acellular foci that contain densely homogenous collagen, which accounts for more than half of the mass (Fig. 5.6a). Conventional DFSP histology may be observed in the remainder of the tumor. The etiology of the sclerosis is unknown, and in these foci the tumor cells may demonstrate nuclear palisading reminiscent of schwannoma (Fig. 5.6b).

Myoid Variant

Myoid differentiation in DFSP is another rare phenomenon, which is characterized by conventional DFSP with scattered to confluent nodules of spindle cells with distinct cytoplasmic boundaries, eosinophilic cytoplasm, and vesicular nuclei (Fig. 5.7). This latter population of cells is negative for CD34 and positive for smooth muscle actin and desmin. Myoid differentiation may

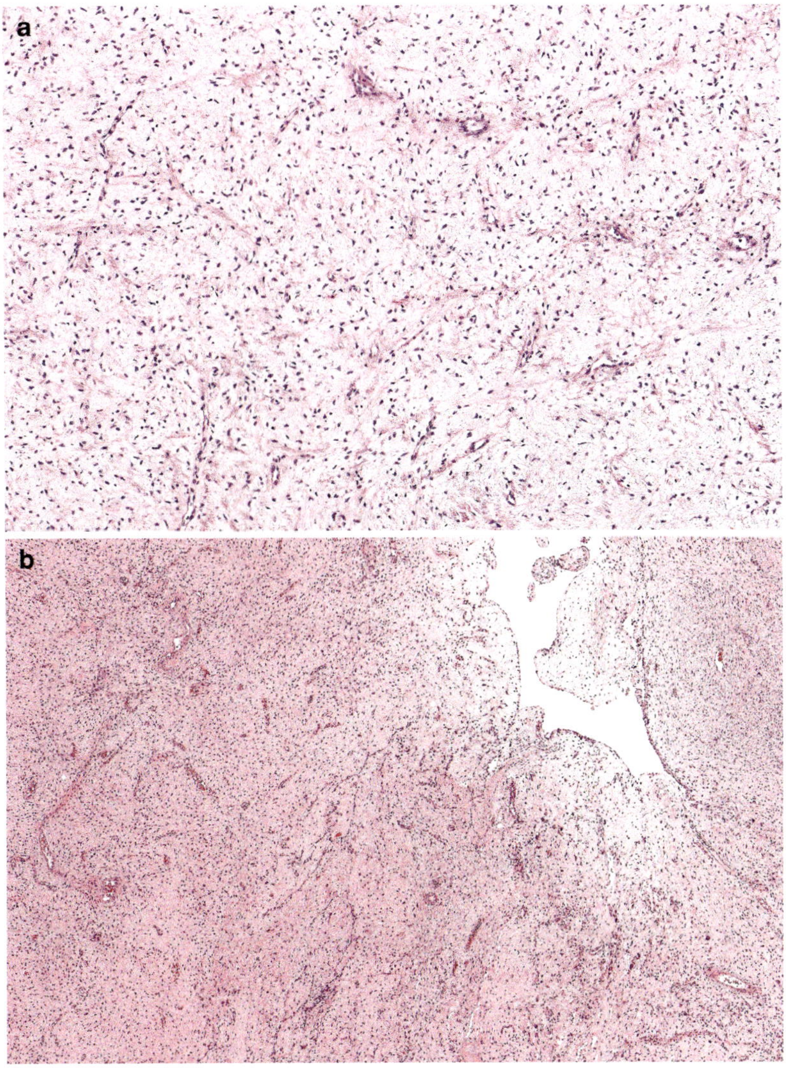

Fig. 5.4 (**a**) Myxoid dermatofibrosarcoma protuberans with uniformly distributed bland stellate and fusiform cells and prominent vascularity. (**b**) Recognition of pseudovascular spaces similar to those seen in GCF can be helpful in the diagnosis of myxoid DFSP

be secondary to hyperplasia of intralesional vascular smooth muscle or the proliferation of pericytes with "myoid" differentiation.

Granular Cell Variant

The granular cell variant is extremely rare, with just four reported cases. Cells with abundant granular cytoplasm, round eccentrically located nuclei, and prominent nucleoli are admixed with conventional DFSP. The granular cells are positive for NKI/C3, but negative for S100 protein, HMB-45, CD34, and keratin.

DFSP with Fibrosarcomatous Transformation

Fibrosarcomatous transformation occurs in 10–20% DFSPs and can arise in all histologic variants (Fig. 5.8a). Sarcomatous change usually resembles conventional fibrosarcoma and is characterized by an expansive growth pattern with a fascicular and herringbone arrangement of atypical spindled tumor cells (Fig. 5.8b). Transformation to high-grade undifferentiated pleomorphic sarcoma is extremely rare. The fusiform tumor cells have enlarged, hyperchromatic and mitotically active nuclei (exceeding four mitotic figures per ten high-power fields) (Fig. 5.8c). CD34 expression may be weak and focal, or absent altogether in fibrosarcomatous areas. The surrounding conventional DFSP retains immunoreactivity for CD34, and this is a useful clue to the diagnosis. *TP53* mutations and p53 protein overexpression have been reported with fibrosarcomatous transformation (Table 5.1).

Differential Diagnosis

Given the numerous variants, the differential diagnosis of DFSP is unsurprisingly broad. Additionally, many of the entities in the differential are also positive for CD34. Conventional DFSP must be differentiated from cellular fibrous histiocytoma, a dermal-based lesion that may

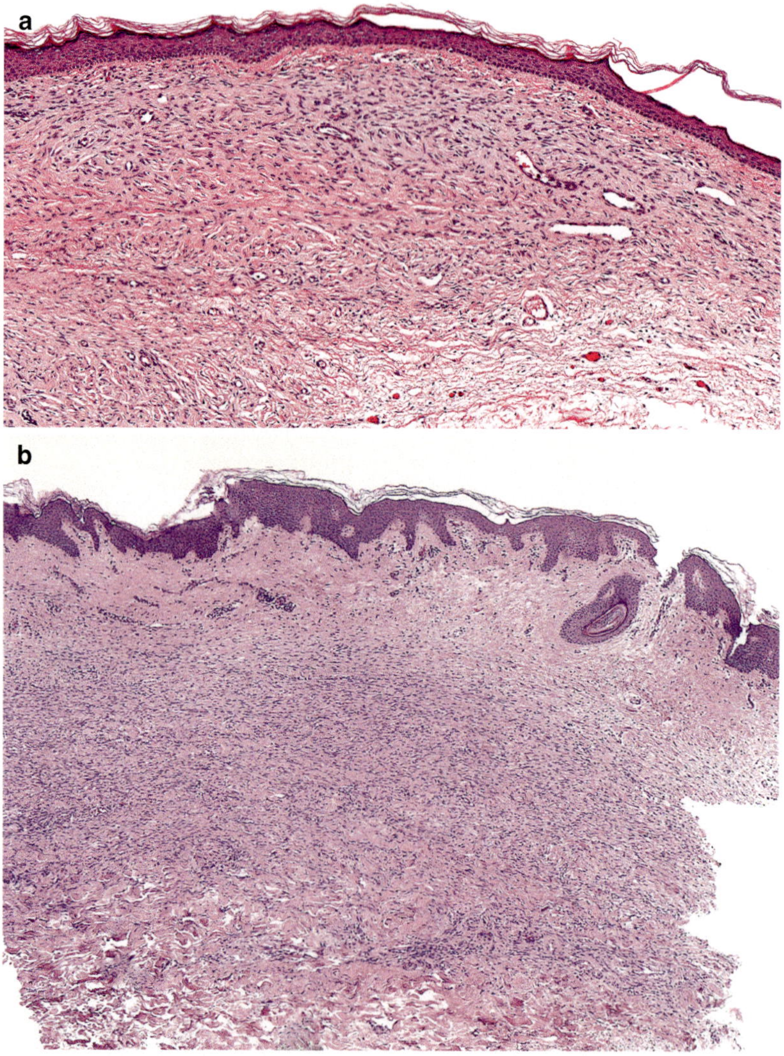

Fig. 5.5 (**a**, **b**) Atrophic DFSP with minimal (**a**) and more extensive plaque-like growth (**b**). Note thinning of the epidermis in example (**a**). (**c**) Higher-power view of parallel arrangement of lesional cells. (Images 5**b**, **c** courtesy of Dr. Thomas Mentzel, Dermatopathology Bodensee, Friedrichshafen, Germany)

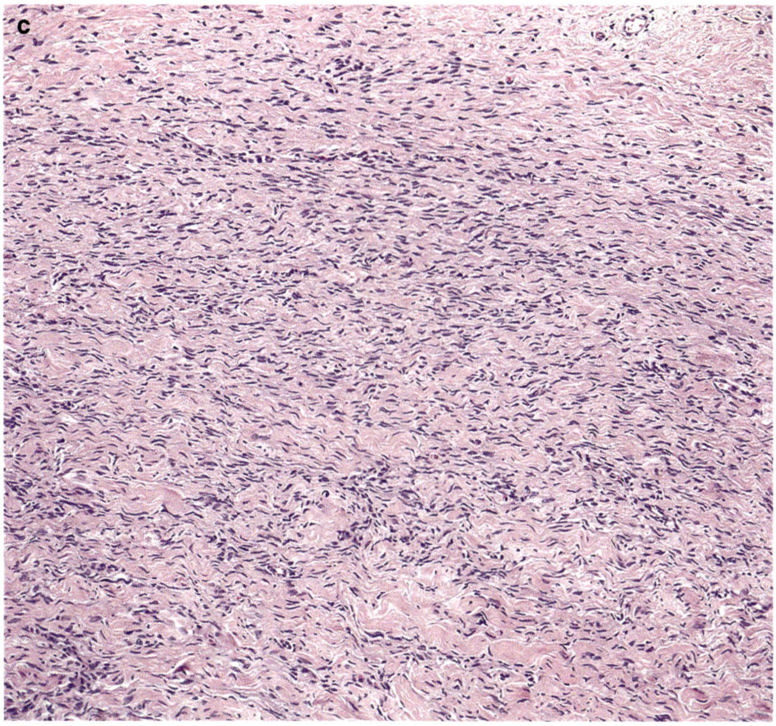

Fig. 5.5 (continued)

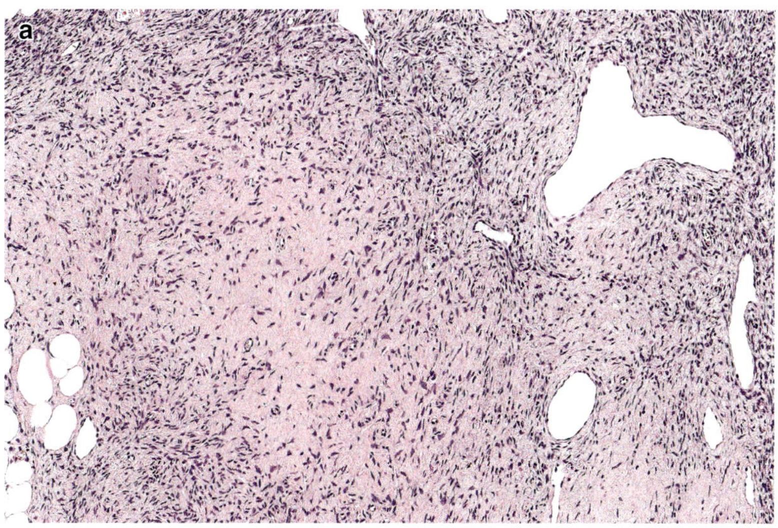

Fig. 5.6 (**a**) Sclerosing DFSP with dense stromal hyalinization. (**b**) Nuclear palisading similar to that seen in schwannoma is sometimes seen in sclerosing DFSP

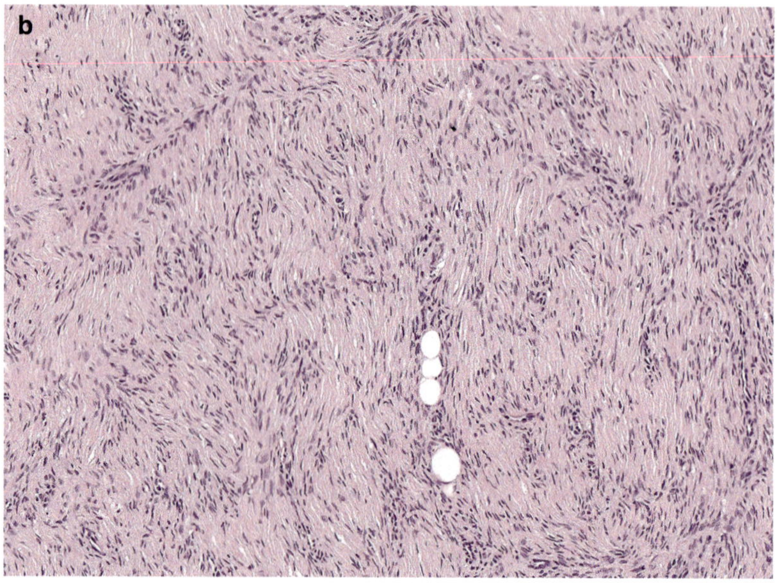

Fig. 5.6 (continued)

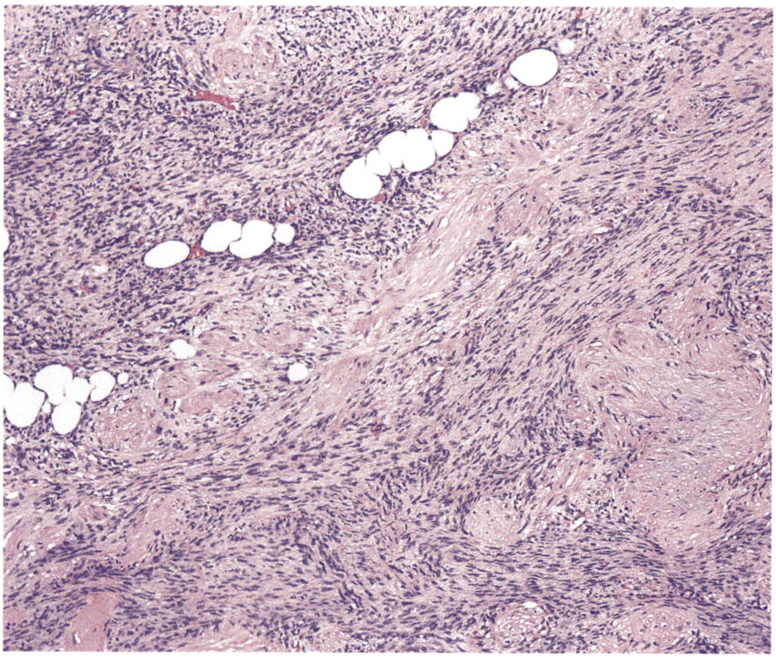

Fig. 5.7 Myoid DFSP with scattered and confluent myoid nodules composed of spindle cells with abundant eosinophilic cytoplasm and indistinct boundaries. (Image courtesy of Dr. Thomas Mentzel, Dermatopathology Bodensee, Friedrichshafen, Germany)

also exhibit storiform growth and can focally extend into the subcutaneous fat. Cellular fibrous histiocytoma will send out short radial extensions into the surrounding fat often accompanied by fat necrosis and an inflammatory infiltrate, unlike the broad front of "honeycomb" fat infiltration seen in DFSP; the latter also typically lacks fat necrosis and inflammation. Additional histologic differences seen in cellular fibrous histiocytoma include hyperplasia of the overlying dermis (in more superficial cases) and the peripheral collagen trapping typical of all benign fibrous histiocytomas. Secondary elements (admixed inflammatory cells, foamy histiocytes, pigment-laden macrophages, Touton-like giant cells) may also be present in small numbers in some cases of

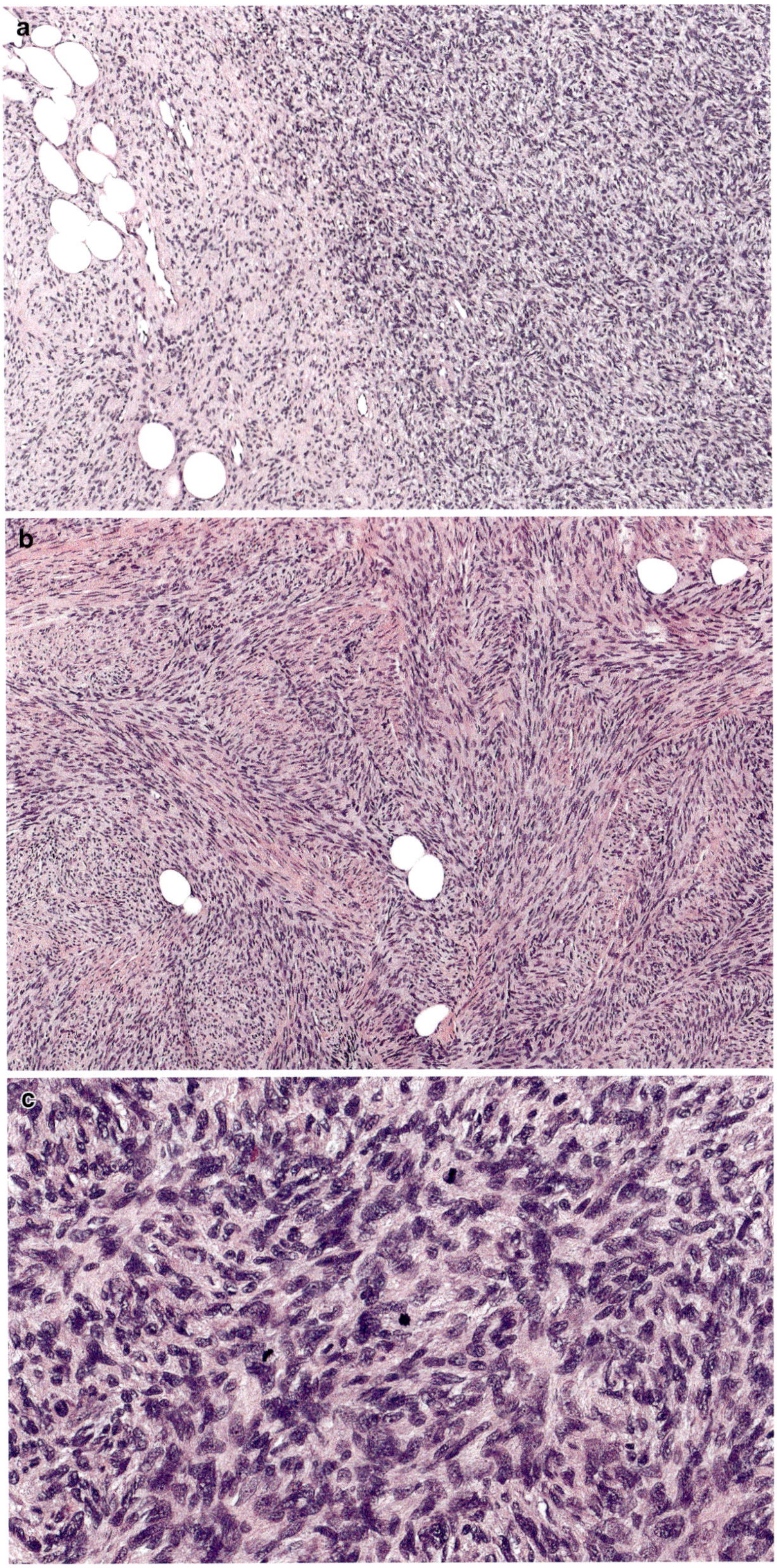

Fig. 5.8 (**a**) Fibrosarcomatous transformation (right) occurring within in conventional DFSP. (**b**) The fibrosarcomatous component is composed of atypical, hyperchromatic spindled cells in a herringbone pattern. (**c**) The fibrosarcomatous component has increased mitotic activity

Table 5.1 Key pathologic features: DFSP and variants

Conventional dermatofibrosarcoma protuberans (DFSP)
Monotonous spindle cells
Storiform growth
Honeycomb infiltration of subcutaneous fat in the absence of fat necrosis and inflammation
Cytologic atypia and mitoses rare
COL1A1-PDGFB fusion
Bednar tumor
Conventional DFSP with melanin-containing, S100-positive dendritic cells
Giant cell fibroblastoma
Spindled and multinucleated cells
Pseudovascular spaces lined by tumor cells
Myxoid change, hemorrhage, and lymphocytes may be present
May have areas of conventional DFSP
Myxoid variant
Myxoid change in more than 50% of tumor
Spindle and stellate cells uniformly distributed in abundant myxoid stroma
Prominent thin-walled vessels
Atrophic variant
Greater than 50% thinning of involved dermis
Parallel arrangement of lesional cells
Need histologic features and clinical, nonprotuberant growth to make the diagnosis
Sclerosing variant
Paucicellular or acellular hyalinized stroma accounts for more than 50% of tumor
May demonstrate nuclear palisading similar to schwannoma
Myoid variant
Conventional DFSP with nodules of cells with distinct cytoplasmic boundaries, eosinophilic cytoplasm, and vesicular nuclei
SMA expression in a myofibroblastic "tram-track" pattern in myoid component
Granular cell variant
Conventional DFSP with admixed cells with abundant granular cytoplasm, round eccentrically located nuclei with prominent nucleoli
Second population of cells may express NKI/C3
Fibrosarcomatous transformation
Usually resembles adult fibrosarcoma with herringbone architecture
Undifferentiated pleomorphic sarcoma rare
Nuclei with hyperchromasia, pleomorphism, and mitotic activity (greater than four mitotic figures per ten high-power fields)
Variable CD34 expression in fibrosarcomatous component (often diminished)
Precursor conventional DFSP often at periphery

cellular fibrous histiocytoma. Cellular fibrous histiocytoma is often positive for FXIIIa (85% of cases), CD68, and SMA (focal "tram-track" pattern) but is generally negative for CD34.

Solitary fibrous tumor is a CD34-positive fibroblastic tumor that may rarely involve the skin. Solitary fibrous tumor is generally well circumscribed, has variable cellularity, demonstrates a haphazard arrangement of tumor cells around hemangiopericytic (staghorn-like) vessels, and is immunoreactive for STAT-6 secondary to a *NAB2-STAT6* gene fusion.

Spindle cell lipoma is also positive for CD34 and has a variable admixture of uniform, bland-appearing spindle cells within a variably myxoid-to-collagenous stroma and mature adipocytes. The tumor cells of spindle cell lipoma may be arranged in short fascicles or a random pattern, but a storiform pattern is not seen. Characteristically, spindle cell lipoma has ropey collagen fibers and loss of retinoblastoma (RB1) protein expression by immunohistochemistry.

Benign peripheral nerve sheath tumors can also be positive for CD34 and may have a fascicular and/or storiform architecture. Schwannoma and sclerotic DFSP have variable cellularity and nuclear palisading in common. However, schwannoma and neurofibroma are diffusely positive for S100 protein and SOX10; have somewhat pleomorphic nuclei, often with degenerative atypia; and contain secondary elements. Perineurioma is positive for CD34 but also immunoreactive for GLUT1, EMA, and claudin-1, unlike DFSP. The pigmented and myxoid variants of the aforementioned entities enter the differential for Bednar tumor and myxoid DFSP, respectively.

Desmoplastic and spindle cell melanomas need to be distinguished from atrophic and sclerosing DFSP variants. Older age, sun-damaged skin, the presence of a junctional component, and expression of S100 protein, SOX-10, and other melanocytic markers (HMB-45, MART-1, etc.) aid in the diagnosis of melanoma. Desmoplastic melanoma is typically only positive for S100 protein and SOX10.

The main differential diagnostic consideration for GCF is angiosarcoma and undifferentiated pleomorphic sarcoma. Young age, the absence of vascular markers (CD31 and ERG), CD34 expression, and, if necessary, molecular confirmation of *COL1A1-PDGFB* fusion aid in differentiating GCF from these entities.

The myxoid variant of DFSP may be confused with superficial angiomyxoma, which can also infiltrate the subcutis and is positive for CD34. However, typical cases of the latter have a lobular and circumscribed growth pattern, less uniform cellularity, and perivascular neutrophils (~50%) and may contain epithelial structures. Low-grade fibromyxoid sarcoma (LGFMS) has uniformly bland spindle cells within a variably collagenous-to-myxoid stroma and has a focally storiform growth pattern, which may lead to confusion with myxoid DFSP. However, LGFMS has negative to weak CD34 expression and is diffusely positive for MUC4, unlike DFSP. Molecular confirmation of the t(7;16)(q13;p11) of LGFMS enables definitive diagnosis in difficult cases. Low-grade myxofibrosarcoma is multinodular and may be CD34-positive, but is more atypical. The tumor cells of myxofibrosarcoma are not uniformly distributed in the myxoid stroma and often condense around curvilinear vessels. Myxoid liposarcoma only rarely arises in the subcutis of the extremities. It is characterized by spindled and stellate cells in a myxoid matrix in association with lipoblasts, mucin pools, and a plexiform or arborizing network of thin-walled vessels. Myxoid liposarcoma is usually CD34-negative and harbors a t(12;16)(q13;p11) *FUS-DDIT3* translocation.

For acral DFSP, epithelioid sarcoma, cellular fibrous histiocytoma, superficial acral fibromyxoma, cellular digital fibroma, and perineurioma enter the differential diagnosis, especially in small biopsies. CD34 expression can be seen in 50–60% of epithelioid sarcoma cases, and there may be foci of spindled growth. However, epithelioid sarcoma has keratin expression, a greater degree of cytologic atypia, and a lack of INI-1 (SMARCB1) protein expression. Superficial acral fibromyxoma occurs in a periungual location on the hands and feet. The lesion is CD34-positive, but the spindle cells are arranged in bands and fascicles within a variably collagenous-to-myxoid stroma. Cellular digital fibroma, considered a cellular version of superficial acral fibromyxoma, is densely cellular, but lacks a storiform architecture.

Myoid DFSP can be distinguished from myofibroma by the lack of diffuse SMA expression and absence of the branching capillary vasculature often present in myofibroma. Myofibromas are also negative for CD34. Myopericytoma occurs in the subcutis of the extremities and has a characteristic concentric growth of "myoid" pericytic cells around vessels, diffuse smooth muscle actin expression, and minimal CD34 expression.

The granular cell variant of DFSP is differentiated from granular cell tumor by the absence of S100 expression and admixed spindle cells.

Areas of fibrosarcomatous transformation, especially if present without a conventional DFSP component, as may occur in small or limited biopsies, need to be differentiated from other malignant monomorphous mesenchymal spindle cell neoplasms. Adult-type fibrosarcoma is a diagnosis of exclusion and is discussed in detail in Chap. 6. Superficial malignant peripheral nerve sheath tumors are frequently associated with neurofibromatosis type 1 and arise in a preexisting benign nerve sheath tumor, generally a neurofibroma. MPNST demonstrates variable and sometimes very limited S100, SOX-10, and GFAP expression. Spindle cell melanoma is also S100- and SOX10-positive and may express other melanocytic markers, but melanoma is CD34-negative, and the surrounding skin often has sequela of sun damage. Monophasic synovial sarcoma rarely presents as a superficial tumor, often around the smaller joints found in the hands and feet and wrists and ankles. Synovial sarcoma is very rarely positive for CD34, but will have diffuse TLE1 and focal keratin and/or EMA expression. Synovial sarcoma has a characteristic t(18;X)(p11.1;q11.2) *SYT-SSX* translocation in the overwhelming majority of cases. Sarcomatoid carcinoma typically has more pleomorphism, is negative for CD34, and has focal keratin and p63 expression.

Plexiform Fibrohistiocytic Tumor

Clinical Features

Plexiform fibrohistiocytic tumor (PFT) is a locally aggressive tumor of children and young adults with a slight female predilection. Three quarters of patients are affected in the first two decades of life. It most often presents as a painless soft tissue mass with contractures. The extremities are the most commonly affected sites, with upper more frequently involved than lower. PFT has a high rate of local recurrence, up to 38%, but low risk of metastasis (<10%). Metastatic lesions typically involve regional lymph nodes and rarely the lungs. Surgical resection is the mainstay of treatment. Radiotherapy may be used to manage large and locally aggressive lesions, but the role of chemotherapy is not well defined.

Pathologic Features

PFT within the skin has a multinodular, poorly circumscribed growth pattern within the deeper dermis and subcutis (Fig. 5.9a). There is a plexiform arrangement of nodules connected to each other by short intersecting fascicles of tumor cells (Fig. 5.9b). Three distinct cell populations are present in varying numbers: fibroblastic spindle cells, mononuclear histiocytoid cells, and multinucleated osteoclast-like giant cells. The histiocytoid and giant cells are located centrally within the nodules, and the fibroblastic cells are found peripherally (Fig. 5.9c). Tumors are subclassified based on the relative amounts of the three cells types: (1) fibroblastic type = comprised predominantly of fascicles of spindle cells, (2) fibrohistiocytic (cellular) type = comprised predominantly of nodules of histiocytoid cells and giant cells in a "cannonball" pattern, and (3) mixed type = comprised of intermixed fascicles and nodules. The mixed type accounts for the majority of cases. The histologic subtype has no bearing on prognosis. Cytologic atypia is generally mild, but may be moderate to be marked in a subset of cases. Rarely, osseous metaplasia is identified. The giant cells are strongly positive for CD68, which is less intensely expressed in the histiocytoid cells. The fibroblastic cells are positive for smooth muscle actin. Additionally, there may be focal CD34 expression limited to the fibroblastic cells, but tumors are usually negative for desmin, S100, FXIIIa, and keratin. No recurrent molecular alterations have been identified in PFT (Table 5.2).

Differential Diagnosis

Various lesions with plexiform growth need to be distinguished from PFT. Plexiform spindle cell nevus contains pigmented cells on closer inspection and is diffusely S100-protein-positive. Plexiform neurofibroma is pathognomonic for type 1 neurofibromatosis, contains cells with

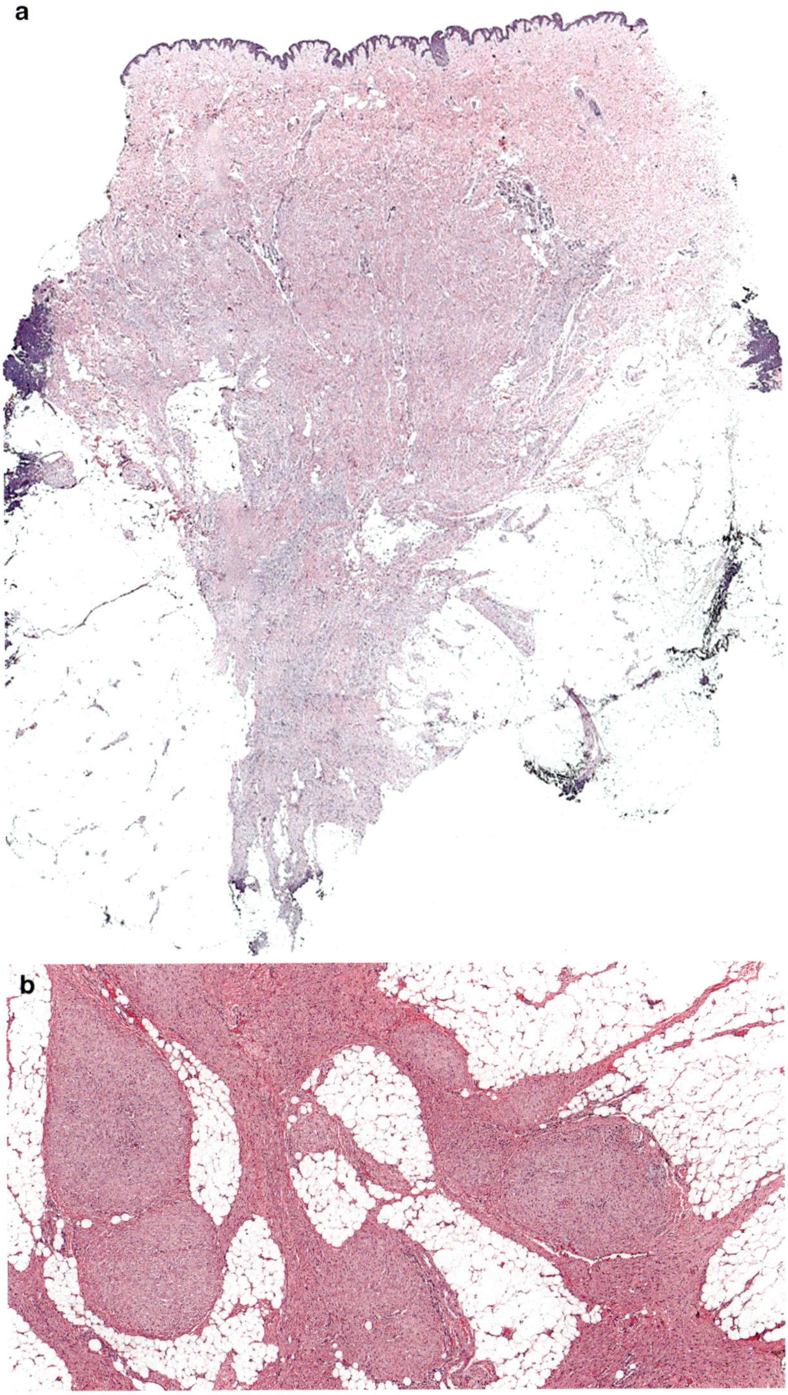

Fig. 5.9 (**a**) Plexiform fibrohistiocytic tumor located in dermis and subcutis with multinodular growth. (**b**) Plexiform arrangement of nodules connected by intersecting fascicles of tumor cells. (**c**) Three distinct cell types: nodules are comprised of histiocytoid and multinucleated giant cells with peripherally arranged fibroblastic cells

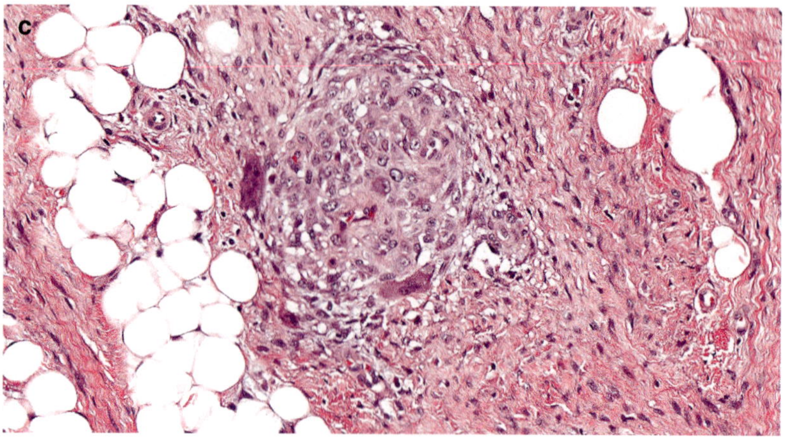

Fig. 5.9 (continued)

Table 5.2 Key pathologic features: plexiform fibrohistiocytic tumor

Plexiform growth pattern with variable amounts of histiocyte-like cells, osteoclast-like giant cells, and spindled fibroblastic cells
Nodules of histiocytes-like cells and osteoclast-like giant cells
Spindle cells at periphery of nodules

wavy nuclei and is S100-protein-positive. Plexiform schwannoma may extend into the subcutis, but will have alternating areas of cellularity with nuclear palisading and is S100-protein-positive.

In addition to various lesions with plexiform growth, the differential diagnoses of PFT also depend on the morphologic variant. The fibrohistiocytic (cellular) nodules share features with juvenile xanthogranuloma, Langerhans cell histiocytosis, granulomata, and cellular neurothekeoma. Juvenile xanthogranuloma contains Touton-like giant cells in comparison with osteoclast-like giant cells, while Langerhans cell histiocytosis contains histiocytes that are positive for S100 protein, CD1a, and langerin. Epithelioid granulomata lack osteoclast-like giant cells and have numerous admixed inflammatory cells. Although some have postulated that cellular neurothekeoma is related to PFT, cellular neurothekeoma lacks the plexiform growth pattern and triphasic histology and has a more uniform population of spindled to epithelioid cells than PFT. Immunohistochemistry has little role in the differential diagnosis of cellular neurothekeoma and PFT, as there is significant immunophenotypic overlap between these entities. The differential diagnosis of soft tissue giant cell tumor is discussed below.

The fibroblastic variant may be difficult to distinguish from reactive myofibroblastic proliferations, sclerotic dermatofibroma, DFSP, and fibromatoses. Reactive myofibroblastic proliferations are generally confined to the dermis with minimal subcutaneous involvement. Dermatofibroma may extend focally into the subcutis, but will have epidermal hyperplasia, peripheral collagen trapping, secondary elements, and FXIIIa immunoreactivity. In contrast to the strong and diffuse staining in DFSP, CD34 is only focally positive in PFT. Fibromatoses have long, broad fascicles rather than the short, plexiform fascicles of PFT. Fibromatoses also typically contain thin-walled vessels and scattered perivascular lymphocytes. Nuclear beta-catenin expression, when present, aids in the diagnosis of the fibromatoses.

The mixed variant has features similar to cellular neurothekeoma, epithelioid granulomata, soft tissue giant cell tumor, and fibrous hamartoma of infancy. As the name would suggest, fibrous hamartoma of infancy is seen within the first 2 years of life, presents on the chest wall and axilla, and lacks CD68-positive histiocytes. The other entities have been or are subsequently addressed.

Angiomatoid Fibrous Histiocytoma

Clinical Features

Angiomatoid fibrous histiocytoma (AFH), previously called angiomatoid malignant fibrous histiocytoma, occurs in the superficial soft tissue of children and young adults, but may be seen at any age. The lesion usually presents as a painless nodule in the deep dermis and subcutis. Visceral and bone lesions have been documented and tend to arise in older age groups. Systemic symptoms, including fever and anemia, can occur secondary to tumoral cytokine production. Rapid growth correlates with intralesional hemorrhage. Local recurrence may occur in 15% of cases, and rare (<5%) cases may metastasize, typically to regional lymph nodes and rarely to the lungs, liver, and brain. Distant metastasis has resulted in patient mortality.

Pathologic Features

AFH is a circumscribed, subcutaneous mass with an incomplete fibrous capsule and peripheral lymphoplasmacytic cuff, which often demonstrates germinal center formation (both present in >80% of cases) (Fig. 5.10a, b). Conventional tumors are comprised of polygonal and spindled

a

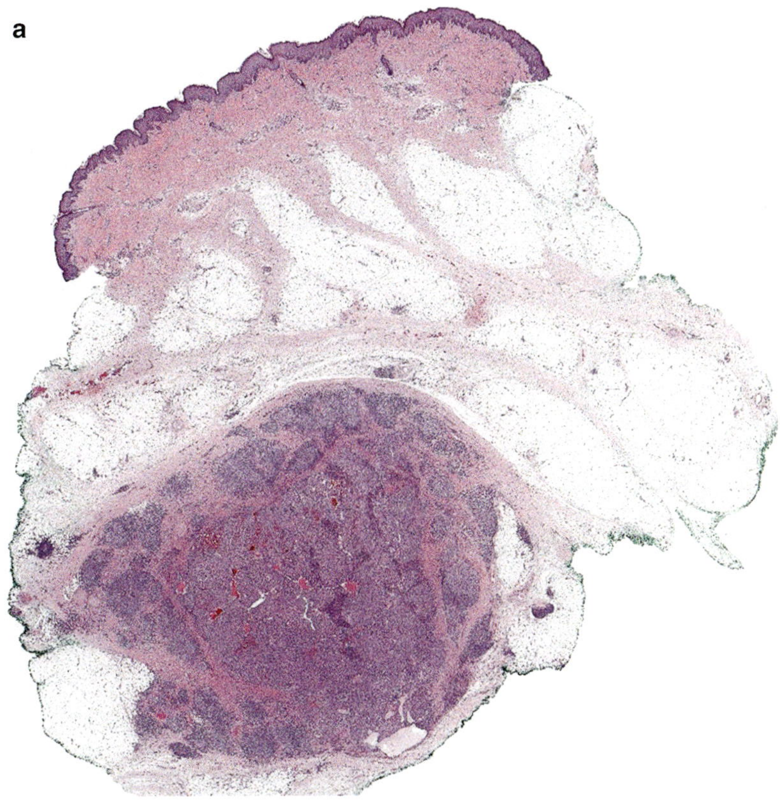

Fig. 5.10 (**a**) Angiomatoid fibrous histiocytoma located within the subcutis. (**b**) Angiomatoid fibrous histiocytoma almost always has a peripheral fibrous pseudocapsule with a lymphocytic cuff. Germinal center formation is commonly present. (**c**) Most angiomatoid fibrous histiocytomas are composed of histiocytoid tumor cells arranged in short intersecting fascicles. (**d**) Pseudovascular spaces with osteoclast-like giant cells. (**e**) Hemorrhage and hemosiderin-laden cells. (**f**) Marked cytologic atypia and/or atypical mitotic figures may be present but do not portend aggressive behavior. (**g**) Reticular and myxoid growth with retained pseudocapsule and peripheral inflammation. (**h**) The reticular/myxoid variant of angiomatoid fibrous histiocytoma is comprised of anastomosing spindle cells within a myxoid stroma. (**i**) Tumor with primitive round cell morphology

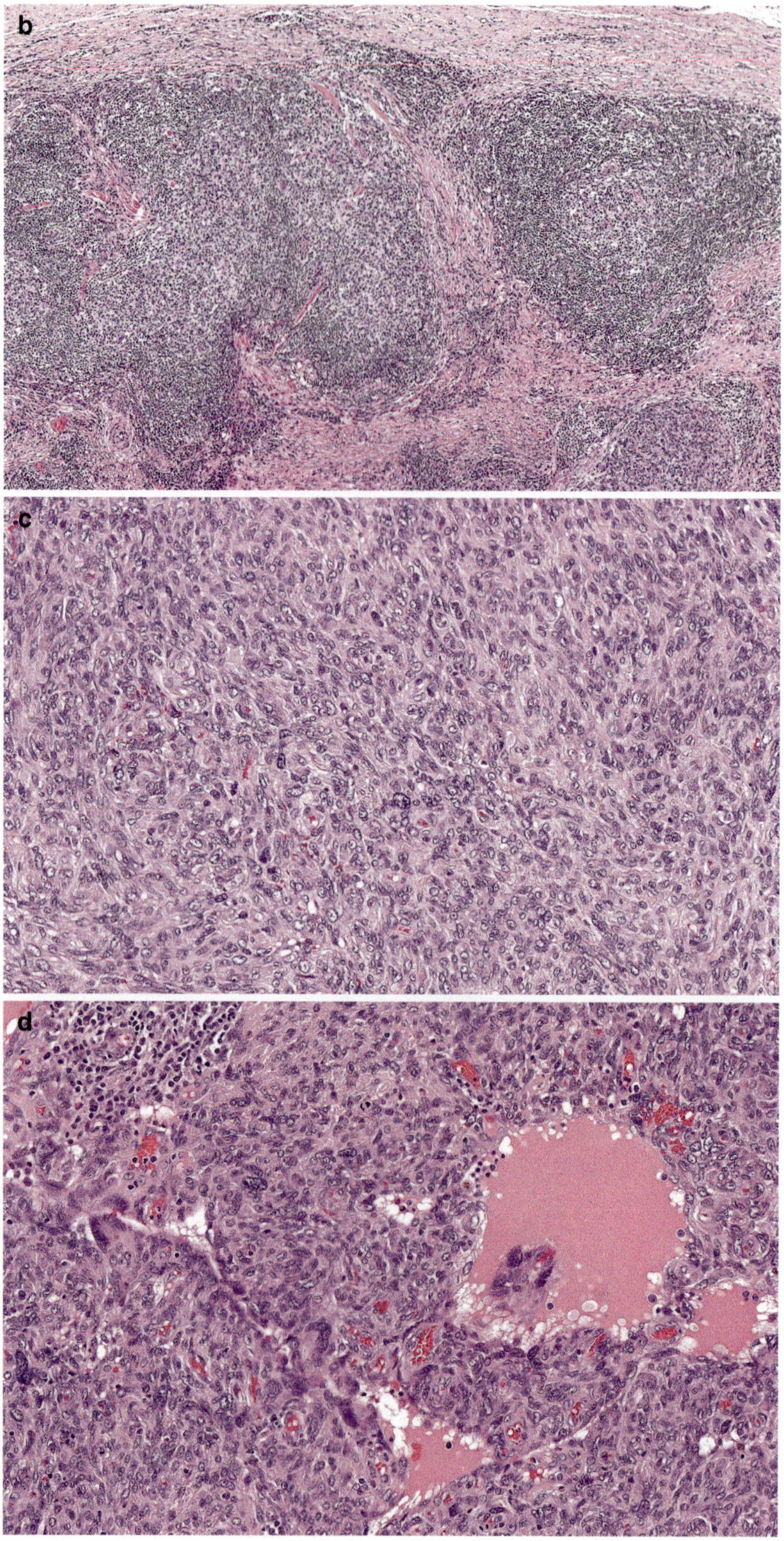

Fig. 10 (continued)

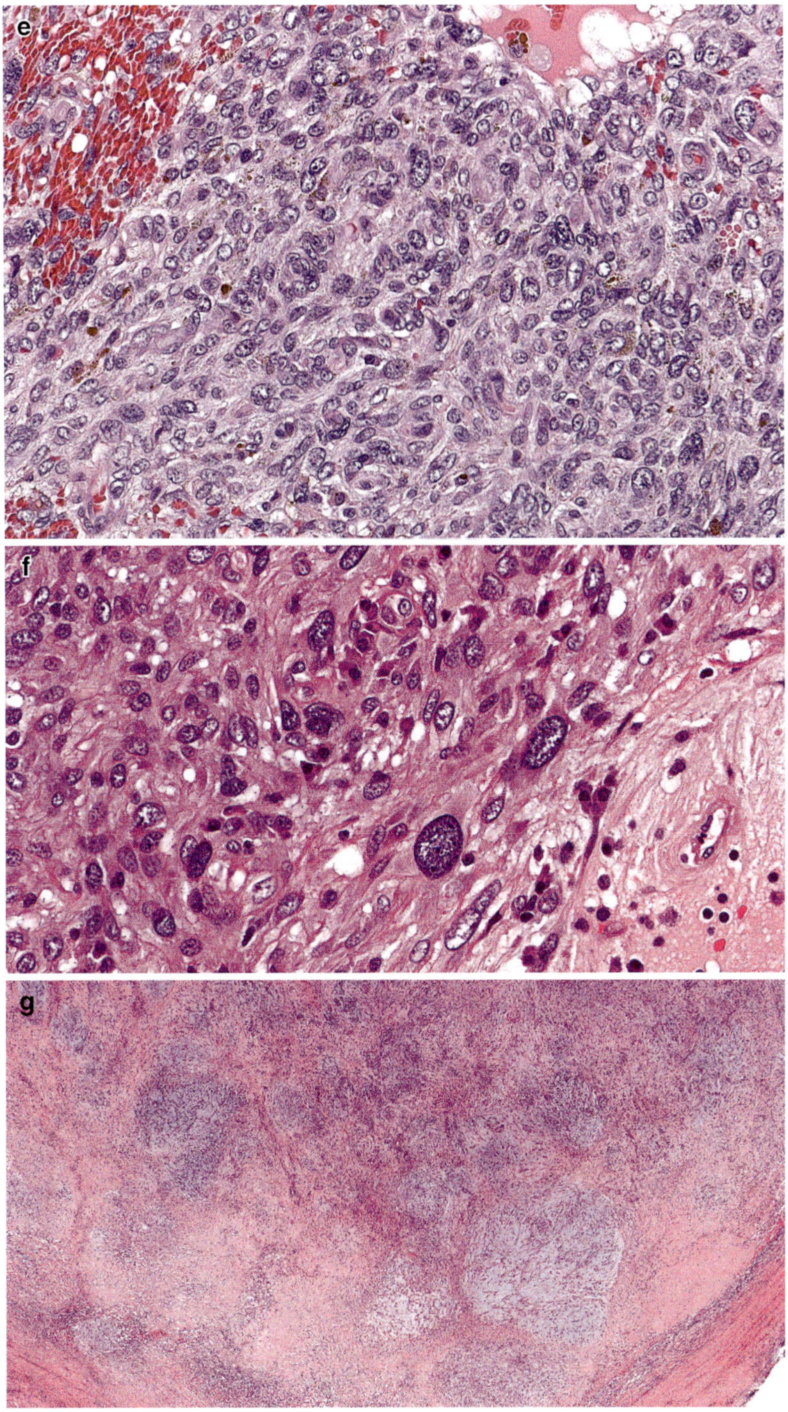

Fig. 10 (continued)

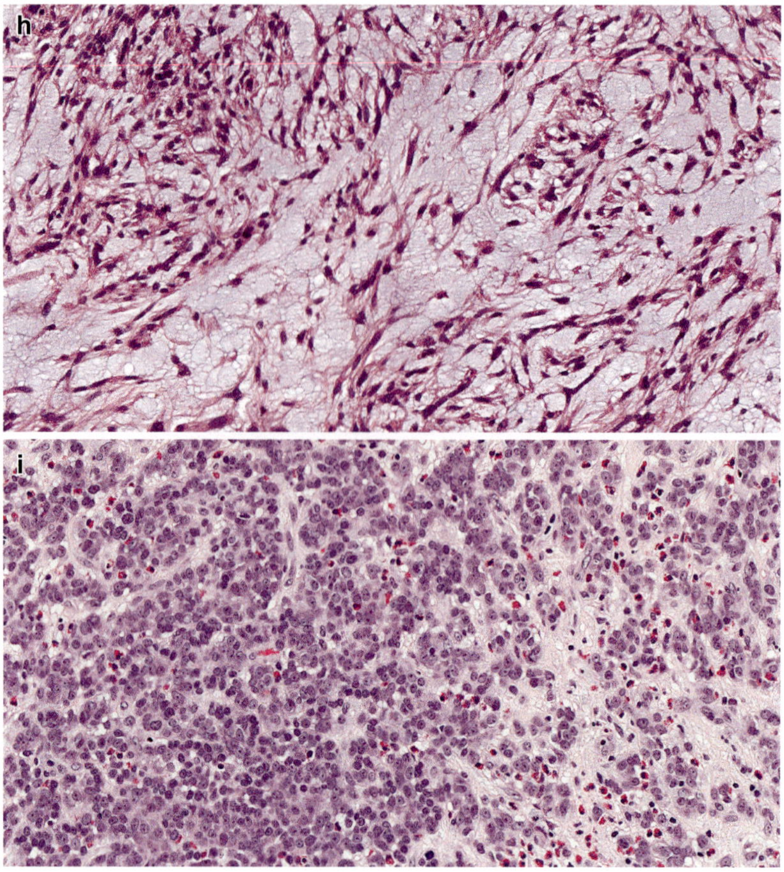

Fig. 10 (continued)

cells with eosinophilic cytoplasm and vesicular nuclei arranged in short, intersecting fascicles or storiform whorls (Fig. 5.10c). Variably sized, blood-filled pseudovascular spaces lined by flattened tumor cells are present in approximately 50% of cases, and in a few cases, these spaces may account for the majority of the tumor volume and be associated with osteoclast-like giant cells (Fig. 5.10d). Scattered hemosiderin-laden histiocytes may be present (Fig. 5.10e), but xanthoma cells are absent. The stroma varies from myxoid to sclerotic to desmoplastic. Marked cytologic atypia and/or atypical mitotic figures may be identified (Fig. 5.10f), but neither is a reliable parameter for predicting more aggressive biological behavior. Several cases with a reticular growth pattern and myxoid background have been described (Fig. 5.10g, h), but these cases still retain the characteristic pseudocapsule, peripheral lymphocytic aggregates, and pseudovascular spaces seen in conventional AFH. Very rare cases may have a small round blue cell morphology (Fig. 5.10i). Approximately 50% of cases are immunoreactive for some combination of desmin, EMA, CD68, and CD99. The tumors are consistently negative for S100 protein, cytokeratin, CD31, CD34, and myogenin. Over 90% of cases have gene fusions involving *EWSR1*; the *EWSR1-CREB1* fusion is more common than the *EWSR1-ATF1* fusion. Less than 10% have an *FUS-ATF1* or other gene fusion (Table 5.3).

Differential Diagnosis

The differential diagnosis of AFH encompasses both benign and malignant lesions. Aneurysmal

Table 5.3 Key pathologic features: angiomatoid fibrous histiocytoma

Fibrous pseudocapsule with lymphoid infiltrate
Histiocytoid and spindle cells in fascicles, whorls, or sheets
Blood-filled spaces lined by tumor cells in 50% cases
Remainder of cases with focal hemorrhage or hemosiderin-laden cells
Rare cases with marked cytologic atypia and mitotic activity
>90% gene fusions involving *EWSR1*

benign fibrous histiocytoma occurs in the extremities of young adults and presents as a hemorrhagic nodule within the dermis. It lacks a fibrous capsule and retains classic features of fibrous histiocytoma, including epidermal hyperplasia, peripheral collagen trapping, and secondary elements.

Vascular tumors enter the differential given the hemorrhage-filled spaces. However, true vascular lesions are positive for CD31 and ERG. Additionally, Kaposi sarcoma is positive for HHV-8.

The peripheral lymphoplasmacytic component may cause confusion with intranodal proliferations or metastases. Intranodal palisaded myofibroblastoma contains thick collagen fibers ("amianthoid fibers"), and inflammatory pseudotumor of lymph node lacks pseudovascular spaces. Follicular dendritic sarcoma occurs within lymph nodes and is positive for CD21 and CD35, but negative for desmin and smooth muscle actin. Stromal desmoplasia raises the possibility of metastatic sarcomatoid carcinoma. Carcinoma is positive for cytokeratin and p63, and careful inspection of the fibrous capsule in AFH will reveal the absence of true subcapsular sinuses.

AFH with reticular growth bears resemblance to myoepithelial neoplasms, extraskeletal myxoid chondrosarcoma, ossifying fibromyxoid tumor, low-grade fibromyxoid sarcoma, and myxoid liposarcoma. In addition to SMA and EMA expression, myoepithelial tumors also express keratins and S100 protein. Deep-seated myoepithelial lesions commonly show *EWSR1* rearrangements, and superficial tumors frequently demonstrate *PLAG1* rearrangements. Extraskeletal myxoid chondrosarcoma lacks a peritumoral lymphoplasmacytic infiltrate, is sometimes positive for EMA, but negative for desmin, and has a *NR4A3* rearrangement. Ossifying fibromyxoid tumor usually has a peripheral rim of mature bone, a distinct cord-like-to-nested pattern of tumor cells, and focal S100 protein expression. Low-grade fibromyxoid sarcoma lacks a fibrous pseudocapsule, hemorrhagic spaces, and peritumoral lymphocytes and is positive for MUC4. Myxoid liposarcoma has scattered lipoblasts, arborizing "chicken-wire" vessels, and *DDIT3* rearrangement.

Round cell change and CD99 expression in AFH overlap with Ewing sarcoma, rhabdomyosarcoma, and poorly differentiated synovial sarcoma. Ewing sarcoma contains alternate *EWSR1* translocations, partnering with *ERG* or *FLI1* in most cases, which can be parsed out with targeted RT-PCR. AFH has desmin expression in 50% of cases, but lacks other markers of skeletal muscle differentiation, including myogenin and MyoD1, which are positive in rhabdomyosarcoma. Synovial sarcoma is TLE-1-positive and has *SYT-SSX* rearrangement, unlike AFH.

Giant Cell Tumor of Soft Tissue

Clinical Features

Giant cell tumor of soft tissue (GCT-ST), also known as soft tissue giant cell tumor or giant cell tumor of low malignant potential, is an uncommon tumor that bears histologic resemblance to its bone counterpart, but occurs in the superficial or deep soft tissues; these lesions are also genetically distinct from one another. All age groups can be affected, though most cases are described in middle-aged adults. Most tumors occur in the extremities as painless nodules. Trunk and head and neck involvement occurs less frequently. Complete resection is the treatment of choice, as there is an up to 20% risk of recurrence and extremely low risk of metastasis and/or death.

Pathologic Features

GCT-ST presents as multiple, well-circumscribed nodules that are separated by collagen bands containing hemosiderin-laden macrophages (Fig. 5.11a). A peripheral rim of metaplastic bone is usually seen at least focally. The nodules are a mixture of polygonal to spindled mononuclear cells and osteoclast-type giant cells (Fig. 5.11b). Both cell types contain lightly amphophilic cytoplasm and oval, occasionally convoluted nuclei with pinpoint nucleoli. The mononuclear cells are variably mitotically active, but even the most briskly active cases will lack nuclear atypia. Occasionally there may be dispersed foci devoid of giant cells that have a storiform arrangement of spindled mononuclear cells. Variable numbers of foamy macrophages may be present. Cystic and hemorrhagic spaces resembling aneurysmal bone cyst can form, but necrosis is rare. Focal vascular invasion is present in 30% of cases (Fig. 5.11c). The mononuclear cells express RANKL, an important protein in osteoclast recruitment and differentiation, and are variably positive for CD68. In contrast, the multinucleated osteoclast-type

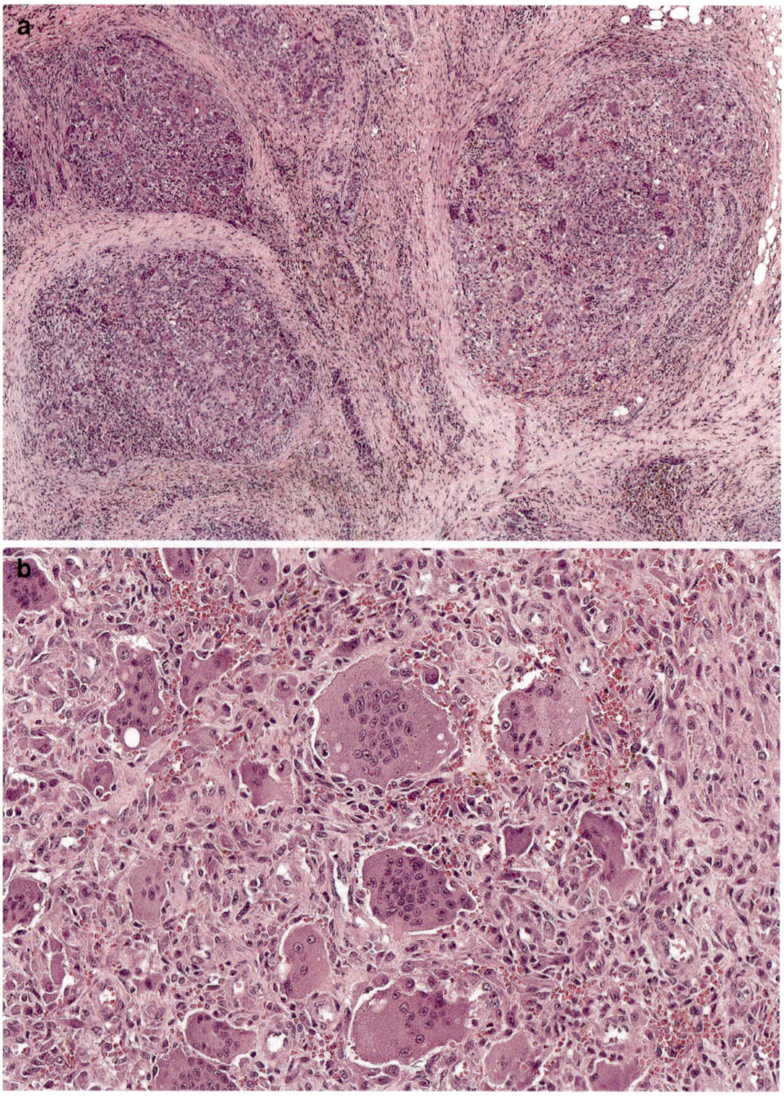

Fig. 5.11 (**a**) Giant cell tumor of soft tissue with multinodular growth with delineating, hemosiderin-containing fibrous bands. (**b**) The tumor is composed of an admixture of mononuclear histiocytoid cells and osteoclast-type giant cells. Mitotic activity is common, but the nuclei are bland. (**c**) Focal vascular invasion may be seen

Fig. 5.11 (continued)

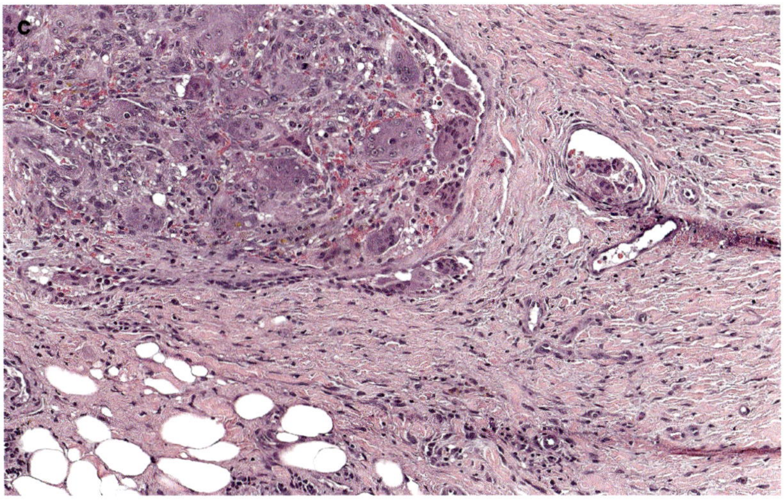

Table 5.4 Key pathologic features: giant cell tumor of soft tissue

Bland mononuclear cells and osteoclast-like giant cells
Mitoses common
Peripheral shell of bone common
Cytologic atypia, necrosis, and atypical mitoses uncommon
Secondary aneurysmal bone cyst-like changes may be seen
May have focal vascular invasion

giant cells strongly express CD68, but are negative for RANKL. No recurrent molecular alterations have been identified in these tumors. Despite the morphologic similarities to its bony counterpart, GCT-ST has a different immunophenotypic and genetic profile. GCT-ST has lower levels of RANKL (corresponding with lower mRNA levels) and SATB2 expression and lacks *H3F3A* mutation (present in greater than 90% of GCT of bone) (Table 5.4).

Differential Diagnosis

GCT-ST is most commonly confused with tenosynovial giant cell tumor (TSGCT). TSGCT typically occurs near joints, especially around the digits, and has a more heterogeneous population with admixed histiocytes and lymphocytes and less evenly dispersed giant cells. Primary aneurysmal bone cyst may rarely occur in the soft tissue. GCT-ST can have ABC-like degeneration, but will still retain solid areas and does not arise in bone. The fibrohistiocytic (cellular) and mixed variants of plexiform fibrohistiocytic tumor (PFT) may also be considered. GCT-ST has a multinodular rather than plexiform growth pattern and has foci of bone formation. PFT has smaller nodules and a biphasic appearance and areas comprised solely of spindle cells lacking a storiform architecture. Rare cases of undifferentiated pleomorphic sarcoma and sarcomatoid carcinoma contain numerous multinucleated cells, but these entities can be ruled out on the basis of their more significant cytologic atypia and presence of positivity for high-molecular-weight cytokeratins in the case of sarcomatoid carcinoma. Epithelioid sarcoma can be excluded by demonstrating keratin expression and lack of INI-1 immunoreactivity.

Superficial CD34-Positive Fibroblastic Tumor

Clinical Features

Superficial CD34-positive fibroblastic tumor is a recently described neoplasm that occurs to date exclusively in adults between the second and seventh decades of life. It arises as a painless mass in the superficial soft tissue of the lower extremities, especially around the knees, but may uncommonly involve the upper extremity, thorax, abdomen, or head and neck. Complete resection is the treatment of choice. Although only a few cases have been described, the limited clinical follow-up data available suggests this lesion has a relatively good outcome, with only a single documented case of regional lymph node metastasis.

Pathologic Features

Superficial CD34-positive fibroblastic tumor has the overall low-power appearance of a circumscribed mass within the deep dermis and subcutis, but on closer inspection has infiltrative edges and may extend into adjacent fascia and skeletal muscle. The moderately cellular to hypercellular proliferation contains spindled to epithelioid cells arranged in fascicles and sheets (Fig. 5.12a).

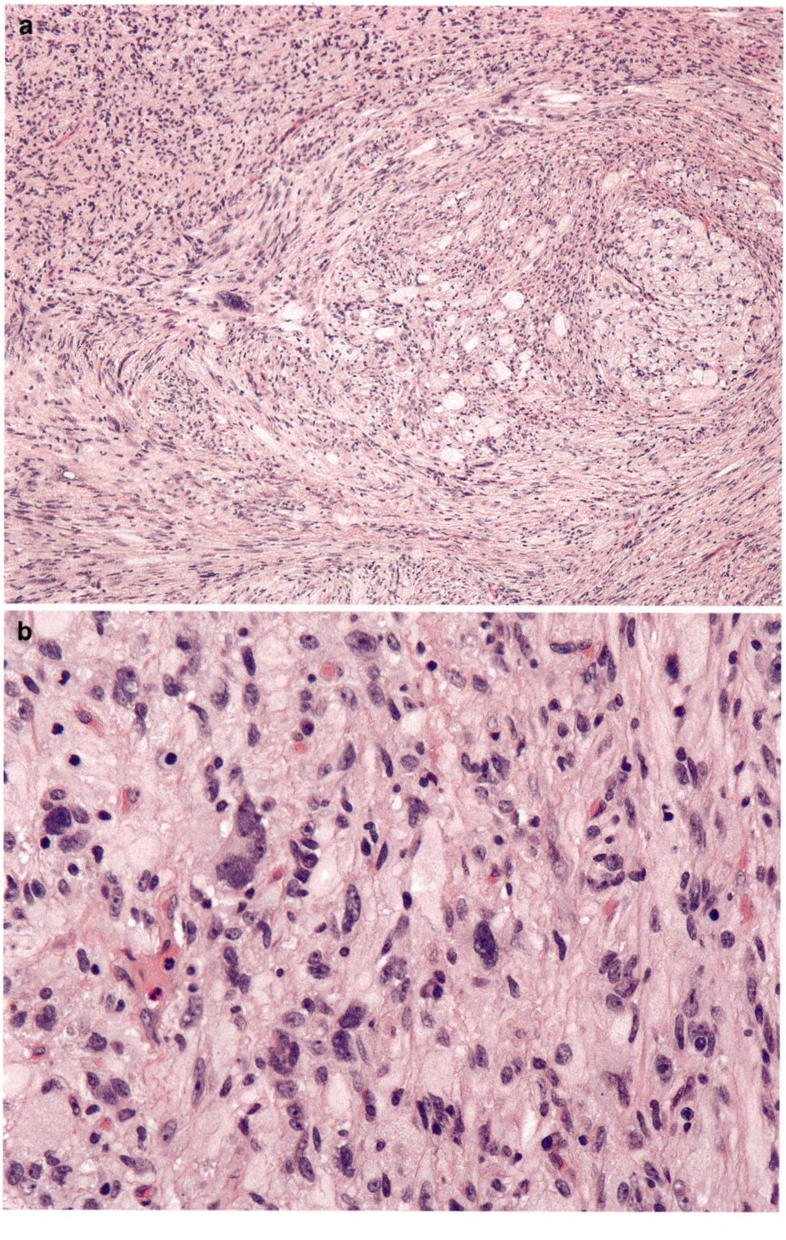

Fig. 5.12 (**a**) Superficial CD34-positive fibroblastic tumor is comprised of spindled to epithelioid cells arranged in fascicles and sheets. Some cells contain abundant granular to glassy eosinophilic cytoplasm, while others have foamy cytoplasm. (**b**) Diffuse cytologic atypia is present, but mitotic figures are absent. (**c**) As the name suggests, tumor cells are diffusely positive for CD34. (**d**) Focal cytokeratin expression is seen in two-thirds of cases. (Images **a**, **b** courtesy of Dr. Andrew Folpe, Department of Laboratory Medicine and Pathology, Mayo Clinic, Rochester, MN)

Fig. 5.12 (continued)

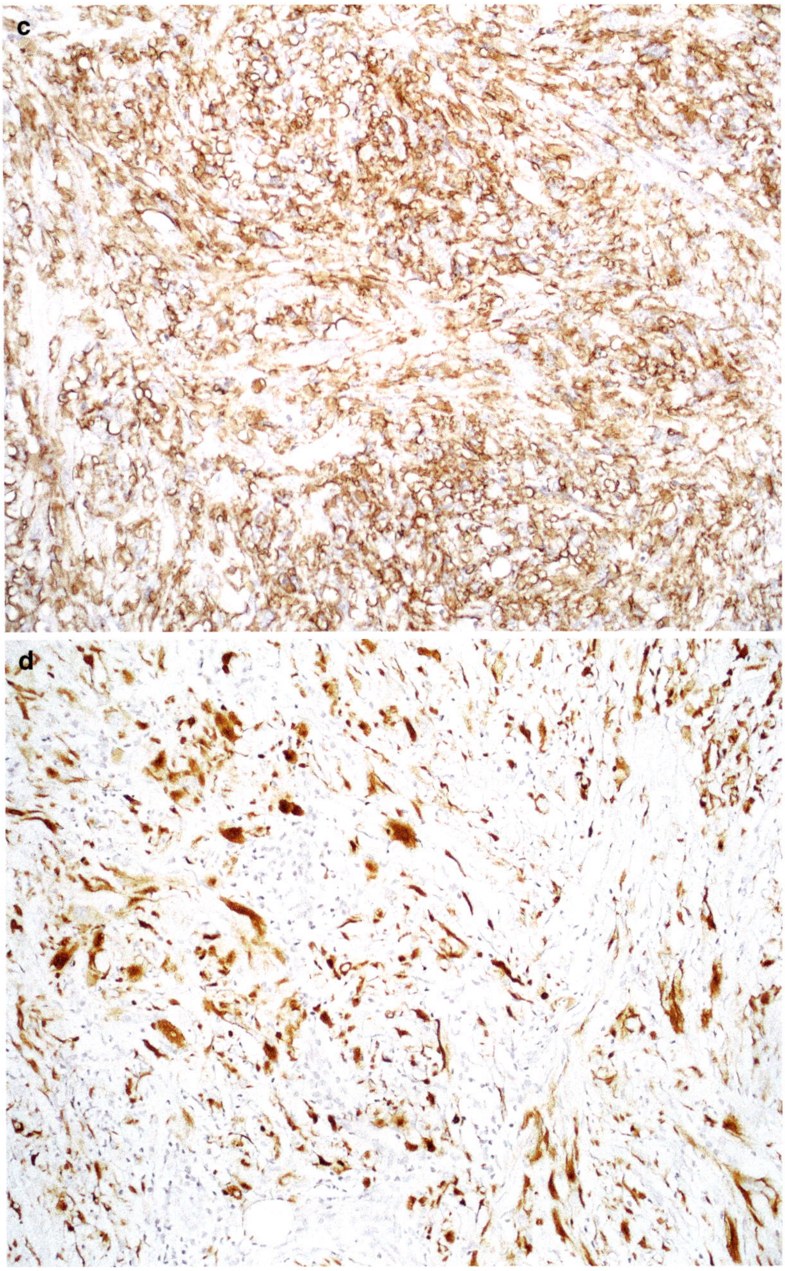

Most cells have abundant granular to glassy eosinophilic cytoplasm, but scattered cells may have foamy cytoplasmic change. Intranuclear pseudoinclusions and chronic inflammation are relatively common. Arborizing thin-walled capillaries are conspicuous in areas with fascicular architecture. The diffuse cytologic atypia of these tumors is characterized by nuclear pleomorphism, convolution, and hyperchromasia (Fig. 5.12b). When not obscured by intranuclear pseudoinclusions, one to multiple prominent nucleoli may be present and are reminiscent of viral cytopathic change. Despite the severe cytologic atypia, mitotic figures are nearly absent, a finding which is supported immunohistochemically by a low Ki-67 proliferation index. As its name suggests, tumor cells strongly and diffusely express CD34, and two-thirds of cases may have focal cytokeratin expression (Fig. 5.12c, d). Desmin, smooth muscle actin, and S100 protein are negative, and TP53 overexpression is absent. No recurrent molecular alterations have been identified in these tumors.

Differential Diagnosis

Superficial location, intranuclear pseudoinclusions, and virocyte-like cells are shared features with pleomorphic hyalinizing angiectatic tumor and myxoinflammatory fibroblastic sarcoma. Pleomorphic hyalinizing angiectatic tumor is also CD34-positive, but contains its namesake hyalinized angiectatic vessels and hemosiderin-laden spindle cells. Myxoinflammatory fibroblastic sarcoma contains admixed inflammatory cells, myxoid foci containing pseudolipoblasts, is negative for CD34, and often has *MGEA5* and *TGFBR3* rearrangements.

DFSP is also positive for CD34 and demonstrates infiltrative growth in the dermis and subcutis, but lacks atypical nuclear features. When fibrosarcomatous transformation is present in DFSP, the diffuse cytologic atypia is accompanied by herringbone architecture and increased mitotic activity. A high proliferation index will separate undifferentiated pleomorphic sarcoma from superficial CD34-positive fibroblastic tumor. Cytologic atypia and keratin expression overlap with epithelioid sarcoma, but INI-1 expression is retained in superficial CD34-positive fibroblastic tumor (Table 5.5).

Table 5.5 Key pathologic features: superficial CD34-positive fibroblastic tumor

Spindled and epithelioid cells in fascicles and sheets
Diffuse cytologic atypia with nuclear pleomorphism and prominent nucleoli
Low mitotic activity
Positive for CD34 and often positive for cytokeratin; INI1 expression is retained

Inflammatory Myofibrolastic Tumor

Clinical Features

Inflammatory myofibroblastic tumors (IMT) can occur at virtually any anatomic site, and rare primary cutaneous cases have been reported under several different names, including cutaneous plasma cell granuloma and inflammatory pseudotumor. IMT most commonly arises in children and young adults, but elderly patients may be affected. Cutaneous lesions generally present as solitary plaques and nodules on the head and neck, although other body sites may be involved. Some cases can have associated systemic signs and symptoms, including fever, malaise, and weight loss. Laboratory abnormalities, such as anemia, thrombocytosis, and elevated erythrocyte sedimentation rate, may be observed. The aforementioned sequelae resolve with tumor excision, which is the treatment of choice. The risk for recurrence is 25%, while metastases are exceedingly rare. Chemotherapy, radiation, and crizotinib, an ALK inhibitor, may be useful in aggressive cases.

Pathologic Features

IMT is a circumscribed nodular or multinodular proliferation of spindled fibroblastic and myofibroblastic cells and inflammatory cells, which demonstrates three histologic patterns. The first pattern resembles nodular fasciitis and consists of a variable loose myxoid and fibrous stroma, small blood vessels, extravagated erythrocytes, hemosiderin, neutrophils, lymphocytes, eosinophils, and few plasma cells (Fig. 5.13a). The second pattern is characterized by a compact fascicular-to-storiform proliferation of spindle cells, some of which have a ganglion-like appearance, in association with a lymphoplasmacytic infiltrate and fibromyxoid stroma (Fig. 5.13b). Germinal centers may occasionally be present. The third pattern is hypocellular and contains an abundance of hyalinized collagen in a plate-like arrangement (Fig. 5.13c). Sparse plasma cells

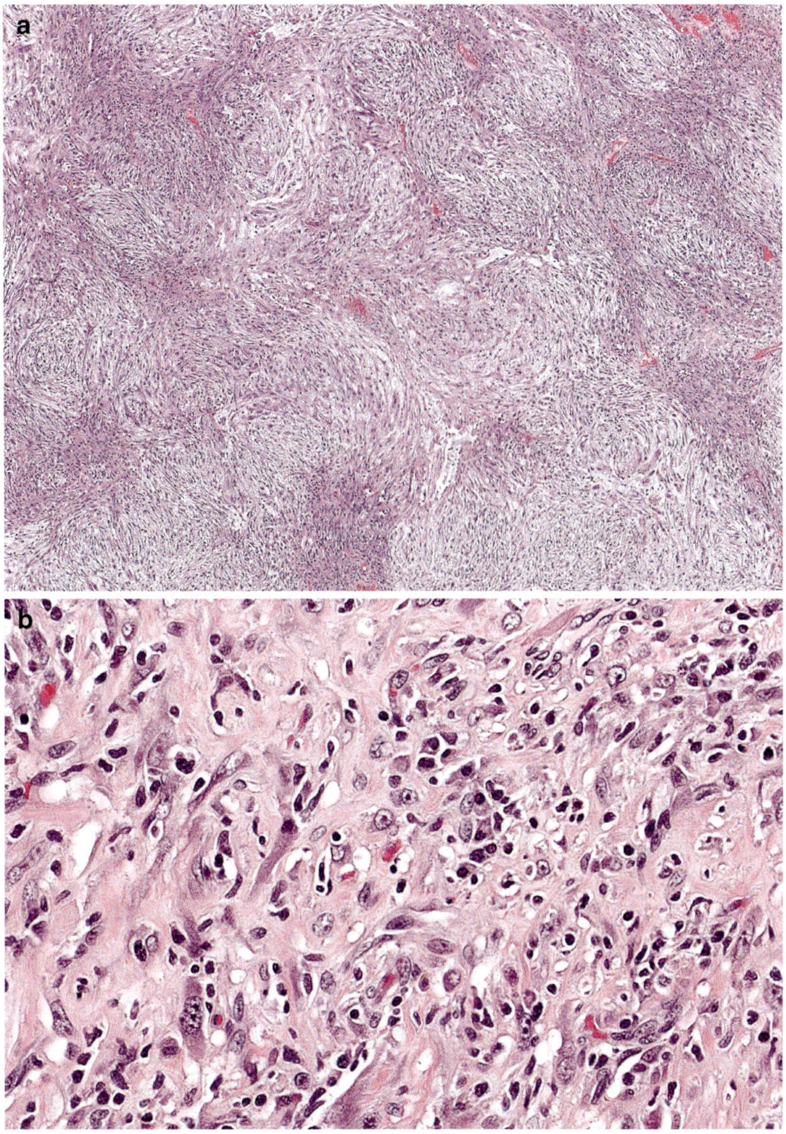

Fig. 5.13 (**a**) Inflammatory myofibroblastic tumor resembling nodular fasciitis. (**b**) Compact variant containing ganglion-like cells and dense lymphoplasmacytic infiltrate. (**c**) Hyalinized, hypocellular variant with plate-like collagen. (**d**) Cytoplasmic ALK expression by immunohistochemistry

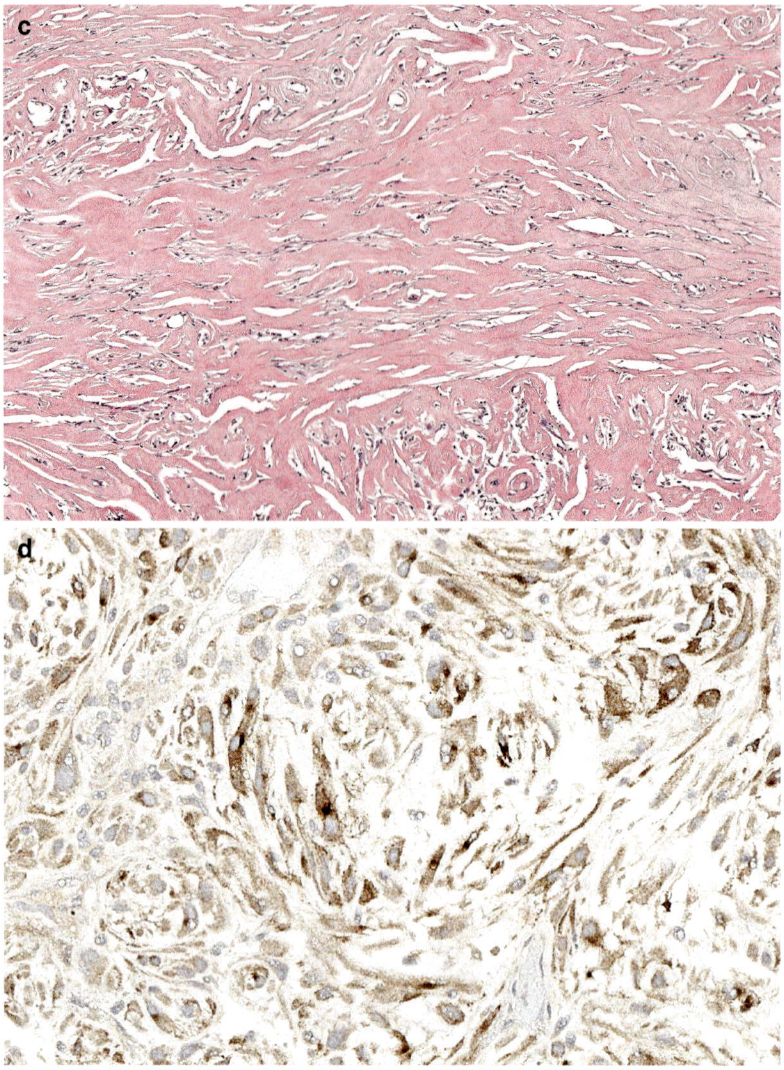

Fig. 5.13 (continued)

and eosinophils comprise the inflammatory component in this variant, and foci of dystrophic calcification and osseous metaplasia may be present. Different patterns may coexist in the same tumor. Mitotic activity may be brisk, but atypical forms are absent. The tumor cells demonstrate variable expression of smooth muscle actin, desmin, keratin, and CD68. Up to 60% of cases have cytoplasmic ALK expression, a finding which correlates well with the presence of an *ALK* (2p23) rearrangement with several partners, including *TPM3*, *TPM4*, *ATIC*, *SEC31L1*, and *CARS* (Fig. 5.13d). Fusion with *RNABP2* is associated with nuclear membrane or perinuclear ALK localization and epithelioid morphology, while fusion with *CLTC* manifests with granular cytoplasmic staining. ALK-negative IMT is associated with a later age of onset, increased cytologic atypia, and higher risk of distant metastases (Table 5.6).

Differential Diagnosis

The differential diagnosis varies for the different histologic patterns of IMT. Myxedematous IMT

Table 5.6 Key pathologic features: inflammatory myofibroblastic tumor

Myofibroblastic and fibroblastic spindle cells with variable inflammatory infiltrate
Nodular fasciitis-like variant with neutrophils, lymphocytes, and eosinophils but rare plasma cells
Cellular variant with ganglion-like cells and numerous plasma cells
Hyalinized variant with few spindled cells, plasma cells, and lymphocytes

resembles nodular fasciitis, but the latter has a less prominent inflammatory element. Compact lesions overlap with inflamed smooth muscle tumors and extranodal interdigitating dendritic cell tumor. Smooth muscle tumors are diffusely positive for smooth muscle actin and desmin and have long intersecting fascicles rather than a storiform arrangement. Interdigitating dendritic cell tumor has whorled architecture and lymphocyte aggregates, but also has diffuse S100 protein expression and is ALK-negative. The sclerotic form of IMT resembles IgG4-related sclerosing inflammatory lesions, but is not associated with an increased number of intratumoral IgG4-positive plasma cells or elevated serum IgG4.

Selected References

1. Bohman SL, Goldblum JR, Rubin BP, Tanas MR, Billings SD. Angiomatoid fibrous histiocytoma: an expansion of the clinical and histological spectrum. Pathology. 2014;46(3):199–204.
2. Carter JM, Weiss SW, Linos K, DiCaudo DJ, Folpe AL. Superficial CD34-positive fibroblastic tumor: report of 18 cases of a distinctive low-grade mesenchymal neoplasm of intermediate (borderline) malignancy. Mod Pathol. 2014;27(2):294–302.
3. Chen G, Folpe AL, Colby TV, Sittampalam K, Patey M, Chen MG, Chan JK. Angiomatoid fibrous histiocytoma: unusual sites and unusual morphology. Mod Pathol. 2011;24(12):1560–70.
4. Coffin CM, Watterson J, Priest JR, Dehner LP. Extrapulmonary inflammatory myofibroblastic tumor (inflammatory pseudotumor). A clinicopathologic and immunohistochemical study of 84 cases. Am J Surg Pathol. 1995;19(8):859–72.
5. Coffin CM, Hornick JL, Fletcher CD. Inflammatory myofibroblastic tumor: comparison of clinicopathologic, histologic, and immunohistochemical features including ALK expression in atypical and aggressive cases. Am J Surg Pathol. 2007;31(4):509–20.
6. de Menezes S, Mar A, Dowling J, Wright A. A case of cutaneous inflammatory Myofibroblastic tumor. Pediatr Dermatol. 2016;33(6):e377–80.
7. Folpe AL, Morris RJ, Weiss SW. Soft tissue giant cell tumor of low malignant potential: a proposal for the reclassification of malignant giant cell tumor of soft parts. Mod Pathol. 1999;12(9):894–902.
8. Gleason BC, Hornick JL. Inflammatory myofibroblastic tumours: where are we now? J Clin Pathol. 2008;61(4):428–37.
9. Guo H, Garcia RA, Perle MA, Amodio J, Greco MA. Giant cell tumor of soft tissue with pulmonary metastases: pathologic and cytogenetic study. Pediatr Dev Pathol. 2005;8(6):718–24. Epub 2005 Nov 21.
10. Inoue T, Misago N, Okawa T, Narisawa Y. Inflammatory myofibroblastic tumor of the skin grossly mimicking squamous cell carcinoma: a case report. J Dermatol. 2012;39(1):107–10.
11. Jacobson-Dunlop E, White CR Jr, Mansoor A. Features of plexiform fibrohistiocytic tumor in skin punch biopsies: a retrospective study of 6 cases. Am J Dermatopathol. 2011;33(6):551–6.
12. Jaffer S, Ambrosini-Spaltro A, Mancini AM, Eusebi V, Rosai J. Neurothekeoma and plexiform fibrohistiocytic tumor: mere histologic resemblance or histogenetic relationship? Am J Surg Pathol. 2009;33(6):905–13.
13. Jha P, Moosavi C, Fanburg-Smith JC. Giant cell fibroblastoma: an update and addition of 86 new cases from the Armed Forces Institute of Pathology, in honor of Dr. Franz M Enzinger. Ann Diagn Pathol. 2007;11(2):81–8.
14. Kuzel P, Mahmood MN, Metelitsa AI, Salopek TG. A clinicopathologic review of a case series of dermatofibrosarcoma protuberans with fibrosarcomatous differentiation. J Cutan Med Surg. 2015;19(1):28–34.
15. Lee JC, Liang CW, Fletcher CDM. Giant cell tumor of soft tissue is genetically distinct from its bone counterpart. Mod Pathol. 2017;30(5):728–33.
16. Liang CA, Jambusaria-Pahlajani A, Karia PS, Elenitsas R, Zhang PD, Schmults CD. A systematic review of outcome data for dermatofibrosarcoma protuberans with and without fibrosarcomatous change. J Am Acad Dermatol. 2014;71(4):781–6.
17. Llombart B, Serra-Guillén C, Monteagudo C, López Guerrero JA, Sanmartín O. Dermatofibrosarcoma protuberans: a comprehensive review and update on diagnosis and management. Semin Diagn Pathol. 2013;30(1):13–28.
18. Maher OM, Prieto VG, Stewart J, Herzog CE. Characterization of metastatic angiomatoid fibrous histiocytoma. J Pediatr Hematol Oncol. 2015;37(4):e268–71.
19. Mancini I, Righi A, Gambarotti M, Picci P, Dei Tos AP, Billings SD, Simi L, Franchi A. Phenotypic and molecular differences between giant-cell tumour of soft tissue and its bone counterpart. Histopathology. 2017;71(3):453–60.
20. Mariño-Enríquez A, Wang WL, Roy A, Lopez-Terrada D, Lazar AJ, Fletcher CD, Coffin CM,

Hornick JL. Epithelioid inflammatory myofibroblastic sarcoma: an aggressive intra-abdominal variant of inflammatory myofibroblastic tumor with nuclear membrane or perinuclear ALK. Am J Surg Pathol. 2011;35(1):135–44.
21. Mentzel T, Schärer L, Kazakov DV, Michal M. Myxoid dermatofibrosarcoma protuberans: clinicopathologic, immunohistochemical, and molecular analysis of eight cases. Am J Dermatopathol. 2007;29(5):443–8.
22. O'Connell JX, Wehrli BM, Nielsen GP, Rosenberg AE. Giant cell tumors of soft tissue: a clinicopathologic study of 18 benign and malignant tumors. Am J Surg Pathol. 2000;24(3):386–95.
23. Oliveira AM, Dei Tos AP, Fletcher CD, Nascimento AG. Primary giant cell tumor of soft tissues: a study of 22 cases. Am J Surg Pathol. 2000;24(2):248–56.
24. Remstein ED, Arndt CA, Nascimento AG. Plexiform fibrohistiocytic tumor: clinicopathologic analysis of 22 cases. Am J Surg Pathol. 1999;23(6):662–70.
25. Salomao DR, Nascimento AG. Plexiform fibrohistiocytic tumor with systemic metastases: a case report. Am J Surg Pathol. 1997;21(4):469–76.
26. Schaefer IM, Fletcher CD. Myxoid variant of so-called angiomatoid "malignant fibrous histiocytoma": clinicopathologic characterization in a series of 21 cases. Am J Surg Pathol. 2014;38(6):816–23.
27. Shah KK, McHugh JB, Folpe AL, Patel RM. Dermatofibrosarcoma protuberans of distal extremities and Acral sites: a Clinicopathologic analysis of 27 cases. Am J Surg Pathol. 2018;42(3):413–9.
28. Shmookler BM, Enzinger FM, Weiss SW. Giant cell fibroblastoma. A juvenile form of dermatofibrosarcoma protuberans. Cancer. 1989;64(10):2154–61.
29. Tanas MR, Rubin BP, Montgomery EA, Turner SL, Cook JR, Tubbs RR, Billings SD, Goldblum JR. Utility of FISH in the diagnosis of angiomatoid fibrous histiocytoma: a series of 18 cases. Mod Pathol. 2010;23(1):93–7.
30. Thway K, Fisher C. Angiomatoid fibrous histiocytoma: the current status of pathology and genetics. Arch Pathol Lab Med. 2015;139(5):674–82.
31. Thway K, Noujaim J, Jones RL, Fisher C. Dermatofibrosarcoma protuberans: pathology, genetics, and potential therapeutic strategies. Ann Diagn Pathol. 2016;25:64–71.
32. Wada N, Ito T, Uchi H, Nakahara T, Tsuji G, Yamada Y, Oda Y, Furue M. Superficial CD34-positive fibroblastic tumor: a new case from Japan. J Dermatol. 2016;43(8):934–6.
33. Zelger B, Weinlich G, Steiner H, Zelger BG, Egarter-Vigl E. Dermal and subcutaneous variants of plexiform fibrohistiocytic tumor. Am J Surg Pathol. 1997;21(2):235–41.

Malignant Fibrous, Fibrohistiocytic, and Myofibroblastic Tumors

6

Aaron M. Udager, Reena Singh, Steven D. Billings, and Rajiv M. Patel

Abstract

This chapter covers fibrous, fibrohistiocytic, and myofibroblastic tumors that have metastatic potential. Congenital/infantile fibrosarcoma is the exception to that rule, as it behaves less aggressively than its adult counterpart. Adult-type fibrosarcoma is a diagnosis in decline due to the recognition of distinct variants: low-grade fibromyxoid sarcoma, sclerosing epithelioid fibrosarcoma, myxofibrosarcoma, low-grade myofibroblastic sarcoma (myofibrosarcoma), and myxoinflammatory fibroblastic sarcoma. Undifferentiated pleomorphic sarcoma may also present as a superficial tumor and will be briefly discussed. The chapter closes with a discussion of undifferentiated pleomorphic sarcomas of the skin, specifically atypical fibroxanthoma and pleomorphic dermal sarcoma.

A. M. Udager · R. M. Patel (✉)
Department of Pathology, University of Michigan Medical School, Ann Arbor, MI, USA
e-mail: rajivpat@med.umich.edu

R. Singh
Department of Pathology, Oregon Health and Science University School of Medicine, Portland, OR, USA

S. D. Billings
Department of Pathology, Cleveland Clinic, Cleveland, OH, USA

Congenital/Infantile Fibrosarcoma

Clinical Features

Congenital/infantile fibrosarcoma (CIFS) is a low-grade sarcoma that almost always presents within the first year of life. One-third of tumors are congenital, and there is a slight male predisposition. Tumors present as painless masses within the superficial and deep soft tissues of the distal extremities, followed by involvement of the trunk, head and neck, retroperitoneum, and rarely, viscera. Due to rapid growth, there may be ulceration of the overlying skin and/or erosion of the underlying bone. Congenital lesions may be apparent on in utero scans. Despite a relatively high rate of local recurrence, CIFS only rarely metastasizes, and the overall mortality rate is low.

Pathologic Features

Tumors grow in infiltrative, cellular sheets of closely packed spindle cells separated by variable amounts of collagen (Fig. 6.1a). Tumors with minimal collagen have a primitive appearance with haphazard or swarming appearance to the cells (medullary type), while tumors with more collagen have regularly intersecting fascicles with a herringbone appearance (desmoplastic type) (Fig. 6.1b, c). Tumor cells are uniformly

S. D. Billings et al. (eds.), *Soft Tissue Tumors of the Skin*,
https://doi.org/10.1007/978-1-4939-8812-9_6

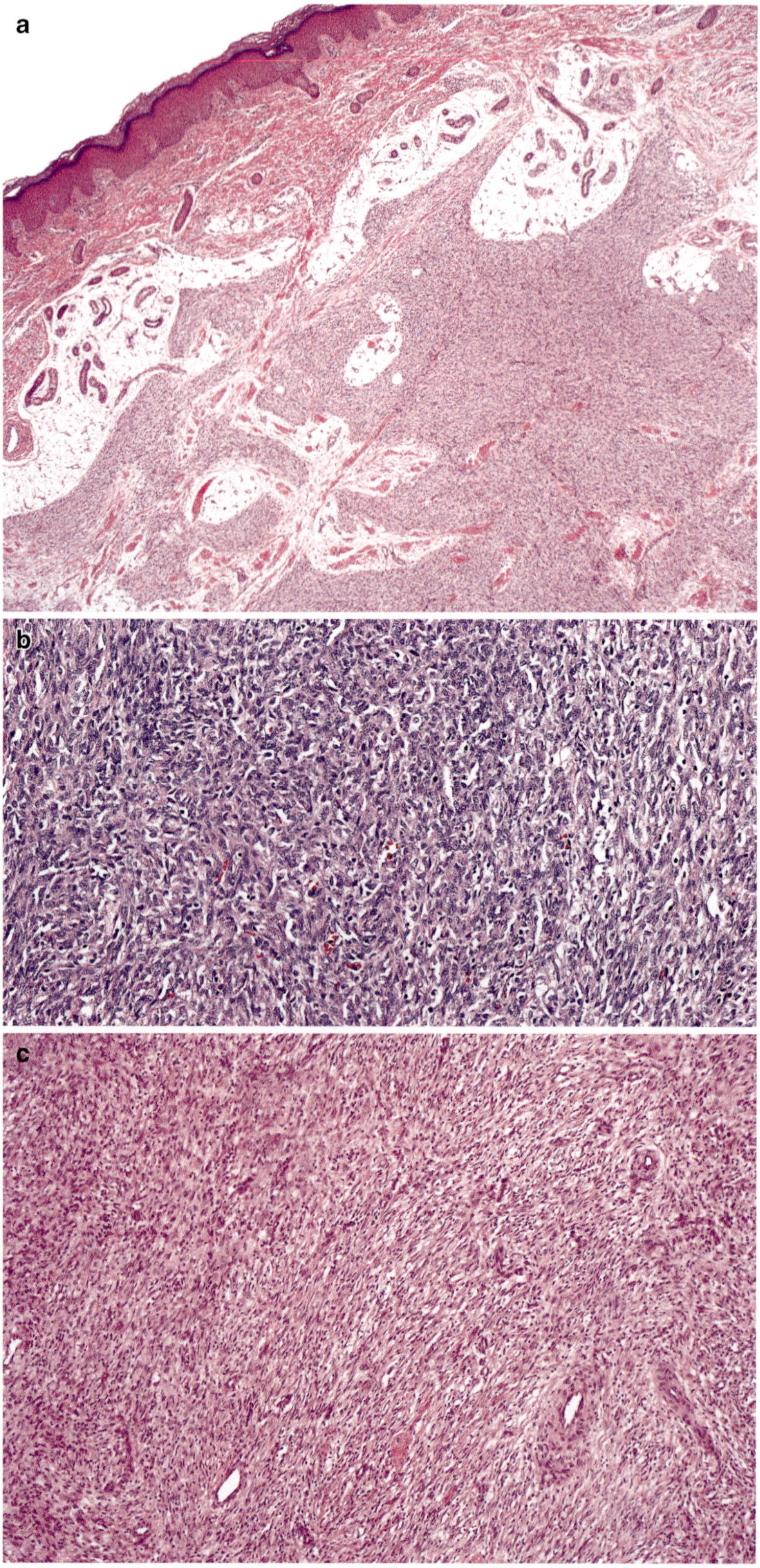

Fig. 6.1 (**a**). Congenital/infantile fibrosarcoma has an infiltrative, sheet-like growth of spindle cells separated by variable amounts of collagen. (**b**). Immature-appearing (medullary type) tumor with sparse collagen and haphazard arrangement of cells. (**c**). Tumors with increased collagen have organized, intersecting fascicles (desmoplastic type). (Images courtesy of Dr. Michael Fritsch, Department of Pathology and Laboratory Medicine, University of Wisconsin School of Medicine, Madison, WI)

atypical with vesicular nuclei. Pleomorphic and multinucleated cells are rare. Lymphocytes may be present diffusely or as small aggregates. The vasculature is variable, ranging from congested and dilated to hemangiopericytomatous (staghorn)-like. Large tumors frequently have necrosis, hemorrhage, and cystic degeneration. The immunophenotype is relatively nonspecific, but muscle markers, including muscle-specific actin and smooth muscle actin, may be focally positive. WT1 (clone 6F-H2) demonstrates strong and diffuse cytoplasmic immunoreactivity. Although WTI is a sensitive marker, it is not specific for CIFS and is similarly positive in infantile fibromatosis. This finding compounds the diagnostic dilemma in recurrent CIFSs, which may be histologically identical to infantile fibromatosis (see Chap. 4). Characteristically, CIFS harbors an *ETV6-NTRK3* gene fusion resulting from t(12;15)(p13;q25) translocation. Recently, *BRAF* rearrangement and *EML4-NTRK3*, *TPM3-NTRK1*, and *LMNA-NTRK1* fusions have been described in *ETV6-NTRK3*-negative cases and in cases with CIFS-like morphology occurring in older children (Table 6.1).

Differential Diagnosis

The differential diagnosis for CIFS includes cellular infantile fibromatosis, myopericytoma, infantile myofibroma, dermatofibrosarcoma protuberans, monophasic synovial sarcoma, spindle cell rhabdomyosarcoma, and malignant peripheral nerve sheath tumor. Despite the significant morphologic and immunophenotypic overlap, CIFS can typically be distinguished from cellular infantile fibromatosis by its herringbone growth pattern, high cellularity, marked mitotic activity, and/or necrosis. Documenting the *ETV6-NTRK3* gene fusion confirms the diagnosis of CIFS in problematic cases. Myopericytoma and myofibroma may represent lesions on a histologic spectrum with CIFS, but both have diffuse smooth muscle actin expression. Myopericytoma has a regular distribution of vessels with branching or staghorn appearance compared to the variable vasculature in CIFS. Myofibroma demonstrates biphasic nodules with peripheral light and central dark staining areas. Dermatofibrosarcoma protuberans has a storiform pattern, diffuse CD34 immunoreactivity, and *PDGFB* rearrangement. Monophasic synovial sarcoma expresses keratins or EMA focally, has diffuse TLE-1 expression, and harbors *SYT-SSX* translocation. Rhabdomyosarcomas can be distinguished by desmin and myogenin immunoreactivity. Superficial malignant peripheral nerve sheath tumor is usually seen arising from a benign peripheral nerve sheath tumor and has variable S100 protein expression.

Table 6.1 Key pathologic features: congenital/infantile fibrosarcoma

Key pathologic features
Cellular spindle cell proliferation with variable collagen
Primitive appearance (medullary type) or herringbone architecture (desmoplastic type)
Minimal nuclear pleomorphism
Numerous mitoses and/or necrosis
Admixed lymphocytes
Variable vasculature with some hemangiopericytoma-like vessels
ETV6-NTRK3 gene fusion in majority

Adult-Type Fibrosarcoma

Clinical Features

Adult-type fibrosarcoma is exceptionally rare and has become a diagnosis of exclusion due to recognition of several distinct entities, which in the past were regarded as fibrosarcoma. Most cases previously diagnosed as fibrosarcoma in the skin likely represent fibrosarcomatous dermatofibrosarcoma protuberans (see Chap. 5). True adult-type fibrosarcoma occurs in the fifth and sixth decades of life. The deep soft tissues of the lower extremities are commonly affected, but occasional tumors may be subcutaneous. Some cases are associated with prior radiation therapy. Local recurrence is common, and there is a significant risk of metastasis and death.

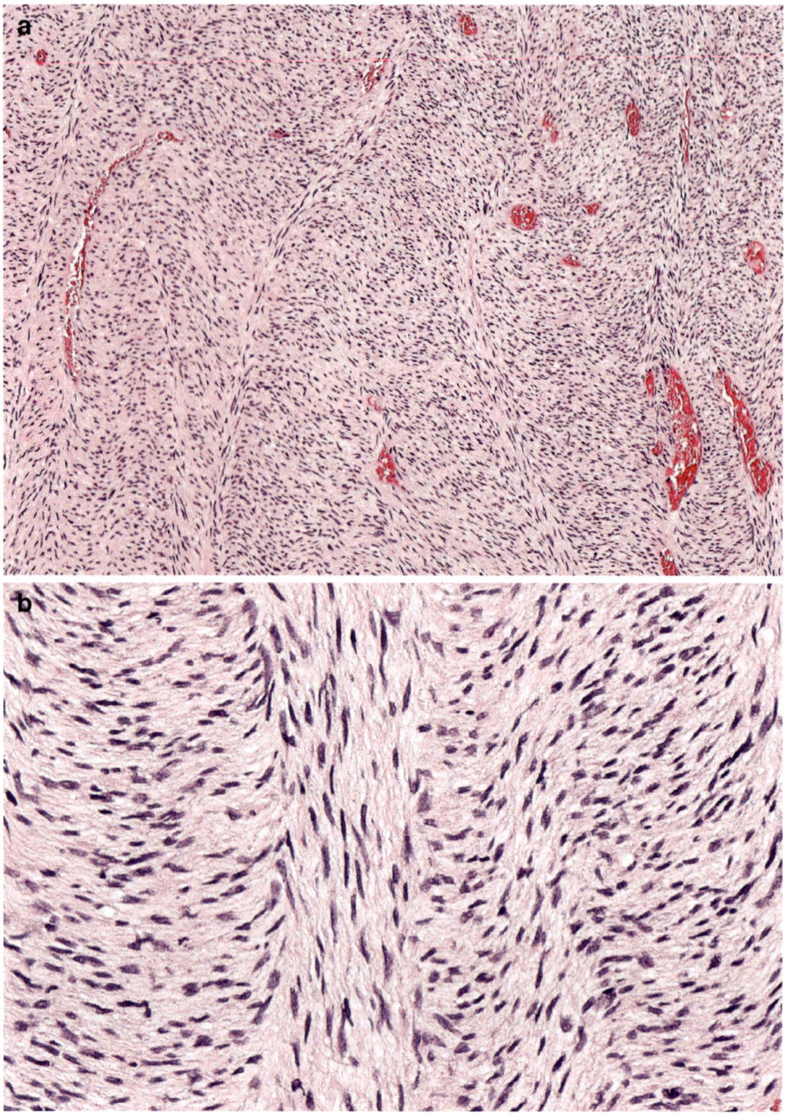

Fig. 6.2 (**a**). Adult-type fibrosarcoma with herringbone architecture. (**b**). The tumor is composed of uniform atypical spindled cells with indistinct cytoplasmic boundaries, mildly pleomorphic nuclei, and variable mitotic figures

Table 6.2 Key pathologic features: adult-type fibrosarcoma

Diagnosis of exclusion (especially consider fibrosarcomatous transformation of dermatofibrosarcoma protuberans)
Uniform proliferation of spindle cells with herringbone arrangement in fibrous stroma
Pleomorphic cells are rare
Higher-grade lesions should be diagnosed as undifferentiated pleomorphic sarcoma
Haphazard arrangement of tumor cells, increased mitoses, and necrosis

Pathologic Features

Adult-type fibrosarcoma is generally well circumscribed and at least partially invested by a fibrous capsule. The fusiform cells are arranged in fascicles with intervening stromal collagen, imparting a herringbone appearance (Fig. 6.2a). The uniform tumor cells have indistinct cytoplasmic boundaries, mildly pleomorphic nuclei, and variable mitotic figures (Fig. 6.2b). Cases with high-grade morphology should be diagnosed as undifferentiated pleomorphic sarcoma, provided that a specific line of differentiation has been adequately ruled out. The tumor is diffusely positive for vimentin and may have focal smooth muscle actin expression. Markers indicative of a particular line of differentiation including keratins, EMA, S100, CD34, and desmin are negative. Complex chromosomal abnormalities have been described, but recurrent genetic aberrations have not (Table 6.2).

Differential Diagnosis

As adult-type fibrosarcoma is a diagnosis of exclusion, it needs to be separated from its many mimics. Leiomyosarcoma has plump cells with distinct cytoplasmic boundaries, blunt-ended nuclei, diffuse smooth muscle actin expression, and also usually expresses desmin. Synovial sarcoma has diffuse TLE-1 staining, focal keratin immunoreactivity, and *SYT-SSX* rearrangement. Malignant peripheral nerve sheath tumor may be associated with a benign peripheral nerve sheath tumor and have S100 protein expression. Spindle cell melanoma is diffusely positive for S100 protein and may have areas of conventional melanoma morphology. Spindle cell rhabdomyosarcoma expresses desmin, myogenin, and MyoD1.

Low-Grade Fibromyxoid Sarcoma

Clinical Features

Low-grade fibromyxoid sarcoma (LGFMS) has a slight male predilection and typically occurs in young to middle-aged adults, but a broad age range may be affected. Children appear to be disproportionately afflicted by superficial LGFMS. In one large series of superficial LGFMS, 37% of cases arose in pediatric patients. Superficial LGFMS most commonly arises in the lower extremities, but may also involve the trunk, upper extremities, and vulvar/inguinal region. LGFMS is relatively indolent in the short term, but this tumor is notorious for the development of late (>5 years from diagnosis) metastasis in close to half of patients. Metastases, commonly to the lungs and pleura, have been reported up to 45 years after initial diagnosis. Mortality is approximately 40%. Dedifferentiated round cell morphology is the only histologic feature associated with more aggressive clinical behavior. Wide local excision with lifelong follow-up is the preferred treatment.

Pathologic Features

LGFMS may be well circumscribed with a fibrous pseudocapsule or infiltrative, although superficial tumors are more commonly circumscribed. Superficial tumors are centered in the subcutis, but may extend into the overlying dermis. Tumors have low to moderate cellularity and are comprised of spindle cells arrayed in swirling to fascicular patterns in a variably fibrous to myxoid stroma. Transition from fibrous to myxoid zones is often abrupt (Fig. 6.3a). The myxoid zones often have conspicuous curvilinear vessels and spindled to stellate-appearing cells (Fig. 6.3b), while the fibrous zones may be paucicellular and hyalinized. The individual tumor cells are relatively bland with scant cytoplasm, dark oval nuclei, and inconspicuous nucleoli (Fig. 6.3c). Other changes include epithelioid cells, foci of intermediate-grade histology with increased mitotic activity, and collagen rosettes, characterized by central collagen cores with peripherally palisading tumor cells (Fig. 6.3d). Tumors with a predominance of rosettes are designated as the hyalinizing spindle cell tumor with giant rosettes (HSCTGR) variant of LGFMS (Fig. 6.3e). Rarely, dedifferentiation into an anaplastic round cell sarcoma may occur. Over 90% of tumors are positive for MUC4, a highly sensitive and specific marker for LGFMS. Focal immunoreactivity for EMA is relatively common. Two-thirds of cutaneous cases are associated with *FUS* gene rearrangements, commonly t(7;16)(q34;p11) *FUS-CREB3L2* and rarely t(11;16)(p11;p11) *FUS-CREB3L1* (Table 6.3).

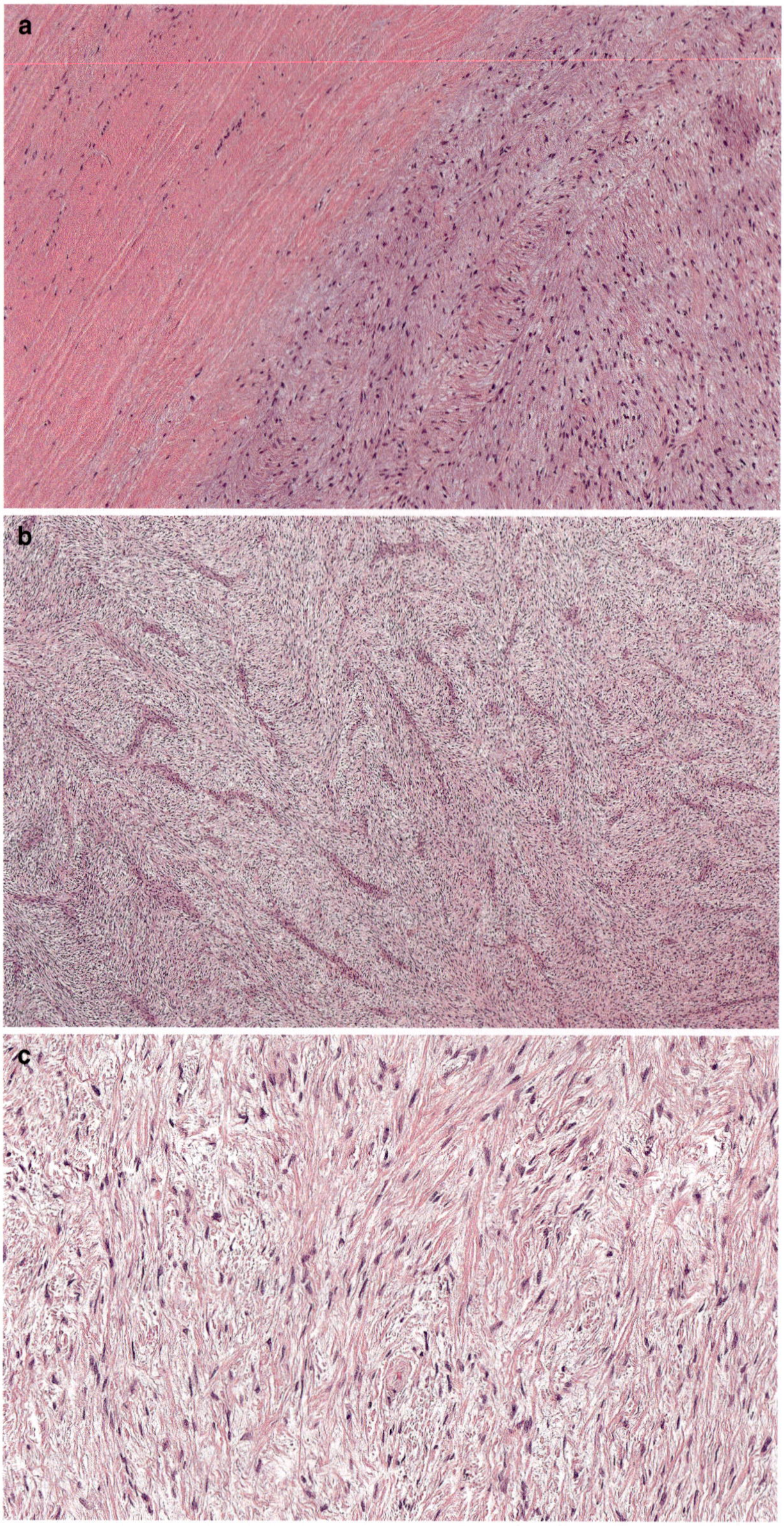

Fig. 6.3 (**a**). Low-grade fibromyxoid sarcoma generally has low cellularity, with alternating fibrous and myxoid zones. Transition from cellular to myxoid zones is often abrupt. (**b**). The myxoid zone often has a conspicuous vasculature. (**c**). The individual tumor cells are hyperchromatic, but bland-appearing with oval nuclei and inconspicuous nucleoli. (**d**). Collagen rosettes with dense cores surrounded by peripherally palisading tumor cells may be present. (**e**). In rare cases the collagen rosettes are numerous (hyalinizing spindle cell tumor with giant rosettes variant)

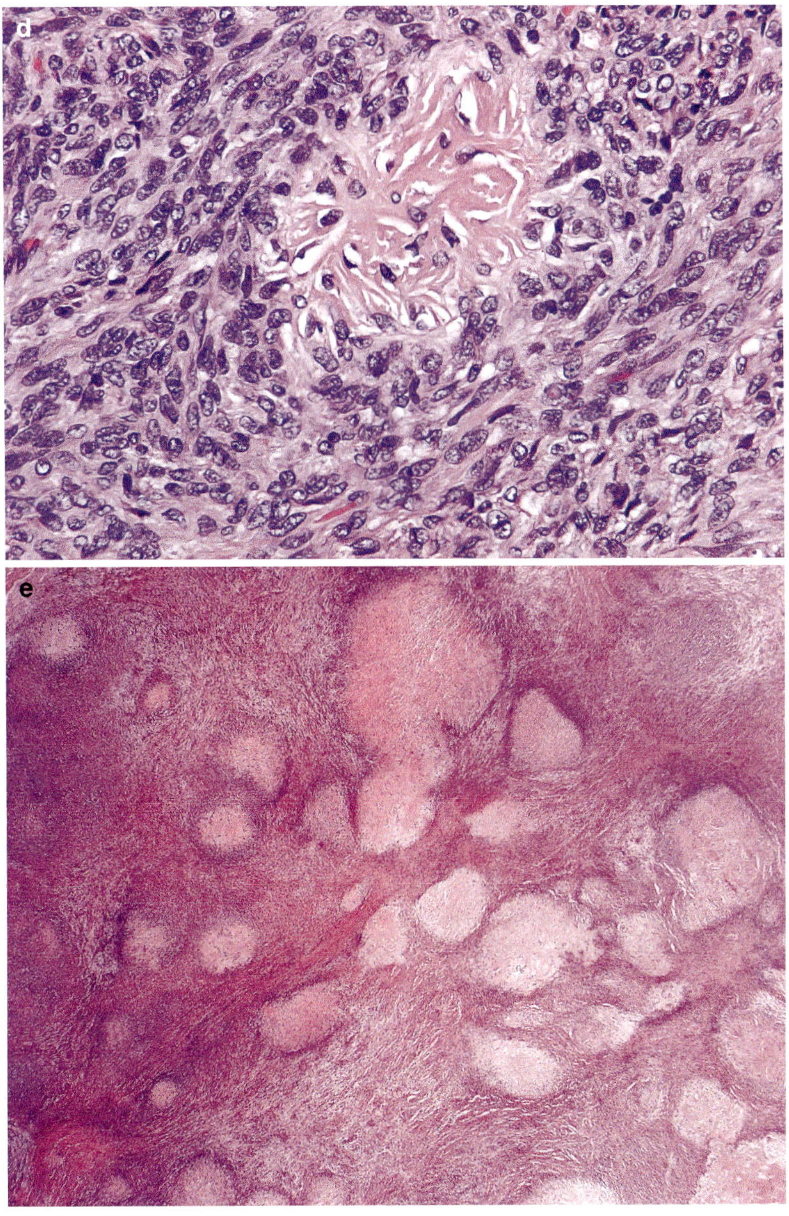

Fig. 6.3 (continued)

Table 6.3 Key pathologic features: low-grade fibromyxoid sarcoma

Bland spindle cells with dark, oval nuclei and low mitotic activity
Variably fibrous and myxoid zones
Transition between myxoid and fibrous zones is often abrupt
Curvilinear or arcuate thin-walled vessels in myxoid zones
Diffuse MUC4 immunoreactivity

Differential Diagnosis

LGFMS may be difficult to distinguish from a variety of tumors, including nodular fasciitis, perineurioma, neurofibroma, fibromatosis, superficial angiomyxoma, dermatofibrosarcoma protuberans, low-grade malignant peripheral nerve sheath tumor, synovial sarcoma, and myxofibrosarcoma. Nodular fasciitis has a "tissue culture-like" arrangement of fibroblasts and myofibroblasts, myxoid degeneration with extravasated erythrocytes, and granulation tissue-like vessels at the periphery of the lesion. Perineurioma is also EMA-positive, but is additionally positive for GLUT-1 and claudin-1. Neurofibroma is positive for S100 protein and CD34, both of which are negative in LGFMS. Superficial fibromatosis does not typically have myxoid change like its deeper counterparts and often demonstrates nuclear beta-catenin localization by immunohistochemistry. Superficial angiomyoma is less cellular than LGFMS and does not have the alternating fibrous zones. Dermatofibrosarcoma protuberans may have any combination of myxoid and hyalinized areas, but recognition of conventional areas with a storiform arrangement, diffuse CD34 expression, and identification of *PDGFB* gene rearrangement all aid in its diagnosis. Low-grade malignant peripheral nerve sheath tumor and synovial sarcoma have a marbled appearance, but can be separated out in the majority of cases by S100 and TLE-1 expression, respectively. LGFMS and myxofibrosarcoma are commonly confused due to their similar nomenclature and histology. Myxoid areas in myxofibrosarcoma tend to form discrete nodules, and in these areas the hyperchromatic and pleomorphic tumor cells aggregate around a well-developed, thin-walled vascular network. HSCTGR resembles neuroblastoma-like schwannoma, but the latter is diffusely positive for S100 protein and has conventional Antoni A and Antoni B areas. None of the aforementioned tumors in the differential diagnosis are positive for MUC4.

Sclerosing Epithelioid Fibrosarcoma

Clinical Features

Sclerosing epithelioid fibrosarcoma (SEF) is an unusual sarcoma that shares clinical, morphologic, immunohistochemical, and molecular features with low-grade fibromyxoid sarcoma. It typically occurs in middle-aged to older adults and does not demonstrate a gender preference. Tumors usually present as an enlarging painless mass on the extremities, limb girdles, thorax, or head and neck. Most cases involve the deep soft tissue. Wide surgical excision and close clinical follow-up are the mainstay of treatment. Recurrence is common, and metastases to the lungs, pleura, bone, and brain occur in up to 80% of cases.

Pathologic Features

SEF is an unencapsulated, but circumscribed tumor, though there may be foci of infiltration into the surrounding fascia, muscle, and periosteum. The neoplastic cells are arranged singly and in variably sized cords, trabeculae, and nests within a densely hyalinized stroma (Fig. 6.4a). Occasional arrangement into alveoli and acini may be observed. Myxoid, chondroosseous, and calcific foci may be noted. The tumor is comprised of bland epithelioid cells with moderate clear to lightly eosinophilic cytoplasm, irregular vesicular nuclei, and small nucleoli (Fig. 6.4b). Most tumors have a low mitotic rate, but some can have prominent nuclear pleomorphism, necrosis, and mitotic activity. Cleft-like spaces at the periphery of the tumor give an impression of angiolymphatic invasion. Areas resembling low-grade fibromyxoid sarcoma with or without collagen rosettes may be present (Fig. 6.4c). Immunohistochemistry demonstrates MUC4 expression in the majority of cases, and tumors may show variable EMA and S100 expression. Stains for keratins, CD34, smooth muscle actin, and desmin are typically negative. *FUS-CREB3L2* fusion is identified in SEF with hybrid features of low-grade fibromyxoid sarcoma, suggesting that some cases of SEF exist along a spectrum with low-grade fibromyxoid sarcoma. However, "pure" SEF uncommonly has the *FUS-CREB3L2* fusion. *EWSR1-CREB3L1* fusion has been documented in a few of the aforementioned cases. Overall, *EWSR1* and *CREB3L1* rearrangements are predominant over *FUS* and *CREB3L2* rearrangements in "pure" SEF. The precise relationship between SEF and low-grade fibromyxoid sarcoma is uncertain (Table 6.4).

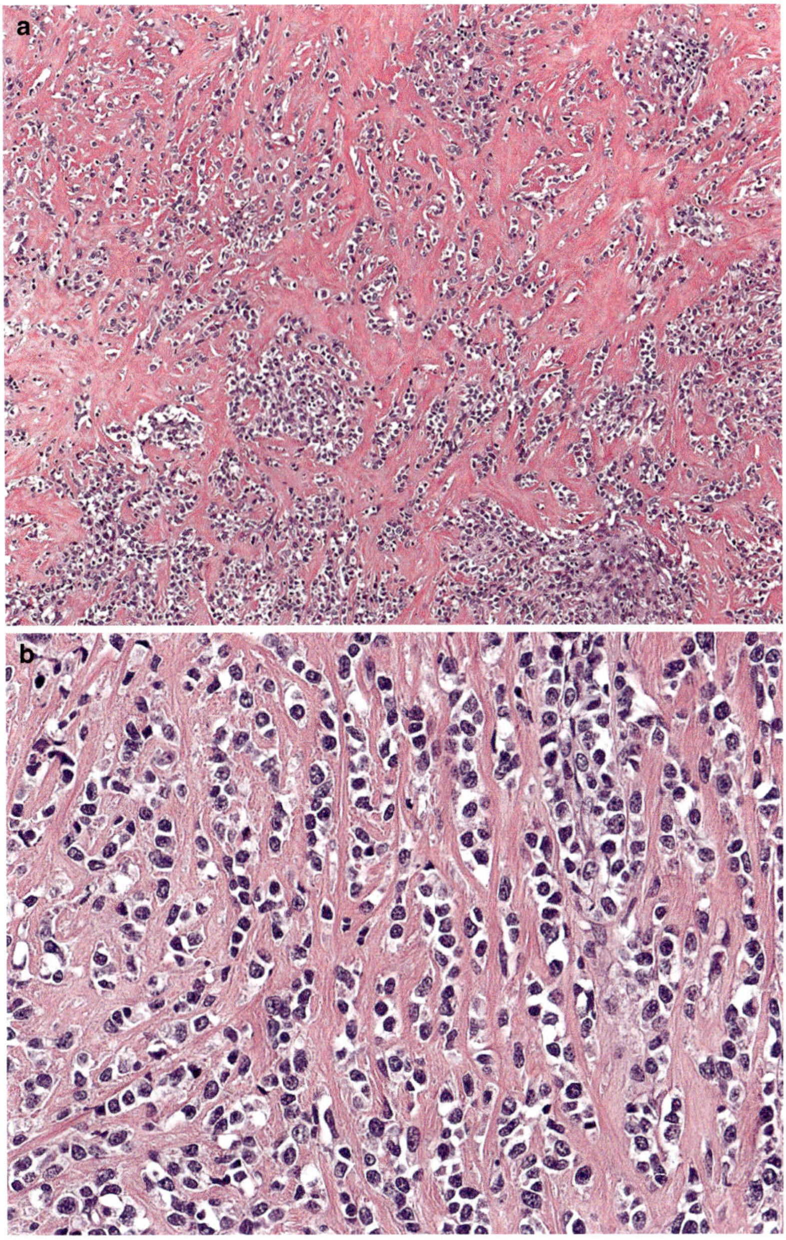

Fig. 6.4 (**a**). Sclerosing epithelioid fibrosarcoma with cords, trabeculae and nests of tumor cells within hyalinized stroma. (**b**). High-power view of the bland epithelioid cells with moderate pale to amphophilic cytoplasm, irregular vesicular nuclei, and small nucleoli. (**c**). Tumor with hybrid features of sclerosing epithelioid fibrosarcoma (left) and low-grade fibromyxoid sarcoma (right)

Differential Diagnosis

SEF is a rare tumor that may be mistaken for ossifying fibromyxoid tumor, sclerosing rhabdomyosarcoma, clear cell sarcoma, sclerosing lymphoma, and infiltrating carcinoma. Ossifying fibromyxoid tumor also has focal S100 protein expression, but most cases have a fibrous pseudocapsule with a peripheral shell of bone and are usually negative or only focally positive for MUC4. Sclerosing rhabdomyosarcoma expresses desmin and myogenin. Clear cell sarcoma expresses melanocytic markers, such as HMB-45 and/or Melan-A in addition to S100 protein. Sclerosing lymphoma and infiltrating carcinoma can be ruled out with hematolymphoid

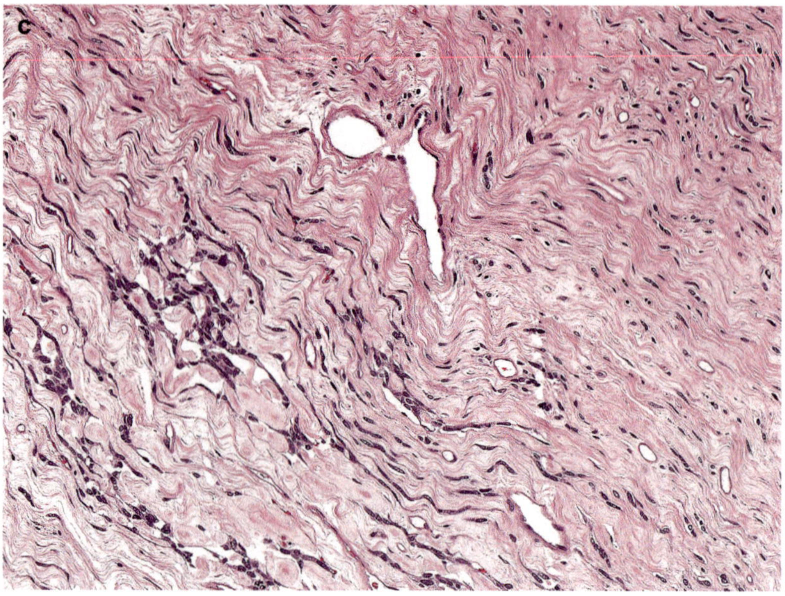

Fig. 6.4 (continued)

Table 6.4 Key pathologic features: sclerosing epithelioid fibrosarcoma

Cords and nests of epithelioid cells with bland features and low mitotic activity
Densely hyalinized stroma
Cases with hybrid features of low-grade fibromyxoid sarcoma have similar immunohistochemical and genetic features
"Pure" SEF predominantly has *EWSR1-CREB3L1* fusion

markers and keratins, respectively. EMA should be utilized cautiously when metastatic carcinoma is in the differential diagnosis, as 50% of SEFs may express EMA.

Myxofibrosarcoma

Clinical Features

Myxofibrosarcoma is a relatively common sarcoma in older adults and shows a slight male predominance. Tumors usually present as enlarging painless masses in the subcutaneous soft tissue of the lower extremities. Other sites include the upper extremities, thorax, and head and neck region. One-third of cases occur in the deep soft tissue. Myxofibrosarcoma is prone to frequent local recurrences. Low-grade lesions have a relatively low risk of metastasis, but metastatic risk increases with higher tumor grade. The rare epithelioid variant is seen mainly in high-grade tumors and has a worse prognosis with a higher rate of metastasis, including to lymph nodes, which is an unusual event for a sarcoma. Myxofibrosarcomas are infiltrative tumors that frequently extend beyond the clinically apparent lesion. Wide excision is required to achieve negative margins.

Pathologic Features

Myxofibrosarcoma has a wide morphologic spectrum, but typically shows multinodular growth and a variably myxoid stroma (Fig. 6.5a). The tumor is centered in the subcutis with frequent extension into the dermis (Fig. 6.5b). Rare cases may be restricted to the dermis. Low-grade tumors are hypocellular and comprised predominantly of spindled to stellate cells with enlarged, hyperchromatic nuclei in a prominent myxoid stroma (Fig. 6.5c). Tumor cells often cluster around curvilinear vessels, and cells with vacuolated cytoplasm ("pseudolipoblasts") may be present. Low-grade cases are devoid of significant mitotic activity or necrosis. In contrast, intermediate- and high-grade tumors demonstrate increased cellularity, pleomorphism, mitotic

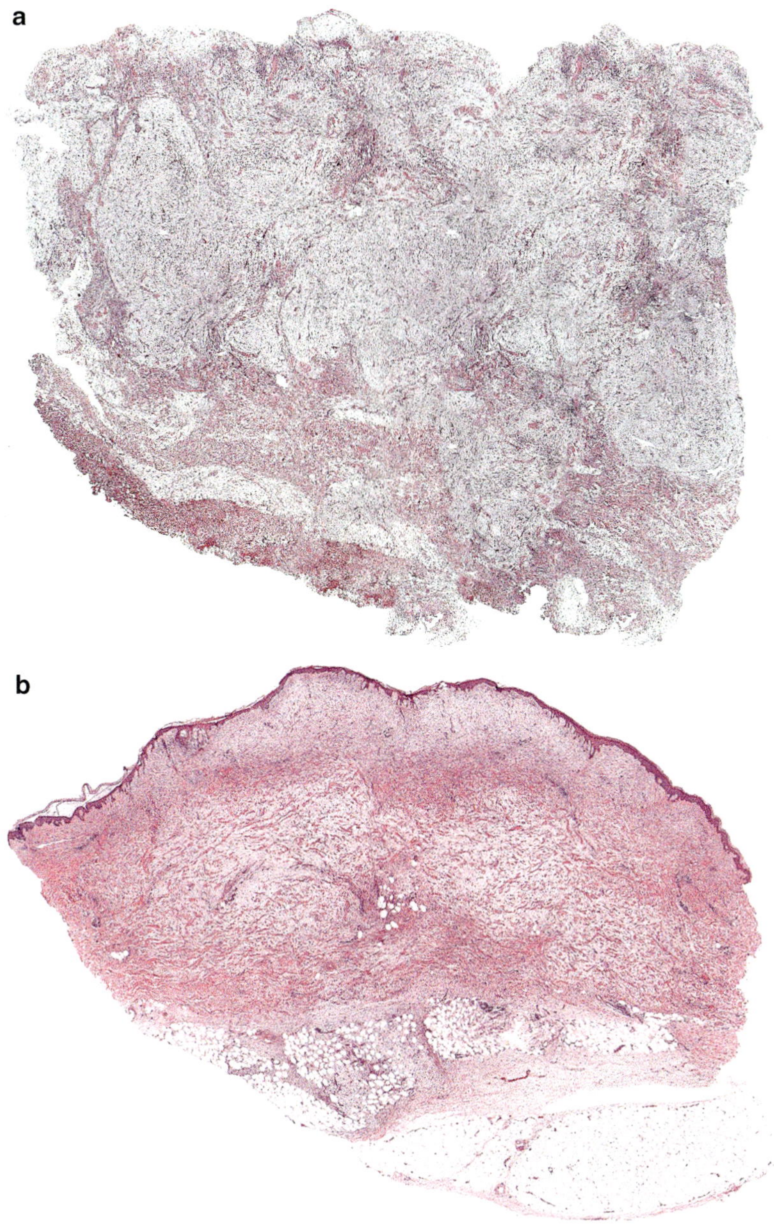

Fig. 6.5 (**a**). Low-power view of low-grade myxofibrosarcoma showing a multinodular, myxoid tumor in the subcutis. (**b**). Myxofibrosarcoma often extends into the dermis. The myxoid stroma may be less conspicuous in the dermis. (**c**). Low-grade tumor with cells condensing around thin-walled arcuate vessels and containing "pseudolipoblasts." (**d**). Low-power view of high-grade tumor with increased cellularity, necrosis, and less myxoid appearance. (**e**). Intermediate- to high-grade myxofibrosarcomas have more marked atypia and can have areas with little to no myxoid stroma. (**f**). Epithelioid variant of myxofibrosarcoma with sheets of atypical epithelioid tumor cells. Areas of conventional myxofibrosarcoma help with the recognition of this variant

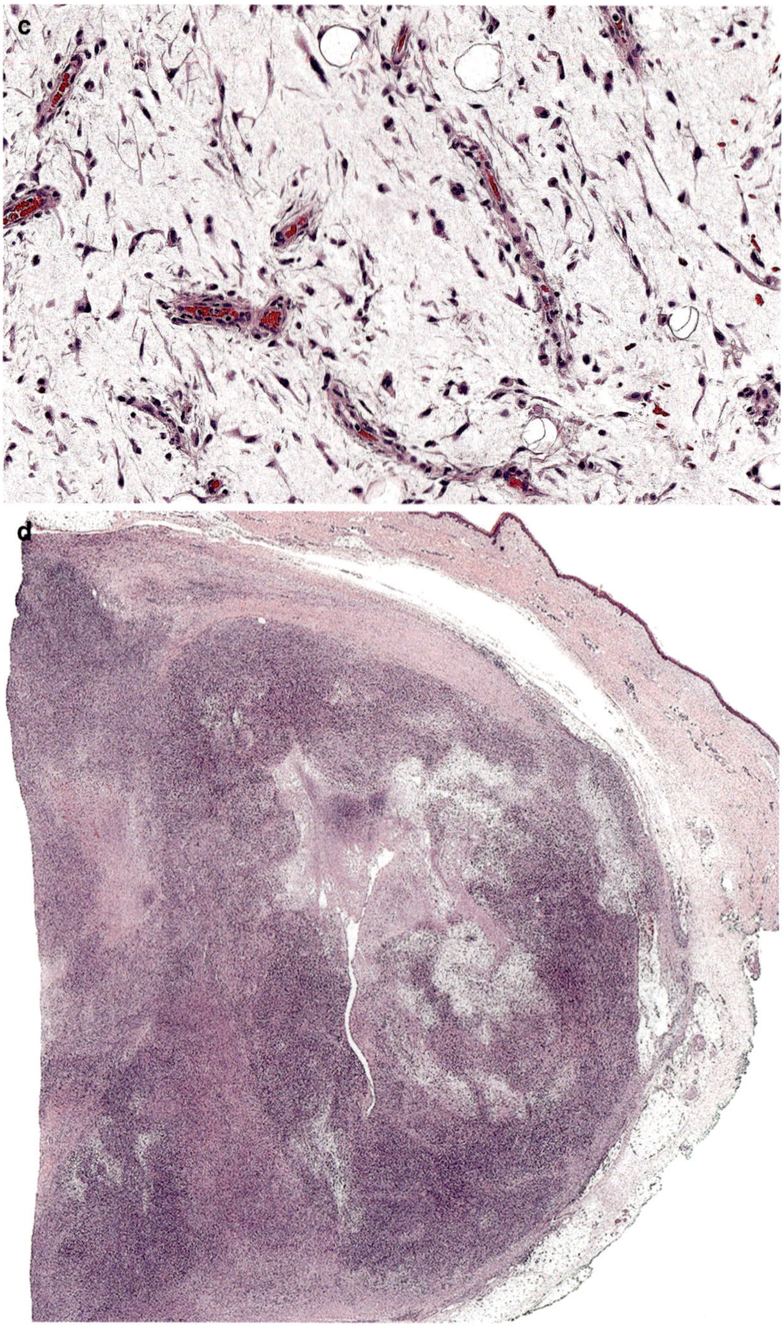

Fig. 6.5 (continued)

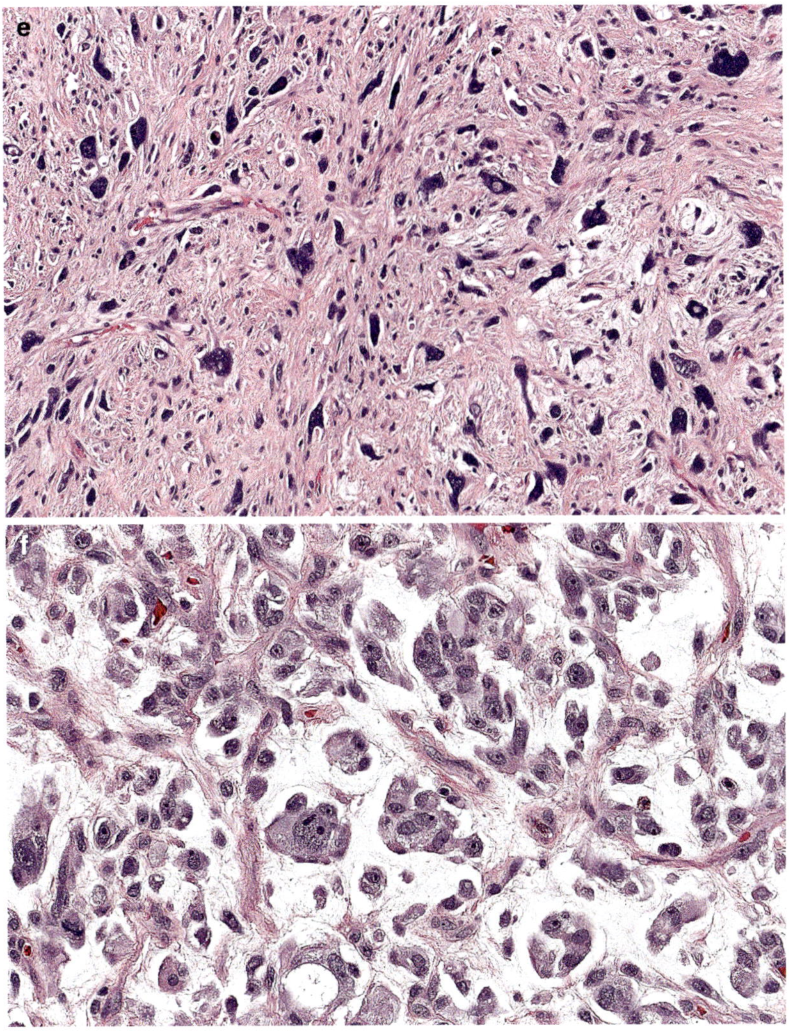

Fig. 6.5 (continued)

activity, and necrosis. The characteristic myxoid stroma and vasculature may be obscured by the increased cellularity (Fig. 6.5d). Intermediate to high-grade tumors may have areas of marked pleomorphism and areas with less myxoid stroma (Fig. 6.5e). Finding areas with myxoid stroma and the characteristic curvilinear vasculature helps establish the diagnosis in higher-grade tumors. It is important to note that myxofibrosarcoma frequently progresses to higher-grade tumors on subsequent recurrences. The epithelioid variant has small clusters of cells with abundant eosinophilic cytoplasm, vesicular nuclei, and prominent nucleoli (Fig. 6.5f).

The immunophenotype is relatively nonspecific, but tumors may show patchy muscle-specific actin, smooth muscle actin, and CD34 expression. Stains for keratin, S100, desmin, and CD68 are typically negative. Myxofibrosarcoma usually shows a highly complex karyotype without highly recurrent molecular alterations. As might be expected from differences in histology and clinical behavior, intermediate- and high-grade tumors demonstrate more complex karyotypes when compared to their low-grade counterparts. These higher-grade tumors are more akin to undifferentiated pleomorphic sarcoma in terms of clinical behavior and encom-

Table 6.5 Key pathologic features: myxofibrosarcoma

Multinodular tumor with myxoid stroma
Cells with enlarged, hyperchromatic nuclei
Tumor cells condense around thin, curvilinear vessels
Admixed pseudolipoblasts
Higher-grade tumors have increased pleomorphism, cellularity, mitoses, and/or necrosis

pass a group that was previously designated as myxoid malignant fibrous histiocytoma (Table 6.5).

Differential Diagnosis

Low-grade myxofibrosarcoma may be difficult to distinguish from a variety of benign and malignant tumors, including nodular fasciitis, myxoma, spindle cell lipoma, nerve sheath myxoma, low-grade fibromyxoid sarcoma, and myxoid liposarcoma. Higher-grade tumors need to be differentiated from sarcomatoid carcinomas, melanoma, pleomorphic leiomyosarcoma, pleomorphic and higher-grade myxoid/round cell liposarcomas, pleomorphic rhabdomyosarcoma, and myxoinflammatory fibroblastic sarcoma. Nodular fasciitis lacks cytologic atypia and has less prominent myxoid stroma. The hypocellularity of myxoma and low-grade myxofibrosarcoma may overlap, but the lesional cells of myxoma lack nuclear hyperchromasia and cytologic atypia. Spindle cell lipoma has bland spindle cells, ropey collagen, and mature fat in varying quantities. Nerve sheath myxoma lacks cytologic atypia and curvilinear vessels, is found commonly on the digits, and is diffusely S100 protein-positive. Myxoid/round cell liposarcoma occurs in deeper locations, has true lipoblasts, an arborizing thin-walled vasculature, and harbors a *DDIT3* translocation. Demonstration of this latter feature is especially helpful in myxoid/round cell liposarcomas with a significant round cell component, as these cases may overlap with epithelioid myxofibrosarcoma. Both the epithelioid and higher-grade variants need to be differentiated from melanoma and carcinoma by a panel of immunohistochemical stains including S100 protein and cytokeratins. Pleomorphic leiomyosarcoma expresses smooth muscle actin diffusely rather than the membranous expression that may be seen in myxofibrosarcoma. Pleomorphic rhabdomyosarcomas demonstrate skeletal muscle differentiation with desmin, myogenin, and/or MyoD1 expression. Pleomorphic liposarcoma demonstrates lipoblasts with pleomorphic nuclei that are scalloped by intracytoplasmic lipid vacuole(s). The differential diagnosis with myxoinflammatory fibroblastic sarcoma is discussed below.

Undifferentiated Pleomorphic Sarcoma

Clinical Features

Undifferentiated pleomorphic sarcoma (UPS) is a pleomorphic soft tissue sarcoma with no definite line of differentiation. It is included in this chapter because it was historically considered of fibrohistiocytic origin and termed malignant fibrous histiocytoma. UPS is an aggressive tumor that commonly arises in the deep soft tissues of the lower proximal extremities but can occur at a variety of sites. Approximately 20% of cases originate in the subcutaneous soft tissue. Adults aged 50–70 are commonly affected. Rare tumors are associated with previous radiation therapy and may have a more aggressive course than sporadic UPS. Local recurrence and metastasis each occur at a rate of approximately 30%. The standard for therapy is wide local resection with or without (neo)adjuvant radiotherapy.

Pathologic Features

UPS has infiltrative edges and a storiform to haphazard arrangement of plump spindle and histiocytoid cells with pleomorphic nuclei (Fig. 6.6a, b). The histiocytoid cells are occasionally multinucleated, but some tumors may have numerous admixed osteoclast-like giant or inflammatory cells. The cytoplasm may be densely eosinophilic or xanthomatous. Mitotic figures are numerous, and atypical forms are

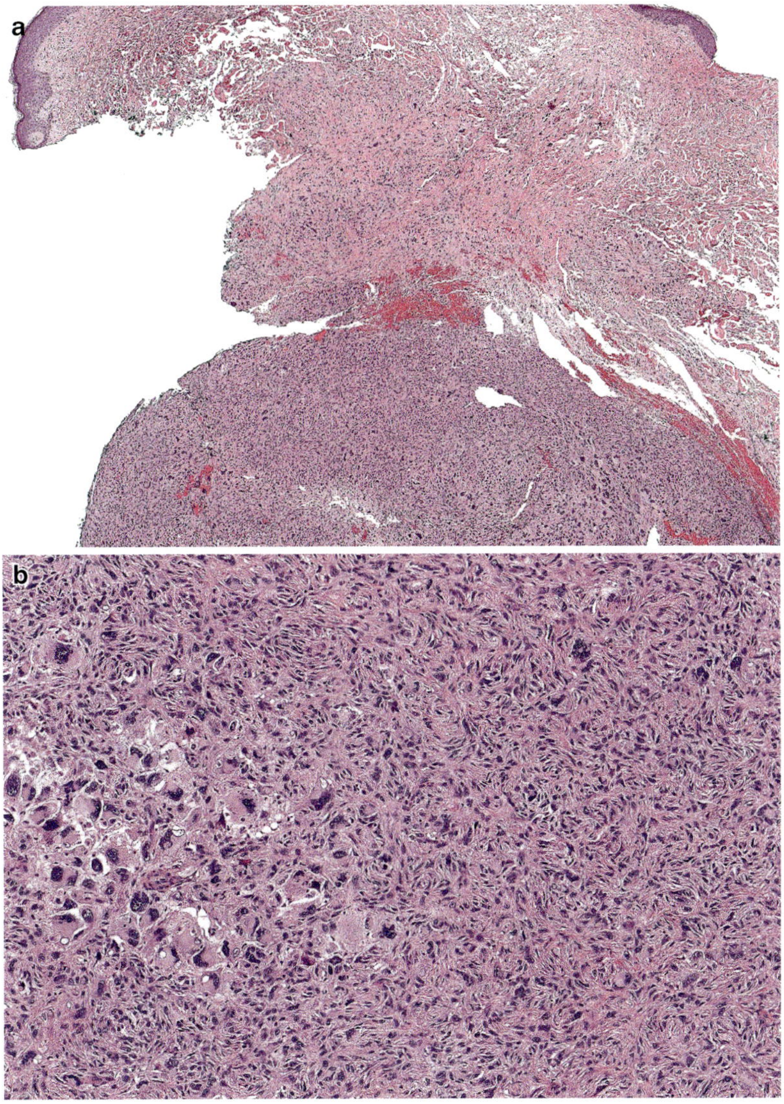

Fig. 6.6 (**a**). Undifferentiated pleomorphic sarcoma may arise in the subcutis. (**b**). Storiform and haphazard arrangement of markedly atypical, plump spindled, and histiocytoid cells

typically present. Necrosis is often seen. Although UPS does not have a characteristic vasculature like myxofibrosarcoma, some tumors may have a prominent hemangiopericytoma (staghorn)-like vasculature. The stroma is usually collagenous, but myxoid change, metaplastic bone, and cartilage may be noted. Some tumors have focal expression of smooth muscle actin in a "tram-track" membranous pattern, but stains for keratins, S100, desmin, myogenin, and hematolymphoid markers are generally negative. UPS has a complex karyotype without recurrent genetic aberrations.

Differential Diagnosis

UPS is a diagnosis of exclusion and needs to be differentiated from both benign and malignant entities. Pleomorphic fibroma has stellate cells with pleomorphic, hyperchromatic nuclei, but lacks the mitotic activity and cellularity of UPS. Pleomorphic lipoma contains bizarre, floret-like, multinucleated giant cells with hyperchromatic nuclei and abundant eosinophilic cytoplasm. In contrast to UPS, pleomorphic lipoma is well-circumscribed with scattered ropey collagen fibers and mast cells. The lesional cells of both pleomorphic fibroma and lipoma are positive for CD34 and may demonstrate a loss of RB1 protein expression. Atypical fibrous histiocytoma contains atypical, multinucleated cells and may have atypical mitotic figures, but recognition of the features of classic benign fibrous histiocytoma, including peripheral collagen trapping, a grenz zone with the overlying dermis, and epidermal hyperplasia will aid in the diagnosis. Wildly pleomorphic cells are often present in sarcomatoid carcinoma and melanoma, which can be excluded by an immunohistochemical panel containing keratins, S100 protein, and melanocytic markers. UPS may have foci of myxoid change that raise consideration of high-grade myxofibrosarcoma, but this should be diagnosed when the classic features of multinodular growth and myxoid foci with curvilinear vessels intimately associated with tumor cells are present. Pleomorphic liposarcoma may occur in superficial locations and has UPS-like areas, but identification of pleomorphic lipoblasts is the key to diagnosis. UPS with prominent osteoclast-like giant cells needs to be differentiated from giant cell tumor of soft tissue. The latter lacks the cytologic atypia of UPS. The differential diagnosis with myxoinflammatory fibroblastic sarcoma is covered below. Finally, UPS can be separated from atypical fibroxanthoma and pleomorphic dermal sarcoma (discussed in detail below) by the dermal origin and occurrence on the sun-damaged skin of the head and neck region of the latter two (Table 6.6).

Table 6.6 Key pathologic features: undifferentiated pleomorphic sarcoma

Infiltrative, deep soft tissue tumor of lower extremities with aggressive clinical course
20% cases may arise in subcutis
Storiform and haphazard arrangement of markedly atypical, pleomorphic tumor cells
Some tumors have prominent osteoclast-like giant cells or inflammation
Atypical mitoses and necrosis are common
May have membranous smooth muscle actin expression but otherwise lacks expression of lineage-specific immunohistohemical markers

Low-Grade Myofibroblastic Sarcoma (Myofibrosarcoma)

Clinical Features

Low-grade myofibroblastic sarcoma (myofibrosarcoma) is an uncommon low-grade sarcoma with a slight male predominance that typically occurs in adults, with only rare reported cases in children. Tumors typically present as an enlarging, painless superficial or deep soft tissue mass on the extremities or head and neck. In general, low-grade myofibroblastic sarcoma is a locally aggressive neoplasm, with high rates of local recurrence, and metastases occuring in about 10% of cases. It should be noted that undifferentiated pleomorphic sarcomas may demonstrate myofibroblastic differentiation, but will display more aggressive behavior than low-grade myofibroblastic sarcoma. Wide excision is the treatment of choice.

Pathologic Features

Low-grade myofibroblastic sarcoma may be infiltrative or have a circumscribed, pushing border (Fig. 6.7a). Some cases may have a multinodular growth pattern. The tumor is comprised of spindle cells with fascicular to storiform growth, eosinophilic cytoplasm, ill-defined cytoplasmic boundaries, and fusiform nuclei. The nuclei vary from plump and vesicular with a pinpoint nucleolus to wavy and dark with evenly dispersed chromatin (Fig. 6.7b). The fibrous stroma may have foci of myxoid change and hemorrhage and contains a network of thin-walled vessels. Both the vessels and stroma may undergo hyalinization. Cytologic atypia and mitotic activity are mild to moderate, but scattered foci of marked atypia and increased proliferation may be present. Immunohistochemistry shows variable smooth muscle actin (in a "tram-tack" pattern) and/or desmin expression, consistent with a myofibroblastic phenotype. Stains for keratins, EMA, CD34, S100, and beta-catenin are negative. There are no known recurrent molecular alterations in low-grade myofibroblastic sarcoma (Table 6.7).

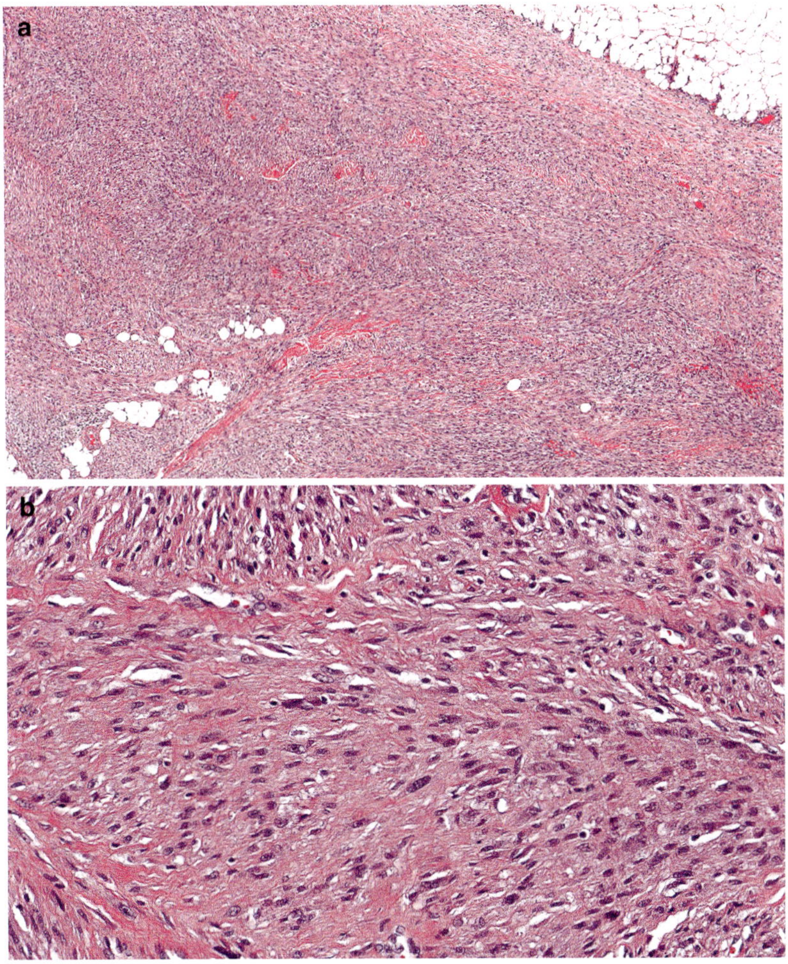

Fig. 6.7 (**a**). Low-grade myofibroblastic sarcoma (myofibrosarcoma) with pushing border and fascicular to storiform arrangement of cells. (**b**). Tumor cells have eosinophilic cytoplasm with indistinct boundaries and nuclei varying from vesicular with pinpoint nucleoli to dark and wavy

Table 6.7 Key pathologic features: low-grade myofibroblastic sarcoma (myofibrosarcoma)

Infiltrative growth or pushing borders
Plump spindle cells with eosinophilic cytoplasm and vesicular to dark nuclei
Smooth muscle actin with tram-track pattern immunoreactivity

Differential Diagnosis

Low-grade myofibroblastic sarcoma is an uncommon tumor and may be difficult to distinguish from other benign and low-grade malignant myofibroblastic tumors. Nodular fasciitis presents with a short history of rapid growth, lacks a diffusely infiltrative architecture, and has less atypia than low-grade myofibroblastic sarcoma. Fibrosarcomatous transformation in dermatofibrosarcoma protuberans demonstrates herringbone architecture, CD34 expression, and *PDGFB* rearrangement. Inflammatory myofibroblastic tumor occurs in younger patients, has a dense inflammatory component, and is often ALK-positive. Leiomyosarcoma has blunt-ended nuclei, diffuse membranous and cytoplasmic smooth muscle actin expression, and marks with additional smooth muscle markers (desmin, calponin, and caldesmon).

Myxoinflammatory Fibroblastic Sarcoma

Clinical Features

Myxoinflammatory fibroblastic sarcoma (MIFS), also known as inflammatory myxohyaline tumor with Reed-Sternberg-like cells or acral myxoinflammatory fibroblastic sarcoma, is a rare low-grade sarcoma without gender predilection that typically occurs in middle-aged adults. Tumors present as a slowly growing, painless soft tissue mass of the distal extremities, particularly the hands and fingers. However, rare cases may occur on the proximal extremities and trunk, and some cases may be locally destructive. These lesions are managed with surgical excision. Local recurrence is common (30–70%), and cases may rarely metastasize to regional lymph nodes.

Pathologic Features

MIFS is a multilobular and poorly circumscribed tumor usually occurring in the subcutis where it extends out along fibrous septa and fascial planes. The proportions of myxoid, hyaline, and inflammatory components vary considerably between and even within tumors (Fig. 6.8a). Despite this heterogeneity, identification of various atypical cells aids in its diagnosis. The hallmark of this tumor is large, epithelioid cells with abundant eosinophilic cytoplasm, vesicular nuclei, and prominent nucleoli, reminiscent of a virocyte or Reed-Sternberg cell (Fig. 6.8b). Various other cells may be present in MIFS: plump spindle cells with fibrillary cytoplasm and moderately atypical nuclei; pleomorphic cells with smudged hyperchromatic nuclei; histiocytes with emperipolesis; pseudolipoblasts, particularly in myxoid areas; ganglion-like cells; and multinucleated giant cells, including Touton-like giant cells (Fig. 6.8c, d). Lymphocytes and plasma cells are the main inflammatory component, but neutrophils and eosinophils may be encountered. Germinal centers and hemosiderin may occasionally be seen. In spite of the marked cytologic atypia, there is a paucity of mitotic activity (<2/50 HPF), and necrosis is absent. The immunophenotype is relatively nonspecific, but tumors may show variable staining for smooth muscle actin, CD34, CD68, and keratin. Importantly, immunohistochemical stains for ALK and CD30 are negative. Most cases of MIFS have *TGFBR3-MGEA5* gene fusion resulting from a t(1:10)(p22;q34). The same genetic aberration is present in hemosiderotic fibrolipomatous tumor (HFLT) and in tumors with hybrid features of MIFS and HFLT. Recently, characterized rearrangements of *TGFBR3* and *MGEA5* by FISH have been described in pleomorphic hyalinizing angiectatic tumor (PHAT). Additionally, the so-called "early PHAT" lesions share clinicopathologic characteristics with HFLT (see Chap. 12). These observations suggest that HFLT, PHAT, and MIFS may be genetically related entities along a morphologic and biologic spectrum (Table 6.8).

Differential Diagnosis

MIFS may be difficult to distinguish from a variety of benign and malignant tumors with overlapping morphologic features, including reactive infectious and inflammatory processes, nodular fasciitis, tenosynovial giant cell tumor, inflammatory myofibroblastic tumor, myxofibrosarcoma, and undifferentiated pleomorphic sarcoma. Rare cases may be confused with cutaneous involvement by classical Hodgkin lymphoma or anaplastic large cell lymphoma. Reactive infectious and inflammatory processes may have virocytes and marked inflammation, but immunohistochemistry and/or RNA in situ hybridization can confirm the presence of various viruses, which should not be present in MIFS. Nodular fasciitis does not have marked cytologic atypia and prominent inflammation. Tenosynovial giant cell tumor occurs in a similar location, has inflammation, multinucleated giant cells, and hemosiderin, but lacks the atypia of MIFS. Inflammatory myofibroblastic tumor has significant inflammation, but lacks the varied and

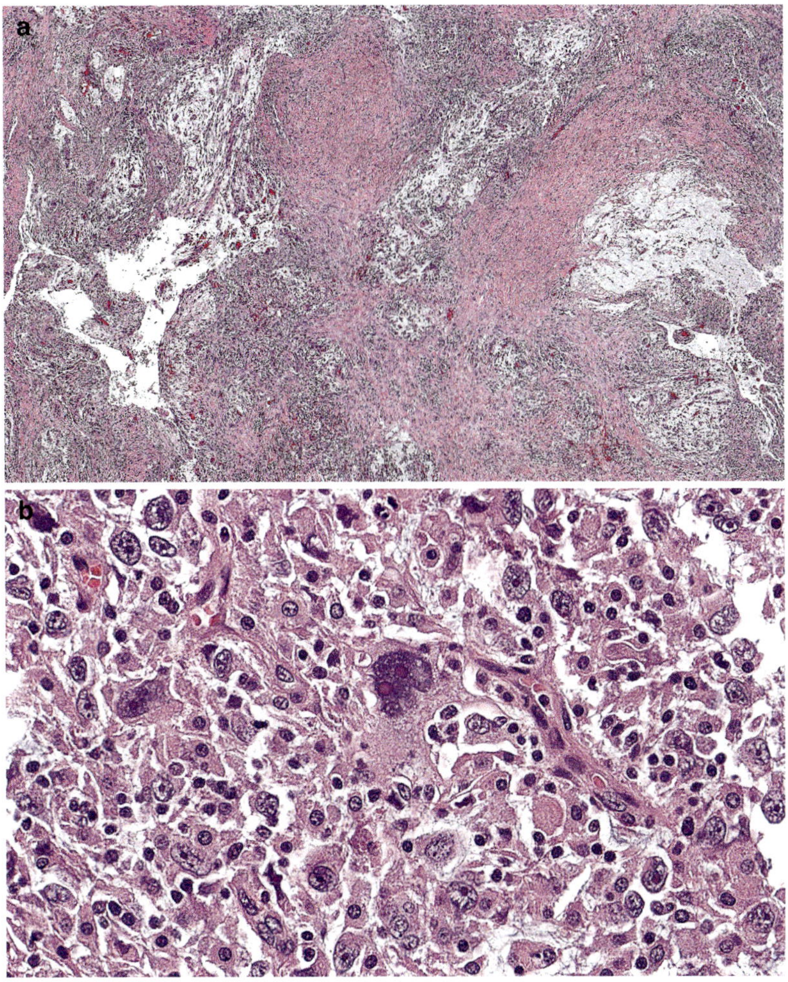

Fig. 6.8 (**a**). Myxoinflammatory fibroblastic sarcoma has variable amounts of myxoid and hyalinized zones admixed with inflammatory cells. (**b**). Reed-Sternberg or virocyte-like cells with prominent intranuclear inclusions are the hallmark of this tumor. (**c**). Numerous atypical spindle cells are present: plump spindled cells with atypical nuclei in hyalined zones (left), cells with degenerating hyperchromatic nuclei (bottom right), and virocyte-like nuclei (top right). Scattered about in the right half are also histiocytes with emperipolesis. (**d**). Myxoid zone with mixed inflammation and pseudolipoblasts

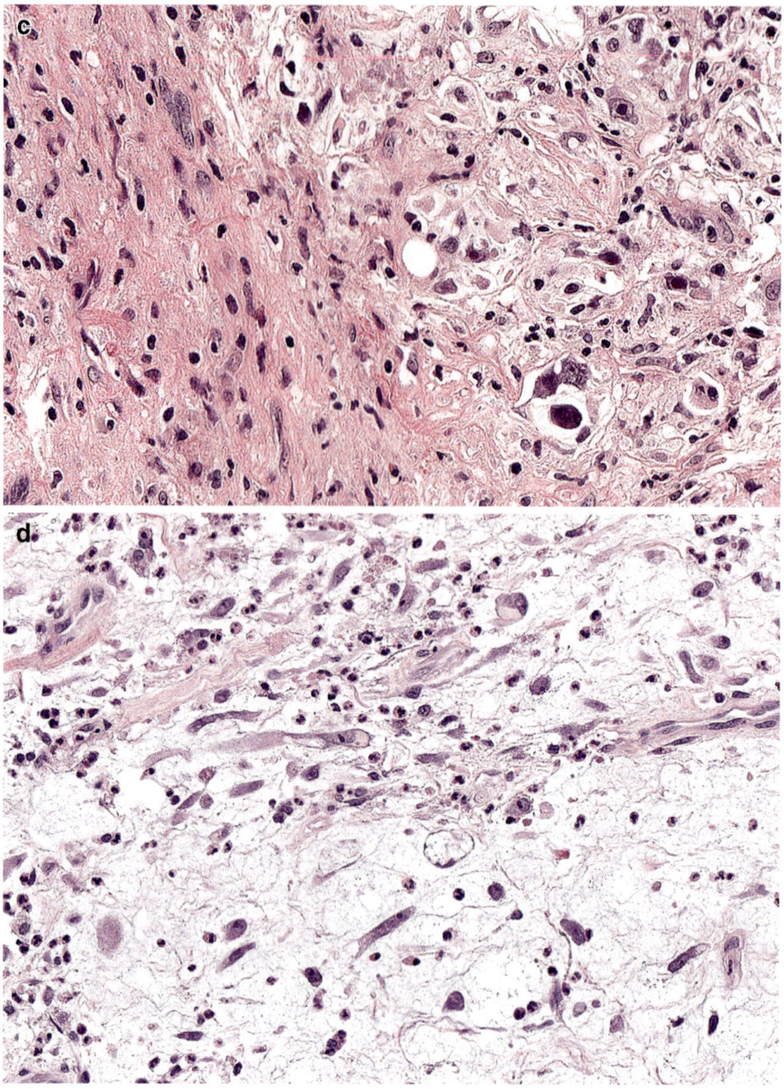

Fig. 6.8 (continued)

Table 6.8 Key pathologic features: myxoinflammatory myofibroblastic sarcoma

Variably hyalinized and myxoid areas
Pleomorphic cells with prominent nuclei resembling Reed-Sternberg cells or virocytes
Plump spindle cells, histiocytes with emperipolesis, multinucleated giant cells, and pleomorphic cells with smudged chromatin also present
Pseudolipoblasts in myxoid areas
Predominantly plasma cells and lymphocytes

markedly atypical cells of MIFS. Furthermore, a significant proportion of inflammatory myofibroblastic tumors demonstrate ALK expression by immunohistochemistry. Myxofibrosarcoma and undifferentiated pleomorphic sarcoma may have significant inflammation, but the presence of marked atypia with concomitant mitotic inactivity would be unusual for these tumors. The clinical location would also be unusual for myxofibrosarcoma and undifferentiated pleomorphic sarcoma. Classical Hodgkin lymphoma will express CD30 and CD15, and anaplastic large cell lymphoma is positive for CD30.

Atypical Fibroxanthoma and Pleomorphic Dermal Sarcoma

Clinical Features

Atypical fibroxanthoma (AFX) and pleomorphic dermal sarcoma (PDS) encompass primary undifferentiated pleomorphic sarcomas of the skin and represent a spectrum of the same neoplasm. These tumors occur on sun-exposed sites in the elderly, especially the head and neck region. A subset of tumors may be secondary to radiation therapy, and young patients with xeroderma pigmentosum may be affected. These tumors present as a rapidly enlarging soft tissue mass. Wide local excision and Mohs microsurgery are the preferred treatment methods. When strict diagnostic criteria (discussed below) are applied, AFX has up to a 10% risk of local recurrence with essentially no risk for metastasis in multiple studies when the tumor is confined to the dermis. There are reports of rare cases of metastasizing AFX, almost all of which showed infiltration into the subcutis. It is our practice to categorize such tumors as PDS. PDS has a higher risk of recurrence (25%) and the potential for metastases (10–20%). Metastases have been documented to the skin, regional lymph nodes, and lungs. Death from PDS has been reported.

Pathologic Features

AFX presents as an expansile nodule confined to the dermis (Fig. 6.9a). While AFX with involvement of the subcutis has been reported, we prefer to restrict the definition to those confined to the dermis (see above). There may be a grenz zone of uninvolved dermis between the tumor and the overlying epidermis, or there may be epidermal atrophy and erosion secondary to mass effect. The tumor is typically composed of hyperchromatic spindled cells and pleomorphic tumor cells typically arranged in an irregular storiform to fascicular growth pattern (Fig. 6.9b). AFX may also have a haphazard, sheet-like growth or herringbone pattern (Fig. 6.9c, d). Mitotic activity is conspicuous and atypical mitotic figures are commonly present. A wide range of histologic features have been described including monomorphous spindle cell and pseudoangiomatous, xanthomatous, granular, clear cell, and keloidal variants (Fig. 6.9e-j).

PDS has significant histologic overlap with AFX and may have the same morphologic variants as described above. PDS differs from AFX by its infiltration into the subcutis (Fig. 6.10a, b) and relatively frequent tumor necrosis (Fig. 6.10c), perineural invasion, and/or lymphovascular invasion. The presence of any of these features supports a diagnosis of PDS over AFX.

Both AFX and PDS have similar immunohistochemical profiles. By definition, they are negative for cytokeratins, S100 protein, and SOX10. They are usually diffusely positive for CD10 and CD68, but these stains are nonspecific and do not aid in the differential diagnosis. Frequently they express SMA in a "tram-track" pattern, indicative of partial myofibroblastic differentiation. Nonspecific staining for EMA, CD99, p63, melanocytic markers (e.g., Melan-A), and CD31may also be observed. The pattern of CD31 immunoreactivity is granular in nature in contrast to crisp membranous staining of endothelial cells. Focal immunoreactivity for ERG may be seen, but they typically lack the diffuse, strong staining seen in vascular neoplasms. The granular cell variant has been reported to express NKI/C3, but this marker is relatively nonspecific. A subset of tumors may have diffuse TP53 protein expression. Immunostains for desmin and CD34 are typically negative. Both tumors show a highly complex karyotype with a high frequency of chromosome 9p and 13q deletions. TERT promoter mutations with a UV signature appear to

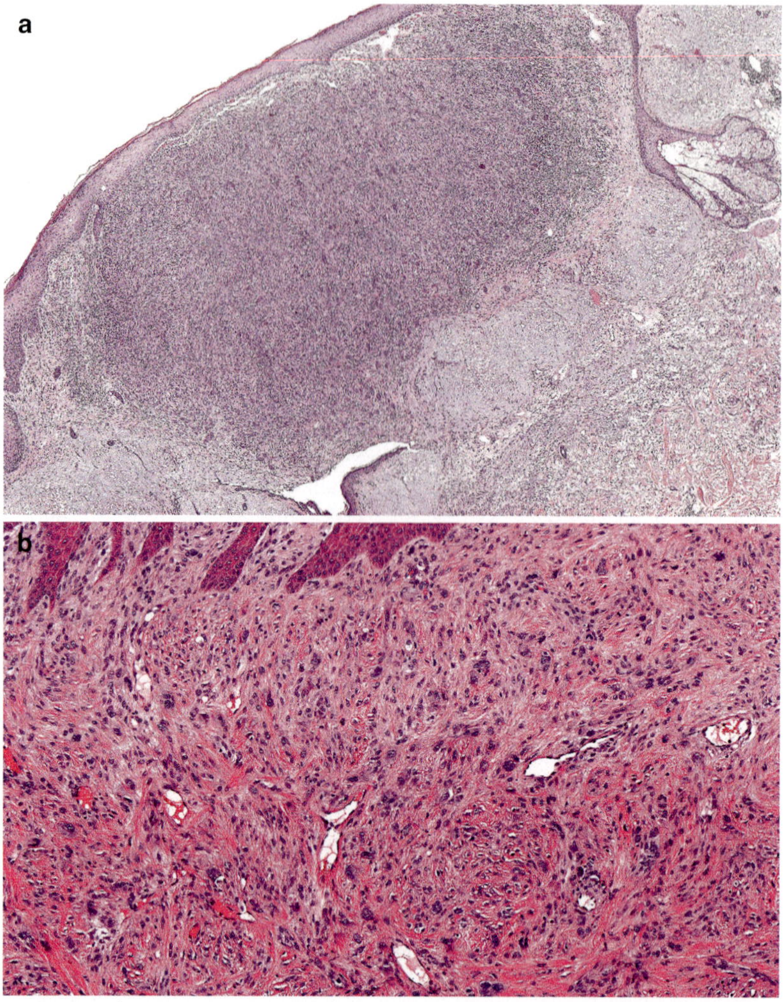

Fig. 6.9 (**a**). Atypical fibroxanthoma is a circumscribed, dermal-based lesion with a pushing border. Note the solar elastosis in the background. (**b**). Atypical fibroxanthoma is typically composed of hyperchromatic to pleomorphic cells arranged in a storiform to fascicular pattern. (**c**). The tumor cells of atypical fibroxanthoma may be arranged in a sheet-like growth pattern. (**d**). Rarely, the tumor cells have a herringbone pattern. (**e**). Atypical fibroxanthoma is sometimes composed of uniform atypical spindled cells with relatively little pleomorphism. (**f**). The pseudoangiomatous variant of atypical fibroxanthoma has large blood-filled spaces and may be confused with angiosarcoma. (**g**). The tumor cells in some cases have abundant foamy cytoplasm imparting a xanthomatous appearance. (**h**). Some atypical fibroxanthomas have dense granular cytoplasm. (**i**). Rare cases have abundant optically clear cytoplasm and can mimic metastatic renal cell carcinoma. (**j**). Atypical fibroxanthoma rarely has prominent keloid-like collagen

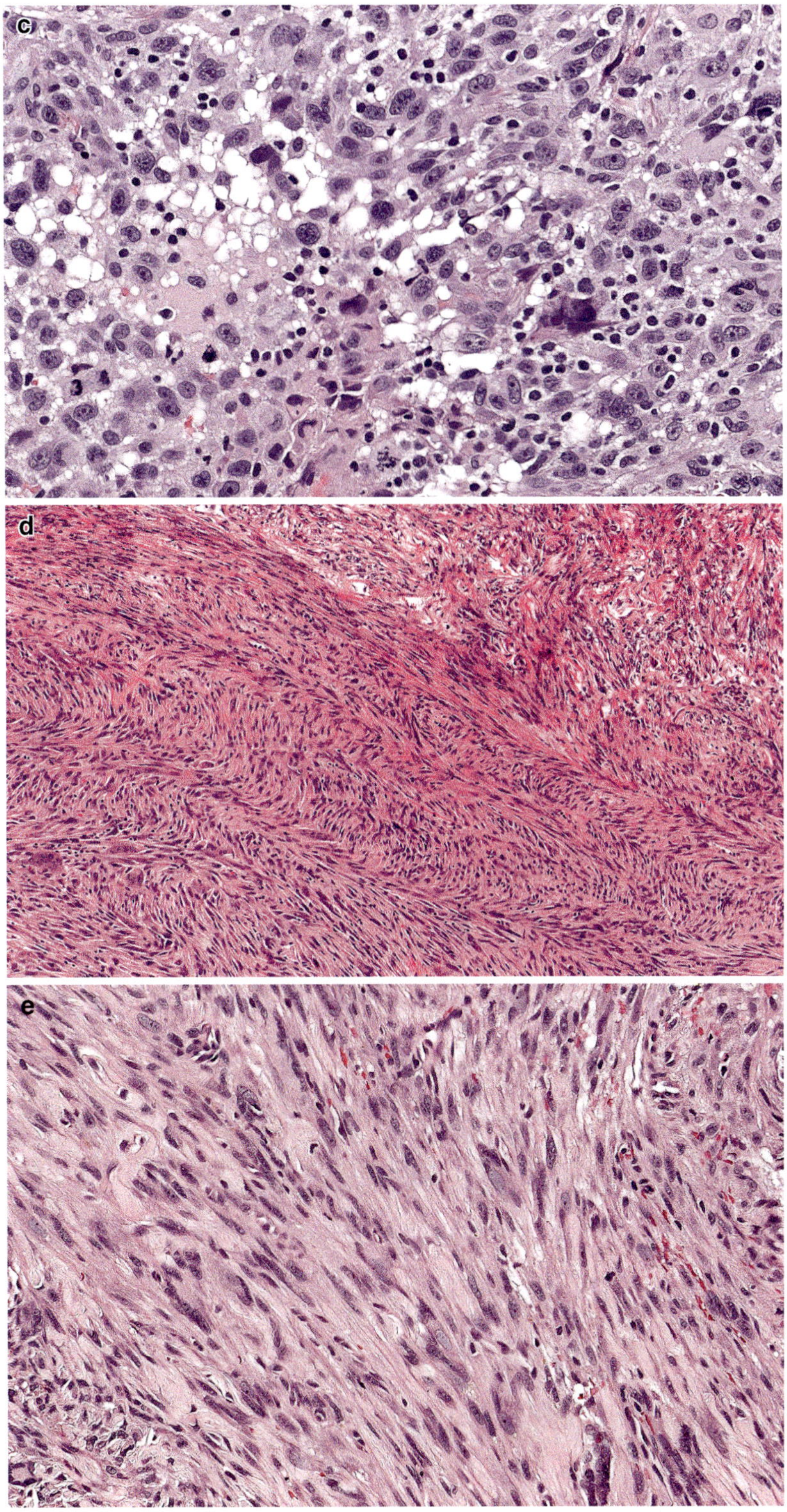

Fig. 6.9 (continued)

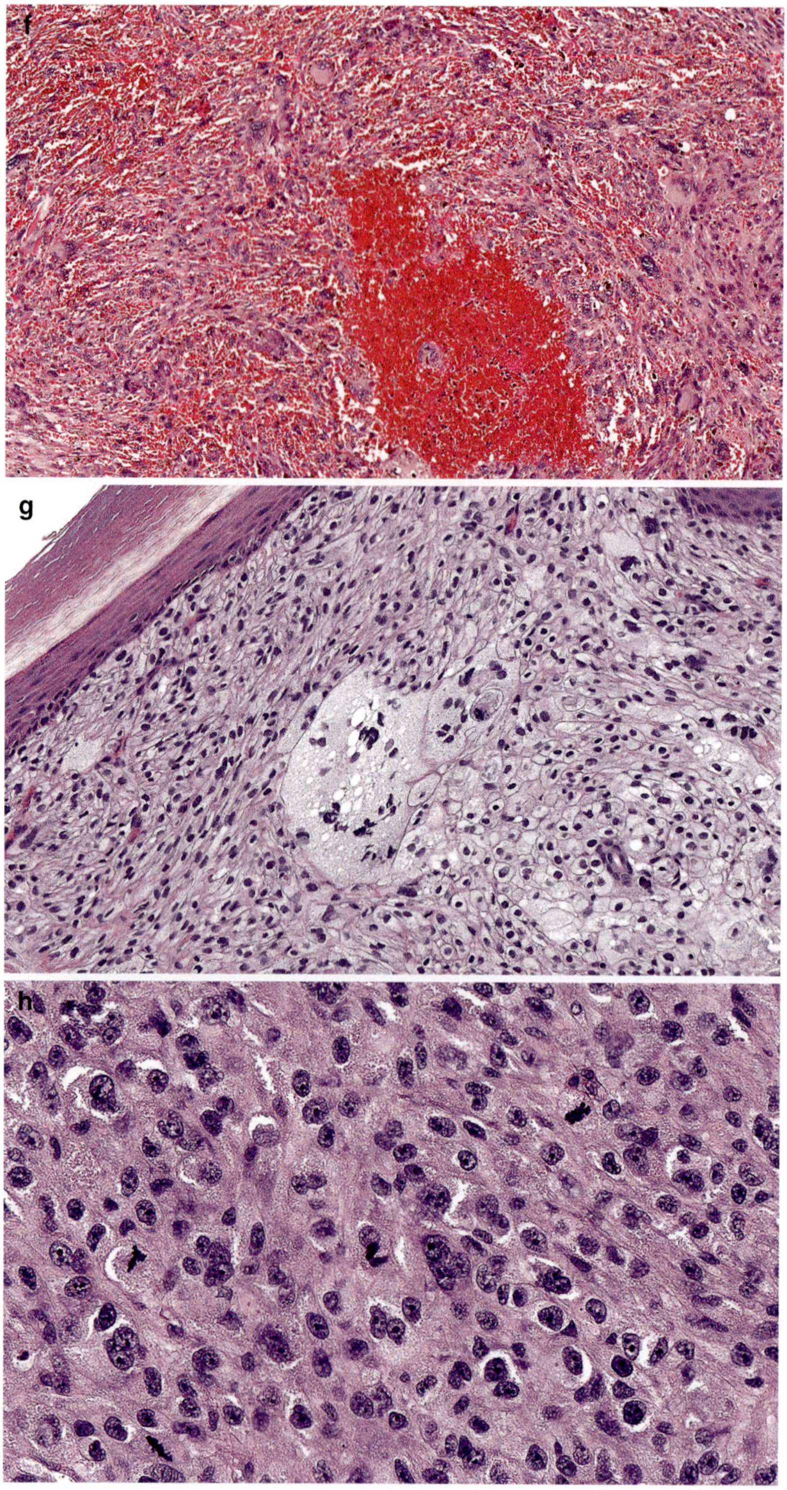

Fig. 6.9 (continued)

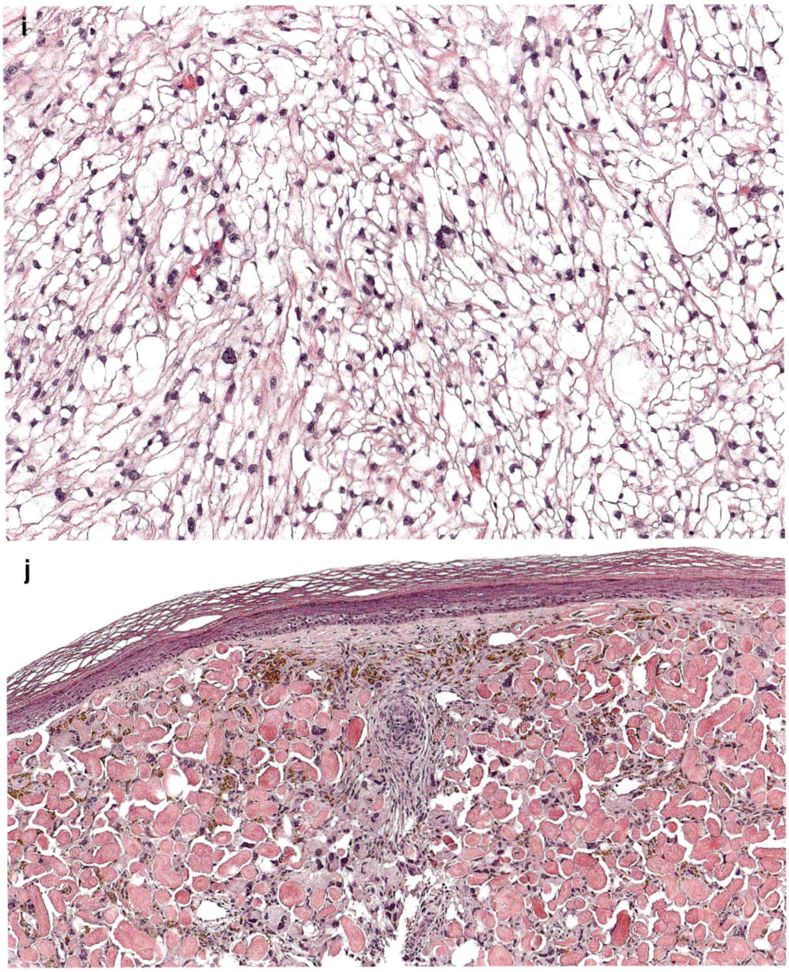

Fig. 6.9 (continued)

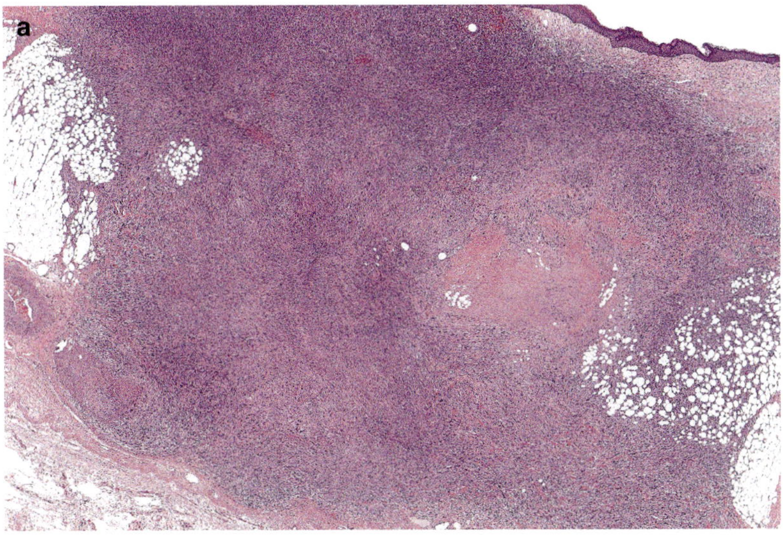

Fig. 6.10 (**a**). Unlike atypical fibroxanthoma, pleomorphic dermal sarcoma infiltrates into the subcutis, and the pattern of infiltration can be quite extensive. (**b**). Higher-power image demonstrating tumor cells of pleomorphic dermal sarcoma infiltrating through the subcutaneous fat. (**c**). Tumor necrosis is often seen in pleomorphic dermal sarcoma

Fig. 6.10 (continued)

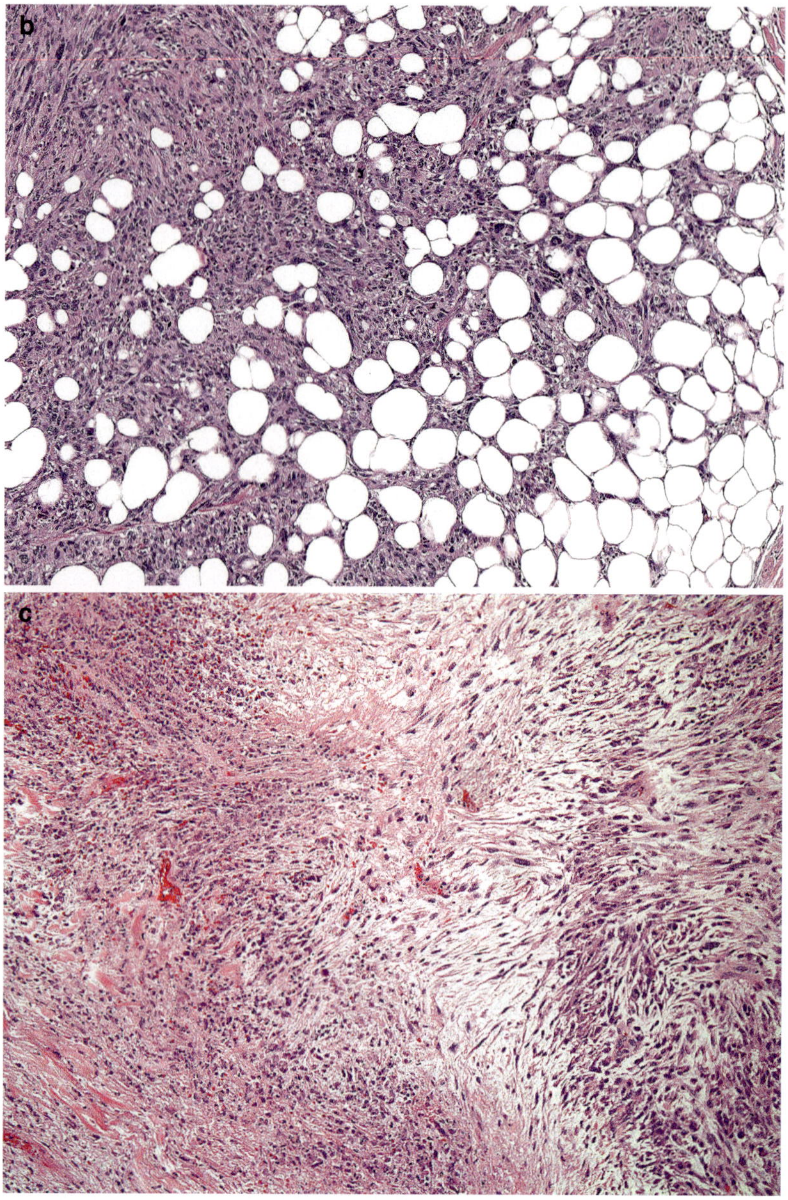

be the most common mutation seen in both AFX and PDS. The genetic and histopathologic similarities support the contention that AFX and PDS are representative entities on a spectrum of the same neoplasm. Mutations of H-, K-, and N-*RAS* genes are found only in PDS, suggesting that these genetic events may contribute to progression from a precursor AFX.

Differential Diagnosis

The primary differential considerations that must be considered in every case of AFX and PDS are sarcomatoid squamous cell carcinoma and spindle cell or desmoplastic melanoma (see Chaps. 2 and 3). Sarcomatoid squamous cell carcinoma will have some evidence of high molecular weight cytokeratin and p63 expression in the vast majority of cases. A precursor in situ component is also sometimes present. Spindle cell and desmoplastic melanoma often have an in situ component and lymphoid aggregates and are positive for S100 protein and SOX10. AFX and PDS with intratumoral hemorrhage may be mistaken for cutaneous angiosarcoma, but the latter expresses CD31 and ERG diffusely and typically has evidence of vasoformation at least focally. Dermal cutaneous leiomyosarcomas rarely present on the head and neck, typically have an intersecting fascicular growth pattern, and are positive for both smooth muscle actin and desmin. Clear cell AFX can be differentiated from metastatic clear cell renal cell carcinoma with PAX-8 and/or CA-IX stains and from cutaneous PEComas with smooth muscle actin and HMB-45 staining. The differentiating features between AFX/PDS and undifferentiated pleomorphic sarcoma were previously discussed.

Benign entities in the differential diagnosis include pleomorphic fibroma, pleomorphic fibrous papule, and atypical fibrous histiocytoma. Both pleomorphic fibroma and pleomorphic fibrous papule contain atypical cells, but lack the cellularity and diffuse marked atypia and mitotic activity of AFX and PDS. Atypical fibrous histiocytoma has admixed hyperchromatic, pleomorphic, and multinucleated cells and may have rare atypical mitoses, but atypical fibrous histiocytoma typically occurs on the extremities and has characteristic pathologic features of benign fibrous histiocytoma, including peripheral collagen trapping and epidermal hyperplasia (see Chap. 4) (Tables 6.9 and 6.10).

Table 6.9 Key pathologic features: atypical fibroxanthoma

Localized to the dermis with pushing border
Less than 2 cm
Lacks infiltration into the subcutis, necrosis, and perineural or lymphovascular invasion

Table 6.10 Key pathologic features: pleomorphic dermal sarcoma

Infiltrates into the subcutaneous tissue and possibly into fascia, muscle, and periosteum
Larger than 2 cm
Necrosis in 50% cases
Perineural and lymphovascular invasion common

Selected References

1. Antonescu CR, Rosenblum MK, Pereira P, Nascimento AG, Woodruff JM. Sclerosing epithelioid fibrosarcoma: a study of 16 cases and confirmation of a clinicopathologically distinct tumor. Am J Surg Pathol. 2001;25(6):699–709.
2. Arbajian E, Puls F, Magnusson L, Thway K, Fisher C, Sumathi VP, Tayebwa J, Nord KH, Kindblom LG, Mertens F. Recurrent EWSR1-CREB3L1 gene fusions in sclerosing epithelioid fibrosarcoma. Am J Surg Pathol. 2014;38(6):801–8.
3. Argani P, Fritsch M, Kadkol SS, Schuster A, Beckwith JB, Perlman EJ. Detection of the ETV6-NTRK3 chimeric RNA of infantile fibrosarcoma/cellular congenital mesoblastic nephroma in paraffin-embedded tissue: application to challenging pediatric renal stromal tumors. Mod Pathol. 2000;13(1):29–36.
4. Bahrami A, Folpe AL. Adult-type fibrosarcoma: a reevaluation of 163 putative cases diagnosed at a single institution over a 48-year period. Am J Surg Pathol. 2010;34(10):1504–13.
5. Billings SD, Giblen G, Fanburg-Smith JC. Superficial low-grade fibromyxoid sarcoma (Evans tumor): a clinicopathologic analysis of 19 cases with a unique observation in the pediatric population. Am J Surg Pathol. 2005;29(2):204–10.
6. Brenn T. Pleomorphic dermal neoplasms: a review. Adv Anat Pathol. 2014;21(2):108–30.
7. Carter JM, Sukov WR, Montgomery E, Goldblum JR, Billings SD, Fritchie KJ, Folpe AL. TGFBR3 and MGEA5 rearrangements in pleomorphic hyalinizing angiectatic tumors and the spectrum of related neoplasms. Am J Surg Pathol. 2014;38(9):1182–992.
8. Choy B, Hyjek E, Montag AG, Pytel P, Haydon R, Luu HH, Zhen CJ, Long BC, Kadri S, Segal JP, Furtado LV, Cipriani NA. High prevalence of MiTF staining in undifferentiated pleomorphic sarcoma: caution in the use of melanocytic markers in sarcoma. Histopathology. 2017;70(5):734–45.
9. Chung EB, Enzinger FM. Infantile fibrosarcoma. Cancer. 1976;38(2):729–39.
10. Clarke LE, Zhang PJ, Crawford GH, Elenitsas R. Myxofibrosarcoma in the skin. J Cutan Pathol. 2008;35(10):935–40.
11. Coffin CM, Dehner LP. Fibroblastic-myofibroblastic tumors in children and adolescents: a clinicopatho-

logic study of 108 examples in 103 patients. Pediatr Pathol. 1991;11(4):569–88.
12. Davis JL, Lockwood CM, Albert CM, Tsuchiya K, Hawkins DS, Rudzinski ER. Infantile NTRK-associated mesenchymal tumors. Pediatr Dev Pathol. 2018;21(1):68–78.
13. de Feraudy S, Mar N, McCalmont TH. Evaluation of CD10 and procollagen 1 expression in atypical fibroxanthoma and dermatofibroma. Am J Surg Pathol. 2008;32(8):1111–22.
14. Dineen SP, Roland CL, Feig R, May C, Zhou S, Demicco E, Sannaa GA, Ingram D, Wang WL, Ravi V, Guadagnolo A, Lev D, Pollock RE, Hunt K, Cormier J, Lazar A, Feig B, Torres KE. Radiation-associated undifferentiated pleomorphic sarcoma is associated with worse clinical outcomes than sporadic lesions. Ann Surg Oncol. 2015;22(12):3913–20.
15. Evans HL. Low-grade fibromyxoid sarcoma. A report of two metastasizing neoplasms having a deceptively benign appearance. Am J Clin Pathol. 1987;88(5):615–9.
16. Evans HL. Low-grade fibromyxoid sarcoma: a clinicopathologic study of 33 cases with long-term follow-up. Am J Surg Pathol. 2011;35(10):1450–62.
17. Fisher C. Myofibrosarcoma. Virchows Arch. 2004;445(3):215–23.
18. Folpe AL, Lane KL, Paull G, Weiss SW. Low-grade fibromyxoid sarcoma and hyalinizing spindle cell tumor with giant rosettes: a clinicopathologic study of 73 cases supporting their identity and assessing the impact of high-grade areas. Am J Surg Pathol. 2000;24(10):1353–60.
19. Griewank KG, Schilling B, Murali R, Bielefeld N, Schwamborn M, Sucker A, Zimmer L, Hillen U, Schaller J, Brenn T, Schadendorf D, Mentzel T. TERT promoter mutations are frequent in atypical fibroxanthomas and pleomorphic dermal sarcomas. Mod Pathol. 2014;27(4):502–8.
20. Guillou L, Benhattar J, Gengler C, Gallagher G, Ranchère-Vince D, Collin F, Terrier P, Terrier-Lacombe MJ, Leroux A, Marquès B, Aubain Somerhausen Nde S, Keslair F, Pedeutour F, Coindre JM. Translocation-positive low-grade fibromyxoid sarcoma: clinicopathologic and molecular analysis of a series expanding the morphologic spectrum and suggesting potential relationship to sclerosing epithelioid fibrosarcoma: a study from the French sarcoma group. Am J Surg Pathol. 2007;31(9):1387–402.
21. Kao YC, Fletcher CDM, Alaggio R, Wexler L, Zhang L, Sung YS, Orhan D, Chang WC, Swanson D, Dickson BC, Antonescu CR. Recurrent BRAF gene fusions in a subset of pediatric spindle cell sarcomas: expanding the genetic Spectrum of tumors with overlapping features with infantile Fibrosarcoma. Am J Surg Pathol. 2018;42(1):28–38.
22. Laskin WB, Fetsch JF, Miettinen M. Myxoinflammatory fibroblastic sarcoma: a clinicopathologic analysis of 104 cases, with emphasis on predictors of outcome. Am J Surg Pathol. 2014;38(1):1–12.
23. Lucas DR. Myxoinflammatory fibroblastic sarcoma: review and update. Arch Pathol Lab Med. 2017;141(11):1503–7.
24. Luzar B, Calonje E. Morphological and immunohistochemical characteristics of atypical fibroxanthoma with a special emphasis on potential diagnostic pitfalls: a review. J Cutan Pathol. 2010;37(3):301–9.
25. Magro G, Salvatorelli L, Vecchio GM, Musumeci G, Rita A, Parenti R. Cytoplasmic expression of Wilms tumor transcription factor-1 (WT1): a useful immunomarker for young-type fibromatoses and infantile fibrosarcoma. Acta Histochem. 2014;116(7):1134–40.
26. Matushansky I, Charytonowicz E, Mills J, Siddiqi S, Hricik T, Cordon-Cardo C. MFH classification: differentiating undifferentiated pleomorphic sarcoma in the 21st Century. Expert Rev Anticancer Ther. 2009;9(8):1135–44.
27. Meis-Kindblom JM, Kindblom LG. Acral myxoinflammatory fibroblastic sarcoma: a low-grade tumor of the hands and feet. Am J Surg Pathol. 1998;22(8):911–24.
28. Meis-Kindblom JM, Kindblom LG, Enzinger FM. Sclerosing epithelioid fibrosarcoma. A variant of fibrosarcoma simulating carcinoma. Am J Surg Pathol. 1995;19(9):979–93.
29. Mentzel T, Calonje E, Wadden C, Camplejohn RS, Beham A, Smith MA, Fletcher CD. Myxofibrosarcoma. Clinicopathologic analysis of 75 cases with emphasis on the low-grade variant. Am J Surg Pathol. 1996;20(4):391–405.
30. Mertens F, Fletcher CD, Antonescu CR, Coindre JM, Colecchia M, Domanski HA, Downs-Kelly E, Fisher C, Goldblum JR, Guillou L, Reid R, Rosai J, Sciot R, Mandahl N, Panagopoulos I. Clinicopathologic and molecular genetic characterization of low-grade fibromyxoid sarcoma, and cloning of a novel FUS/CREB3L1 fusion gene. Lab Investig. 2005;85(3):408–15.
31. Michal M, Kazakov DV, Hadravský L, Kinkor Z, Kuroda N, Michal M. High-grade myxoinflammatory fibroblastic sarcoma: a report of 23 cases. Ann Diagn Pathol. 2015;19(3):157–63.
32. Mihic-Probst D, Zhao J, Saremaslani P, Baer A, Oehlschlegel C, Paredes B, Komminoth P, Heitz PU. CGH analysis shows genetic similarities and differences in atypical fibroxanthoma and undifferentiated high grade pleomorphic sarcoma. Anticancer Res. 2004;24(1):19–26.
33. Miller K, Goodlad JR, Brenn T. Pleomorphic dermal sarcoma: adverse histologic features predict aggressive behavior and allow distinction from atypical fibroxanthoma. Am J Surg Pathol. 2012;36(9):1317–26.
34. Mirza B, Weedon D. Atypical fibroxanthoma: a clinicopathological study of 89 cases. Australas J Dermatol. 2005;46(4):235–8.

35. Montgomery E, Goldblum JR, Fisher C. Myofibrosarcoma: a clinicopathologic study. Am J Surg Pathol. 2001;25(2):219–28.
36. Nascimento AF, Bertoni F, Fletcher CD. Epithelioid variant of myxofibrosarcoma: expanding the clinicomorphologic spectrum of myxofibrosarcoma in a series of 17 cases. Am J Surg Pathol. 2007;31(1):99–105.
37. Patel RM, Downs-Kelly E, Dandekar MN, Fanburg-Smith JC, Billings SD, Tubbs RR, Goldblum JR. FUS (16p11) gene rearrangement as detected by fluorescence in-situ hybridization in cutaneous low-grade fibromyxoid sarcoma: a potential diagnostic tool. Am J Dermatopathol. 2011;33(2):140–3.
38. Pritchard DJ, Soule EH, Taylor WF, Ivins JC. Fibrosarcoma--a clinicopathologic and statistical study of 199 tumors of the soft tissues of the extremities and trunk. Cancer. 1974;33(3):888–97.
39. Roland CL, Wang WL, Lazar AJ, Torres KE. Myxofibrosarcoma. Surg Oncol Clin N Am. 2016;25(4):775–88.
40. Sakamoto A, Oda Y, Itakura E, Oshiro Y, Nikaido O, Iwamoto Y, Tsuneyoshi M. Immunoexpression of ultraviolet photoproducts and p53 mutation analysis in atypical fibroxanthoma and superficial malignant fibrous histiocytoma. Mod Pathol. 2001a;14(6):581–8.
41. Sakamoto A, Oda Y, Itakura E, Oshiro Y, Tamiya S, Honda Y, Ishihara A, Iwamoto Y, Tsuneyoshi M. H-, K-, and N-ras gene mutation in atypical fibroxanthoma and malignant fibrous histiocytoma. Hum Pathol. 2001b;32(11):1225–31.
42. Scoccianti G, Ranucci V, Frenos F, Greto D, Beltrami G, Capanna R, Franchi A. Soft tissue myxofibrosarcoma: A clinicopathological analysis of a series of 75 patients with emphasis on the epithelioid variant. J Surg Oncol. 2016;114(1):50–5.
43. Sheng WQ, Hisaoka M, Okamoto S, Tanaka A, Meis-Kindblom JM, Kindblom LG, Ishida T, Nojima T, Hashimoto H. Congenital-infantile fibrosarcoma. A clinicopathologic study of 10 cases and molecular detection of the ETV6-NTRK3 fusion transcripts using paraffin-embedded tissues. Am J Clin Pathol. 2001;115(3):348–55.
44. Smith SC, Poznanski AA, Fullen DR, Ma L, McHugh JB, Lucas DR, Patel RM. CD34-positive superficial myxofibrosarcoma: a potential diagnostic pitfall. J Cutan Pathol. 2013;40(7):639–45.
45. Tardío JC, Pinedo F, Aramburu JA, Suárez-Massa D, Pampín A, Requena L, Santonja C. Pleomorphic dermal sarcoma: a more aggressive neoplasm than previously estimated. J Cutan Pathol. 2016;43(2):101–12.
46. Tjarks BJ, Ko JS, Billings SD. Myxofibrosarcoma of unusual sites. J Cutan Pathol. 2018;45(2):104–10.
47. Variend S, Bax NM, van Gorp J. Are infantile myofibromatosis, congenital fibrosarcoma and congenital haemangiopericytoma histogenetically related? Histopathology. 1995;26(1):57–62.
48. Vernon SE, Bejarano PA. Low-grade fibromyxoid sarcoma: a brief review. Arch Pathol Lab Med. 2006;130(9):1358–60.
49. Weiss SW, Enzinger FM. Malignant fibrous histiocytoma: an analysis of 200 cases. Cancer. 1978;41(6):2250–66.
50. Willems SM, Mohseny AB, Balog C, Sewrajsing R, Briaire-de Bruijn IH, Knijnenburg J, Cleton-Jansen AM, Sciot R, Fletcher CD, Deelder AM, Szuhai K, Hensbergen PJ, Hogendoorn PC. Cellular/intramuscular myxoma and grade I myxofibrosarcoma are characterized by distinct genetic alterations and specific composition of their extracellular matrix. J Cell Mol Med 2009;13(7):1291–1301. doi: https://doi.org/10.1111/j.1582-4934.2009.00747.x. Epub 2009 Mar 13.

Cutaneous Vascular Lesions

7

Darya Buehler and Steven D. Billings

Abstract

Cutaneous vascular lesions comprise a wide spectrum of entities. Most are benign, but vascular tumors of intermediate malignancy, with a propensity for recurrence but limited metastatic potential, and fully malignant vascular neoplasms are encountered. Many of these vascular proliferations demonstrate significant histologic overlap. However, careful attention to histomorphology and in some cases, the application of ancillary diagnostic tests, usually result in proper classification in all but the most difficult of cases. This chapter will review the wide range of vascular lesions encountered in dermatopathology practice.

Benign Vascular Proliferations of the Skin

A number of benign vascular lesions present primarily in the skin. Some are defined more by their clinical presentations than their histologic features. For example, distinctive cutaneous capillary vascular malformations, such as port wine stain or salmon patch are clinically distinctive and easily recognized. Microscopically, they all consist of a proliferation of dilated capillaries and small veins that cannot be distinguished from one another based upon histopathologic features alone. For this reason, they are essentially never biopsied to establish the diagnosis. Thus, these vascular lesions will not be discussed in this chapter. Likewise, complex vascular malformations and malformations seen in association with genetic syndromes require a largely clinical and radiologic approach to diagnosis, are rarely biopsied, and are therefore beyond the scope of this chapter. Rather, the focus is on vascular lesions in which histologic examination is common and crucial for establishing the diagnosis. The terminology for a subset of these lesions has been updated to reflect the 2014 International Society for The Study of Vascular Anomalies (ISSVA) classification.

Capillary Hemangioma (Cherry Hemangioma or Campbell De Morgan Spot)

Clinical Features

Cherry hemangiomas are very common acquired vascular lesions that arise in middle-aged and older patients. Clinically, they present as asymptomatic, slightly raised to polypoid bright red pap-

D. Buehler (✉)
Pathology and Laboratory Medicine, University of Wisconsin School of Medicine and Public Health, Madison, WI, USA
e-mail: buehler2@wisc.edu

S. D. Billings
Department of Pathology, Cleveland Clinic, Cleveland, OH, USA

S. D. Billings et al. (eds.), *Soft Tissue Tumors of the Skin*,
https://doi.org/10.1007/978-1-4939-8812-9_7

ules, located most commonly, but not exclusively, on the extremities. Cherry hemangiomas may be numerous. When traumatized, they may turn a blue-black color due to thrombosis, resulting in a clinical resemblance to a melanocytic tumor. These lesions are universally benign.

Pathologic Features

Microscopically, cherry hemangiomas are vaguely polypoid and consist of thin-walled, dilated capillaries in the papillary dermis lined by flat endothelial cells, which lack cytologic atypia, multilayering, and mitotic figures (Fig. 7.1). They lack the distinctly crowded lobular architecture and mitotic activity of lobular capillary hemangioma (pyogenic granuloma) (discussed below). Occasional cases will show intravascular organizing thrombi, sometimes with associated intravascular papillary endothelial hyperplasia (Masson tumor). Older or traumatized lesions may show stromal hyalinization (Table 7.1). Typically, we use the term "hemangioma" or "capillary hemangioma" when encountering these lesions, although their etiology is unclear and they might be more appropriately classified as telangiectasias. The term cherry hemangioma is a clinical descriptor reflecting the bright red color of these lesions seen during dermatologic examination.

Differential Diagnosis

Pyogenic granulomas have a more distinctly crowded, lobular architecture and are often ulcerated. Lymphatic malformations can occasionally contain intravascular erythrocytes, giving them a similar appearance to capillary hemangiomas. The irregular outlines of the lymphatic channels, presence of intravascular valves, and the expression of lymphatic markers such as podoplanin (D2–40) can aid in this distinction, though immunostains are not typically necessary. Lymphatic proliferations often contain collections of lymphocytes within their septa, which are not present in capillary hemangiomas. Capillary and venulocapillary malformations may appear very similar in superficial biopsies, but are distinguished based on their clinical presentation.

Pyogenic Granuloma

Clinical Features

Pyogenic granuloma, or lobular capillary hemangioma, is one of the most common vascular proliferations encountered by dermatopathologists. The term "pyogenic granuloma" is a misnomer as these lesions have neither an infectious etiology nor

Table 7.1 Key pathologic features: capillary hemangioma

Dilated thin-walled capillary or capillary-venular vessels in the papillary dermis
No atypia or multilayering of endothelial cells, lacks mitotic activity
Stromal hyalinization common in older lesions

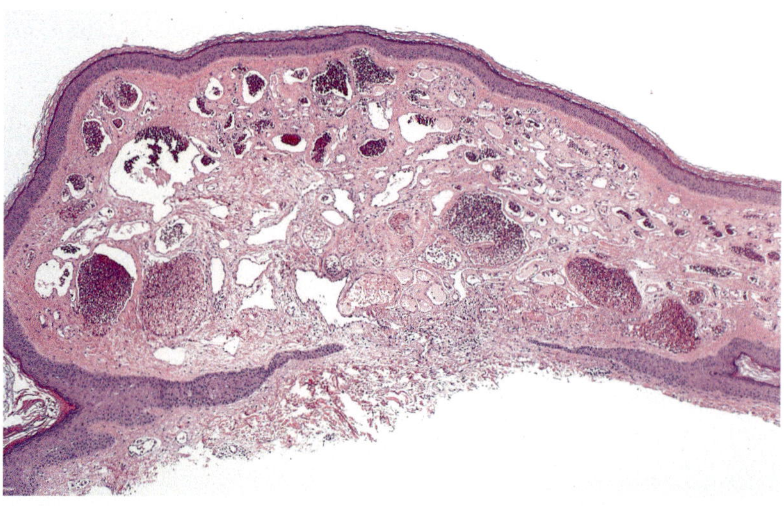

Fig. 7.1 Capillary hemangioma or Campbell De Morgan spot. Polypoid collection of thin-walled dilated capillaries in the papillary dermis without endothelial cytologic atypia, multilayering, or mitotic activity

granulomatous inflammation. That being said, the morphologically accurate descriptor "lobular capillary hemangioma" is not terribly specific, since several distinctive pediatric hemangiomas (such as infantile hemangioma, congenital nonprogressive hemangioma, and tufted angioma) also have lobular capillary architecture. For this reason, the term pyogenic granuloma is preferred, especially in children where the distinction between different types of hemangiomas has important treatment implications. Pyogenic granuloma is an acquired, most likely reactive proliferative lesion that occurs at any age, most commonly on the head and neck (including the oral and nasal mucosa) and the extremities. They are typically solitary, with only rare multiple/eruptive forms described, sometimes in association with highly active antiretroviral therapy (HAART), retinoid treatment or other medications. They present as a polypoid, often ulcerated, erythematous to violaceous nodules. Clinically, they may occasionally resemble a melanocytic tumor. The so-called granuloma gravidarum is a variant that arises in the gingiva of pregnant women and resolves after delivery.

Pathologic Features

Microscopically, pyogenic granulomas are composed of distinct lobules of closely packed capillaries, often surrounding larger feeder vessels (Fig. 7.2a). Superficial lesions often have an epidermal collarette, and if ulcerated will show an associated brisk inflammatory reaction and granulation tissue. In more cellular examples, it can be difficult to appreciate the vascular lumina because the capillaries are so tightly packed (Fig. 7.2b). Pyogenic granuloma is a mitotically active lesion, but atypical mitotic figures are not a feature. Rare examples show mild nuclear atypia with enlargement and hobnail morphology of endothelial cells. The stroma is fibrous or fibromyxoid, with a variable number of inflammatory cells. Intravascular pyogenic granulomas consist of closely packed capillaries arising within a wall of a vein (Fig. 7.3). They tend to arise in the deeper dermis or subcutis. The lesional circumscription and recognition of the pre-existing vessel wall at the periphery establish the diagnosis. Inflammation is not a prominent feature in intravascular cases (Table 7.2).

Differential Diagnosis

The diagnosis of pyogenic granuloma in adults is rarely difficult. Capillary hemangiomas (see above) can have an epidermal collarette but lack the closely packed vessels and inflammation often seen in pyogenic granuloma. Rarely, exuberant pyogenic granulomas in sun-damaged skin can be confused with angiosarcoma, in part because of the brisk mitotic rate, cellularity, and mild cytologic atypia. Recognition of the lobular architecture and the lack of infiltrative growth help to exclude angiosarcoma. The presence of a pericytic layer that can be highlighted by an SMA stain is also helpful for making this distinction.

Bacillary angiomatosis, caused by *Bartonella henselae* and *quintana* bacterial microorganisms, is associated with a reactive vascular proliferation that can resemble pyogenic granuloma. The associated cytoplasmic amphophilic granular material containing the microorganism, and the epithelioid nature of the endothelial cells allows for its distinction. The organisms can be highlighted by a Warthin-Starry or Giemsa stain. Bacillary angiomatosis is most commonly seen in the setting of AIDS, but with advent of effective antiretroviral medications, it has become uncommon, at least in the United States.

Rare cases of Kaposi sarcoma can show morphologic overlap with pyogenic granuloma. These cases often have more solid, spindled areas and occur in the setting of AIDS or other immunocompromised states. Nuclear immunoreactivity for the HHV8 latent nuclear antigen can readily identify cases of Kaposi sarcoma.

The differential diagnosis of pyogenic granuloma in infants and children is discussed below.

Infantile Hemangioma

Clinical Features

Infantile hemangioma, formerly known as *juvenile hemangioma* or *cellular hemangioma of infancy*, is the most common pediatric soft tissue tumor, seen in approximately 4% of children. It is more common in fair-skinned individuals, affecting about 10% of Caucasians with a female predilection. Infantile hemangiomas can present as cutaneous or subcutaneous tumors, most often in

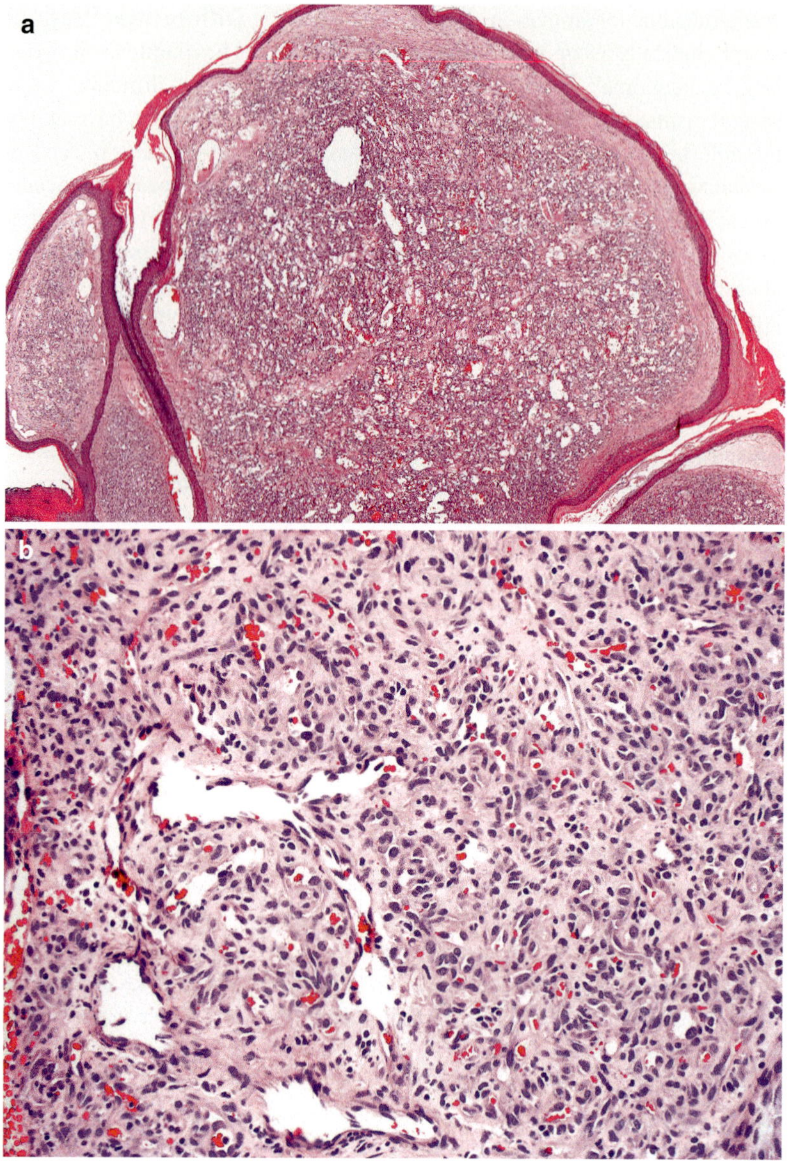

Fig. 7.2 Cutaneous pyogenic granuloma. (**a**) Polypoid vascular proliferation with epidermal collarette composed of closely packed capillaries surrounding dilated feeder vessels. (**b**) Higher power image demonstrating closely packed capillaries

the head and neck area; genital or visceral tumors often involve the liver, GI tract, or upper aerodigestive tract. Segmental infantile hemangioma of the face may be associated with PHACES syndrome. Interestingly, deep skeletal muscle is spared. All share a similar clinical course. They present shortly after birth, usually starting as an red to bluish macule, undergo rapid growth during the first year of life (proliferative phase), and then involute slowly over the course of several years (involution phase). Rare cases present at birth and may involute rapidly. The clinical presentation varies dramatically from clinically innocuous lesions that regress spontaneously without treatment to lesions causing life-threatening complications or cosmetic and functional deformities. Some patients present with consumptive hypothyroidism due to the expression of type 3 iodothyronine deiodinase by the lesional cells. By imaging, they are high-flow lesions that lack the shunting that typifies arteriovenous malformations. Infantile hemangiomas are infrequently biopsied except in clinically ambiguous cases. Accurate histologic diagnosis is very important as infantile hemangioma uniquely responds to treatment with propranolol.

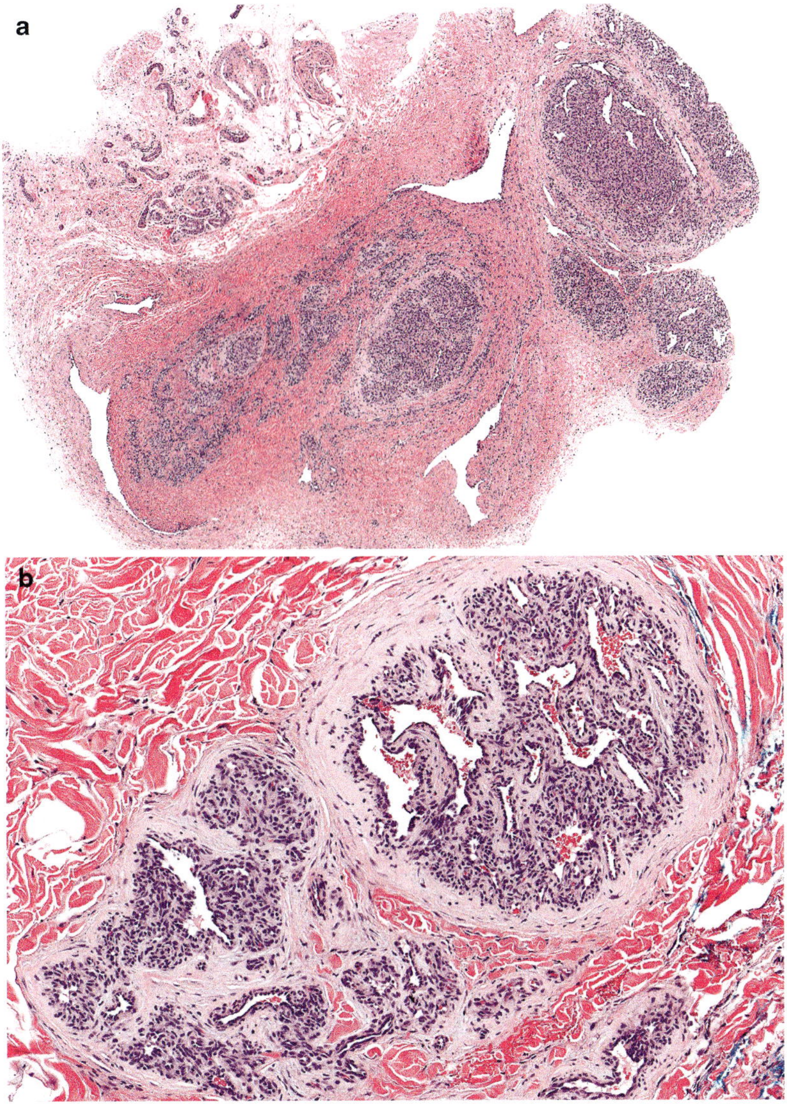

Fig. 7.3 Intravascular pyogenic granuloma. (**a**) Intravascular proliferation arising from the wall of a vein in the deep dermis/subcutis. (**b**) Lobular capillary proliferation filling and expanding the vascular lumen. Inflammation is inconspicuous

Table 7.2 Key pathologic features: pyogenic granuloma

Lobular proliferation of closely packed capillaries
Epidermal collarette in superficial lesions
Variable ulceration and inflammatory infiltrate
Intravascular pyogenic granuloma
Closely packed capillaries within a pre-existing vessel
Lack of substantial inflammation

Pathologic Features

While infantile hemangioma generally fits the generic label of "lobular capillary hemangioma," the lesions have a very distinctive histologic appearance that depends upon the phase in which the lesion is biopsied. In the proliferative phase, infantile hemangioma consists of lobules of densely packed, plump, mitotically active capillaries surrounded by pericytes and separated by delicate fibrous septa or normal tissue elements like adipose tissue, adnexal structures, nerves, or skeletal muscle fibers (Fig. 7.4). The growth is nondestructive, and reactive stromal changes such as fibrosis, myxoid change, or granulation tissue that characterize pyogenic granuloma and congenital nonprogressive hemangioma do not occur in infantile hemangioma.

The capillaries are surrounded by a thin basement membrane and form small rounded lumina which can be obscured by rapidly proliferating endothelial cells (Fig. 7.5a). The base of the lobule can show feeding arteries and draining veins. In the involutional phase, the endothelial cells and pericytes become more attenuated, resulting in open capillary lumina, while the basement membranes become thick and hyalinized. Characteristic features include the presence of apoptotic dust within the basement membrane and an increased number of perivascular mast cells (Fig. 7.5b). Features of both the proliferative and involutional phases often coexist within the same lesion. In end-stage lesions, residual capillaries become completely hyalinized (so-

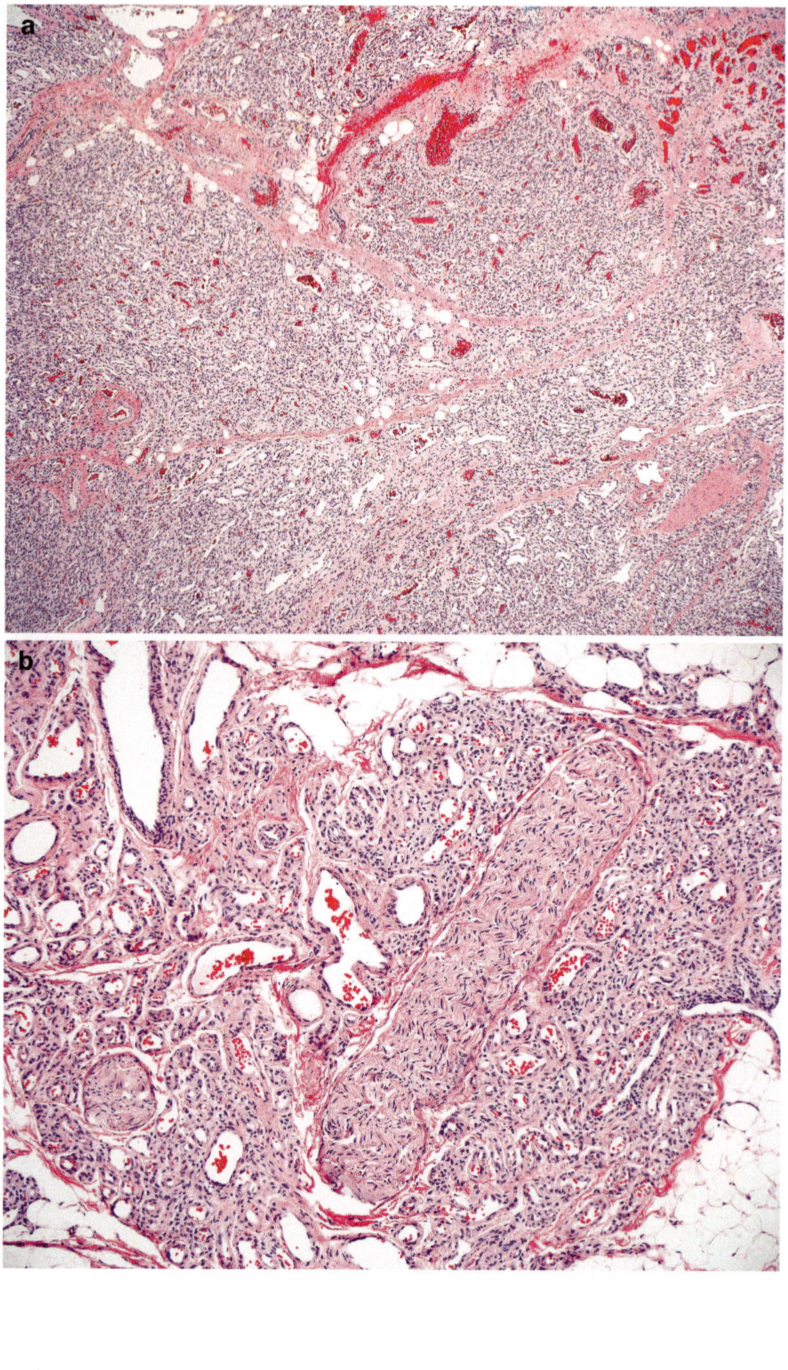

Fig. 7.4 Infantile hemangioma. (**a**) Lobular arrangement of small capillaries separated by thin fibrous septa. (**b**) The capillaries envelop normal tissue elements like nerves, adipose tissue, or adnexa

called ghost vessels), while the large feeding and draining vessels persist (Fig. 7.6a) mimicking a vascular malformation.

Infantile hemangiomas have a unique immunophenotype shared only by the placental vasculature including expression of GLUT1, an erythrocyte glucose transporter protein, Lewis-Y antigen, CCR6, CD15, and FcYRII. The basement membranes in these capillaries express merosin. Since GLUT1 is not expressed in reactive vascular proliferations, other benign hemangiomas, and most vascular malformations (with rare exceptions, such as verrucous hemangioma), it is a very useful immunohistochemical marker for the diagnosis of infantile hemangioma and is expressed in all stages of this lesion (Fig. 7.6b) (Table 7.3).

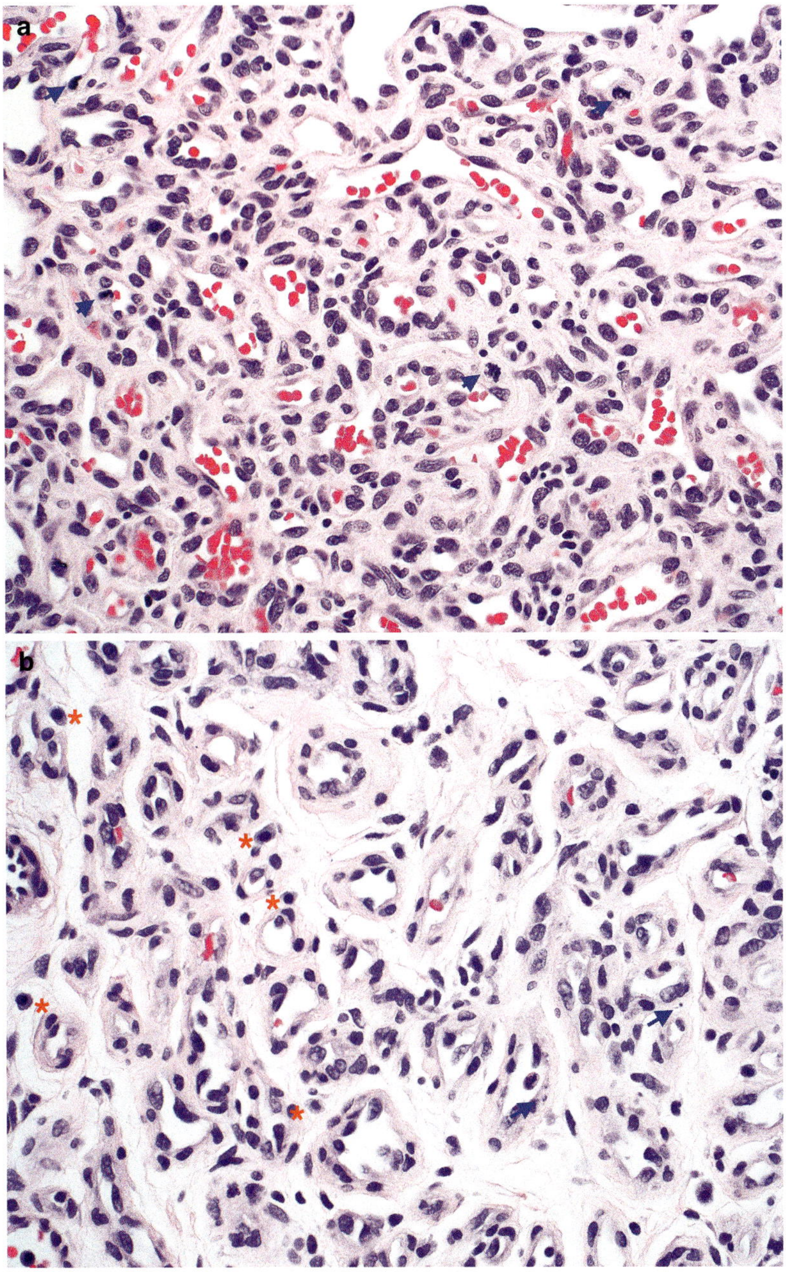

Fig. 7.5 (**a**) Infantile hemangioma, proliferative stage. Tightly packed capillaries are composed of plump endothelial cells and pericytes and form small rounded lumina. Mitotic figures, highlighted by arrows, are common. (**b**) Infantile hemangioma, involutional stage. The capillaries "open up" due to attenuation of endothelial cells and pericytes. The basement membranes are thick and hyalinized, and contain apoptotic dust. Mitotic activity is not seen. Conspicuous mast cells are present, as indicated by asterisks

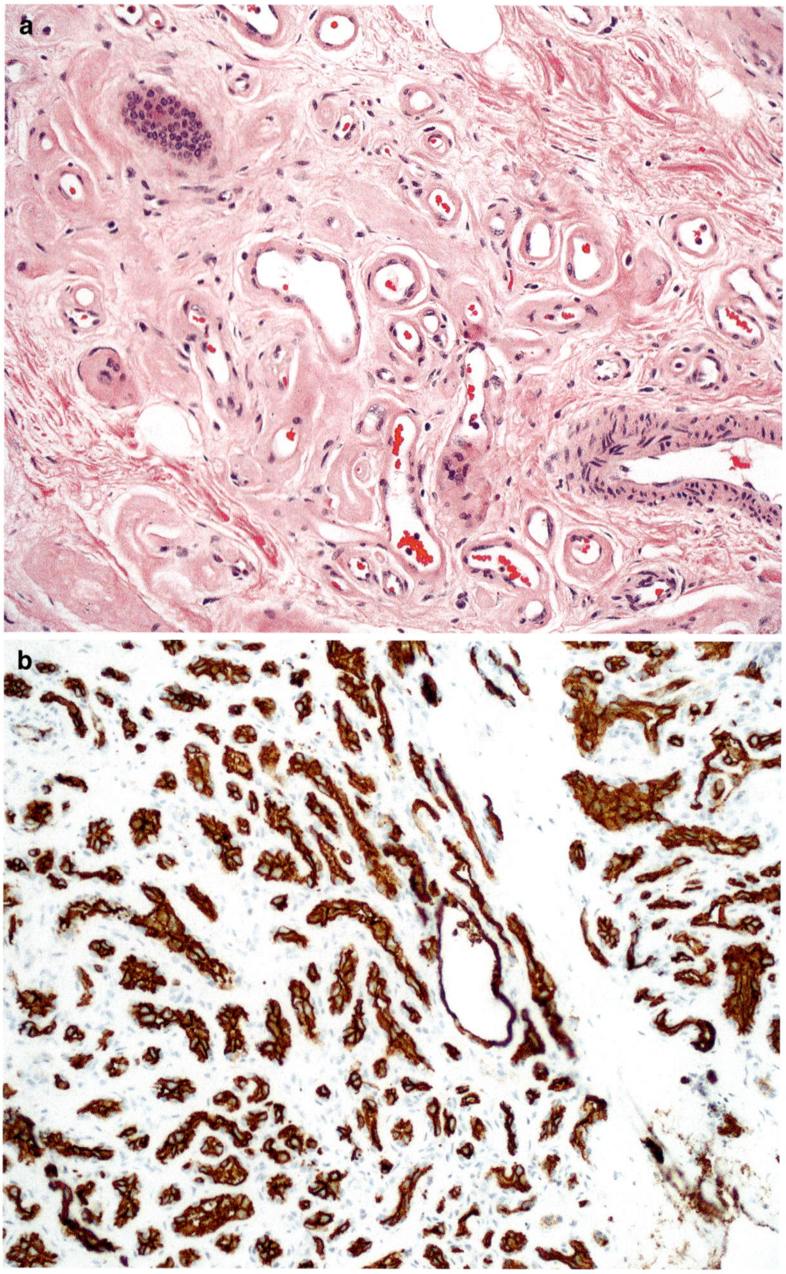

Fig. 7.6 (**a**) Infantile hemangioma, end-stage. Hyalinized residual capillaries in a fibrous background surrounding a large feeding vessel that persists. (**b**) Strong GLUT1 immunoreactivity in infantile hemangioma; intravascular red blood cells are also positive for GLUT1 and serve as an internal control

Differential Diagnosis

The differential diagnosis usually involves congenital nonprogressive hemangiomas (so-called RICH and NICH, discussed below) and pyogenic granuloma. The latter can be distinguished from infantile hemangioma based on its thick fibrous stroma with reactive changes separating tumor lobules and the lack of GLUT1 immunoreactivity. Highly cellular proliferative phase examples can be mistaken for a more aggressive neoplasm such as kaposiform hemangioendothelioma-tufted angioma (KHE/TA, discussed below) or angiosarcoma. Pediatric angiosarcomas are very rare and can be distinguished based on complex architecture, infiltrative growth pattern, greater nuclear atypia, and the lack of a pericytic layer.

Table 7.3 Key pathologic features: infantile hemangioma

Lobules of small capillaries separated by thin fibrous septa or normal tissue elements
Proliferative phase:
Plump capillaries and pericytes with small round lumina
Frequent mitotic figures
Thin basement membrane
Involutional phase:
Open capillaries with flattened endothelial cells
Few or absent mitotic figures
Thickened hyalinized basement membranes with apoptotic dust
Conspicuous mast cells
End-stage lesions retain feeding and draining vessels and can mimic vascular malformations
GLUT1 immunoreactivity present in all stages

Immunohistochemically, angiosarcomas often express podoplanin (D2–40), which is uncharacteristic of infantile hemangioma. An important diagnostic pitfall is the frequent expression of GLUT1 in angiosarcomas. Separation of end-stage examples of infantile hemangioma from vascular malformations is best accomplished by correlation with the clinical and radiologic findings and immunohistochemistry for GLUT1.

Congenital Nonprogressive Hemangioma

Clinical Features

In contrast to infantile hemangioma, congenital nonprogressive hemangiomas are fully formed at birth; subsequently, they may either rapidly involute, usually within the first 6 months of life, partially involute, or persist without any involution. Based on their clinical pattern of involution, these lesions are subclassified as rapidly involuting congenital hemangioma (RICH), partially involuting congenital hemangioma (PICH), and non-involuting congenital hemangioma (NICH). This distinction is largely clinical as these lesions show the same histomorphologic characteristics. Like infantile hemangioma, congenital nonprogressive hemangiomas tend to occur in the dermis, subcutis, and viscera, sparing deep skeletal muscle. There is no gender predilection. By imaging, these are also high-flow lesions without arteriovenous shunting.

Pathologic Features

Congenital nonprogressive hemangiomas are composed of capillary lobules separated by fibrous stroma. The lobules are arranged around a fibrous core containing prominent large interlobular feeding and draining vessels that can resemble vascular malformations (Fig. 7.7). Within the lobules, there are somewhat stellate or crescent-shaped thin-walled draining vessels (Fig. 7.8). At high power, the capillaries have a distinctive appearance with open lumina lined by small, rounded, slightly hyperchromatic "hobnailed" nuclei without significant atypia or mitotic activity (Fig. 7.9a). In the NICH variant, the hobnailed nuclei and large interlobular draining vessels are more common, but the morphologic features of all variants are essentially identical. The stroma is fibrous or myxoid, and, in contrast to infantile hemangioma, adnexal structures are typically destroyed. Calcifications, thrombi, hemosiderin deposits, and extramedullary hematopoiesis are common (Fig. 7.9b) (Table 7.4). Regressed lesions leave a scar. Both RICH and NICH lesions are negative for GLUT1 expression. Recently, *GNAQ* and *GNA11* mutations were identified in congenital nonprogressive hemangiomas of both RICH and NICH subtypes.

Differential Diagnosis

Pyogenic granuloma is perhaps the closest morphologic mimicker of congenital nonprogressive hemangioma, as it is also composed of well-defined lobules of small capillaries in a fibrous stroma. Clinical presentation is very helpful in this distinction as pyogenic granuloma is an acquired, eruptive vascular proliferation. Stellate intralobular and large interlobular draining vessels are not characteristic of pyogenic granuloma. Infantile hemangioma lacks the intralobular stellate vessels of congenital non-progressive hemangioma and shows no fibrous stromal response. The capillaries of infantile hemangioma are also quite different showing plump, oval, mitotically active endothelial cells

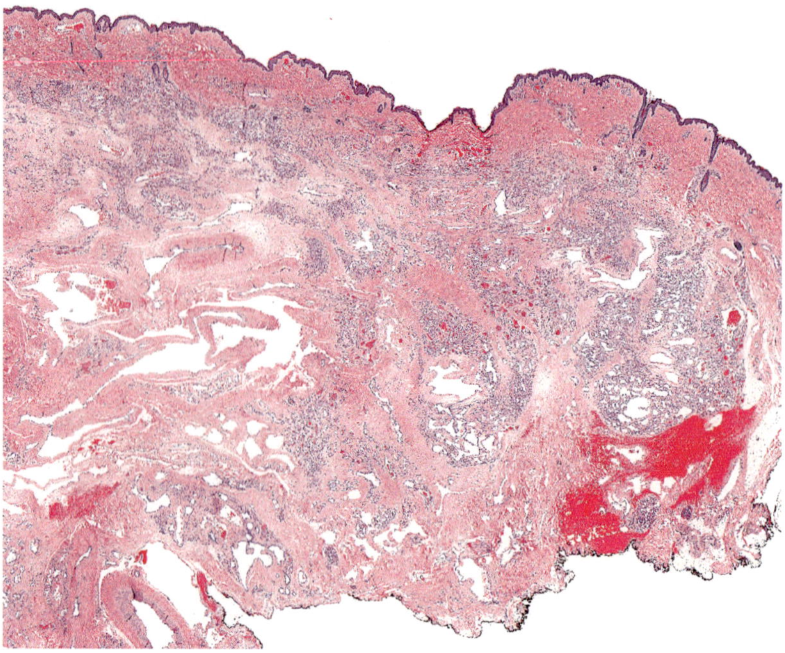

Fig. 7.7 Congenital nonprogressive hemangioma. Well-formed capillary lobules arranged around a fibrous core containing prominent interlobular draining and feeding vessels

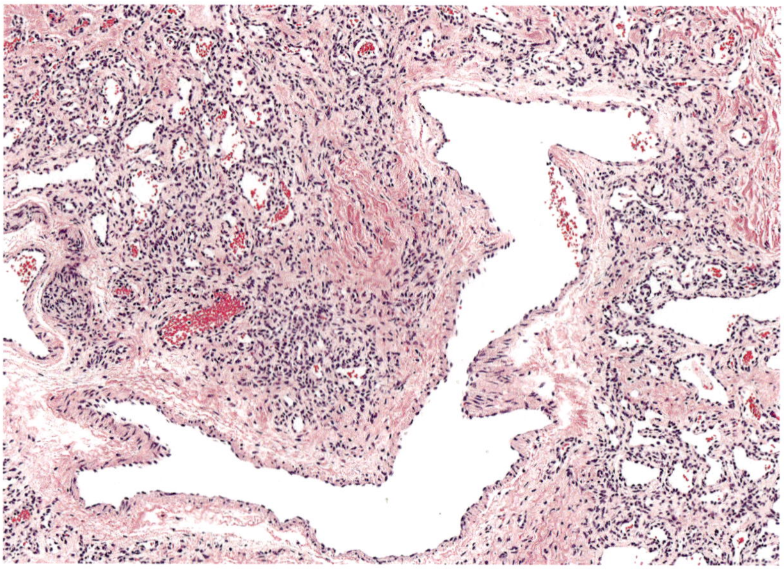

Fig. 7.8 Congenital nonprogressive hemangioma. Stellate or crescent-shaped draining vessels are also present within the capillary lobules, often in the center

during the proliferative phase and flattened endothelium with thick, hyalinized basement membranes containing apoptotic dust during the involutional phase. The clinical history and immunophenotype (GLUT1+) of infantile hemangioma are also very helpful features for making this distinction. Large interlobular feeding and draining vessels in congenital nonprogressive hemangioma can resemble an arteriovenous malformation (AVM), especially since both lesions show a high-flow pattern by Doppler imaging. However, arteriovenous shunting is not characteristic of congenital nonprogressive hemangioma. Stromal fibrosis, myxoid change, and reactive vascular proliferation are common in AVMs, but these vessels do not form well-

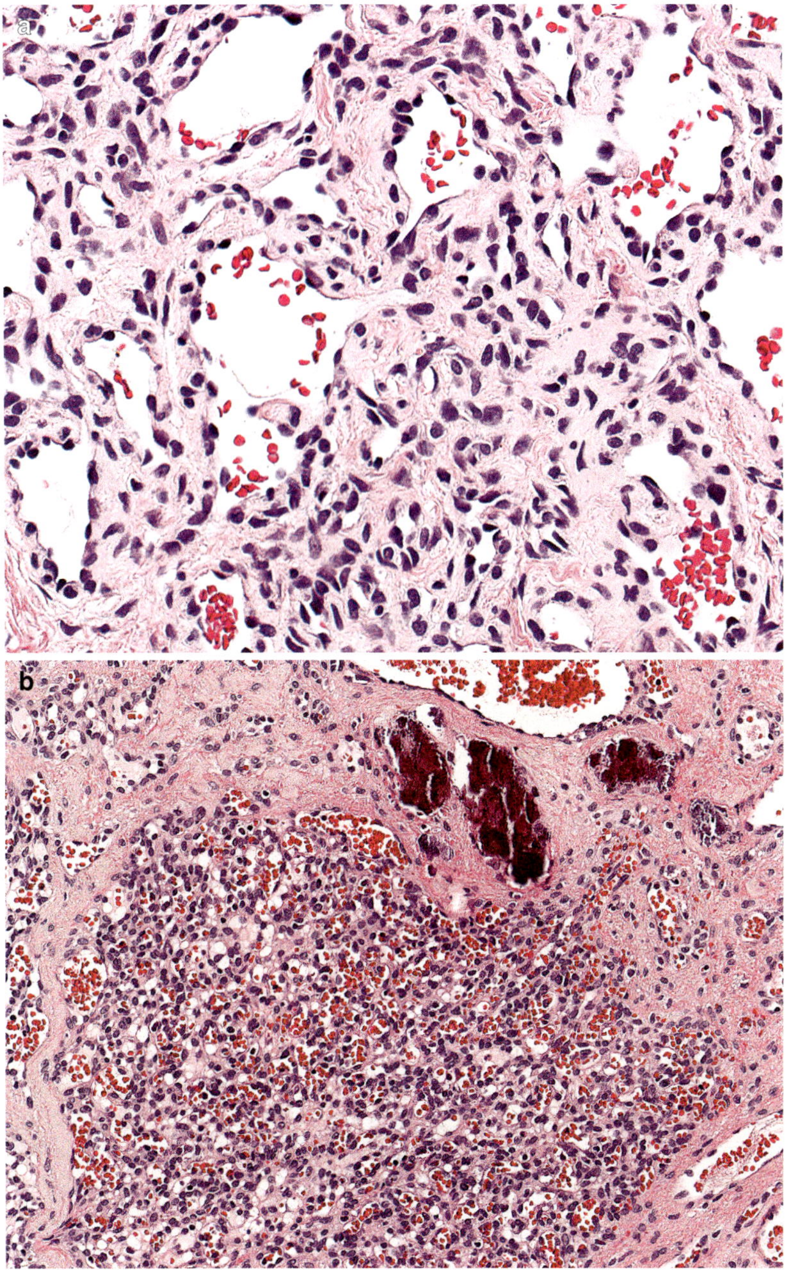

Fig. 7.9 Congenital nonprogressive hemangioma. (**a**) Capillaries lined by uniform rounded endothelial cells with slightly hyperchromatic "hobnailed" nuclei. These features are more conspicuous in the NICH variant. (**b**) Another example showing strikingly uniform dark endothelial cells in a lobular configuration and dystrophic calcifications. Note the lack of mitotic activity

defined capillary lobules and lack the distinctive dark hobnailed endothelial cells seen in congenital nonprogressive hemangioma. That being said, all of the above lesions show some degree of histomorphologic overlap, especially in superficial and core needle biopsies. A multidisciplinary approach is the key to establishing the correct diagnosis.

Venous Malformation (So-Called Cavernous/Sinusoidal Hemangioma)

Clinical Features

The term "cavernous hemangioma" is ubiquitously used by pathologists to describe a lesion composed of multiple dilated vascular channels lined by cytologically bland, mitotically quiescent

Table 7.4 Key pathologic features: congenital nonprogressive hemangioma

Lobules of small capillaries separated by thick fibrous bands
Stellate intralobular and large interlobular draining vessels
Round, slightly hyperchromatic hobnailed endothelial cells without mitotic activity
Fibrosis and myxoid stroma with destruction of adnexal structures
GLUT1 negative
RICH, NICH, and PICH subtypes are defined clinically and have the same histomorphologic features
RICH: rapid involution within the first 6 months to a year
PICH: initial involution similar to RICH but failure to regress completely
NICH: no involution

endothelial cells and often filled with erythrocytes. Regrettably, this descriptive term is nosologically very uninformative for two reasons. First, most of these lesions are not hemangiomas. Recent efforts by the International Society for the Study of Vascular Anomalies (ISSVA) have resulted in a more biologically accurate classification of vascular anomalies that considers the clinical, histopathologic, and genetic/molecular findings together. In the core of this classification is the concept that the term "hemangioma" is only applicable to lesions with proliferative activity (e.g., mitotic figures or immunohistochemical markers such as Ki-67 or WT-1), whereas mitotically quiescent nonproliferative vessels are classified as "malformations" implying errors in vascular development. Under the 2014 ISSVA classification, most of the so-called cavernous hemangiomas would now be classified as venous malformations, either sporadic (most common) or associated with syndromes. This taxonomic placement is also supported by the recent identification of somatic mutations in TIE2, a vascular protein kinase implicated in pathogenesis of familial cutaneomucosal venous malformation (VMCM) syndrome, in sporadic venous malformations. Second, vascular ectasias imparting a cavernous appearance histologically are not unique to venous malformations. They can be seen in many other lesions – other vascular malformations, hemangiomas, and telangiectasias – and even in organizing thrombi. From this standpoint, the term "cavernous hemangioma" is more of a histologic pattern than a distinct clinicopathological entity, and its use as a diagnostic term should be avoided.

Sinusoidal hemangioma, originally described as a distinctive subtype of cavernous hemangioma, presents as a solitary subcutaneous or deep dermal nodule or plaque on the trunk, breasts, or extremities. However, this "sinusoidal hemangioma" pattern can also be observed in a variety of unrelated vascular anomalies, including malformations. The lack of proliferative endothelium in these lesions also supports the contention that they do not represent true hemangiomas. Definitive diagnostic criteria defining "sinusoidal hemangioma" as an entity *sui generis* is currently lacking.

Pathologic Features

The so-called "cavernous hemangioma" pattern consists of a well-circumscribed collection of multiple, ectatic thin-walled vessels, lined by bland mitotically inactive endothelial cells. Upon close examination, these vessels most often contain a variable amount of irregular, disorganized smooth muscle and lack internal elastic lamina, consistent with veins. Oftentimes, there are asymmetric fibromyxoid intimal "bumpers" in the walls of these veins, as well as organizing thrombi and dystrophic calcifications due to slow flow. These features allow us to correctly classify most of the "cavernous hemangiomas" as venous malformations (Fig. 7.10a). Subcutaneous venous malformations, often mislabeled in the past as "venous hemangiomas" are recognized as ill-defined collections of large, dilated veins admixed with adipose tissue and skeletal muscle (Fig. 7.10b). The intervening stroma in venous malformations shows little fibrous response, myxoid change, or reactive capillary proliferation since these are slow-flow lesions. However, organizing thrombi often undergo papillary endothelial hyperplasia (Masson tumor) (discussed below), which may lead to consideration of a proliferative lesion (heman-

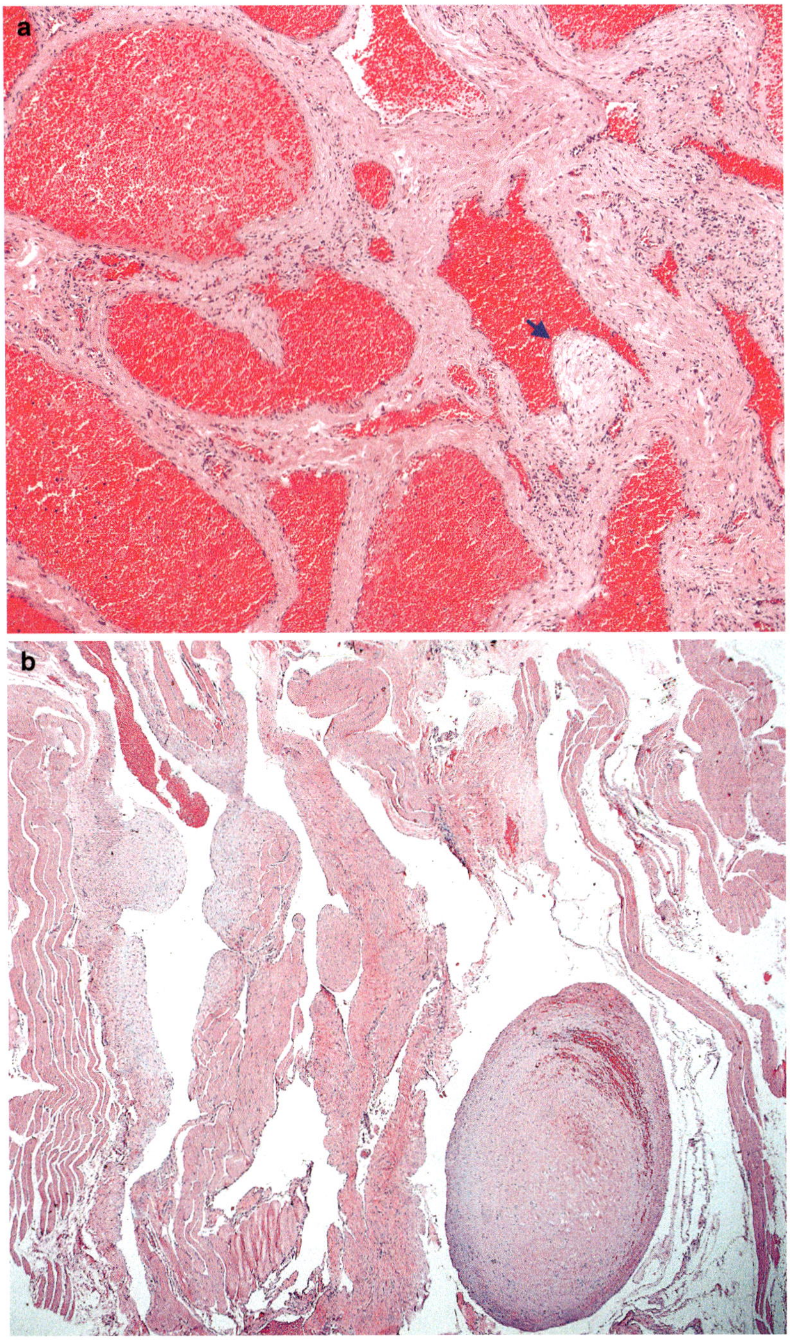

Fig. 7.10 Venous malformations commonly mislabeled in the past as "cavernous hemangioma." (**a**) Superficial venous malformation composed of a well-circumscribed collection of thin dilated veins with a monolayer of bland, mitotically inactive endothelial cells. Asymmetric fibromyxoid intimal "bumpers" are present, as indicated by the arrow. (**b**) Subcutaneous venous malformation composed of irregular, dilated veins admixed with adipose tissue and skeletal muscle, and containing organizing thrombi

gioma) or angiosarcoma. The "sinusoidal hemangioma" pattern shows a circumscribed collection of markedly attenuated interanastomosing channels imparting a sieve-like appearance at low power. Pseudopapillary projections may be seen, due to tangential sectioning (Fig. 7.11). Thrombosis and calcifications are also relatively common (Table 7.5).

Differential Diagnosis

Recognition of cavernous or sinusoidal areas in a vascular lesion is rarely difficult, and many

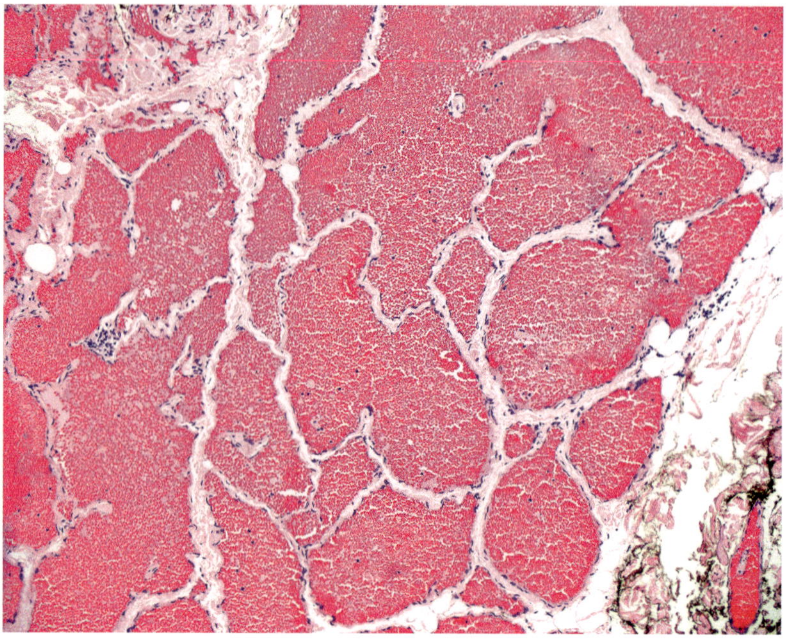

Fig. 7.11 So-called "sinusoidal hemangioma" pattern displaying markedly attenuated interanastomosing vascular channels imparting a sieve-like appearance and containing pseudopapillary projections. The underlying lesion is a sporadic venous malformation

Table 7.5 Key pathologic features: venous malformation (so-called "cavernous/sinusoidal hemangioma")

A non-specific pattern seen in a variety of hemangiomas and vascular malformations, rather than a specific diagnostic entity
Most lesions represent venous malformations
Large ectatic thin-walled vessels lined by attenuated mitotically quiescent endothelium
Organized thrombi are common due to slow blood flow
Interanastomosing channels and pseudopapillary projections may be seen in the "sinusoidal hemangioma" pattern
No significant cytologic atypia or infiltrative growth

lesions can be readily diagnosed as venous malformations based on the above features. However, many other lesions including venolymphatic and capillary malformations, the involutional stage of infantile hemangioma, verrucous hemangioma, angiokeratoma, and spindle cell hemangioma (discussed below) can show cavernous areas. Therefore, classification of a vascular lesion with this appearance should be based on the more specific morphologic features of the abovenamed entities and may require a multidisciplinary approach for diagnosis. The more complex architecture of sinusoidal hemangioma may occasionally raise the question of an angiosarcoma, but angiosarcomas are infiltrative rather than well-circumscribed, and exhibit nuclear atypia and multilayering of endothelial cells, features not seen in sinusoidal hemangioma.

Hyperkeratotic Vascular Lesions:

Angiokeratoma

Clinical Features

There are five clinically distinctive variants of this benign acquired cutaneous vascular lesion with different anatomic predilections. The *Fordyce* type occurs in middle-aged to older men as solitary or multiple red-to-violaceous-to-black papules most commonly on the scrotum. They can also occur on the penis, inner thighs, and lower abdomen and less commonly on the vulva. The *Mibelli* type presents as a warty-appearing lesion over bony prominences on the hands and feet of children and adolescents, suggesting a possible association with trauma. The related *solitary* variant of angiokeratoma is the most common form and pres-

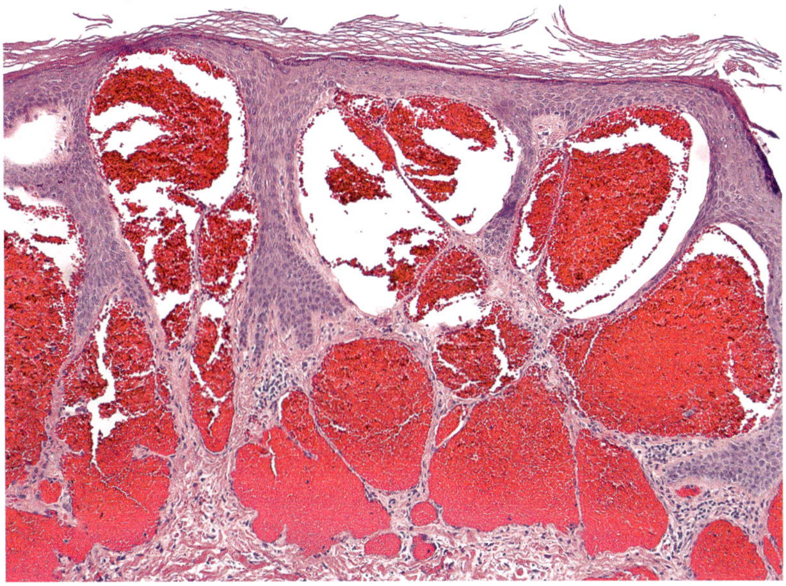

Fig. 7.12 Angiokeratoma. Ectatic, thin-walled vessels with flat endothelial lining fill the upper dermis and protrude into the dermal papillae creating an impression of "intraepithelial" vessels. The epidermis is acanthotic and hyperkeratotic

ents as a single papule on the lower limbs of young males and is also thought to be associated with trauma. *Angiokeratoma circumscriptum* is rare, presenting as a group of coalescing papules or plaques on the extremities of children and, in contrast to the acquired nature of other angiokeratomas, is present at birth. *Angiokeratoma corporis diffusum* presents as multiple papules, predominantly in a "bathing suit" distribution. It is often, though not always, associated with Fabry disease, an X-linked deficiency of α-galactosidase A. Deficiencies in L-fucosidase, β-mannosidase, neuraminidase, β-galactosidase, and α-*N*-acetylgalactosaminidase have also been linked to this variant.

Pathologic Features

Microscopically, all angiokeratomas are similar showing proliferation of ectatic, thin-walled vessels lined by flat, nonproliferative endothelium. The vessels are limited to the superficial dermis in association with an acanthotic, hyperkeratotic epidermis. The vessels typically herniate into the overlying epidermis resulting in the appearance that the vessels are trapped within the epidermis (Fig. 7.12) (Table 7.6).

Table 7.6 Key pathologic features: angiokeratoma

Often occur in frictional areas and may be related to trauma
Acanthotic and hyperkeratotic epidermis
Dilated thin-walled vessels in the upper dermis
Vessels herniate into the overlying epidermis

Differential Diagnosis

The differential diagnosis includes other hyperkeratotic vascular lesions: verrucous venulocapillary malformation (also known as verrucous hemangioma) and cutaneous lymphatic malformation (formerly "lymphangioma circumscriptum"). Both are discussed later in this chapter. Histologically these lesions share the appearance of an acanthotic, hyperkeratotic epidermis and ectatic thin-walled vessels in the papillary dermis. Both can have vessels herniating into the dermal papillae, and may appear nearly identical in superficial biopsies. The primary histologic difference is the depth of the vascular proliferation. The vessels in angiokeratomas are restricted to the upper dermis. In verrucous venulocapillary malformations, the vessels are of the capillary type and involve the subcutis and spare the reticular dermis. In lymphatic malformations, the vessels also extend deeper into papillary dermis and may involve the reticular dermis and subcutis. Cutaneous lymphatic malformation, at least in part, shows features characteristic of a lymphatic phenotype – irregularly angled vessels without significant smooth muscle containing pale proteinaceous material, occasional lymphocytes and valve structures, and expression of podoplanin (D2–40) and other lymphatic markers.

Verrucous Venulocapillary Malformation (Verrucous Hemangioma)

Clinical Features

Verrucous venulocapillary malformation (VVM) is a sporadic vascular anomaly that presents as multiple striking violaceous to blue warty lesions on the distal extremities of children and is typically present at birth. The precise etiology of this lesion is somewhat controversial. In the 2014 ISSVA classification, it is placed within the "unclassified vascular anomaly" category, and the historic term "verrucous hemangioma" is maintained for the time being. However, their clinical and morphological features and, more recently, the identification of *MAP3K3* somatic mutation in lesions indicate that they represent a verrucous venulocapillary or venous malformation.

Pathologic Features

Microscopically, VVMs have two components: (1) superficial ectatic thin-walled, dilated vessels filling the papillary dermis and herniating into an acanthotic, hyperkeratotic epidermis (very similar to angiokeratoma), imparting a verrucous appearance (Fig 7.13a, b), and (2) capillary or venule-sized vessels in a lobular configuration that largely spare the reticular dermis and involve the subcutis (Fig. 7.14a, b). These capillaries show a flat endothelial lining, thick basement membrane, and a pericytic layer. Immunohistochemistry for lymphatic markers is usually negative, which helps to distinguish these lesions from cutaneous lymphatic malformations as discussed above. However, these capillaries can show weak expression of GLUT1 (Table 7.7).

Differential Diagnosis

The differential diagnosis with other cutaneous verrucous lesions is discussed above. A potential pitfall is mistaking the capillary component of verrucous hemangioma for the involutional stage

Fig. 7.13 Verrucous venulocapillary malformation (VVM). (**a**) At low power, superficial dermal and subcutaneous components are noted. (**b**) Superficial dilated thin-walled vessels fill the papillary dermis and protrude into the acanthotic and hyperkeratotic dermal papillae, very similar to angiokeratoma

a

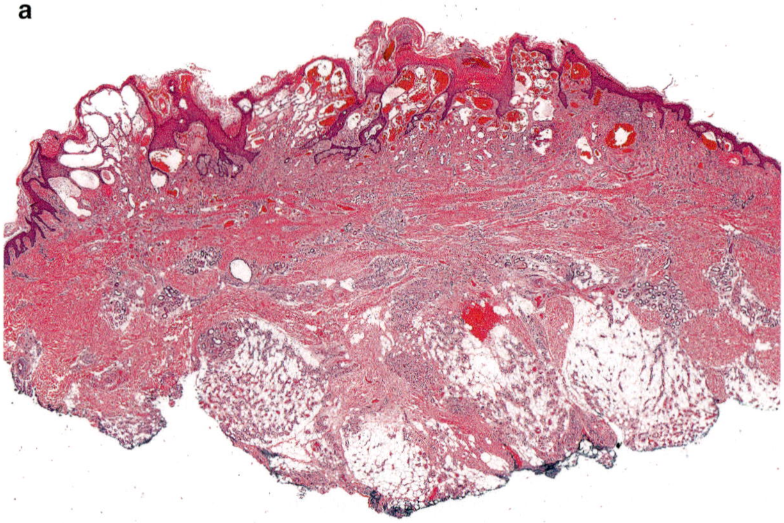

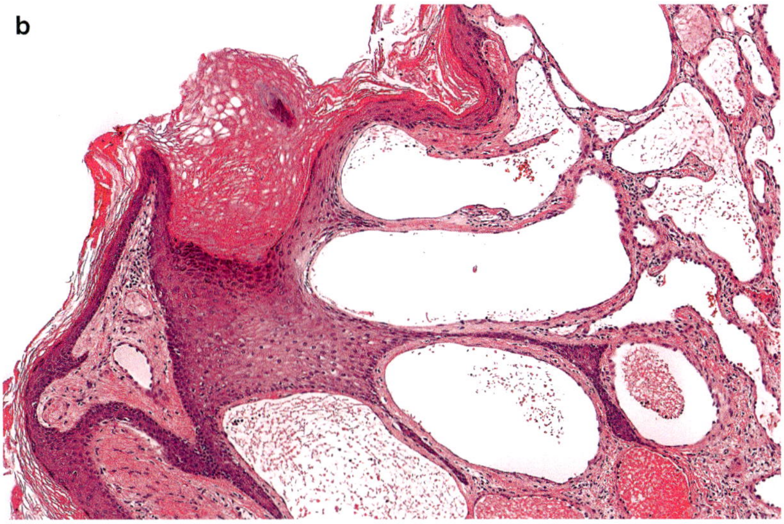

Fig. 7.13 (continued)

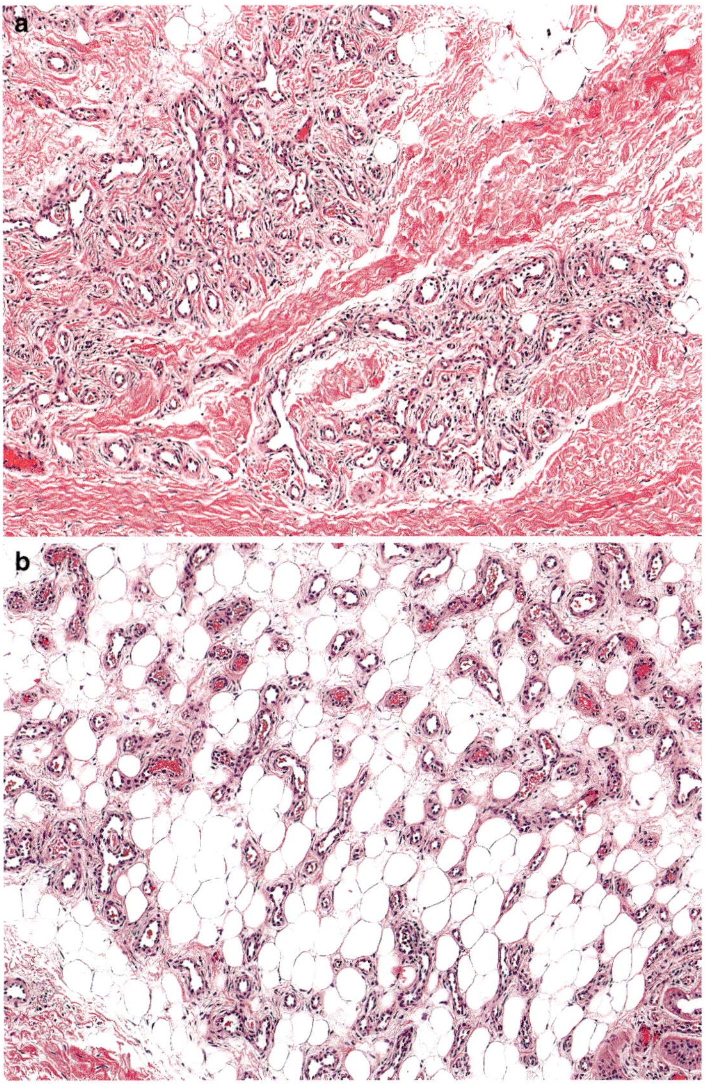

Fig. 7.14 Verrucous venulocapillary malformation (VVM). Subcutaneous capillary or venule-sized vessels with flat endothelial lining, a thick basement membrane, and a pericytic layer. The capillaries involve the subcutis in a lobular (**a**) or more diffuse (**b**) configuration but generally spare the reticular dermis

Table 7.7 Key pathologic features: verrucous venulocapillary malformation (verrucous hemangioma)

Acanthotic, papillomatous epidermis
Ectatic thin-walled superficial vessels extending into dermal papillae, similar to angiokeratoma
Capillary or venular component involving the subcutis and sparing the reticular dermis
Weak GLUT1 immunoreactivity

of infantile hemangioma, particularly in view of the weak GLUT1 immunoreactivity. However, infantile hemangiomas do not show the superficial verrucous component or dilated vascular channels, and have a different clinical presentation.

Arteriovenous Hemangioma (Acral Arteriovenous Tumor) and Arteriovenous Malformations

Clinical Features

Two types of lesions that histologically show a complex admixture of arterial and venous type vessels can be encountered by dermatopathologists. Both are often labeled as "arteriovenous hemangioma." One of them represents a superficial component of more deeply seated true arteriovenous malformations (AVMs). A comprehensive discussion of AVMs is beyond the scope of this chapter, but clarification of the diagnostic terminology is important. In the 2014 ISSVA scheme, these lesions are firmly classified as AVMs rather than hemangiomas since they are present at birth (although the clinical manifestations of arteriovenous shunting may not occur until adolescence or adulthood), grow slowly and proportionally with the child, and lack the proliferative activity (i.e., mitotic figures) that typifies hemangiomas. AVMs usually present as solitary lesions in the skin and subcutis but may also involve the soft tissue, bone, and viscera. The cutaneous manifestation of AVM is that of a warm, raised, possibly pulsating nodule in the head and neck area, scalp, or extremities. By imaging, AVMs are high-flow lesions with evidence of shunting. These are clinically significant lesions that can be complicated by life-threatening hemorrhage or tissue ischemia. Because of the advances in imaging techniques, AVMs are biopsied less and less often, and the diagnosis is best made in consultation with a multidisciplinary team.

By contrast, the other so-called arteriovenous hemangiomas are acquired, small papules on the face or distal extremities of middle-aged adults, although they can also occur in children and older adults. These lesions are well-circumscribed, limited to the dermis and are composed of thick- and thin-walled veins and indeterminate-type vessels that resemble arteries. The etiology of these lesions is uncertain. They lack the clinical and morphologic manifestations of arteriovenous shunting and therefore do not represent AVMs. Their vessels are mitotically quiescent, and, for that reason, they are unlikely to represent hemangiomas. In contrast to AVMs, these lesions are clinically indolent, although bleeding can occur. Simple excision is curative. Another term often used to describe these lesions is "cirsoid aneurysm," but this might also create confusion since historically, the term "cirsoid aneurysm" was introduced to denote large and cosmetically disfiguring AVMs of the scalp. Finally, the name "acral arteriovenous tumor" has been proposed for these lesions, and it is perhaps the least confusing option given the lesion's uncertain pathogenesis. That being said, this term has not gained wide acceptance, so "arteriovenous hemangioma" will be maintained in this text for the time being.

Pathologic Features

Arteriovenous hemangiomas (acral arteriovenous tumors) show a well-circumscribed collection of veins with thick fibromuscular walls, thin-walled vessels, and indeterminate-type vessels resembling arteries in the superficial dermis (Fig. 7.15); arguably, they may lack a true arterial component altogether. In contrast to AVMs, these lesions may contain intravascular thrombi, a sign of a low-flow lesion. The stroma is fibrous. The lack of an arterial component can be demonstrated by elastic staining (Table 7.8).

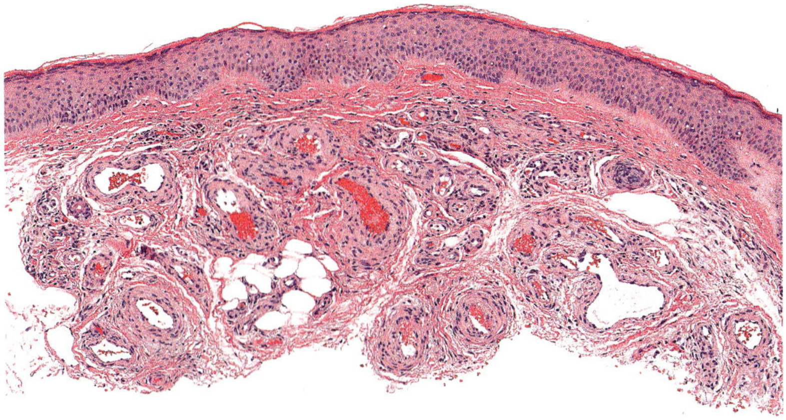

Fig. 7.15 Arteriovenous hemangioma (acral arteriovenous tumor). A well-circumscribed dermal collection of thick- and thin-walled veins and indeterminate-type vessels. The vessels are lined by flat, mitotically quiescent endothelium. There is no reactive tissue response to these vessels

Table 7.8 Key pathologic features: arteriovenous hemangioma/acral arteriovenous tumor

Small superficial collection of thick- and thin-walled veins and indeterminate-type vessels
Lack of a true arterial component
Restricted to the upper dermis
Minimal reactive stromal response

Differential Diagnosis

The principal differential diagnosis is with genuine AVMs. AVMs usually involve the dermis and subcutis and, possibly, underlying structures. They show a combination of thick-walled, larger caliber arteries and veins in a floridly proliferative background of smaller vascular channels that can include capillaries, arterioles, and venules (Fig. 7.16a, b). In response to the high-flow environment with arteriovenous shunting, tissue ischemia, and arterial embolization prior to resection, the stroma shows striking fibromyxoid change and often has a superimposed reactive capillary-type proliferation resembling granulation tissue, pyogenic granuloma, or acroangiodermatitis (Fig. 7.17). The latter phenomenon associated with an underlying AVM has been termed Stewart-Bluefarb syndrome. Organizing thrombi, a sign of a slow-flow vascular anomaly, are uncharacteristic of AVMs.

Venous Lake

Clinical Features

Venous lakes present as red to violaceous papules in the sun-damaged skin of older patients. Classically, they present on the lips, but may arise in other locations as well. Due to their clinical presentation in older patients, they may resemble angiosarcoma or melanoma.

Pathologic Features

A venous lake consists of an ectatic venule in the superficial dermis with surrounding solar elastosis. The ectatic vessel is lined by bland endothelial cells (Fig. 7.18) (Table 7.9). These lesions most likely represent localized vascular ectasia secondary to a lack of stromal support from chronic actinic damage, rather than true hemangiomas.

Differential Diagnosis

Venous lakes rarely pose a diagnostic challenge. Clinically, they may be mistaken for a ganglion cyst or mucocele (if on the lip), but the vascular nature of the lesion can be readily confirmed with immunohistochemistry for vascular markers. Acquired elastotic hemangiomas also occur in sun-damaged skin, but are composed of a band-like proliferation of blood vessels rather than a single ectatic vessel. Thrombosed venous lakes with florid papillary endothelial hyperplasia might raise suspicion for angiosarcoma. This differential diagnosis is discussed below.

Acquired Elastotic Hemangioma

This recently described hemangioma variant, like venous lakes, occurs on the sun-damaged skin of older patients, principally on the arms and neck.

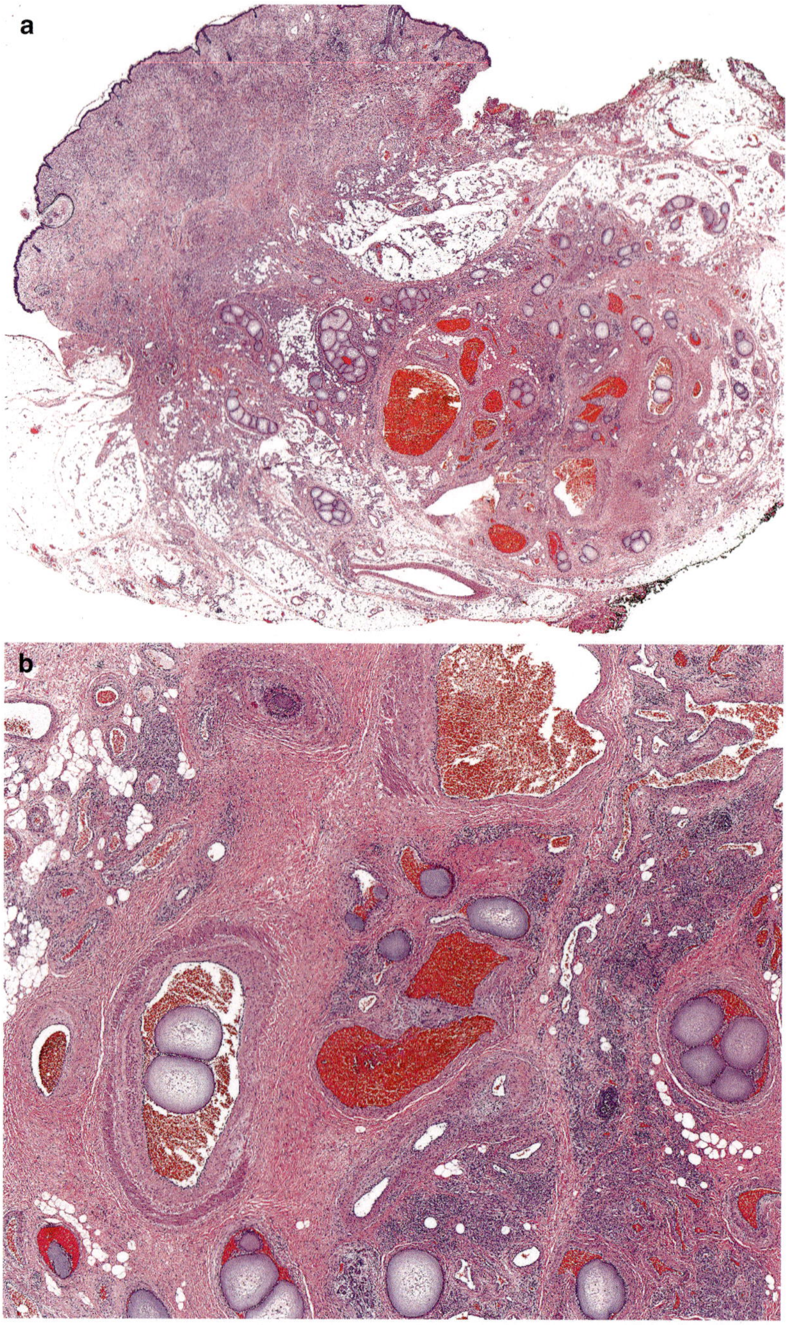

Fig. 7.16 Arteriovenous malformation. (**a**) The lesion is deeper-seated in contrast to arteriovenous hemangioma (acral arteriovenous tumor), which is limited to the dermis. (**b**) Subcutaneous collection of thick-walled abnormal arteries and veins containing embolization material. The stroma shows reactive fibromyxoid change (Case courtesy of Dr. Ivan Damjanov, University of Kansas Medical Center)

Clinically, these lesions present as slowly growing erythematous plaques.

Pathologic Features

Microscopically, acquired elastotic hemangiomas consist of a band-like proliferation of well-formed capillary-like blood vessels in the upper reticular dermis in a background of solar elastosis (Table 7.10). A narrow grenz zone is characteristically present. The blood vessels are lined by bland, slightly hobnailed endothelial cells that protrude into the vessel lumen. Atypia and mitotic activity are absent. Occasional cases may have an accompanying mild lymphocytic infiltrate (Fig. 7.19).

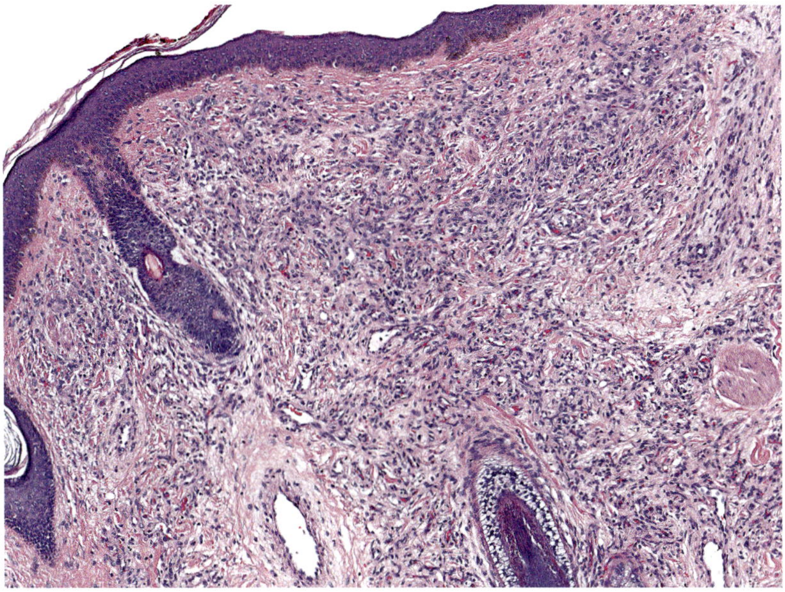

Fig. 7.17 Arteriovenous malformation. Superimposed exuberant reactive capillary-type proliferation in the upper dermis resembling acroangiodermatitis (Stewart-Bluefarb syndrome) (Case courtesy of Dr. Ivan Damjanov, University of Kansas Medical Center)

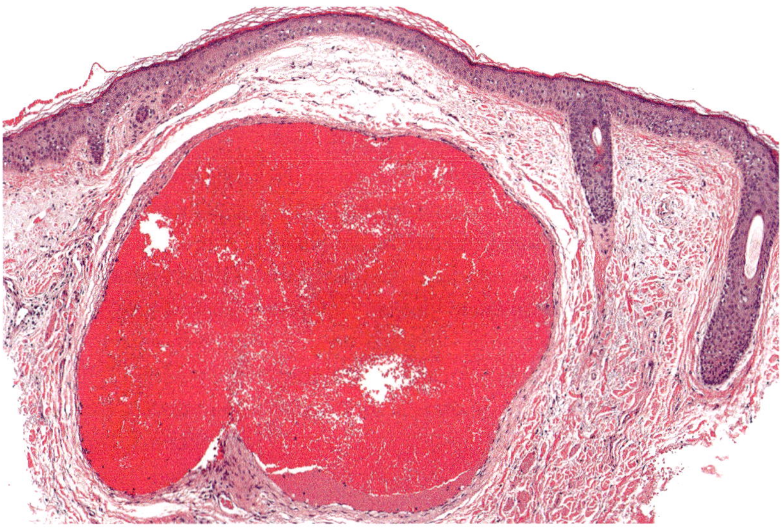

Fig. 7.18 Venous lake. A single dilated vascular channel in the upper dermis lined by attenuated endothelial cells in a background of solar elastosis

Table 7.9 Key pathologic features: venous lake

Solitary ectatic vessel in the upper dermis
Background solar elastosis

Table 7.10 Key pathologic features: acquired elastotic hemangioma

Band-like proliferation of well-formed vessels in the upper reticular dermis
Bland hobnailed endothelial cells
Background solar elastosis

Some studies have demonstrated that up to 90% express podoplanin (D2–40), although at least one study demonstrated conflicting results.

Differential Diagnosis

The band-like growth pattern and background solar elastosis help to distinguish acquired elastotic hemangiomas from other vascular tumors. Hobnail hemangioma is probably the closest mimic (see below). This entity has a wedge-shaped growth pattern, more compressed slit-like vessels

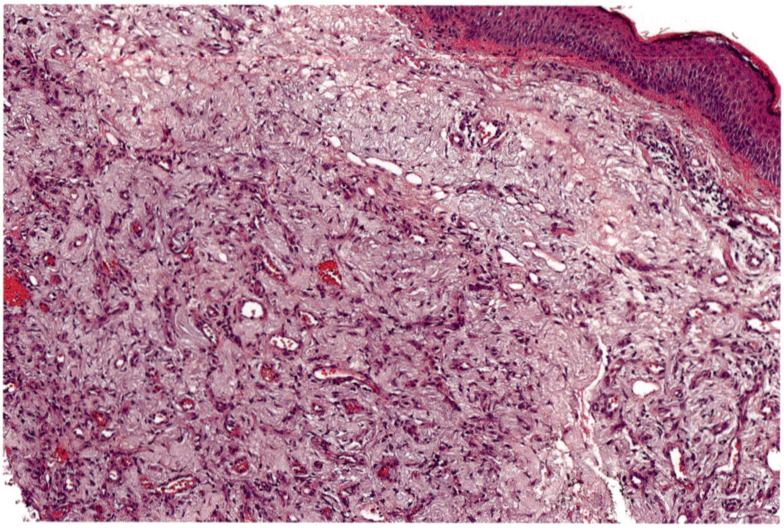

Fig. 7.19 Acquired elastotic hemangioma. Plaque-like proliferation of thin-walled vessels in sun-damaged skin

in the deeper aspects of the tumor, and a consistent lymphocytic infiltrate. Hobnail hemangioma (hobnail lymphatic malformation) tends to present in younger to middle-aged adults, and clinically may have a targetoid appearance. Kaposi sarcoma can be distinguished based on a more infiltrative growth pattern, irregular vessels, a spindle cell component, and the presence of plasma cells. Immunostaining for HHV8 is very helpful in difficult cases. Cutaneous angiosarcomas are more architecturally complex lesions with an infiltrative growth pattern and greater nuclear atypia. Radiation-associated atypical vascular lesions may appear similar morphologically (see below) but can be readily ruled out on clinical grounds.

Microvenular Hemangioma

Clinical Features

Microvenular hemangiomas occur in young adults, usually as solitary lesions, but the occurence of multiple lesions in one patient has been described. Individual lesions are not clinically distinctive, presenting as red to violaceous papules.

Pathologic Features

Microvenular hemangiomas consist of thin-walled, irregular, compressed venules and capillaries that infiltrate between the collagen bundles of the reticular dermis imparting some degree of architectural complexity (Fig. 7.20a). However, at low power, microvenular hemangioma has a relatively symmetric wedge-shaped silhouette. A striking feature is the prominent pericyte layer that invests the vessels (Fig. 7.20b). The vessels commonly infiltrate into arrector pili muscles. The endothelial cells are cytologically bland and express CD31, CD34, and ERG by immunohistochemistry, but are negative for podoplanin (D2–40). The pericytes can be highlighted by an SMA stain (Table 7.11).

Differential Diagnosis

Microvenular hemangiomas are often confused with the patch stage of Kaposi sarcoma. Although the vessels of microvenular hemangiomas are infiltrative, they lack the degree of complexity seen in Kaposi sarcoma, and promontory sign is not observed. The spindle cell component and lymphoplasmacytic infiltrate of Kaposi sarcoma are also not characteristic of microvenular hemangioma. Kaposi sarcoma lacks pericytic investment of vessels and demonstrates nuclear expression of HHV8 latent nuclear antigen by immunohistochemistry.

Hobnail Lymphatic Malformation (Hobnail Hemangioma, Targetoid Hemosiderotic Lymphatic Malformation, Targetoid Hemosiderotic Hemangioma)

Clinical Features

Formerly called hobnail hemangioma or targetoid hemosiderotic hemangioma, this lesion pres-

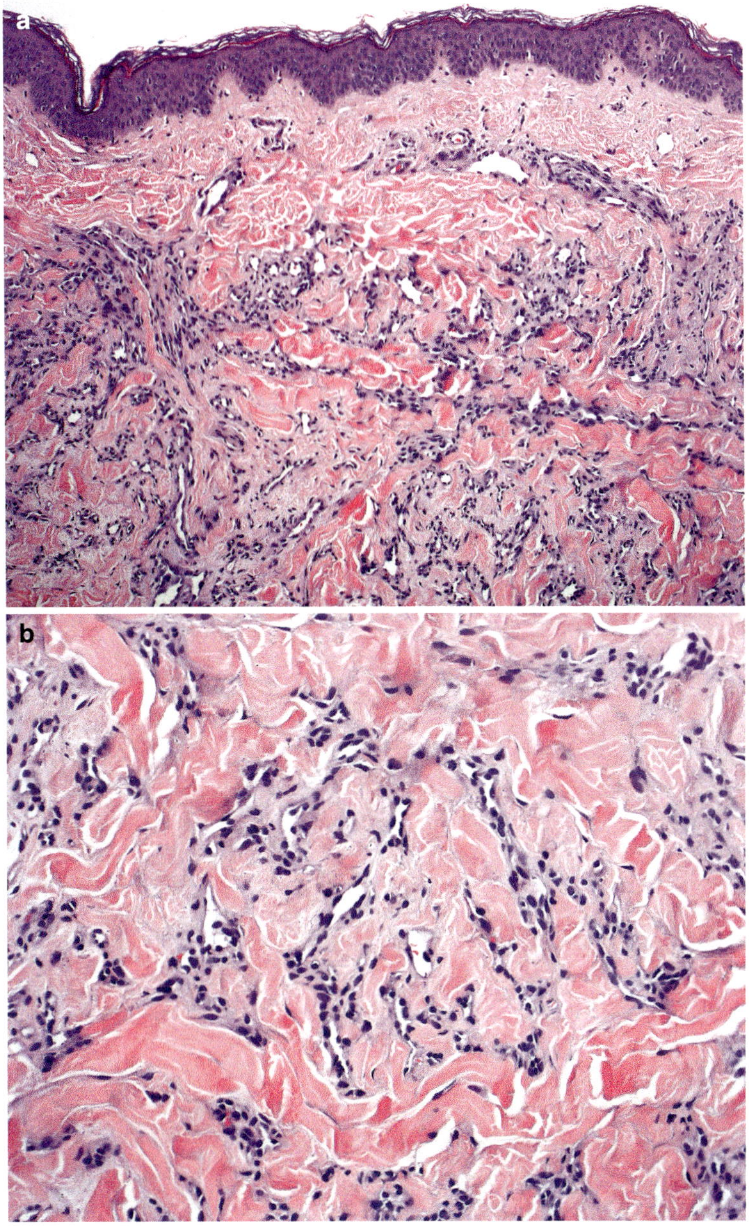

Fig. 7.20 Microvenular hemangioma. (**a**) Proliferation of thin vessels that dissects between collagen bundles of the reticular dermis. (**b**) Higher power view demonstrating the conspicuous pericyte layer investing the vessels

Table 7.11 Key pathologic features: microvenular hemangioma

Well-formed compressed venules or capillaries infiltrating through the dermis
Prominent pericyte layer that can be highlighted by SMA stain
Negative for HHV8

ents on the extremities of young to middle-aged adult patients. Lesions in women have been reported to vary with menstruation. The classic clinical presentation is a central erythematous macule or papule surrounded by a pale ring and an ecchymotic halo, which fades with time. However, as this classic presentation is not very common, the "hobnail hemangioma" term is used more often. Recent studies indicate that these lesions lack the significant proliferative activity that typifies hemangiomas (i.e., a lack of mitotic figures and immunoreactivity for WT-1). Based on this data, this lesion has been reclassified as hobnail (or targetoid hemosiderotic) lymphatic malformation.

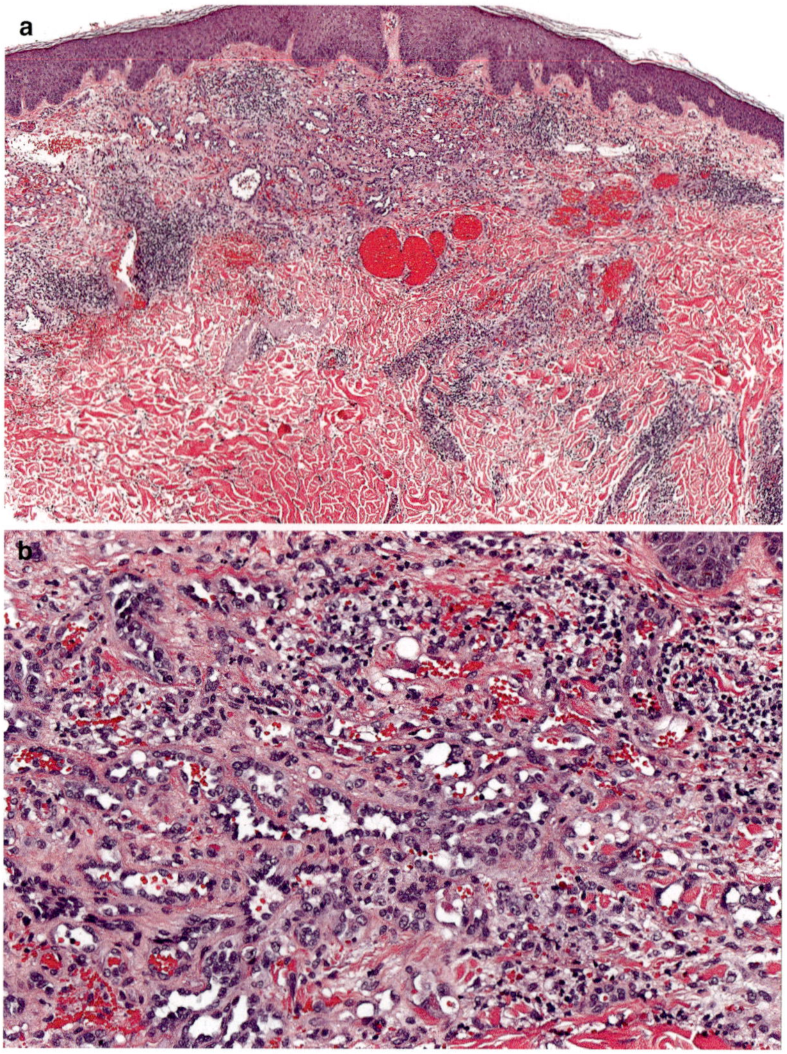

Fig. 7.21 Hobnail/targetoid hemosiderotic lymphatic malformation. (**a**) A superficial wedge-shaped dermal lesion composed of thin dilated vessels lined by cytologically banal hobnailed endothelium associated with a lymphocytic infiltrate. (**b**) Higher power image of vessels lined by hobnail endothelial cells

Pathologic Features

At scanning magnification, these are wedge-shaped tumors with the point of the wedge directed downward (Fig. 7.21a). The superficial component is composed of dilated vessels lined by bland, hobnail endothelial cells with scant cytoplasm, which lack mitotic activity (Fig. 7.21b). Focal intravascular papillae are common. Pericytes are absent. The vessels become more compressed and slit-like with increasing dermal depth and may demonstrate a somewhat dissecting growth pattern in the reticular dermis. A mild scattered lymphocytic infiltrate is commonly present, and extravasated red blood cells and hemosiderin deposits are common. By immunohistochemistry, the vessels demonstrate lymphatic differentiation with expression of podoplanin (D2–40) (Table 7.12).

Table 7.12 Key pathologic features: hobnail lymphatic malformation/hobnail hemangioma

Superficial ectatic lymphatic vessels lined by hobnail endothelial cells
Vessels compressed in the deeper aspect of the reticular dermis
Lymphocytic infiltrate, extravasated red blood cells, and hemosiderin deposition
Lacks mitotic figures and pericytes

Differential Diagnosis

The hobnail morphology can cause confusion with the family of hobnail hemangioendotheliomas including retiform hemangioendothelioma and papillary intralymphatic angioendothelioma (PILA/Dabska tumor) because of the presence of hobnail endothelial cells common to all of these entities. The vessels in hobnail lymphatic malformations lack the complex branching pattern seen in retiform hemangioendothelioma. Similarly, hobnail lymphatic malformation lacks the intravascular growth pattern and prominent papillae of papillary intralymphatic angioendothelioma. There is a variant of radiation-induced atypical vascular lesion that can closely resemble hobnail lymphatic malformation. This entity occurs in previously irradiated skin, usually in the setting of treatment for breast cancer. Angiosarcoma has greater architectural complexity, multilayering of endothelial cells, and nuclear atypia.

Tufted Angioma

Clinical Features

Tufted angioma is an acquired sporadic lesion, which occurs in children and young adults as a solitary erythematous to violaceous plaque or nodule. There is considerable clinical and morphologic overlap between tufted angioma and kaposiform hemangioendothelioma. Kasabach-Merritt phenomenon, a consumptive coagulopathy typically seen in patients with kaposiform hemangioendothelioma, can rarely manifest in association with tufted angioma. For this reason, tufted angioma and kaposiform hemangioendothelioma are often considered to represent lesions in the same disease spectrum.

Pathologic Features

Tufted angiomas are characterized by closely packed round lobules of small basophilic capillaries dispersed in the dermis apart from each other in a so-called "cannonball" pattern. These arcades of capillaries bulge into a crescent-shaped, thin-walled dilated vessel at the periphery of the lobule (Fig. 7.22a). Occasional platelet-trapping microthrombi may be present. The capillaries are cytologically bland with minimal-to-absent spindling, and mitotic figures are rare (Fig. 7.22b). By immunohistochemistry, tufted angioma focally expresses markers of lymphatic differentiation such as podoplanin (D2–40), LYVE-1, and Prox1 (more on this to follow) (Table 7.13).

Differential Diagnosis

Kaposiform hemangioendothelioma is the main lesion in the differential diagnosis. This distinction may be largely academic since, as alluded to previously, tufted angioma likely represents a small superficial kaposiform hemangioendothelioma rather than a distinct entity. In kaposiform hemangioendothelioma the capillary nodules coalesce to form large infiltrative masses deep in the subcutis and have a prominent Kaposi sarcoma-like spindle cell component, which is often arranged in fascicles. Stromal fibrosis and hemosiderin deposits are common. These features are typically not seen in superficial tufted angioma. That being said, on a case-by-case basis, it may be impossible to draw a line of distinction between these two lesions histologically. For this reason, the final diagnosis needs to be correlated with the clinical and radiologic features. The term tufted angioma may be acceptable for a patient with small superficial tumors confined to dermis; however, clinically aggressive lesions (particularly in the setting of consumptive coagulopathy) are best considered to represent kaposiform hemangioendothelioma, irrespective of the predominance of tufted angioma or kaposiform hemangioendothelioma-like features. Kaposiform hemangioendothelioma is discussed below.

In young children, tufted angiomas can also closely resemble congenital nonprogressive hemangiomas (RICH, PICH and NICH), as both have discrete lobules of lesional capillaries. In congenital nonprogressive hemangiomas, a feeding vessel is usually in the center of the lobules, whereas tufted angioma and kaposiform hemangioendothelioma have a crescent-shaped vessel at the lobule periphery. Large interlobular feeding and draining vessels are not seen in tufted angioma. In difficult cases, an immunohistochemical stain for podoplanin (D2–40) is very helpful, as congenital nonprogressive hemangiomas do not

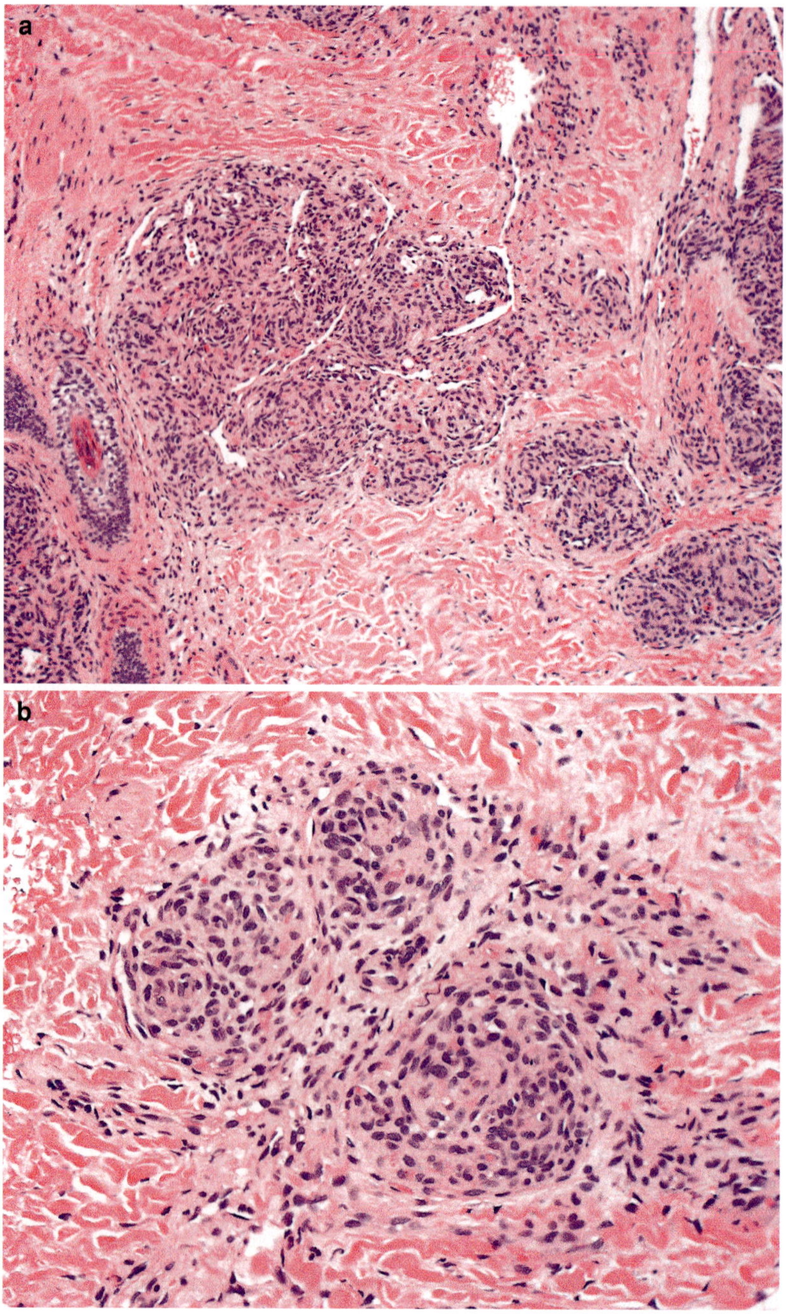

Fig. 7.22 Tufted angioma. (**a**) Discrete nodules of spindled cells with a peripheral ectatic vessel in the dermis. (**b**) Higher power image of nodules of bland spindled endothelial cells

Table 7.13 Key pathologic features: tufted angioma

Lobules of capillaries dispersed in the dermis in a "cannonball" pattern
Crescent-shaped thin-walled dilated vessel at the periphery of capillary lobules
Lymphatic immunophenotype

have lymphatic differentiation. Pyogenic granulomas have more loosely packed capillary lobules and lack the peripheral crescent-shaped vessels and lymphatic differentiation seen in tufted angioma. The proliferative phase of infantile hemangioma can resemble tufted angioma;

this differential diagnosis can be resolved by a combination of D2–40 and GLUT1 immunohistochemical stains, which will label tufted angioma and infantile hemangioma, respectively.

Spindle Cell Hemangioma

Clinical Features

Spindle cell hemangioma is a benign vascular tumor that was originally considered a low-grade vascular tumor of intermediate malignancy (hemangioendothelioma) and labeled "spindle cell hemangioendothelioma." It has since been reclassified as a benign vascular tumor. It generally presents on the distal extremities of adult patients as red to violaceous, often multiple nodules. Spindle cell hemangiomas can arise sporadically or in association with Maffucci syndrome. The majority of both sporadic and Maffucci syndrome-associated cases have mutations in the isocitrate dehydrogenase (*IDH*) gene, more commonly *IDH1* than *IDH2*; this mutation is highly specific for this hemangioma subtype. Spindle cell hemangiomas are benign, but frequently recur, likely secondary to intravascular extension beyond the affected segment of the afflicted vessel.

Pathologic Features

Spindle cell hemangioma is irregular, architecturally complex, and composed of a variety of elements; however, in general, two zones can be discerned. One zone shows prominent cavernous vascular spaces lined by bland endothelium, often with thrombosis and phlebolith formation (Fig. 7.23a, b). The second zone is more cellular and is composed of compressed spindled and mitotically active endothelial cells (arranged in a somewhat fascicular fashion reminiscent of Kaposi sarcoma), pericytes, and vacuolated epithelioid endothelial cells (so-called "blister" cells) (Fig. 7.24). Most spindle cell hemangiomas are at least partially intravascular, and a pre-existing vessel wall is often present at the periphery (Table 7.14). Immunostains for vascular markers, like ERG and CD31, will highlight compressed vessels. An SMA stain will highlight the pericytes within the tumor. Spindle cell hemangiomas also express markers of lymphatic differentiation, such as podoplanin (D2–40) and Prox1.

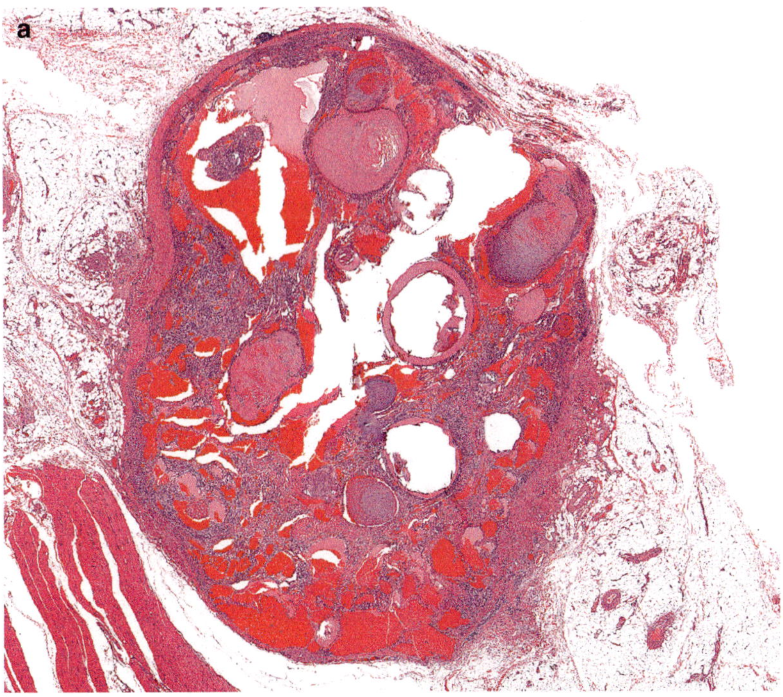

Fig. 7.23 Spindle cell hemangioma. (**a**) Lower power view showing an architecturally complex, intravascular lesion containing numerous calcified organized thrombi (phleboliths). (**b**) Cavernous areas containing thin dilated vessels lined by flat endothelial cells

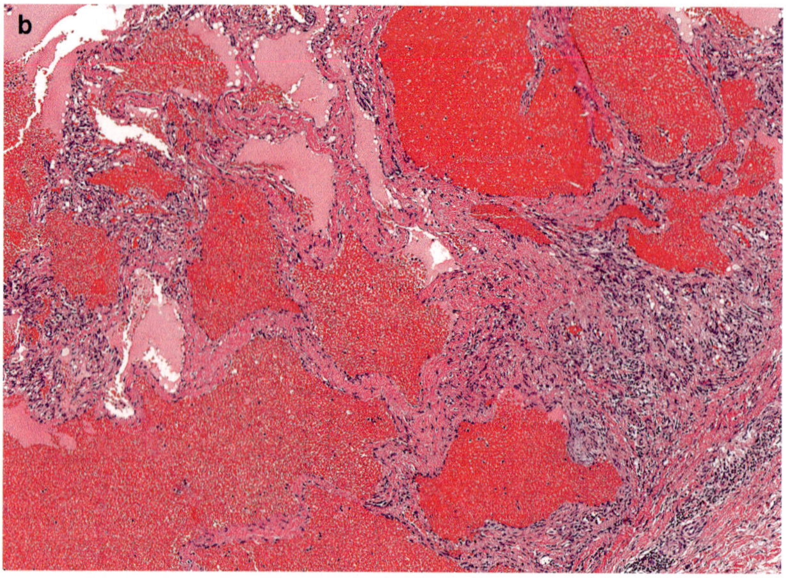

Fig. 7.23 (continued)

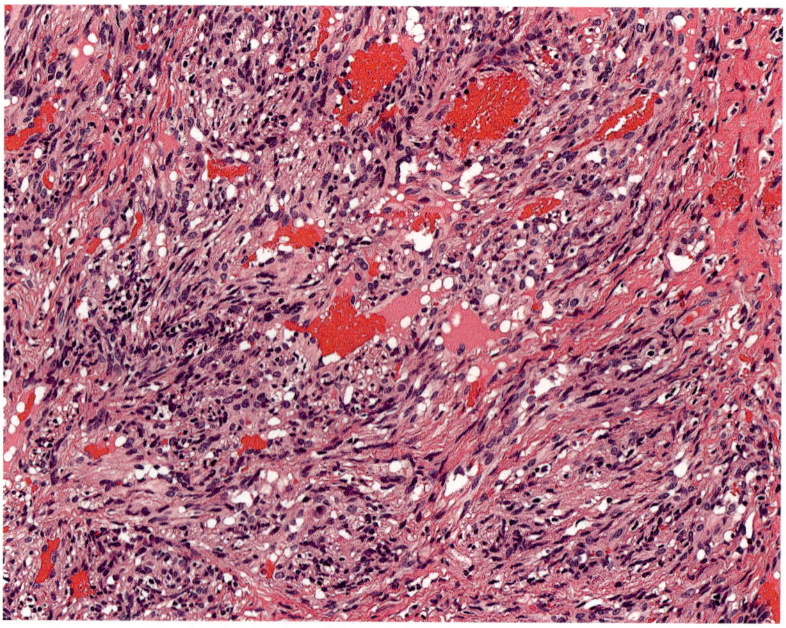

Fig. 7.24 Spindle cell hemangioma has cellular areas composed of fascicles and sheets of spindled endothelial cells, pericytes, and vacuolated endothelial cells

Differential Diagnosis

Because of the prominent spindle cell component, spindle cell hemangioma needs to be distinguished from Kaposi sarcoma. Kaposi sarcoma does not have the varying combinations of histologic features seen in spindle cell hemangioma, usually lacks dilated cavernous spaces and phleboliths, and is positive for HHV8.

Table 7.14 Key pathologic features: spindle cell hemangioma

Combination of:
Compressed spindle cells
Vacuolated epithelioid endothelial cells
Cavernous vascular spaces, often containing phleboliths
Peripheral vessel wall often present
Negative for HHV8
Mutations in *IDH* (*IDH1* > *IDH2*)

Epithelioid Hemangioma (Angiolymphoid Hyperplasia with Eosinophilia)

Clinical Features

Epithelioid hemangiomas usually occur in young to middle-aged adults and are more common in women. The head and neck region is the typical cutaneous location, especially around the posterior ear. However, they can occur in a wide variety of locations including bone and viscera. A purely intravascular form was originally described under the rubric of "intravascular atypical vascular proliferation." Clinically, cutaneous examples present as solitary or multiple pink to erythematous plaques and nodules, often associated with pruritus. Epithelioid hemangioma is benign, although local recurrence occurs in up to one third of cases. There is no risk of metastasis.

Pathologic Features

The microscopic features of epithelioid hemangioma are variable. The classic form has a lobular architecture with closely packed capillaries associated with a larger feeder vessel, which may show evidence of trauma. Admixed with the vascular proliferation is an inflammatory infiltrate of lymphocytes, eosinophils, and histiocytes. In some cases, the infiltrate can be quite brisk with germinal center formation (Fig. 7.25a). This appearance is most predominant in cutaneous locations and is typically the one referred to as angiolymphoid hyperplasia with eosinophilia (ALHE). The capillary vessels are lined by plump polygonal (often referred to as "tombstone-like") endothelial cells with abundant eosinophilic cytoplasm that can fill the vessels' lumina. The nuclei are slightly enlarged with fine chromatin, and often have a distinct but not prominent nucleolus (Fig. 7.25b). Particularly in superficial cutaneous cases, the background inflammatory infiltrate may be so prominent that it obscures the epithelioid endothelium-lined vessels (Fig. 7.25c). Mitotic figures are relatively common, but atypical mitotic figures are not a feature. Cases of epithelioid hemangioma involving deep soft tissue, bone, or the penis typically have a less prominent inflammatory component (although some admixed eosinophils are often present). Additionally, these cases tend to have a more solid growth pattern (Fig. 7.26a) with only a few well-formed capillaries in the center of the lesion. However, a population of small, well-formed vascular channels in a somewhat myxoid stroma is usually identified at the periphery of

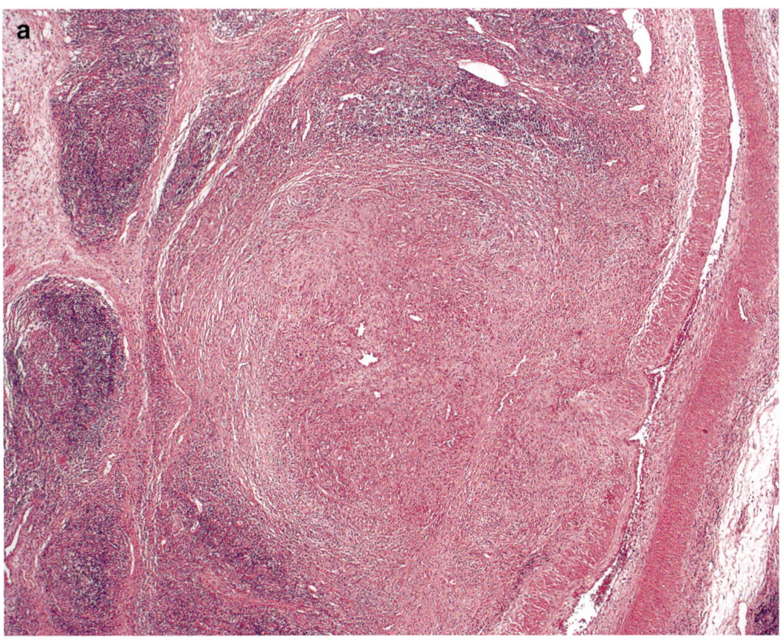

Fig. 7.25 Epithelioid hemangioma. (**a**) A lobular proliferation of capillaries associated with a vessel and a florid peripheral inflammatory infiltrate with germinal center formation. (**b**) The capillaries are lined by polygonal epithelioid ("tombstone-like") endothelial cells with abundant eosinophilic cytoplasm. (**c**) The inflammatory infiltrate may obscure the underlying vascular nature of the lesion

Fig. 7.25 (continued)

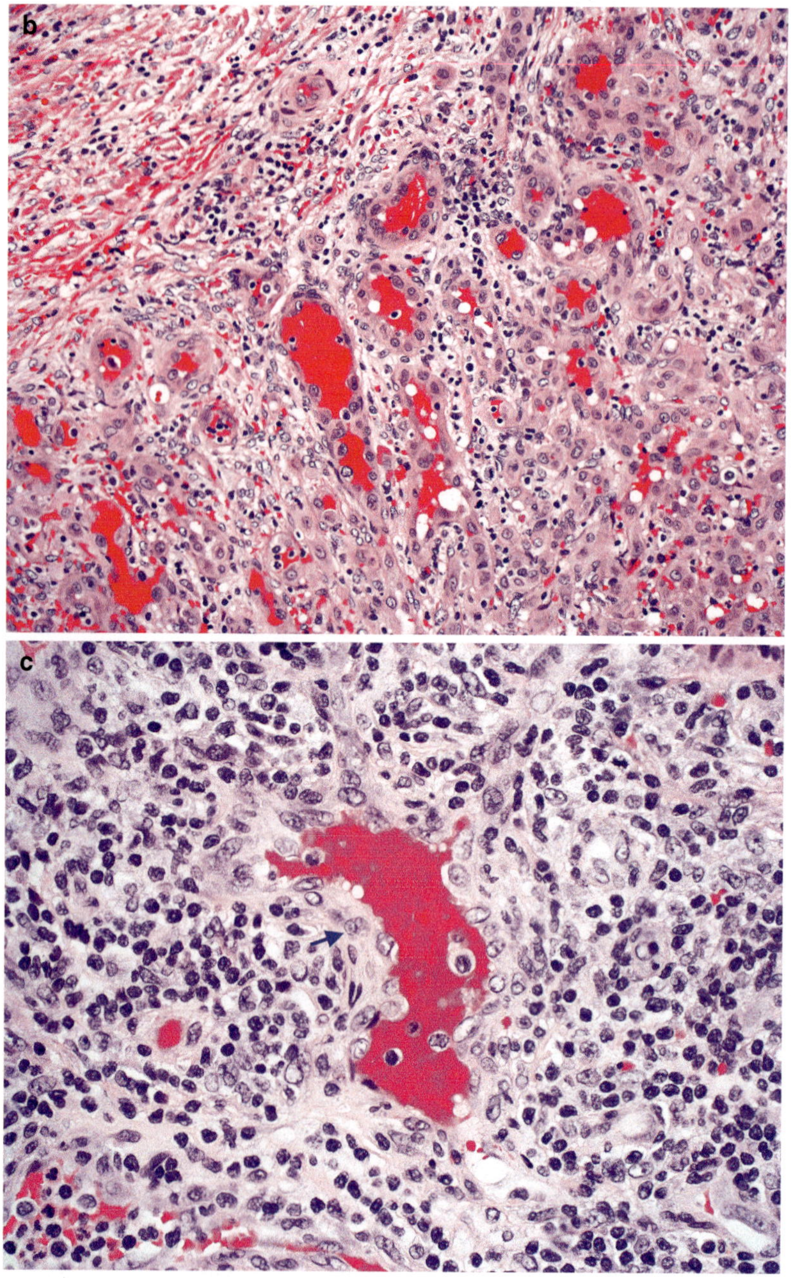

these solid lesions, and is a very helpful diagnostic feature (Fig. 7.26b). Occasionally, epithelioid hemangioma can present as an intravascular tumor analogous to intravascular pyogenic granuloma. The intravascular form often shows a solid growth pattern and usually has less inflammation, with only scattered eosinophils and lymphocytes (Fig. 7.27) (Table 7.15).

Immunohistochemistry is not typically necessary to make the diagnosis. In cellular or intravascular examples, which can mimic other epithelial neoplasms, immunostaining for endothelial markers such as ERG, CD31, or CD34 can be helpful. Like other epithelioid vascular tumors, epithelioid hemangiomas can express cytokeratins. Rearrangements of the *FOS* gene have been

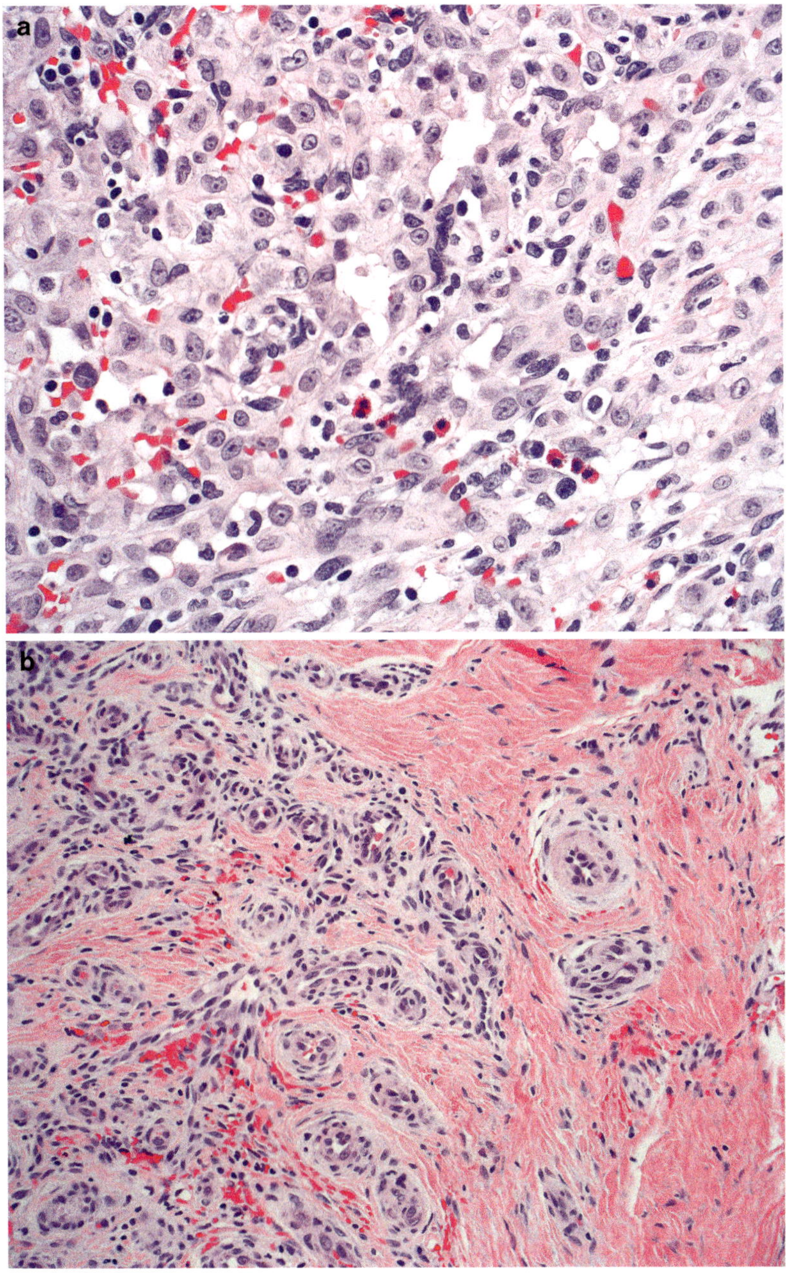

Fig. 7.26 Epithelioid hemangioma. (**a**) More solid growth pattern in epithelioid hemangioma lacking well-formed vessels. Inflammation is sparse but clusters of eosinophils are often present. (**b**) A distinctive population of well-formed small vessels in a fibromyxoid stroma at the periphery of solid epithelioid hemangioma

identified in approximately 30% of cases, but cutaneous lesions with the appearance of ALHE appear to lack this genetic finding.

Differential Diagnosis

The differential diagnosis of epithelioid hemangioma, especially multifocal lesions or those with a solid growth pattern, includes other epithelioid vascular tumors discussed later in this chapter. Epithelioid hemangioendothelioma may also be associated with a vessel but has a characteristic angiocentric, infiltrative growth pattern with cells arranged in cords and nests within a prominent myxohyaline stroma. Eosinophils are usually absent. Vasoformative architecture is not seen in typical epithelioid hemangioendotheli-

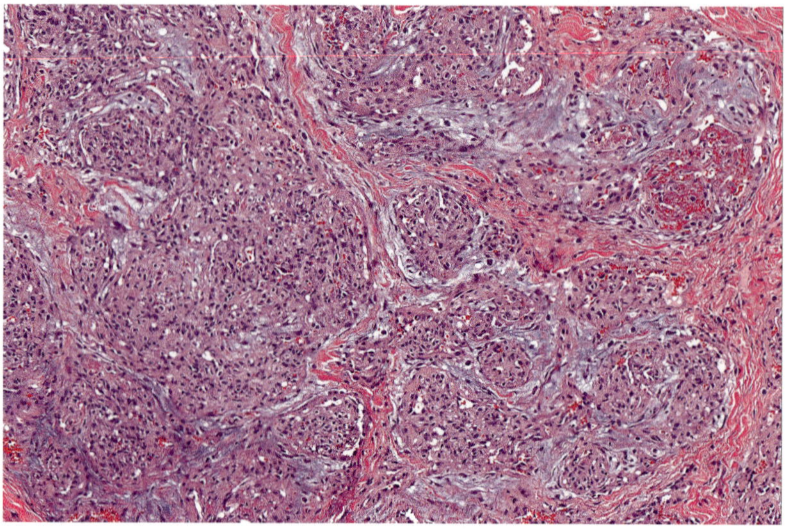

Fig. 7.27 Intravascular epithelioid hemangioma showing solid sheets of epithelioid endothelial cells filling the vascular lumen. The inflammatory component is minimal

Table 7.15 Key pathologic features: epithelioid hemangioma

Capillaries lined by plump polygonal epithelioid endothelial cells that fill vessel lumina
Solid central growth pattern with well-formed small vascular channels at the periphery
Prominent inflammatory component
Eosinophils
Often associated with a traumatized vessel

oma; instead, the cells demonstrate small intracytoplasmic vacuoles possibly representing abortive lumen formation. Occasional similar appearing vacuolated cells can be seen in epithelioid hemangioma, but they are a minority in the context of an overall vasoformative lesion. A recently identified subset of EHEs with *YAP1-TFE3* fusion more closely resembles epithelioid hemangioma due to its more overtly vasoformative appearance and abundant eosinophilic cytoplasm. These tumors have greater cytologic atypia than classic epithelioid hemangioma and express TFE3 by immunohistochemistry, which can be utilized in diagnostically challenging cases. Immunohistochemistry can also help in the distinction of epithelioid hemangioma from classic epithelioid hemangioendothelioma, since the latter expresses CAMTA1 protein, a product of *WWRT1-CAMTA1* fusion unique to these tumors. Epithelioid angiosarcomas are more architecturally complex and infiltrative tumors, and have much greater cytologic atypia than epithelioid hemangioma. Pseudomyogenic hemangioendothelioma/epithelioid sarcoma-like hemangioendothelioma grows in solid sheets, does not form vascular channels, and has a distinctive myoid spindle cell component. Cutaneous epithelioid angiomatous nodule, likely a solid variant of epithelioid hemangioma, is discussed below.

Epithelioid hemangioma with prominent inflammation (the angiolymphoid hyperplasia with eosinophilia variant) is often confused with Kimura disease. The latter appears to be a separate, distinct entity. Kimura disease is prevalent in Asian male patients and is characterized by lymphadenopathy, often around the ears, in association with peripheral eosinophilia without a distinct soft tissue mass. The affected lymph nodes may contain numerous eosinophils and an associated vascular proliferation, but the telltale vessels of epithelioid hemangioma containing plump polygonal cells with abundant eosinophilic cytoplasm, filling vascular lumina, are not characteristic of Kimura disease. In contrast, the latter typically has more flattened, reactive angioproliferative-type capillaries. Other inflammatory and neoplastic processes associated with florid cutaneous lymphoid hyperplasia, such as IgG4-related sclerosing diseases or primary cutaneous follicular center-cell lymphoma, also lack the distinctive epithelioid endothelial cells seen in EH.

Epithelioid hemangiomas differ from cutaneous angiomatous nodule by the presence of more vasoformative elements and often more prominent inflammation (see below).

Cutaneous Epithelioid Angiomatous Nodule

Clinical Features

Cutaneous epithelioid angiomatous nodule (CEAN) was first described in 2004 as a distinctive lesion on the trunk or extremities of middle-aged adults, but it may occur in children and elderly patients and involve any anatomic location. CEAN presents as a small (<1.0 cm), solitary erythematous to violaceous papule or nodule. Multiple or eruptive forms are rare but have been described.

Pathologic Features

Microscopically, CEAN is a circumscribed dermal tumor composed of a largely solid sheet-like proliferation of epithelioid endothelial cells with abundant eosinophilic cytoplasm (Fig. 7.28a). Recognizable vascular channel formation is usually absent or focal in nature, but intracytoplasmic vacuoles are often present. The endothelial nuclei do not show significant pleomorphism, but they typically are somewhat enlarged with a conspicuous but small nucleolus, similar to that seen in epithelioid hemangioma (Fig. 7.28b). These are mitotically active tumors that may have up to five mitotic figures per ten high-power fields, but atypical forms are not seen. The inflammatory infiltrate is usually sparse and includes lymphocytes, histiocytes, and rare eosinophils (Table 7.16).

Differential Diagnosis

The key differential diagnostic considerations include epithelioid hemangioma and epithelioid angiosarcoma. The more conspicuous vascular channel formation, myxoid stroma and prominent inflammatory component of epithelioid hemangioma facilitate its distinction from CEAN. Whether CEAN represents a morphologic variant of epithelioid hemangioma is still debated. Epithelioid hemangioendothelioma can be distinguished from CEAN based on its cord-like growth pattern and distinctive myxohyaline stroma, neither of which are present in CEAN. Epithelioid angiosarcoma is an architecturally more complex lesion characterized by an infiltrative growth pattern and a greater degree of nuclear atypia. Pseudomyogenic hemangioendothelioma/epithelioid sarcoma-like hemangioendothelioma is composed of a combination of spindled and epithelioid cells, has a more infiltrative growth pattern, and usually lacks intracytoplasmic vacuoles. A *SERPINE1-FOSB* fusion is present in pseudomyogenic hemangioendothelioma/epithelioid sarcoma-like hemangioendothelioma that has not been found in CEAN. The presence of this gene fusion can be confirmed by FISH or immunohistochemistry for FOSB, although most cases of CEAN can be distinguished based on histomorphology alone.

Cutaneous Lymphatic Malformation (Lymphangioma Circumscriptum)

Clinical Features

"Lymphangioma circumscriptum" is an outdated term for a localized cutaneous lymphatic malformation. Analogous to other types of malformations, the term "lymphangioma" is no longer biologically accurate in the classification of these lesions, though it is still often used in clinical practice. Cutaneous lymphatic malformations are most often sporadic and manifest at birth or in infancy as groups of hyperkeratotic papules or vesicles that vary in hue from yellow-orange to red. The appearance has been compared to frog spawn. The lesions tend to localize in one area and usually involve the limb girdles, buttocks, or oral cavity, but any site can be affected. Local recurrences are common.

Pathologic Features

All lymphatic malformations, regardless of location, can be divided based on the size of the dilated vascular channels into microcytic (<1 cm), macro-

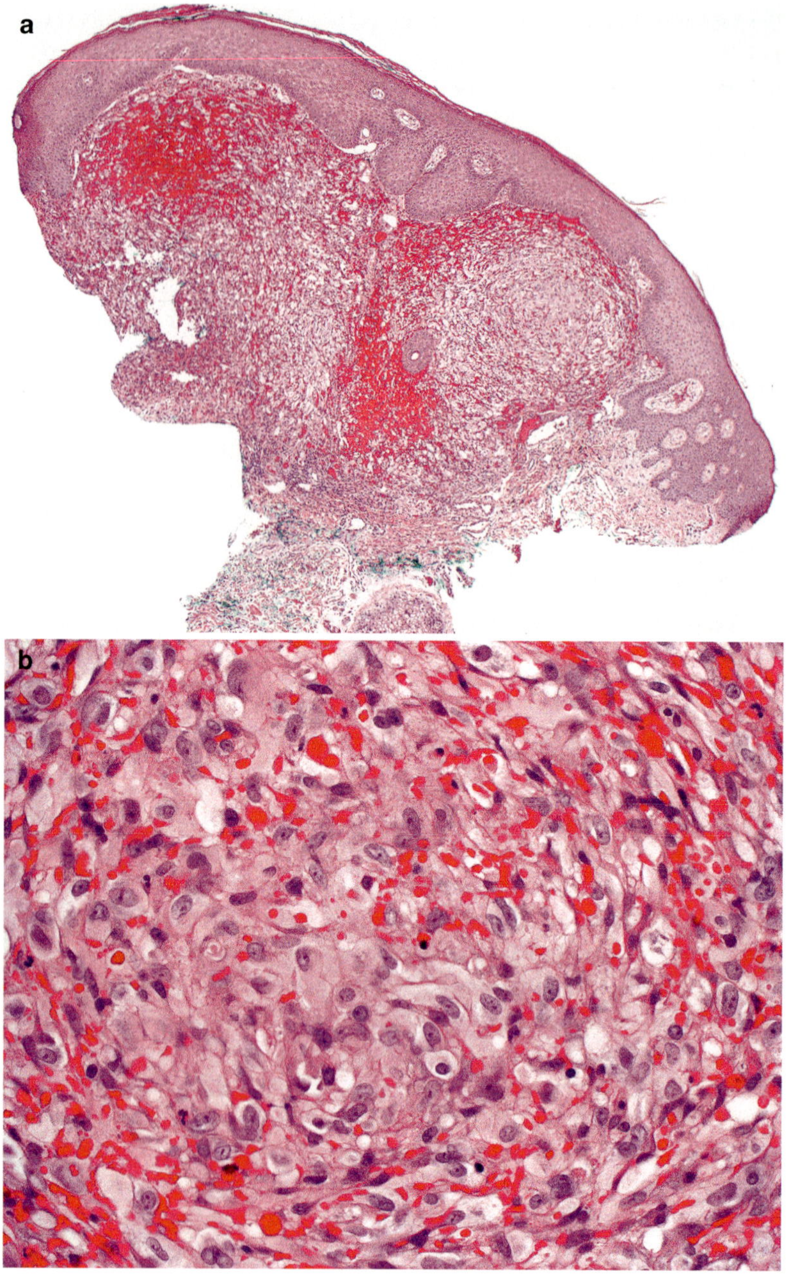

Fig. 7.28 Cutaneous epithelioid angiomatous nodule. (**a**) A well-circumscribed polypoid nodule confined to the upper dermis. (**b**) Solid sheets of plump, mildly atypical epithelioid endothelial cells with abundant eosinophilic cytoplasm and intracytoplasmic vacuoles. Well-formed vascular channels and inflammatory infiltrates are not seen

Table 7.16 Key pathologic features: cutaneous epithelioid angiomatous nodule

Well-circumscribed dermal based nodule
Solid sheets of epithelioid endothelial cells
Intracytoplasmic vacuoles
Vascular channel formation absent to rare

cytic ($\geq$1 cm), or combined subtypes. Cutaneous and subcutaneous lymphatic malformations are usually microcystic. Microscopically, these lesions consist of angulated thin-walled lymphatic channels in the dermis and subcutis. The channels are lined by a flattened or hobnail endothelium and variably contain pale eosinophilic proteinaceous material or lymphocytes (Fig. 7.29a). Thin intravascular projections representing lymphatic valves are sometimes noted. Lymphoid aggregates are common at the periphery of these vessels (Fig. 7.29b). Lymphatic channels may contain red blood cells or organizing thrombi. These relate to trauma or hemorrhage or from communication with the venous channels and thus can mimic venous malformations. The overlying epidermis is

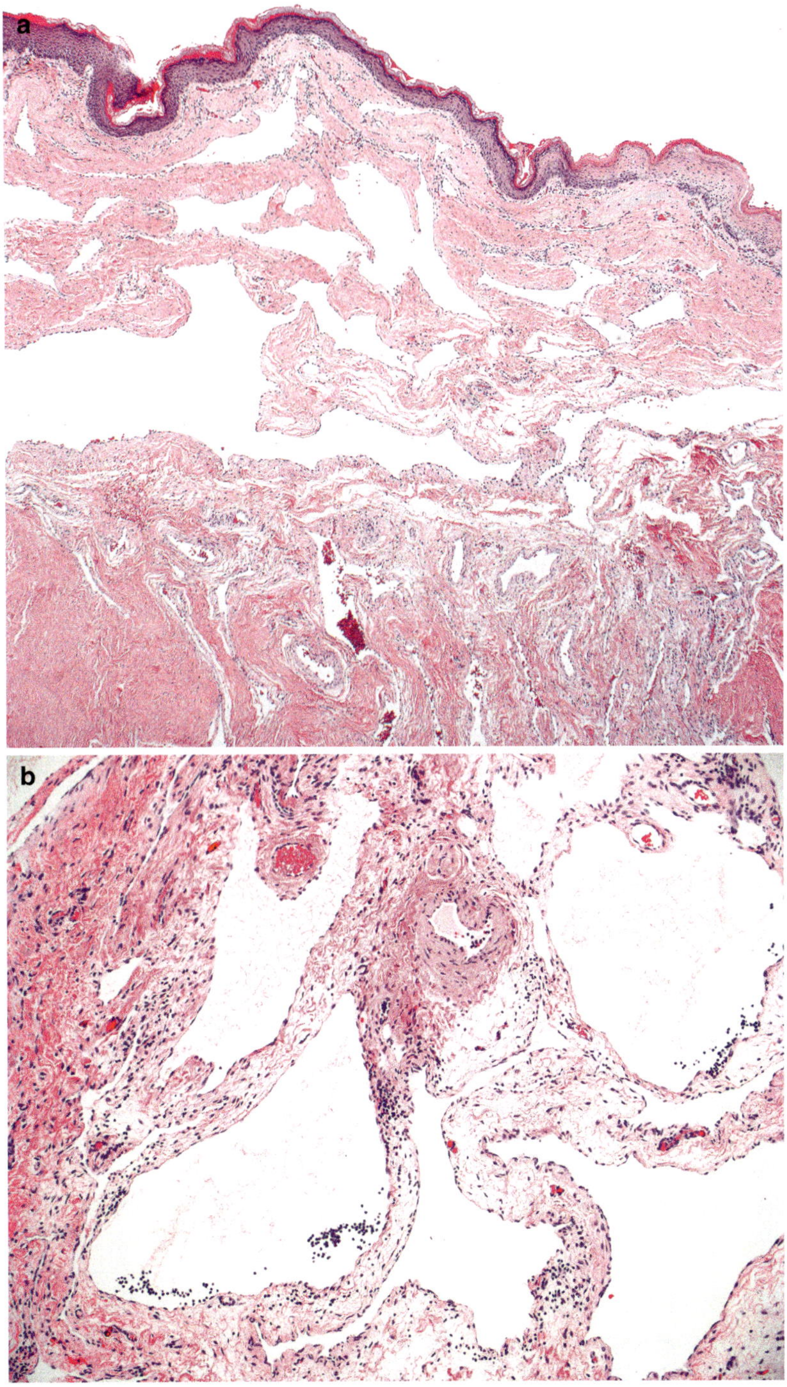

Fig. 7.29 Cutaneous lymphatic malformation (formerly, "lymphangioma circumscriptum"). (**a**) Thin-walled angulated lymphatic channels in the upper dermis. (**b**) The lymphatics often contain pale eosinophilic proteinaceous material and/or lymphocytes

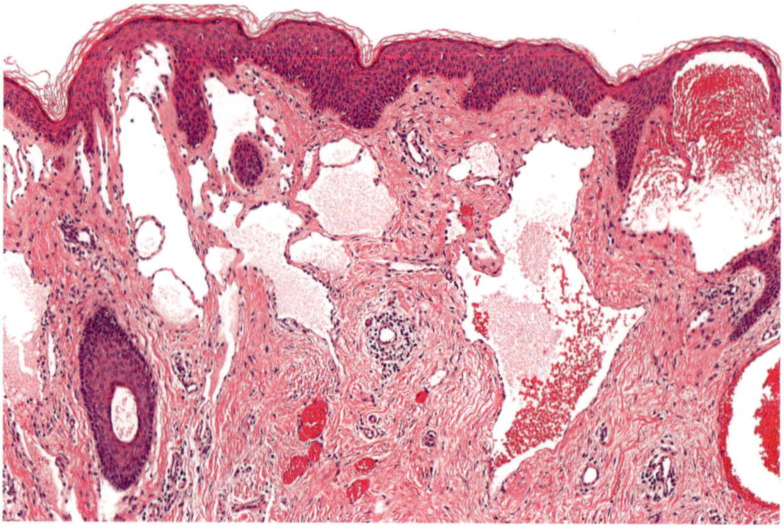

Fig. 7.30 Cutaneous lymphatic malformation (formerly, "lymphangioma circumscriptum"). The superficial lymphatic channels herniate into hyperkeratotic and acanthotic dermal papillae. The lymphatics contain pale eosinophilic proteinaceous material and have evident valves

Table 7.17 Key pathologic features: cutaneous lymphatic malformation

Ectatic angulated vascular spaces within the dermis and subcutis
Intravascular proteinaceous material, occasional lymphocytes, and lymphatic valves
Variable presence of red blood cells in vessels
Superficial vessels extending into dermal papillae, similar to angiokeratoma
Lymphatic immunophenotype: Podoplanin (D2–40), Prox1, LYVE-1, VEGFR3

often acanthotic and hyperkeratotic, and the superficial lymphatic channels may herniate into the dermal papillae and appear trapped within the epidermis (Fig. 7.30). This verrucous appearance is shared with angiokeratoma and verrucous hemangioma (verrucous venulocapillary malformation) discussed above. It is worth noting that cutaneous lymphatic malformation can represent the superficial component of deeper-seated malformations, especially the venous subtype. Consultation with a multidisciplinary vascular malformation team is very valuable in this context. By immunohistochemistry, the endothelial cells express markers of lymphatic differentiation: podoplanin (D2–40), Prox1, LYVE-1, and VEGFR3 (Table 7.17).

Differential Diagnosis

The differential diagnosis of cutaneous lymphatic malformation includes venous malformation, which can be distinguished based on the thicker caliber vessels with more prominent smooth muscle walls, and lack of expression of markers of lymphatic differentiation. The lymphatic immunophenotype is helpful for distinguishing lymphatic malformations from venulocapillary malformations and angiokeratomas. The differential diagnosis with these hyperkeratotic vascular lesions is described above (see angiokeratoma).

Acquired Progressive Lymphangioma ("Benign Angioendothelioma")

Clinical Features

Acquired progressive lymphangioma, also called benign lymphangioendothelioma, is a solitary lesion that most commonly involves the extremities in both children and adults. It presents as an erythematous to brown macule or plaque and can be quite large.

Pathologic Features

Acquired progressive lymphangioma consists of a proliferation of irregular thin-walled vessels involving the dermis and subcutis. The lesional vessels grow in a dissecting pattern parallel to the dermal collagen bundles (Fig. 7.31a). Cytologically, the vessels show a single layer of bland endothelial cells resembling small lymphatics. Focally, papillary projections can be seen reminiscent of hobnail lymphatic malformation (hobnail hemangioma) (Fig. 7.31b). The endothelial cells are positive for podoplanin (Table 7.18).

Differential Diagnosis

Due to the dissecting growth pattern, the primary differential diagnosis includes well-differentiated cutaneous angiosarcoma and patch stage

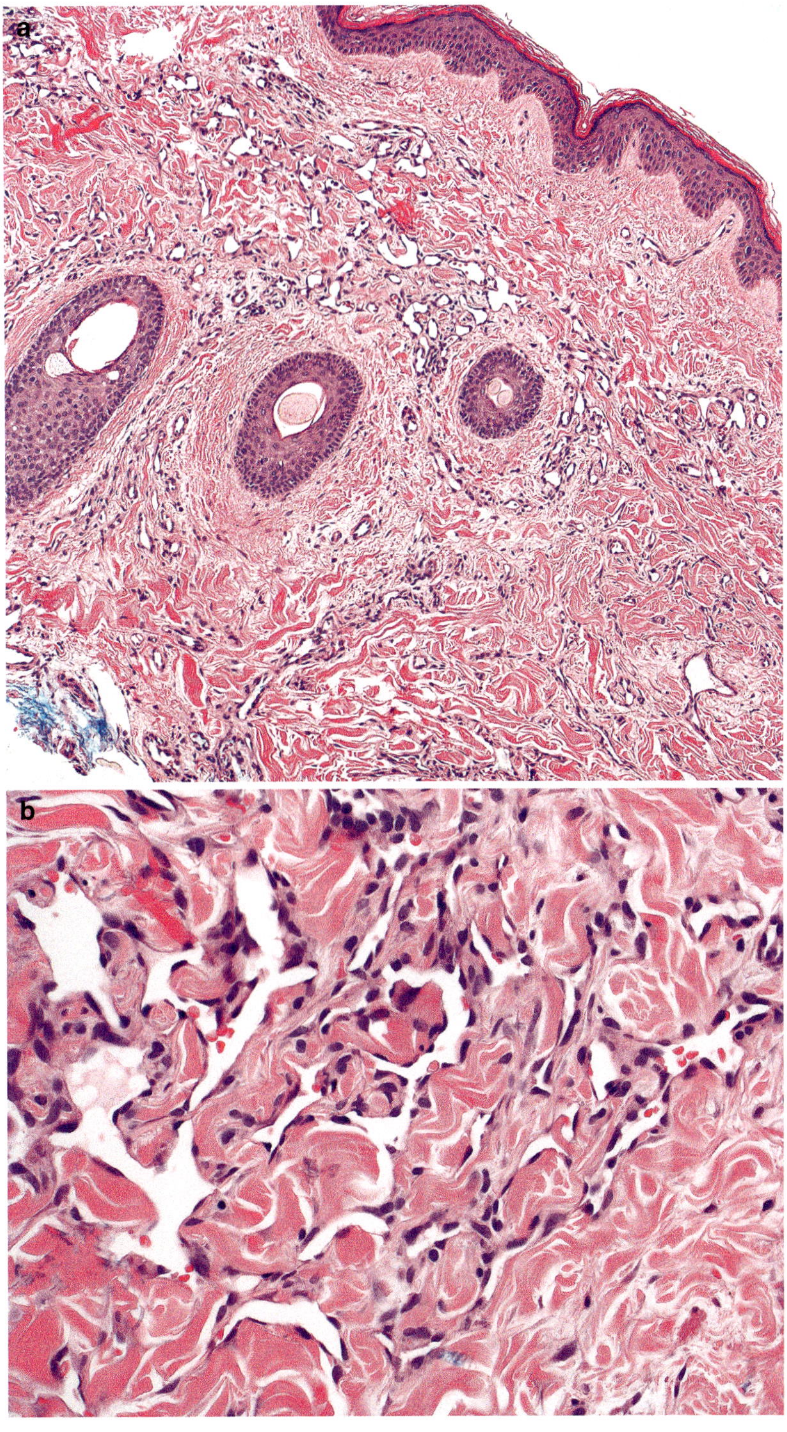

Fig. 7.31 Acquired progressive lymphangioma. (**a**) Irregular small vessels percolate through the dermis parallel to the collagen bundles and wrap around appendages. (**b**) Papillary structures reminiscent of hobnail lymphatic malformation (hobnail hemangioma) may be present

Table 7.18 Key pathologic features: acquired progressive lymphangioma

Horizontally oriented vessels dissecting through dermal collagen
Single layer of flat or slightly hobnail endothelial cells
Positive for podoplanin and CD31
Negative for HHV8

Kaposi sarcoma. Acquired progressive lymphangioma generally lacks the atypia, endothelial multilayering and mitotic activity seen in angiosarcoma. It also lacks the promontory sign of patch stage Kaposi sarcoma; the latter is also positive for HHV8 (latent nuclear antigen-1). Hobnail vascular lesions (retiform hemangioendothelioma, PILA/Dabska tumor, and hobnail hemangioma/hobnail lymphatic malformation) can also enter the differential diagnosis. It is worth remembering that immunostaining for podoplanin does not help in this distinction as all of the above lesions including angiosarcoma and Kaposi sarcoma can be positive for this marker.

Papillary Hemangioma

Clinical Features

Papillary hemangioma was first described as a clinicopathologic entity in 2007. Typically, it presents as a solid sporadic lesion, arises in all age groups, and has a marked predilection for the head and neck area. Even though papillary hemangioma somewhat resembles glomeruloid hemangioma, it is a different lesion and not associated with POEMS syndrome or any other systemic disease. These lesions are benign and recur rarely.

Pathologic Features

Papillary hemangioma has a very striking appearance. At low power, these lesions show seemingly discontinuous intravascular growth of branching papillary fronds that are anchored to the vessel wall (Fig. 7.32a, b). The fibrovascular cores of these papillae contain small, somewhat stellate capillary vessels with thick basement membranes. These are surrounded by prevalent pericytes and lined by uniform, slightly hyperchromatic, mitotically inactive endothelial cells, features resembling congenital nonprogressive hemangioma. The endothelial cells of the dilated dermal vessel in which these papillary structures originate have a flattened, banal appearance. However, the endothelial cells lining the papillary structures look very different and prominently display numerous intracytoplasmic eosinophilic hyaline globules that can be highlighted by PAS-D stain (Fig. 7.33). Ultrastructurally, these globules represent giant lysosomes containing remnants of cellular organelles. By immunohistochemistry, these lesions express vascular and pericytic markers, but lack evidence of lymphatic differentiation (Table 7.19).

Differential Diagnosis

In pediatric patients, papillary hemangioma can be confused with congenital nonprogressive hemangioma (NICH or RICH), since both lesions show small stellate capillary vessels lined by slightly hyperchromatic, mitotically inactive endothelial cells. However, distinctive intravascular growth and intracytoplasmic hyaline globules are not seen in congenital nonprogressive hemangioma. Papillary hemangioma must also be distinguished from other vascular lesions with intravascular growth: glomeruloid hemangioma, papillary intravascular angioendothelioma (PILA/Dabska tumor), and intravascular papillary endothelial hyperplasia (Masson tumor). Glomeruloid hemangioma (discussed below) may appear very similar due to intravascular growth and the presence of intracytoplasmic hyaline globules. Glomeruloid hemangioma usually develops on the trunk and lower extremities and almost always arises in patients with POEMS syndrome or multicentric Castleman disease. Papillary hemangiomas are sporadic and have marked predilection for the head and neck. Glomeruloid hemangioma forms closely packed capillary loops resembling renal glomeruli and lacks the well-developed papillary structures, fibrovascular cores, and larger capillaries of papillary hemangioma. PILA occurs in the subcutis and is uncommon in the head and neck area. The intraluminal papillary structures in PILA have thin hyalin-

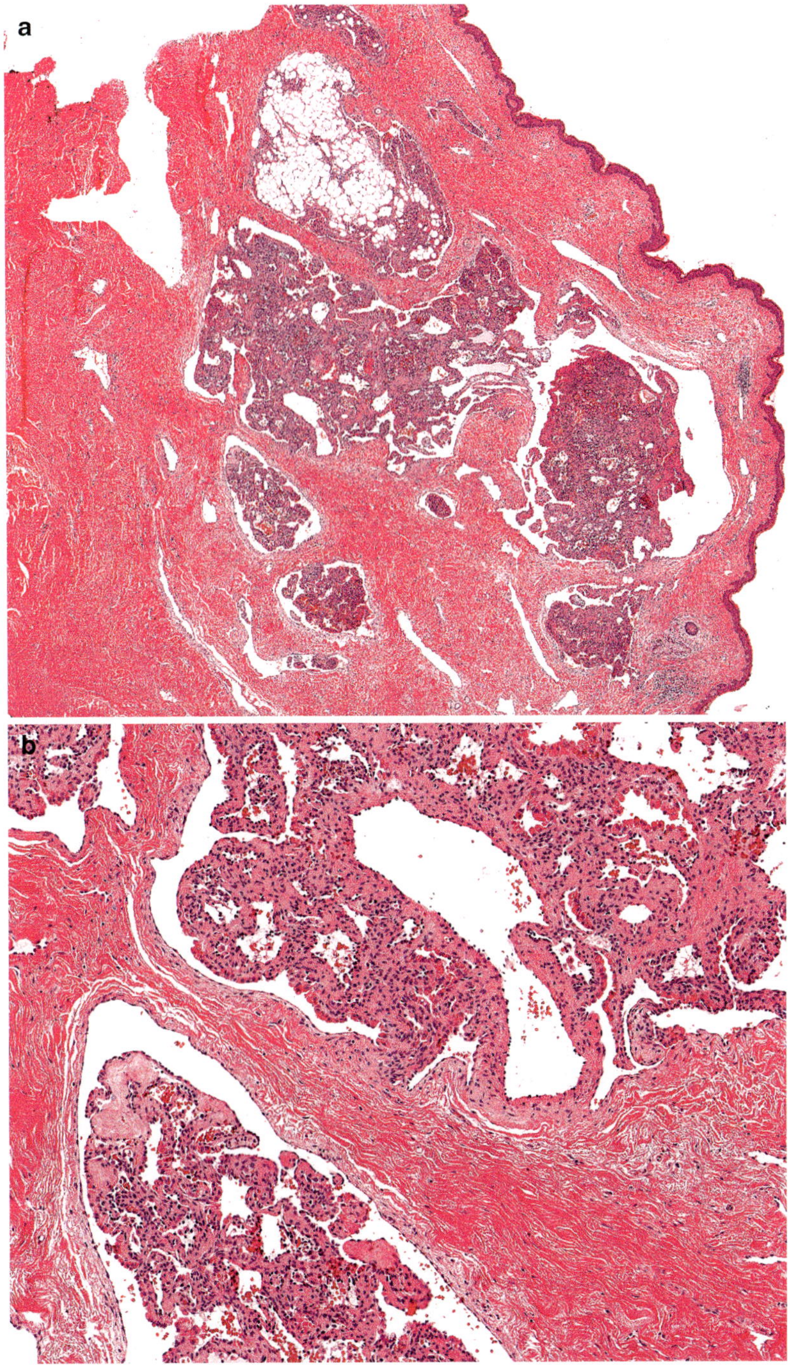

Fig. 7.32 Papillary hemangioma. (**a**) Intravascular growth of well-circumscribed papillary fronds. (**b**) These fronds are seen anchored to the vessel wall or floating freely within the vessel in tangential cuts

ized cores or lack cores altogether and are covered by a mildly atypical cuboidal to columnar hobnailed endothelium. PILA expresses markers of lymphatic differentiation not seen in papillary hemangioma. The pseudopapillary structures in intravascular papillary endothelial hyperplasia are acellular, contain fibrin or collagen, and are lined by a single layer of banal endothelial cells, which lack intracytoplasmic hyaline globules.

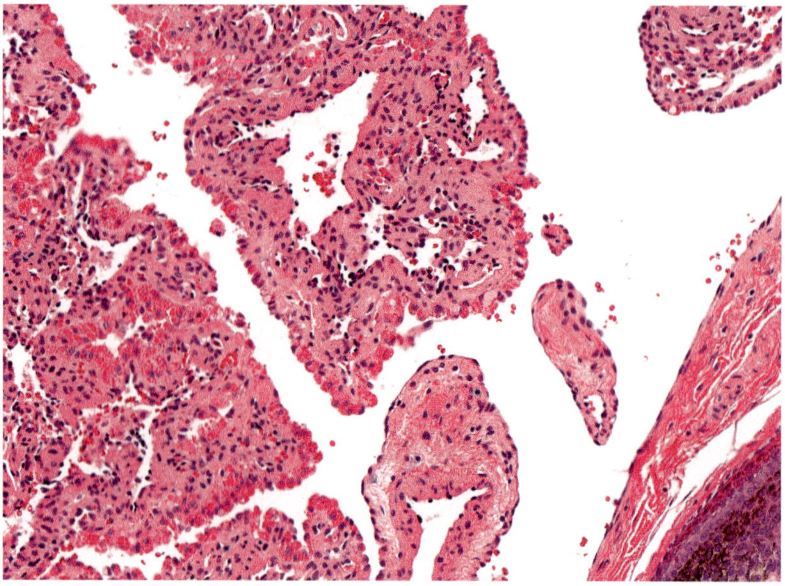

Fig. 7.33 Types of endothelium seen in papillary hemangioma. The fibrovascular cores contain small vessels lined by uniform, slightly hyperchromatic mitotically inactive endothelium and surrounded by pericytes. The wall of the host vessel (lower right) is lined by flat normal endothelium. Endothelium lining the papillary structures shows swollen cytoplasm containing numerous eosinophilic hyaline globules

Table 7.19 Key pathologic features: papillary hemangioma

Intravascular growth of branching papillary fronds anchored to the vessel wall
Three types of endothelial cells
Papillary cores contain capillaries lined by uniform, slightly hyperchromatic endothelium
Outer vessel wall lined by flattened normal endothelium
Papillary surfaces lined by endothelium with intracytoplasmic hyaline globules
No cytologic atypia or significant mitotic activity

Reactive Vascular Lesions

Intravascular Papillary Endothelial Hyperplasia (Masson Tumor)

Clinical Features

Intravascular papillary endothelial hyperplasia occurs most frequently on the head and neck, trunk, and distal extremities, especially the hands. It presents as an erythematous to violaceous or nondescript, small nodule. Although trauma may play a role in the development, such a history is rarely elucidated from the patient.

Pathologic Features

Intravascular papillary endothelial hyperplasia is a reaction pattern consisting of an endothelial proliferation associated with a thrombus; it can occur in any vascular lesion with large dilated vessels and slow flow of blood. Rarely, it occurs in an organizing hematoma. At low power, it is well-circumscribed due to its occurrence within a vessel, though the lesion can sometimes spill out into adjacent soft tissue (Fig. 7.34a). The appearance can vary based on the phase of the process captured histologically. Early on, there is ingrowth of endothelial cells into a thrombus. As the lesion becomes more organized, it takes on the characteristic papillary architecture with a single layer of endothelial cells lining the papillae. The fibrin within the papillae is replaced by collagen over time. The border is outlined by the host vessel (Fig. 7.34b). Mitotic activity is quite common, but atypical mitotic figures are not seen (Table 7.20).

Differential Diagnosis

Due to the architectural complexity of the papillae, intravascular papillary endothelial hyperplasia can be difficult to distinguish

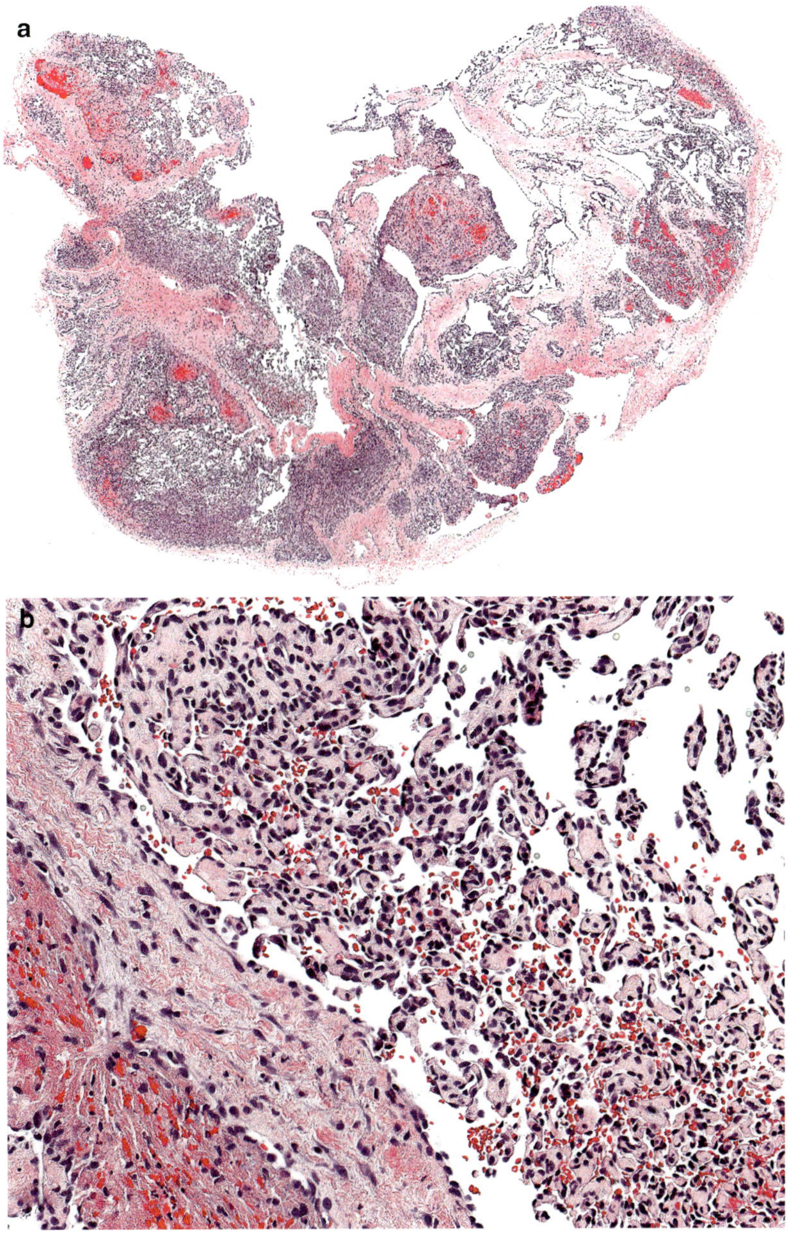

Fig. 7.34 Intravascular papillary endothelial hyperplasia (Masson tumor). (**a**) A small venous malformation with organizing thrombi and a florid papillary proliferation filling the lumen. (**b**) The papillary structures are confined within the vessel wall and show avascular cores containing fibrin or collagen lined by a monolayer of cytologically bland endothelial cells

Table 7.20 Key pathologic features: intravascular papillary endothelial hyperplasia

At least partially intravascular
Florid papillary architecture without infiltrative growth
Lack of atypia or endothelial multilayering
Mitotic activity common, but no atypical forms

from a well-differentiated angiosarcoma, especially in small biopsies. The overall well-circumscribed nature of the lesion without tissue infiltration and lack of endothelial multilayering and overt cytologic atypia help in the distinction.

Reactive Angioendotheliomatosis

Clinical Features

Reactive angioendotheliomatosis is a reactive hyperplastic vascular proliferation that has been described in a number of systemic and inflammatory conditions including systemic infections, hypercoagulable states, cryoglobulinemia, connective tissue diseases, hematopoietic disorders, and severe atherosclerotic peripheral vascular disease. Reactive angioendotheliomatosis has also been described in end-stage renal disease patients with iatrogenic hemodialysis fistulas and evidence of arteriovenous "steal" syndrome; in women with large, pendulous breasts; and in pregnancy. Smoking also appears to be a risk factor. It is thought that tissue ischemia results in localized production of proangiogenic factors leading to the endothelial proliferation. Reactive angioendotheliomatosis can also be related to intravascular histiocytosis. Clinically, these lesions present as purpuric ulcerated plaques, sometimes with a livedoid pattern, and tend to involve the extremities.

Pathologic Features

Microscopically, there is a lobular, intravascular or diffuse dermal proliferation of bland spindled endothelial cells forming small capillaries and wrapping around dermal vessels and adnexal structures (Fig. 7.35a). The diffuse growth pattern (diffuse dermal angiomatosis) appears to be particularly worrisome at scanning magnification as it shows a diffuse proliferation of slit-like vessels dissecting dermal collagen. Lymphocytes, acute inflammation, and microthrombi may be present. Reactive angioendotheliomatosis may superficially involve the subcutis, typically at the periphery of the fat lobules, resembling septal panniculitis (Fig. 7.35b). The endothelial cells are bland but may contain normal mitotic figures (Table 7.21).

Differential Diagnosis

The most important differential diagnosis, especially in diffuse lesions, is with patch stage Kaposi sarcoma. Well-formed capillaries and microthrombi are not usually seen in Kaposi sarcoma, whereas promontory sign, a spindle cell proliferation, intracytoplasmic hyaline globules, and plasma cells are not characteristic of reactive angioendotheliomatosis. HHV8 immunostaining is helpful but should be used with caution as some investigators have noted HHV8 expression in rare reactive angioendotheliomatosis cases. Cutaneous angiosarcomas display greater architectural complexity and show endothelial multilayering and overt cytologic atypia. An immunohistochemical stain for SMA may help to highlight the diffuse pericytic investment of the lesional capillaries in reactive angioendotheliomatosis – a feature not seen in Kaposi sarcoma or angiosarcoma.

Glomeruloid Hemangioma

Clinical Features

This unusual vascular proliferation is, with rare exceptions, seen in the setting of Castleman disease or POEMS (polyneuropathy, organomegaly, endocrinopathy, M-protein, and skin changes) syndrome. Patients present with multiple erythematous papules involving the trunk and extremities. Whether this lesion represents a reactive vascular proliferation or a true vascular neoplasm has been the subject of debate, though most consider it a reactive condition.

Pathologic Features

Glomeruloid hemangioma has a very distinctive appearance consisting of discrete dilated vessels within the dermis containing an intravascular proliferation of densely packed capillaries, resembling a renal glomerulus (so-called glomeruloid tufts) (Fig. 7.36a, b). Within the densely packed capillaries, there are eosinophilic, PAS-positive hyaline globules composed of polyclonal immunoglobulin (Table 7.22). Despite an association with multicentric Castleman disease, glomeruloid hemangiomas do not express HHV-8 (latent nuclear antigen-1).

Differential Diagnosis

Glomeruloid hemangiomas are so distinctive that there is rarely confusion with other entities. Basophilic cellular nodules of tufted angioma

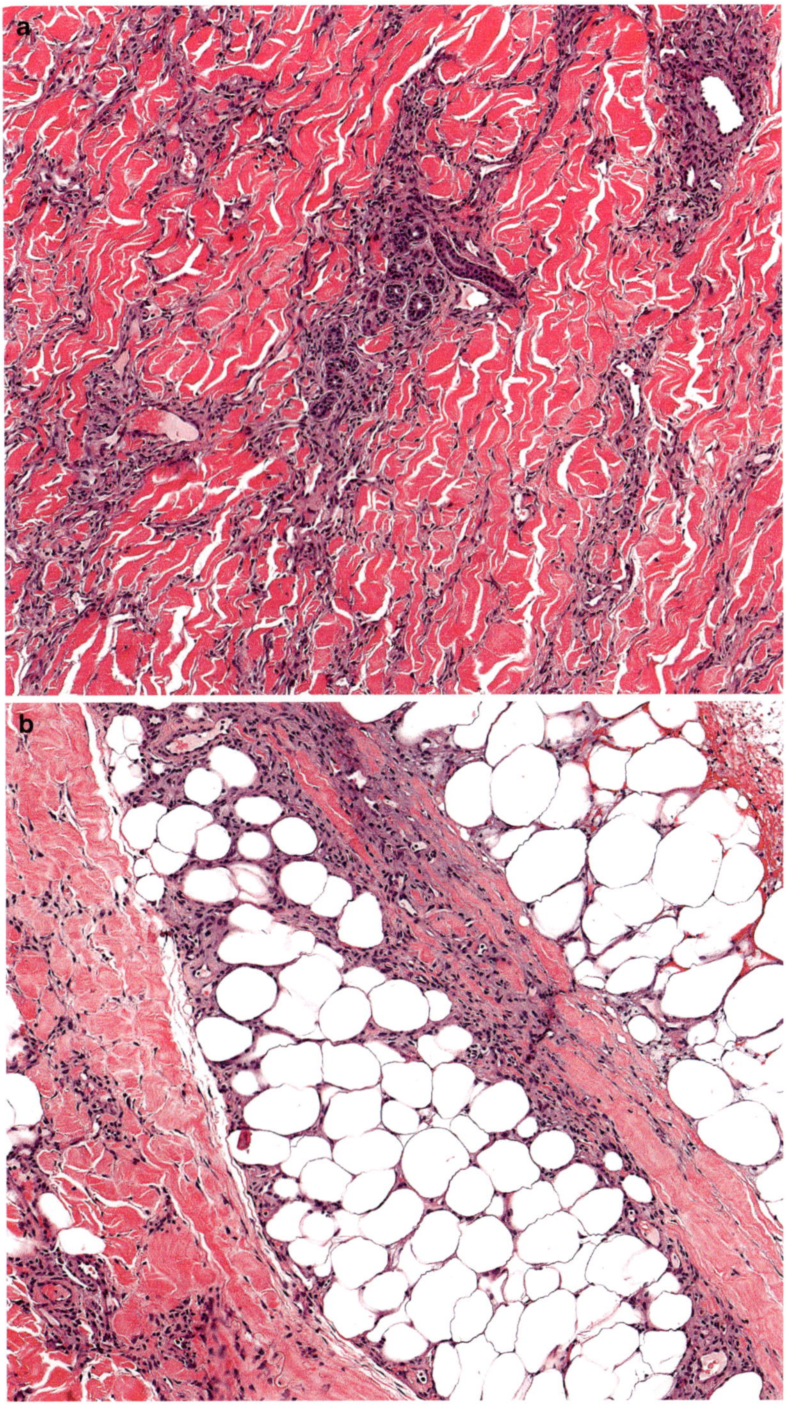

Fig. 7.35 Diffuse dermal angioendotheliomatosis. (**a**) Diffuse dermal proliferation of bland spindled endothelial cells forming slit-like capillaries wrapping around dermal vessels and adnexal structures. (**b**) Involvement of subcutis occurs at the periphery of fat lobules

and kaposiform hemangioendothelioma can bear some resemblance to glomeruloid hemangioma at low magnification. However, the endothelial cells in these lesions are more tightly packed and often undergo spindling. Although both tufted angioma and kaposiform hemangioendothelioma have a distinctive crescent-shaped vessel at the periphery of the capillary nodule, these lesions

Table 7.21 Key pathologic features: reactive angioendotheliomatosis

Lobular or diffuse dermal involvement by thin-walled proliferating capillaries
Microthrombi, acute and chronic inflammation and reactive stromal changes
Lack of architectural complexity and cytologic atypia

do not have true intravascular growth. Microthrombi can be seen in tufted angioma and kaposiform hemangioendothelioma, but intracytoplasmic hyaline globules are not characteristic. Immunohistochemistry for podoplanin (D2–40) is very helpful as tufted angioma and kaposiform hemangioendothelioma are positive, while glo-

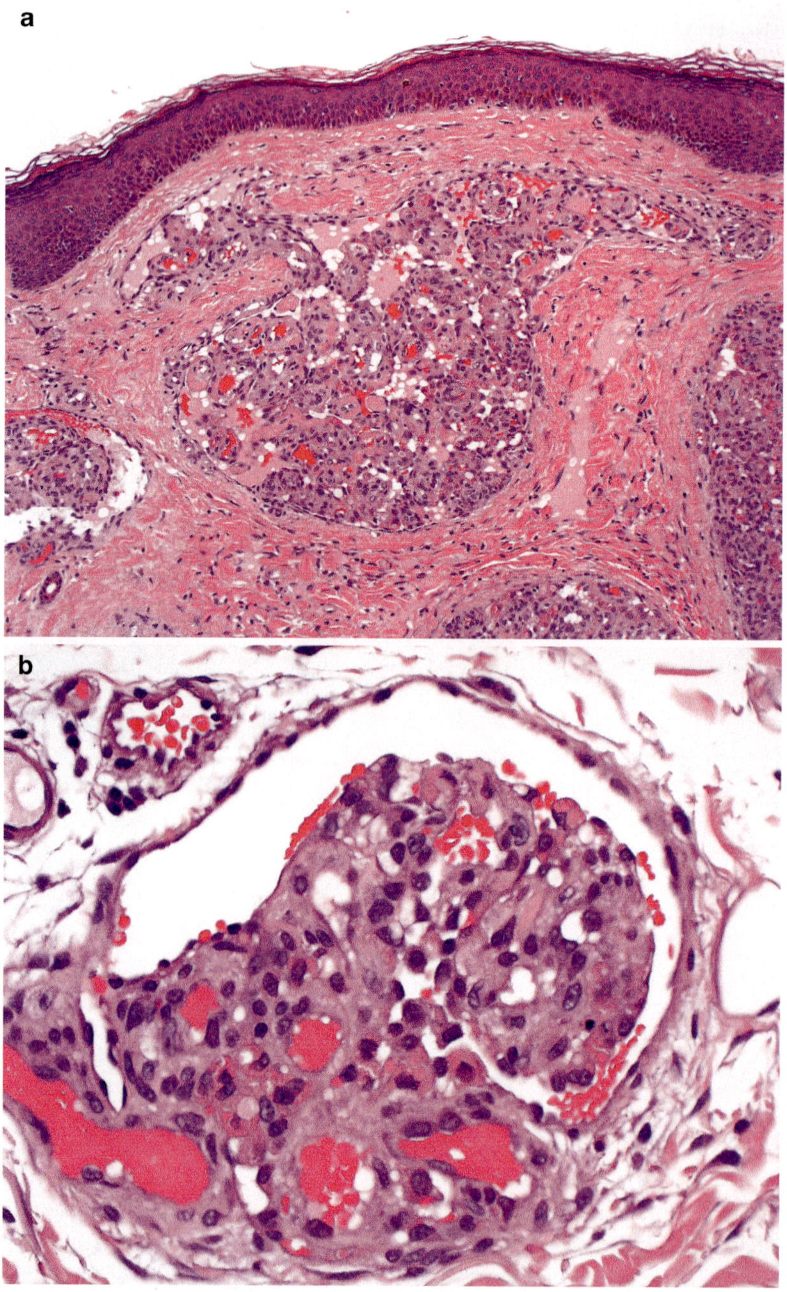

Fig. 7.36 Glomeruloid hemangioma. (**a**) Medium power image demonstrating intravascular growth pattern. (**b**) Higher power image demonstrating intravascular proliferation of capillaries resembling a renal glomerulus

Table 7.22 Key pathologic features: glomeruloid hemangioma

Multiple nodules in the dermis
Intravascular proliferation of small capillaries forming glomeruloid tufts
PAS+ eosinophilic intracytoplasmic hyaline globules
Majority associated with POEMS syndrome or multicentric Castleman disease

meruloid hemangiomas are negative for this marker. The differential diagnosis with papillary hemangioma is discussed above.

Bacillary Angiomatosis

Clinical Features

Bacillary angiomatosis is caused by infection with the gram-negative bacteria *Bartonella henselae* and *Bartonella quintana*. It is seen almost exclusively in the setting of AIDS in the United States. With the advent of effective antiretroviral medications, this condition is quite rare. When it does occur, it presents as multiple red papules. Clinically it can be confused with pyogenic granuloma.

Pathologic Features

Bacillary angiomatosis consists of capillary lobules with plump, clear endothelial cells admixed with neutrophils, lymphocytes, histiocytes, and clumps of amphophilic material that represent clusters of the organism (Fig. 7.37a). The organism is best demonstrated with a Warthin-Starry stain, but can also be highlighted with Giemsa and GMS stains (Fig. 7.37b) (Table 7.23).

Differential Diagnosis

Bacillary angiomatosis is most likely to be confused with epithelioid hemangioma due to the shared epithelioid morphology of the endothelial cells. The presence of the amphophilic clusters of organisms and different constituents of the background inflammatory infiltrate should allow distinction. Pyogenic granulomas can have a similar inflammatory background in ulcerated examples, and a lobular growth pattern, but they lack the epithelioid endothelial cells and amphophilic granular material of bacillary angiomatosis. Knowledge of the clinical setting of AIDS also helps in recognition of bacillary angiomatosis.

Kaposi Sarcoma

Clinical Features

While long considered a true sarcoma, it is now recognized that Kaposi sarcoma is a multiclonal reactive process related to infection with human herpesvirus 8 (HHV-8), and not a clonal neoplasm. This was demonstrated in a landmark study that demonstrated multiple different HHV-8 clones from different lesions within the same patients. In that regard, it should be considered a reactive rather than neoplastic vascular lesion. Kaposi sarcoma occurs in two distinct settings: endemic or classic Kaposi sarcoma and Kaposi sarcoma in the setting of immunosuppression. The endemic form typically presents on the lower extremities, usually in older patients from certain geographic regions: sub-Saharan Africa, the Mediterranean, and parts of Eastern Europe. Immunosuppression-related Kaposi sarcoma most commonly occurs in the setting of AIDS but also occurs in other clinical settings such as organ transplantation or treatment with immunosuppressive medications. In the immunocompromised population, the disease is often multifocal and widespread, involving the skin and visceral organs. Kaposi sarcoma is less commonly seen since the onset of effective anti-HIV retroviral medications and more nuanced approaches to immunosuppression in organ transplant patients.

Regardless of the underlying demographics, Kaposi sarcoma has a similar clinical presentation. The lesions usually start as red patches that can over time develop into red, brown or violaceous plaques, nodules, and tumors, often following skin cleavage lines. Both cutaneous and mucosal involvement are common. Occasional lesions undergo spontaneous regression. Although strictly speaking not a true sarcoma, Kaposi sarcoma can result in mortality if vital structures are involved or if the patient does not respond to antiretroviral therapy or reduction of immunosuppressive medications.

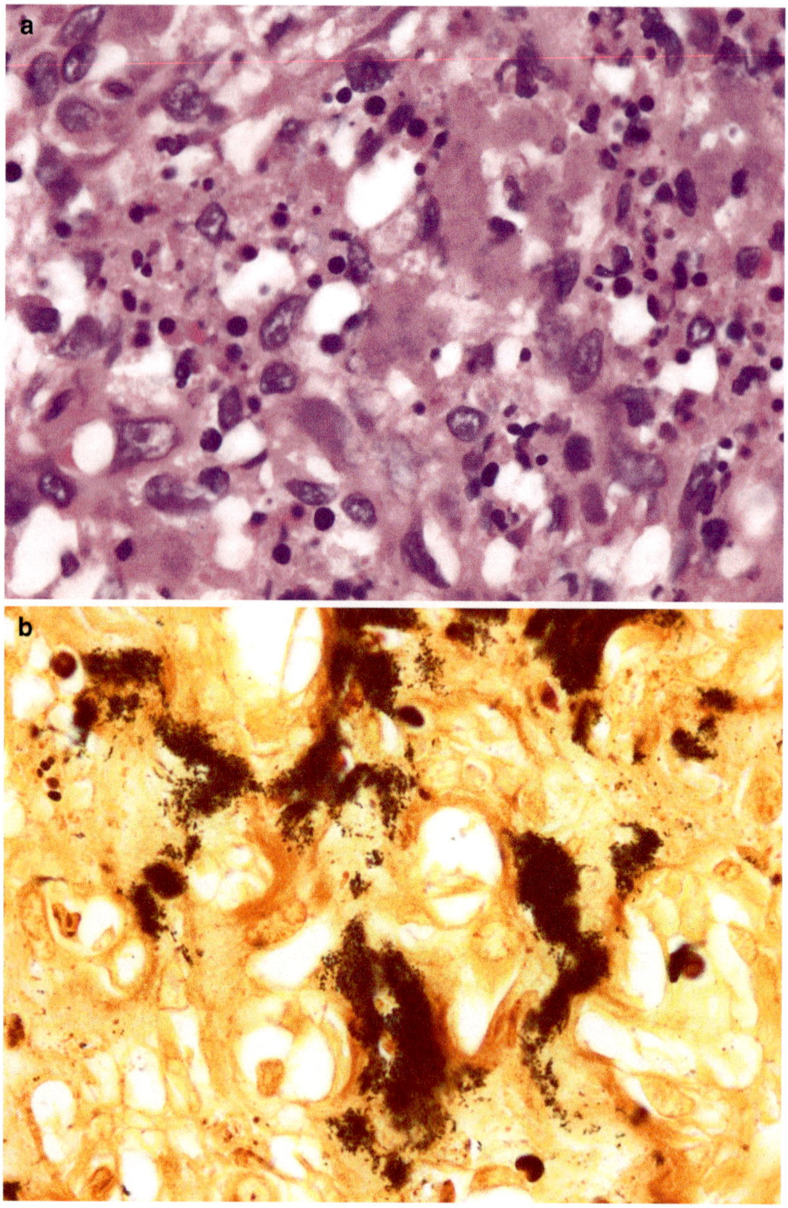

Fig. 7.37 Bacillary angiomatosis. (**a**) Lobular proliferation of plump, mildly atypical epithelioid endothelial cells admixed with stromal neutrophils and cellular debris. (**b**) Warthin Starry stain highlighting the bacterial organisms (Image courtesy of Dr. Wayne Grayson, Ampath National Laboratories, Johannesburg, South Africa)

Table 7.23 Key pathologic features: bacillary angiomatosis

Lobular growth pattern
Capillaries with epithelioid endothelial cells
Amphophilic granular material consisting of clusters of bacteria
Highlighted by Warthin-Starry, Giemsa, or GMS stains
Associated with AIDS

Pathologic Features

Kaposi sarcoma undergoes an evolution in microscopic features that correlates with the clinical presentation. In the patch stage, it is composed of complex infiltrating vessels that dissect between collagen bundles of the dermis, often surrounding pre-existing dermal structures (the so-called promontory sign) (Fig. 7.38). These vessels are lined by a single layer of bland endothelial cells without multilayering. As the tumor evolves into

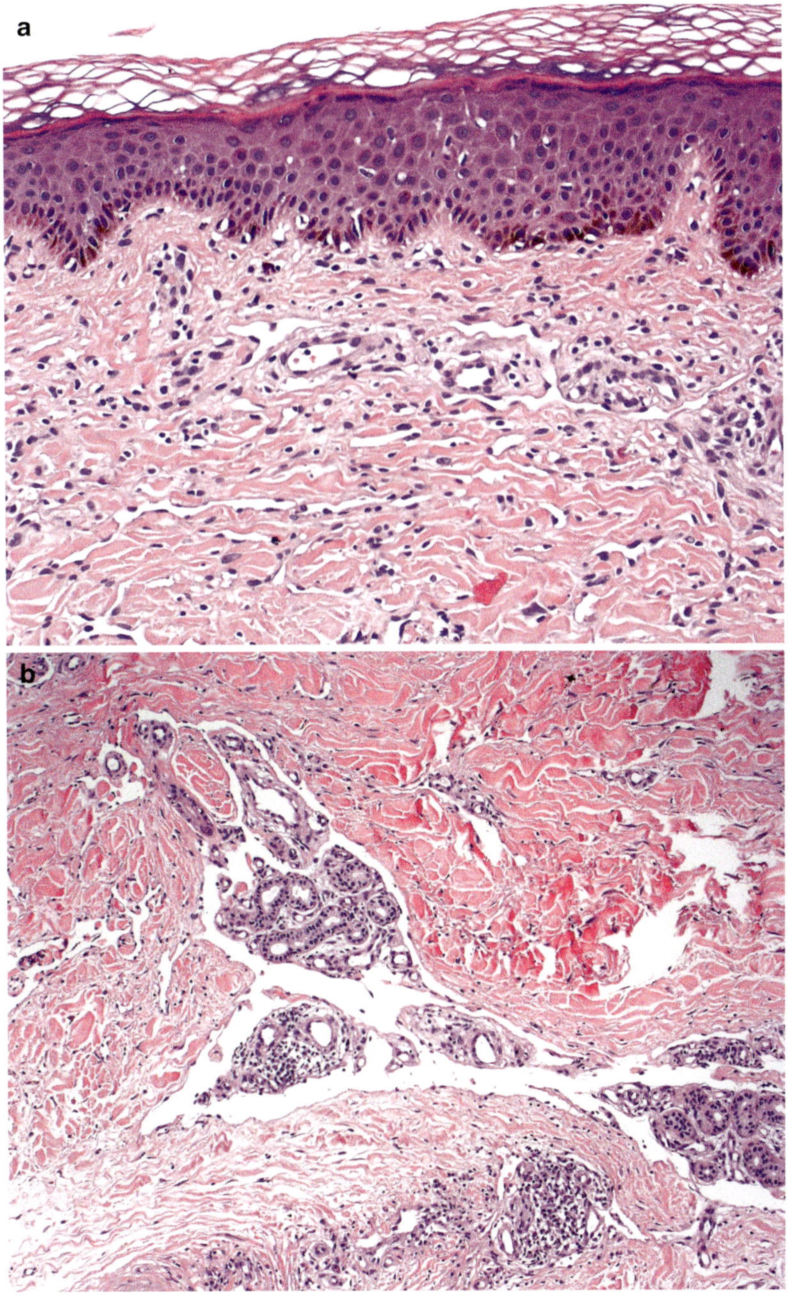

Fig. 7.38 Kaposi sarcoma. (**a**) In the patch stage, there are thin-walled-vessels lined by small, hyperchromatic endothelial cells dissecting through the dermis. (**b**) The neoplastic vessels can surround pre-existing dermal structures resulting in the promontory sign

the plaque and nodular/tumor phases, the lesion becomes more cellular with fascicles of spindled cells with slit-like vascular spaces and extravasated erythrocytes (Fig. 7.39).

A number of histologic variants have been described. Probably the most commonly encountered histologic variant in the United States is the pyogenic granuloma-like variant in which the lesion is exophytic and has an epidermal collarette (Fig. 7.40). The pyogenic granuloma variant still has areas composed of spindled cells resembling those seen in classic Kaposi sarcoma, but superimposed granulation tissue resembling pyogenic granuloma may be present in traumatized lesions. Other described variants include lymphangiomatous (or lymphangioma-like) Kaposi

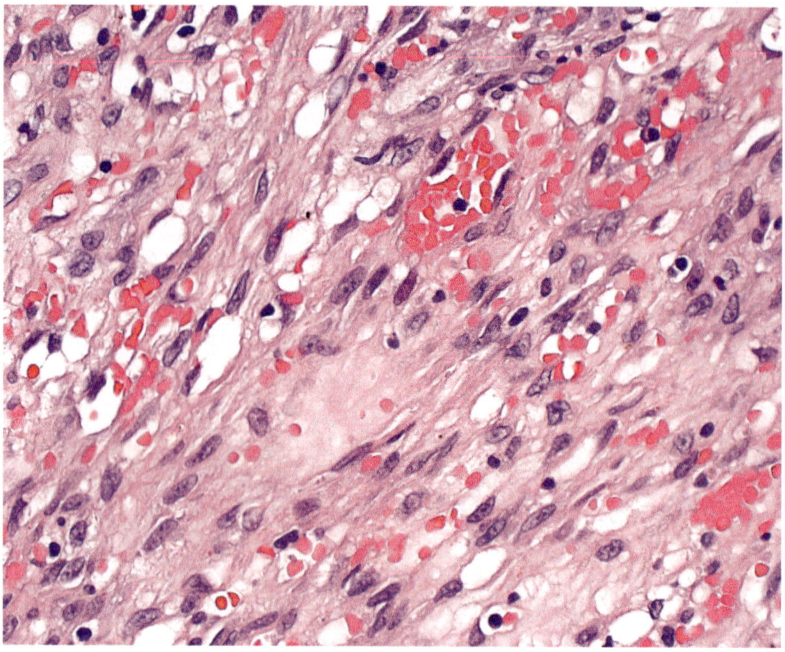

Fig. 7.39 Kaposi sarcoma with fascicles of spindled cells with slit-like vascular lumens and extravasated erythrocytes

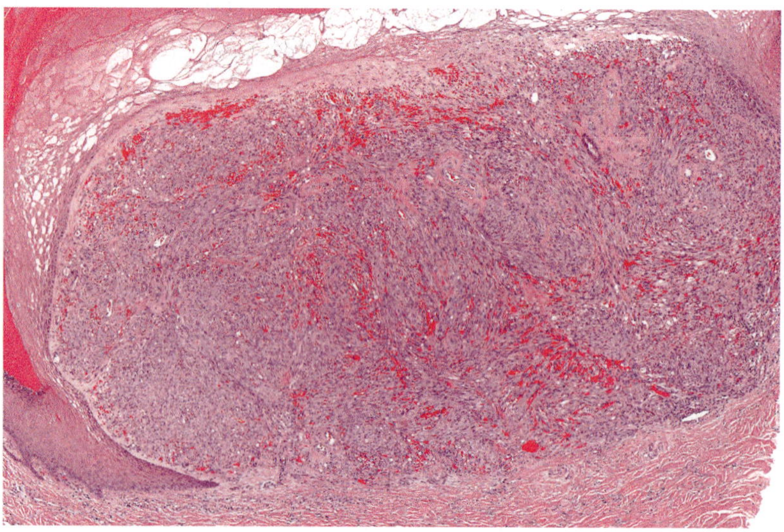

Fig. 7.40 Pyogenic granuloma-like Kaposi sarcoma with epidermal collarette

sarcoma (Fig. 7.41), Kaposi sarcoma with myoid nodules (Fig. 7.42), pleomorphic Kaposi sarcoma (Fig. 7.43) as well as lymphangiectatic, telangiectatic, verrucous, keloidal, and micronodular Kaposi sarcoma. Kaposi sarcoma is positive for vascular markers including CD31, CD34, and ERG. The most valuable immunostain to confirm the diagnosis is the stain for HHV-8 latent nuclear antigen-1, which is consistently positive in essentially all cases (Table 7.24).

Differential Diagnosis

The differential diagnosis varies somewhat based on the stage of Kaposi sarcoma. In the patch stage, the differential diagnosis includes microvenular hemangioma and well-differentiated angiosarcoma. The vessels of microvenular hemangioma are less complex and have a well-developed pericyte layer, as discussed previously. Well-differentiated angiosarcoma usually has more atypia, multilayering of endothelial cells and

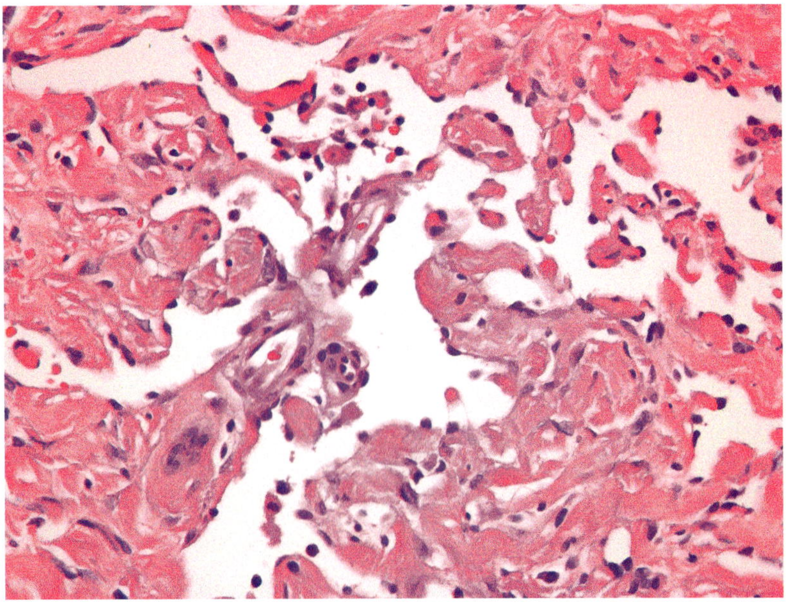

Fig. 7.41 Lymphangioma-like Kaposi sarcoma composed of irregular ectatic vessels resembling lymphatics (Image courtesy of Dr. Wayne Grayson, Ampath National Laboratories, Johannesburg, South Africa)

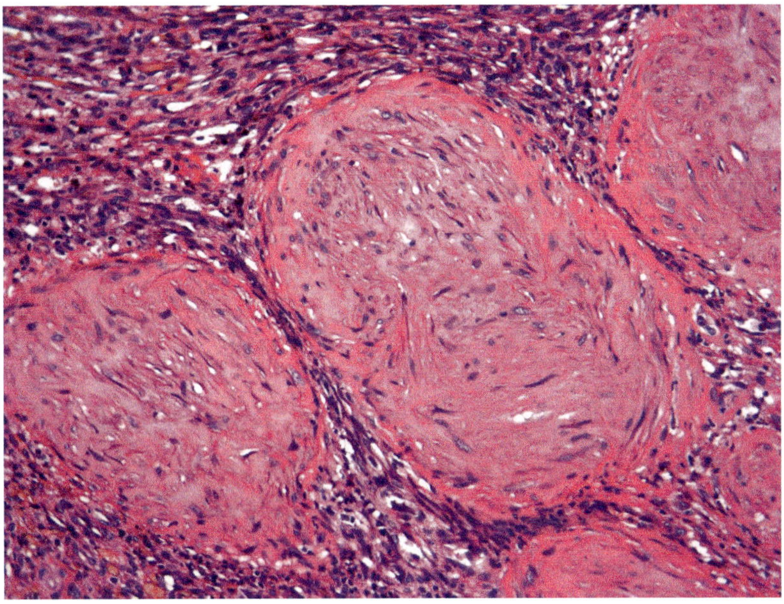

Fig. 7.42 Kaposi sarcoma with myoid nodules (Image courtesy of Dr. Wayne Grayson, Ampath National Laboratories, Johannesburg, South Africa)

presents in sun-damaged skin of the head and neck of elderly Caucasian patients. In the plaque and nodule/tumor phases of Kaposi sarcoma, the differential diagnosis includes spindle cell hemangioma, kaposiform hemangioendothelioma, and angiosarcoma with a solid spindle cell growth pattern. In contrast to spindle cell hemangioma, Kaposi sarcoma is only rarely intravascular and usually lacks ectatic vascular spaces and vacuolated endothelial cells. Kaposiform hemangioendothelioma presents in infants, and the nodules of spindled cells often have an ectatic vessel at the periphery. Angiosarcoma may have areas with a solid proliferation of spindled endothelial cells, but the spindled cells are more atypical, and conventional vasoformative angiosarcoma is often present at the periphery. None of the vascular tumors in the differential diagnosis are positive for HHV-8.

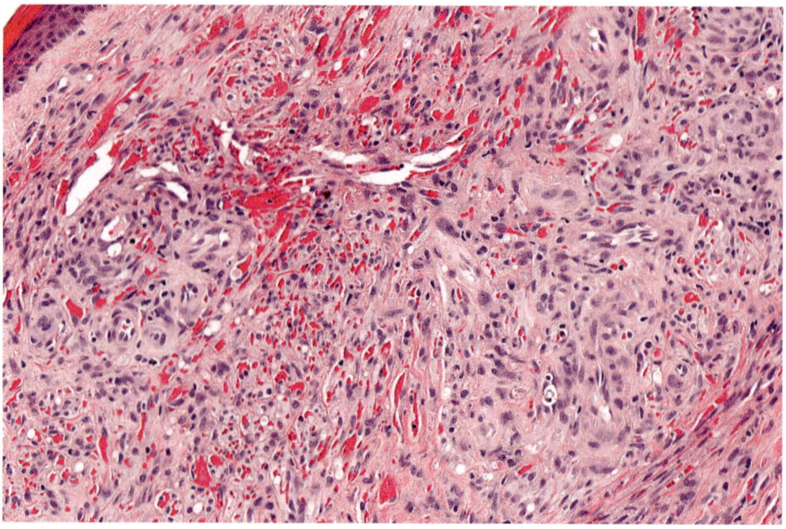

Fig. 7.43 Pleomorphic Kaposi sarcoma with enlarged atypical nuclei

Table 7.24 Key pathologic features: Kaposi sarcoma

Associated with immunosuppression
Caused by HHV-8 infection
Patch stage
Irregular thin-walled vessels dissecting through dermal collagen
Promontory sign
Plaque/tumor stage
Fascicles of spindled cells with slit-like lumens
Extravasated erythrocytes
Positive for CD31, CD34, ERG, podoplanin, HHV-8

Vascular Tumors of Intermediate Malignancy

Kaposiform Hemangioendothelioma

Clinical Features

Kaposiform hemangioendothelioma is an aggressive vascular tumor of intermediate malignancy that typically occurs in the first 2 years of life and may be congenital. KHE usually occurs in the dermis and subcutis, but the deep soft tissues, spleen, and bone may also be involved. Superficial tumors present as red to violaceous masses and can be quite large at presentation. The most common deep soft tissue site is the retroperitoneum. Kaposiform hemangioendothelioma is often associated with a profound thrombocytopenia (Kasabach-Merritt syndrome) secondary to the development of platelet microthrombi within tumor vessels. This is especially true in large, deep-seated tumors, where consumptive coagulopathy may be the presenting feature. Kaposiform hemangioendotheliomas are prone to local recurrence, do not regress without therapy, and may occasionally spread to lymph nodes. However, distant metastases and malignant transformation in KHE do not occur. Mortality is almost invariably due to complications from the underlying coagulopathy, which may result in life-threatening hemorrhage. Treatment is multimodal and includes surgery for small superficial lesions. A variety of medical treatment options have demonstrated limited success including conventional chemotherapy, intralesional or systemic interferon alpha 2a, antiplatelet agents, corticosteroids, intra-arterial embolization, and radiation. More recently, sirolimus has emerged as the most promising treatment agent, as it has been shown to rapidly reverse the thrombocytopenia and reduce the size of lesions by ≥75%, allowing excision of previously unresectable tumors. Platelet transfusions in kaposiform hemangioendothelioma paradoxically increase platelet trapping and worsen any thrombocytopenia. As discussed earlier in this chapter, it is believed that the tufted angioma belongs to the same disease spectrum and likely represents a smaller, more superficial example of kaposiform hemangioendothelioma.

Pathologic Features

Microscopically, kaposiform hemangioendothelioma is a cellular, ill-defined, infiltrative neoplasm composed of coalescing nodules of plump spindled endothelial cells. Similar to tufted angioma, a distinctive crescent-shaped thin-walled dilated vessel is seen at the periphery of capillary nodules. The stroma can also contain these dilated vessels (Fig. 7.44a). The endothelial cells form fascicles and slit-like capillary vessels resembling Kaposi sarcoma, which predominate at the periphery of the nodules (Fig. 7.44b); the central portions contain more epithelioid endothelial cells surrounded by pericytes and often containing platelet microthrombi (Fig. 7.45). The endothelial cells demonstrate

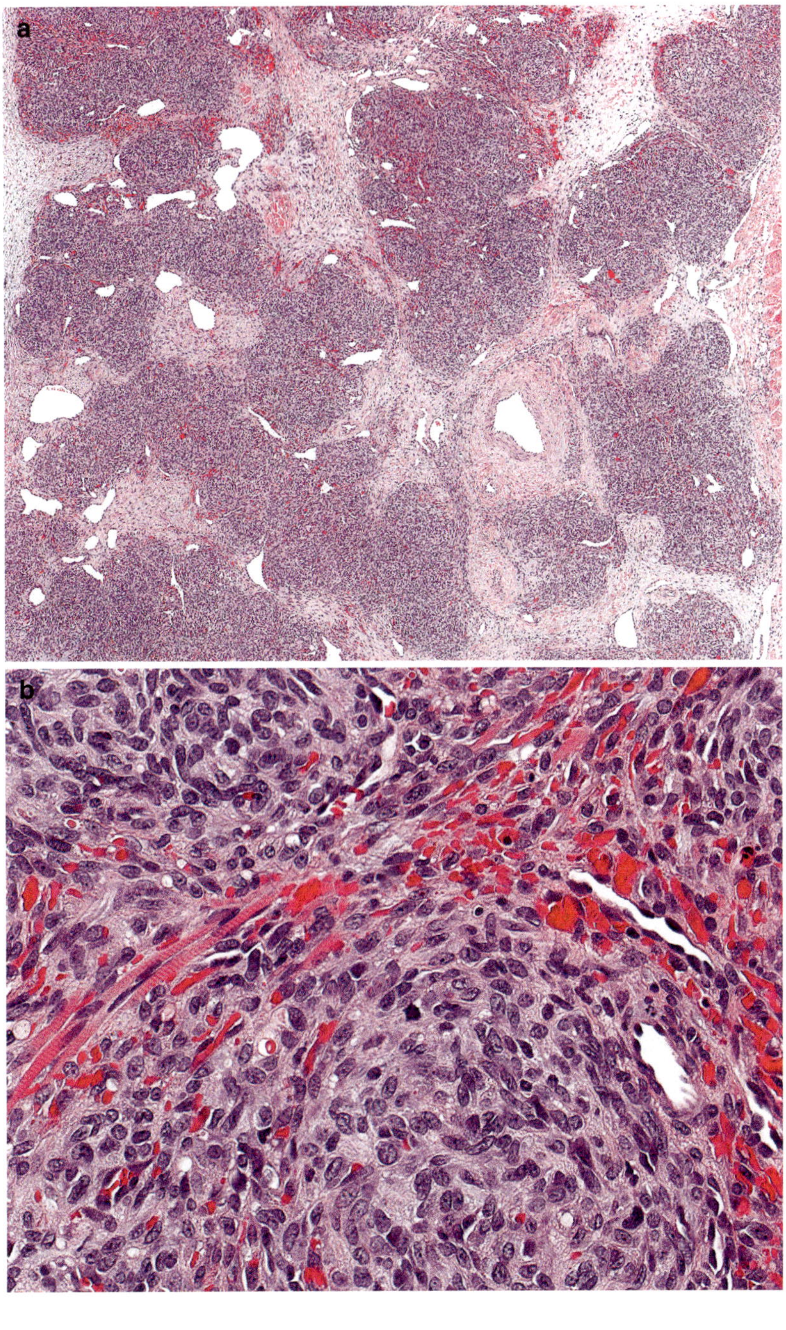

Fig. 7.44 Kaposiform hemangioendothelioma. (**a**) Numerous vascular nodules with a distinctive crescent-shaped vessel at the periphery. (**b**) In the periphery of the cellular areas, the endothelial cells form fascicles and slit-like capillary vessels with bland, mitotically active endothelial cells resembling Kaposi sarcoma

bland vesicular nuclei and amphophilic cytoplasm. Mitotic figures can be seen, and extravasated red blood cells and hemosiderin deposits are common. The spindled endothelial cells and the peripheral crescent-shaped vessels in KHE are positive for lymphatic markers podoplanin (D2–40), LYVE-1, and Prox1. More epithelioid in appearance capillaries in the center of the lobules do not express lymphatic markers resulting in a distinctive and diagnostically helpful pattern (Fig. 7.46) (Table 7.25). GLUT1 is negative in this lesion.

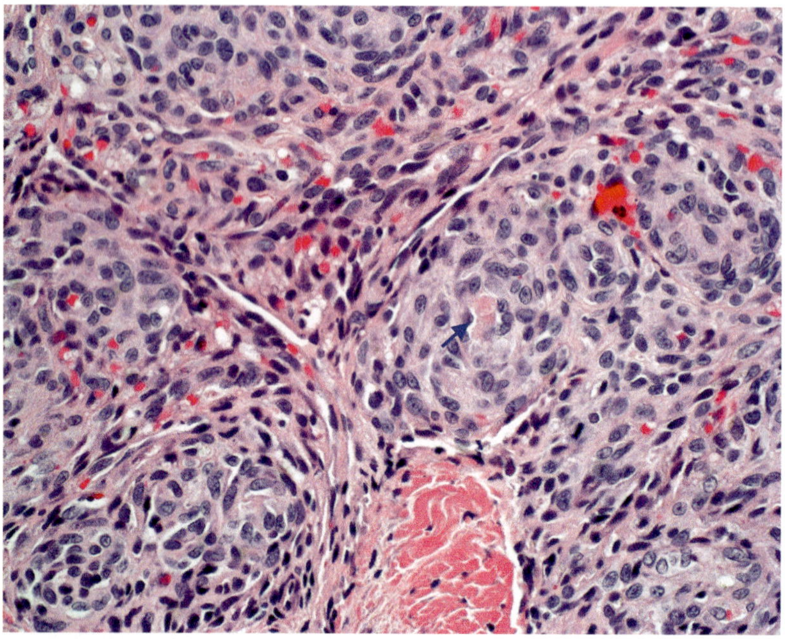

Fig. 7.45 The central portions of the nodules of kaposiform hemangioendothelioma often contain more epithelioid endothelial cells and platelet microthrombi (arrow) and are rich in pericytes

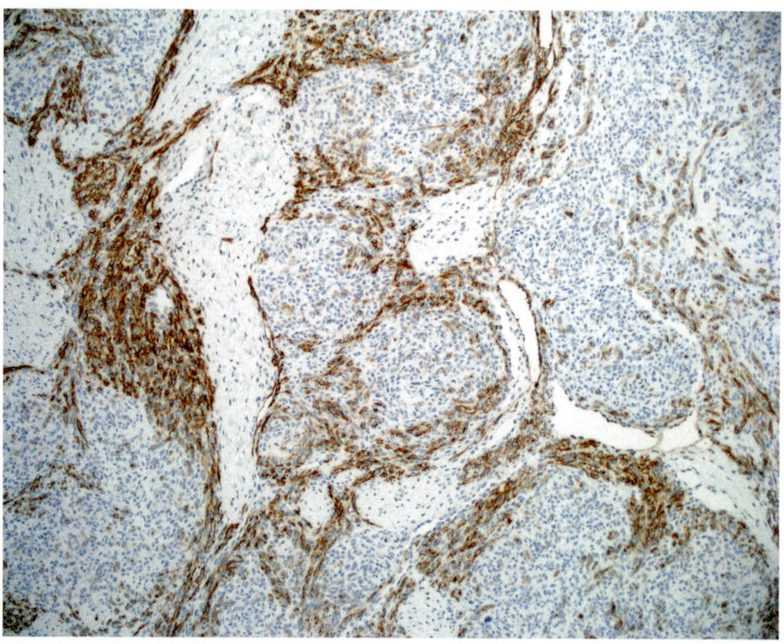

Fig. 7.46 Distinctive pattern of podoplanin (D2–40) immunoreactivity in kaposiform hemangioendothelioma. The periphery of the nodule, where spindle cells predominate and the stellate draining vessels reside, are positive for podoplanin. The center of the nodule with more epithelioid cells is negative

Table 7.25 Key pathologic features: kaposiform hemangioendothelioma

Multiple coalescing nodules of spindled endothelial cells with peripheral ectatic vessels
Spindled cells forming fascicles and slit-like capillaries at the nodule periphery
Epithelioid capillaries with pericytes and platelet microthrombi in the center of the nodule
Minimal atypia, mitotic figures common
Distinctive pattern of podoplanin immunoreactivity

Differential Diagnosis

Kaposiform hemangioendothelioma morphologically overlaps to some extent with Kaposi sarcoma due to the kaposiform spindled endothelial cells. However, Kaposi sarcoma is extraordinary rare in infants and would not have the lobular architecture with peripheral crescent-shaped lymphatic channels, or the epithelioid component containing platelet microthrombi that are seen in KHE. Plasma cell infiltrates and HHV-8 expression do not occur in KHE. As it is most common in infants, KHE can be confused with the highly cellular proliferative phase of infantile hemangioma. Infantile hemangioma lacks a spindled endothelial component and the distinctive perilobular crescentic vessels. Difficult cases can be resolved by utilizing a combination of GLUT1 (positive in infantile hemangioma, negative in kaposiform hemangioendothelioma/tufted hemangioma) and D2–40 (positive in kaposiform hemangioendothelioma/tufted hemangioma, negative in infantile hemangioma) immunostains. Kaposiform hemangioendothelioma/tufted angioma can also closely resemble congenital nonprogressive hemangiomas (RICH and NICH) as both have discrete lobules of lesional capillaries and fibrous stroma containing large irregular stromal vessels. Helpful morphologic features include the lack of a spindle cell component, platelet microthrombi and mitotic activity in congenital nonprogressive hemangiomas, and location of the feeding vessel. In congenital nonprogressive hemangiomas, the feeding vessel is usually in the center of the lobules, whereas kaposiform hemangioendotheliomas have a crescent-shaped vessel at the lobule periphery. In difficult cases, immunostaining for D2–40 is very helpful, as congenital nonprogressive hemangiomas do not demonstrate lymphatic differentiation.

The distinction between kaposiform hemangioendothelioma and tufted hemangioma may be largely academic; as discussed above, tufted angioma likely represents a small superficial kaposiform hemangioendothelioma rather than a distinct entity. In kaposiform hemangioendothelioma the capillary nodules coalesce to form large infiltrative masses deep in the subcutis and have a more prominent spindle cell component, often arranged in fascicles, as well as stromal fibrosis and hemosiderin deposits. These features are typically not seen in superficial tufted angiomas. On a case-by-case basis, it may be impossible to make a distinction between these two lesions. It is imperative that the final diagnosis be correlated with the clinical and radiologic findings. The term tufted angioma may be acceptable for a patient with small superficial tumors confined to dermis; however, clinically aggressive lesions, particularly in the setting of consumptive coagulopathy, are best considered to represent kaposiform hemangioendothelioma, irrespective of the predominance of tufted angioma or kaposiform hemangioendothelioma-like morphology.

Hobnail Hemangioendotheliomas

Clinical Features

The hobnail hemangioendothelioma family includes retiform hemangioendothelioma and papillary intralymphatic angioendothelioma, also known as Dabska tumor; both entities are architecturally complex vascular lesions characterized by hobnail appearance of the endothelial cells and lymphatic phenotype. Both lesions most commonly present on the distal extremities. Classically, papillary intralymphatic angioendothelioma is more common in children, while retiform hemangioendothelioma affects mostly young adults. Both tumors have a potential for local recurrence that can make local control difficult to obtain, but lymph node spread is rare, and bona fide distant metastases do not occur. Therefore these tumors are classified as vascular tumors of borderline malignant potential, although most of these cases behave in a benign fashion if amenable to complete excision.

Pathologic Features

Many cases have overlapping histologic features of both papillary intralymphatic angioendothelioma and retiform hemangioendothelioma, and it is often difficult to separate tumors with mixed morphology into the well-defined ends of the spectrum, especially in a limited biopsy specimen. That being said, they probably represent distinct entities based on their different clinical presentations and evidence of lymphatic differentiation and clear-cut intravascular growth that is seen in papillary intralymphatic angioendothelioma, but not in retiform hemangioendothelioma. Papillary intralymphatic angioendothelioma is characterized by thin, dilated vessels with intraluminal papillary projections containing thin hyalinized cores lined by cuboidal-to-columnar, uniform, hobnailed endothelial cells (Fig. 7.47). Some of the papillae can appear to float within vascular lumina due to tangential sectioning. The surrounding stroma is fibrotic and contains lymphoid aggregates. Retiform hemangioendothelioma has architecturally complex stellate-shaped branching vessels reminiscent of the rete testis lined by uniform, slightly hyperchromatic hobnail endothelial cells (Fig. 7.48a, b). Intravascular projections are not as well developed as those seen in papillary intralymphatic angioendothelioma. An associated lymphocytic infiltrate is often present. The nuclear atypia is mild, and the mitotic activity in these lesions is very low. Both tumors are positive for the vascular markers CD31, CD34, and ERG and interestingly express the neuroendocrine marker synaptophysin. Expression of lymphatic markers is typical in papillary intralymphatic angioendothelioma, but retiform hemangioendotheliomas rarely demonstrate lymphatic differentiation, despite earlier reports (Table 7.26).

Differential Diagnosis

The differential includes hobnail lymphatic malformation (hobnail hemangioma) and angiosarcoma. Hobnail lymphatic malformations are very superficial lesions that are limited

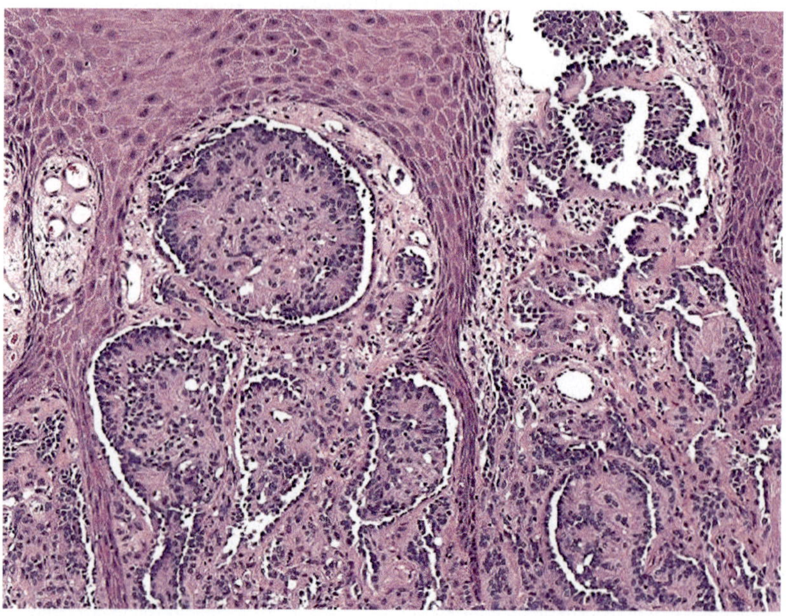

Fig. 7.47 Papillary intralymphatic angioendothelioma composed of intravascular papillae lined by hobnail endothelial cells

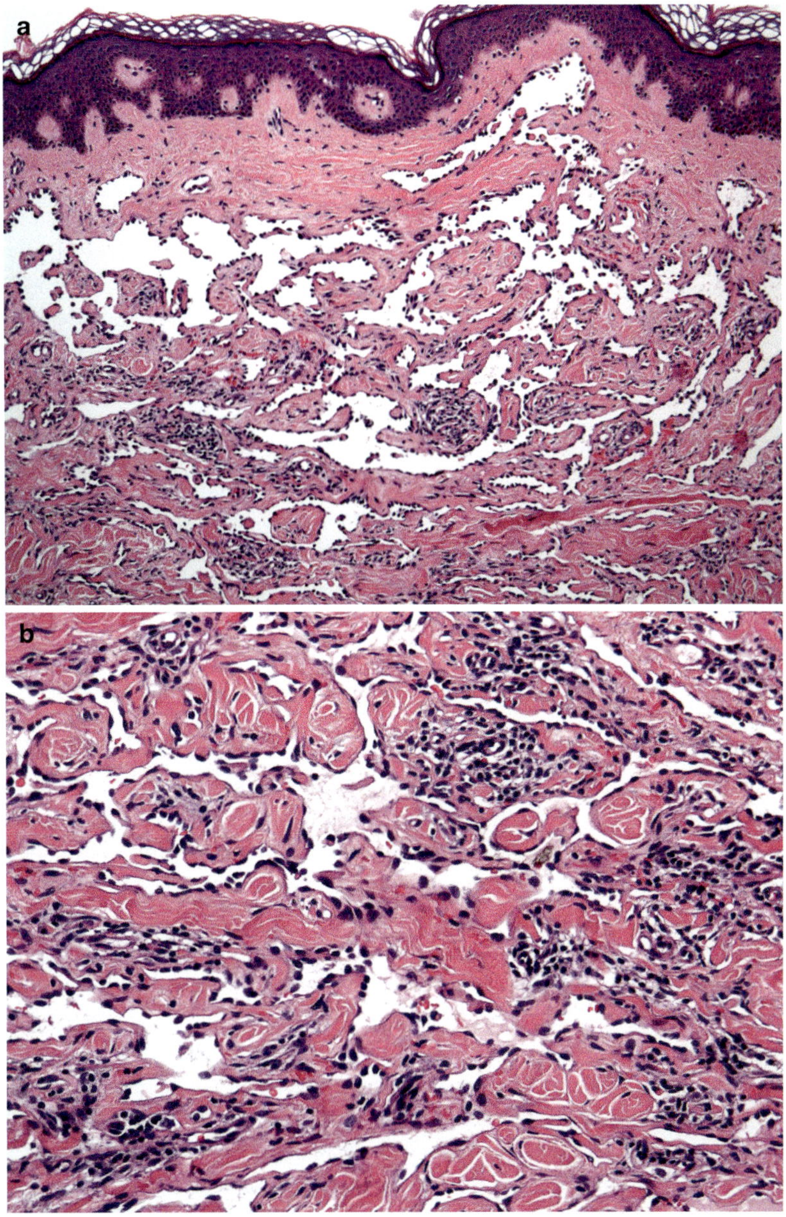

Fig. 7.48 Retiform hemangioendothelioma. (**a**) Dermal proliferation of stellate branching vessels reminiscent of rete testis. (**b**) The vessels are lined by endothelial cells with small, hobnail nuclei. A perivascular lymphocytic infiltrate is often present

to the dermis, and lack the intravascular growth pattern and prominent papillae of papillary intralymphatic angioendothelioma. Hobnail lymphatic malformation can be distinguished from retiform hemangioendothelioma based on its superficial location, relative lack of architectural complexity, and lymphatic immunophenotype, less common in the latter. The differential diagnosis of papillary intralymphatic angioendothelioma with glomeruloid hemangioma and papillary hemangioma is discussed above. The architectural complexity of retiform hemangioendothelioma may raise suspicion for angiosarcoma. Angiosarcomas occur in the sun-damaged skin of elderly patients and cytologically have greater nuclear atypia, endothelial multilayering, and mitotic activity. The vessels of angiosarcoma show a greater variety of architectural

Table 7.26 Key microscopic features: hobnail hemangioendotheliomas

Retiform hemangioendothelioma
Elongated, complex branching vessels resembling rete testis
Hobnail endothelial cells
Stromal fibrosis and lymphoid aggregates
Rare expression of lymphatic markers
Papillary intralymphatic angioendothelioma
Intravascular papillae with thin hyalinized stalks
Cuboidal to columnar hobnailed endothelial cells
Expression of lymphatic markers

patterns within the same tumor including vasoformative, solid, papillary, and spindled growth, but they do not typically share the morphologic resemblance to the rete testis with retiform hemangioendothelioma.

Composite Hemangioendothelioma

Clinical Features

Composite hemangioendothelioma is a very rare form of hemangioendothelioma defined as a vascular neoplasm of intermediate malignancy composed of an architecturally complex admixture of histologically distinct vascular elements. This rare tumor typically occurs in the skin and subcutis of adults and is very rare in children. Deep locations have been reported. Similar to hobnail hemangioendotheliomas discussed above, composite hemangioendothelioma is characterized by a high rate of local recurrence, small risk of lymph node spread, and rare distant metastases. However, a recent study of 11 cases suggests that they may behave more aggressively than previously thought, with metastasis in up to 50% of the cases.

Pathologic Features

Although it seems logical to think of composite hemangioendothelioma as a tumor with combined features of retiform hemangioendothelioma and papillary intralymphatic angioendothelioma, this is not the case. Although very diverse morphologically, most composite hemangioendotheliomas consistently display two components: a retiform component resembling retiform hemangioendothelioma (Fig. 7.49a) and an epithelioid component reminiscent of epithelioid hemangioendothelioma. The latter pattern is composed of nests or sheets of plump epithelioid endothelial cells with eosinophilic cytoplasm often containing an intracytoplasmic vacuole (Fig. 7.49b). Other components described in this lesion include solid spindled cell areas, vasoformative areas with low-grade nuclei reminiscent of well-differentiated angiosarcoma, papillary intralymphatic angioendothelioma-like morphology (Fig. 7.49c), and ectatic vascular channels lined by bland endothelial cells reminiscent of spindle cell hemangioma (Fig. 7.49d), sinusoidal hemangioma, or venous malformation. These tumors variably express markers of lymphatic differentiation. Composite hemangioendotheliomas from the study referenced above, showed expression of neuroendocrine marker synaptophysin, a feature shared with retiform hemangioendothelioma and papillary intralymphatic angioendothelioma, but not with any other vascular neoplasms (Table 7.27). All of the synaptophysin-positive composite hemangioendotheliomas in that study had retiform areas suggesting that composite hemangioendotheliomas may represent a more clinically aggressive variant of retiform hemangioendothelioma.

Differential Diagnosis

Epithelioid hemangioendothelioma (discussed below) and angiosarcoma are the most important differential diagnostic considerations. Epithelioid hemangioendothelioma has similar epithelioid vacuolated endothelial cells, but they are usually arranged in a corded growth pattern or singly in a prominent myxohyaline matrix; this distinctive stroma is not seen in composite hemangioendotheliomas. There is also no evidence of a *WWTR1-CAMTA1* fusion in composite hemangioendotheliomas, either

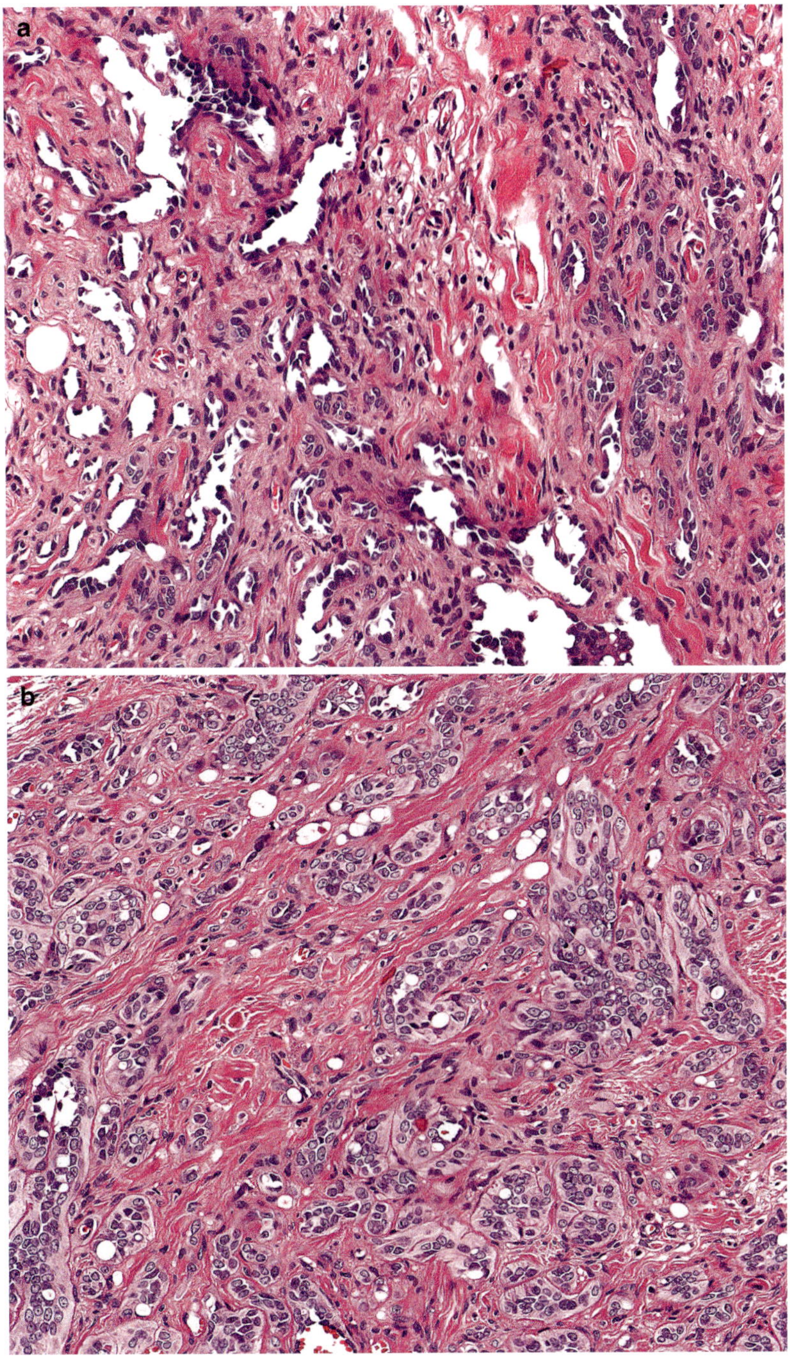

Fig. 7.49 Composite hemangioendothelioma. (**a**) Retiform component showing angulated branching vessels lined by slightly hyperchromatic hobnailed endothelial cells resembling retiform hemangioendothelioma. (**b**) Epithelioid component showing nests of plump epithelioid endothelial cells with abundant eosinophilic cytoplasm and intracytoplasmic vacuoles. This pattern resembles epithelioid hemangioendothelioma but lacks the distinctive myxohyaline stroma. (**c**) Dilated vessels with intravascular papillary structures lined by hobnailed epithelium adjacent to epithelioid component. (**d**) Epithelioid area adjacent to ectatic vessels

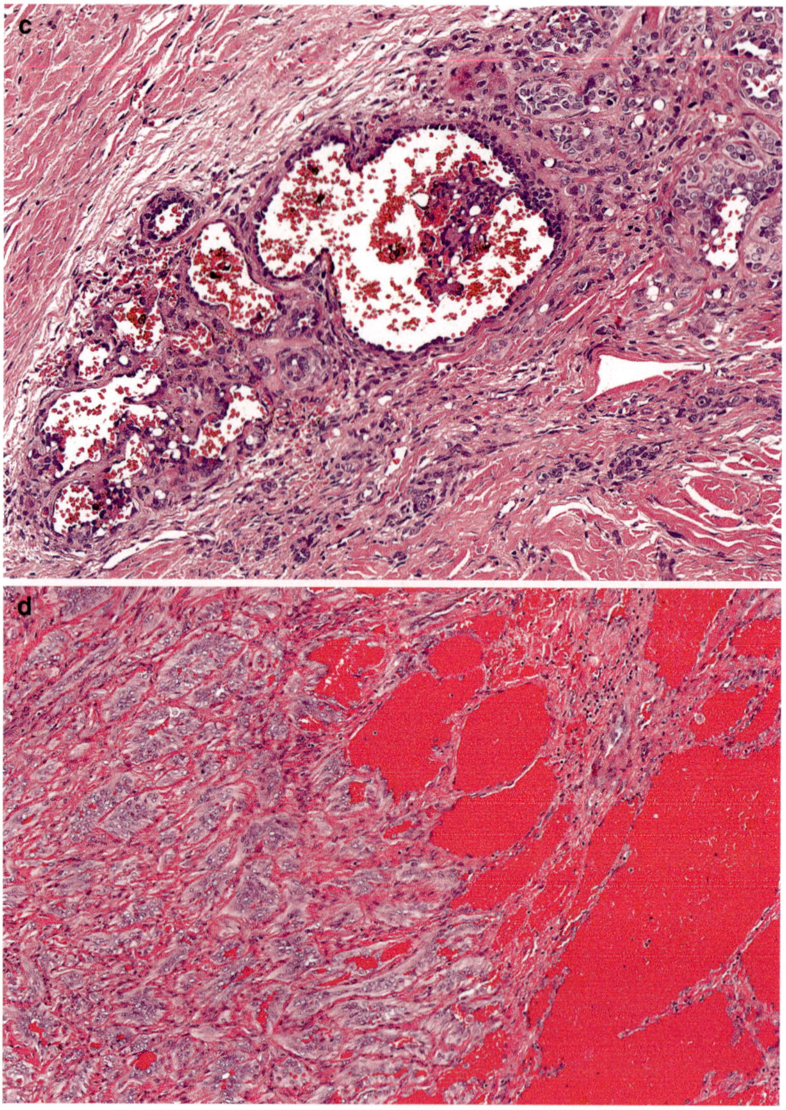

Fig. 7.49 (continued)

Table 7.27 Key pathologic features: composite hemangioendothelioma

Branching retiform pattern that resembles retiform hemangioendothelioma
Solid or nested epithelioid pattern with intracytoplasmic vacuoles resembling EHE
Solid spindled cell component
Distinctive expression of synaptophysin (similar to papillary intralymphatic angioendothelioma and retiform hemangioendothelioma, but not other vascular tumors)

by immunohistochemistry, FISH, or RT-PCR. Distinction from angiosarcomas can be extraordinarily challenging. Angiosarcomas have overt cytologic atypia, endothelial multilayering, mitotic activity, and necrosis and lack the distinctive synaptophysin expression of retiform hemangioendothelioma and papillary intralymphatic angioendothelioma.

Pseudomyogenic (Epithelioid Sarcoma-Like) Hemangioendothelioma

Clinical Features

Epithelioid sarcoma-like hemangioendothelioma was initially described in 2003 as a rare vascular tumor of intermediate malignancy that was frequently misdiagnosed as epithelioid sarcoma. It was subsequently described under the name pseudomyogenic hemangioendothelioma in 2011. It typically occurs on the extremities of adults, especially males, most commonly on the lower extremities. The majority are multifocal at presentation, often involving multiple different tissue planes, including underlying bone. The clinical presentation is variable. They may present as skin-colored nodules and may be ulcerated. They do not clinically resemble a vascular tumor. This neoplasm has a high rate of local recurrence, but lymph node metastasis is uncommon and distant metastases are rare. Surgery is the treatment of choice, but may be very difficult or impossible in selected cases due to multifocal presentation.

Pathologic Features

Pseudomyogenic hemangioendothelioma is composed of sheets of epithelioid to spindled endothelial cells with dense eosinophilic cytoplasm (Fig. 7.50a, b). Vascular differentiation is inconspicuous, with only rare intracytoplasmic vacuole/lumen formation. The tumor nuclei are uniform and exhibit mild to moderate nuclear atypia. The mitotic rate is typically low (<1 MF/10 HPFs). Admixed neutrophils are seen in about 50% of cases and represent a helpful clue to the diagnosis (Fig. 7.50c).

This tumor has a unique immunophenotype. It is consistently positive for cytokeratin (AE1/3) and nuclear markers Fli1 and ERG (both positive in endothelial cells), and has retained INI1 (SMARCB1) expression. Immunoreactivity for CD31 is variable, ranging from 50 to 80% of cases. Immunoreactivity for CD34 is consistently absent. Recently, a recurrent t(7;19) resulting in a *SERPINE-FOSB* fusion has been described in this tumor. Immunostains to detect nuclear expression of FOSB are positive, but it should be pointed out that some epithelioid hemangiomas are also immunoreactive for this marker (Table 7.28).

Differential Diagnosis

The primary differential diagnosis is epithelioid sarcoma, and this distinction is often quite difficult. Epithelioid sarcoma tends to be composed of small nodules, while pseudomyogenic (epithelioid sarcoma-like) hemangioendothelioma has a sheet-like growth pattern and a predominantly spindled morphology, which is less common in epithelioid sarcoma. Epithelioid sarcoma usually has more nuclear atypia. By immunohistochemistry epithelioid sarcoma is positive for cytokeratin, positive for CD34 in 50–60% of cases, and is negative for CD31 and Fli-1. A significant subset of epithelioid sarcomas show some immunoreactivity for ERG if an antibody against the amino terminus is used, so this marker should be utilized with caution in this differential diagnosis. Epithelioid sarcoma demonstrates loss of INI1 (SMARCB1) in over 90% of cases, which is retained in pseudomyogenic (epithelioid sarcoma-like) hemangioendothelioma.

Cutaneous leiomyosarcoma could be considered in the differential diagnosis. Epithelioid sarcoma-like hemangioendothelioma does not have the intersecting fascicles characteristic of smooth muscle tumors, and is negative for markers of true smooth muscle differentiation (e.g., desmin).

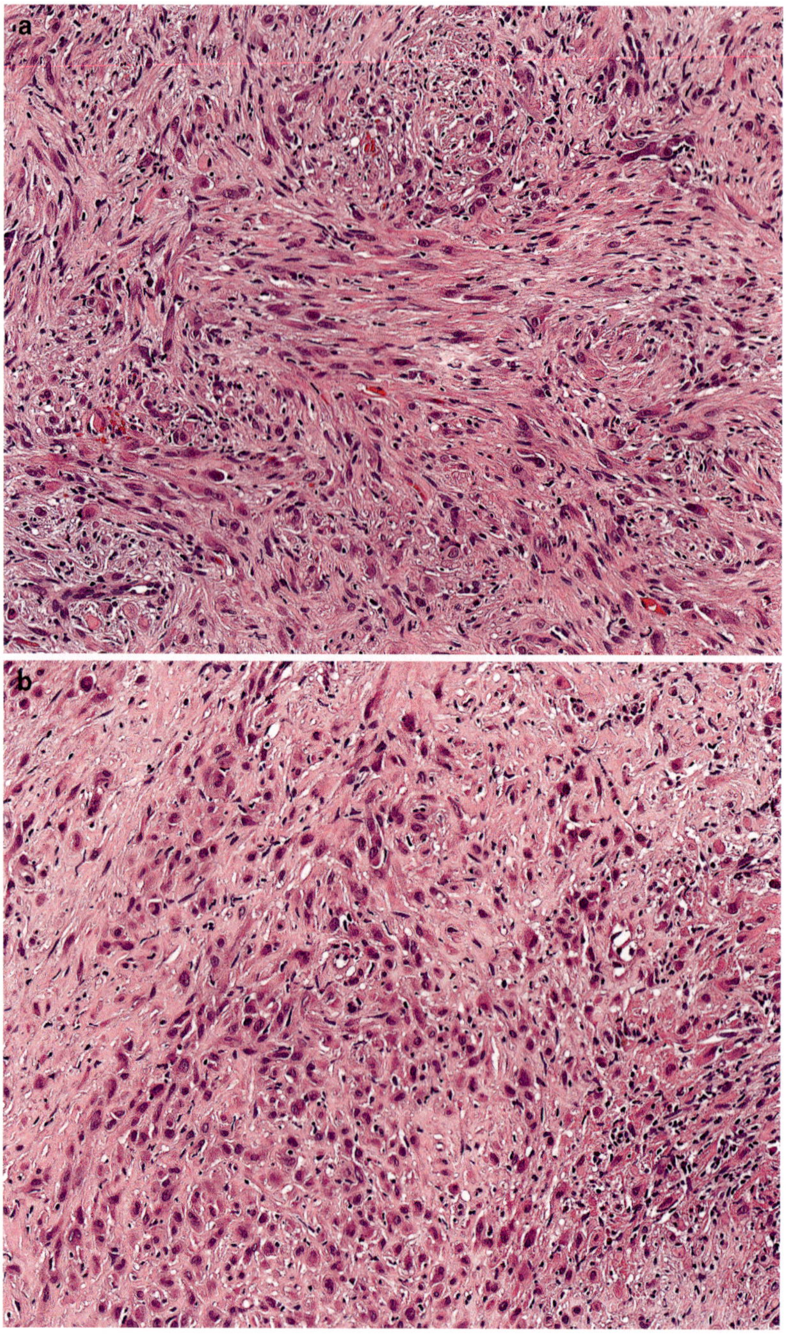

Fig. 7.50 Pseudomyogenic/epithelioid sarcoma-like hemangioendothelioma. (**a**) Vague fascicles of spindled endothelial cells with bland nuclei and abundant eosinophilic cytoplasm imparting a myoid appearance. (**b**) Sheets of epithelioid endothelial cells resembling epithelioid sarcoma set in a fibromyxoid background containing inflammatory cells. (**c**) Neutrophils are commonly present within the tumor

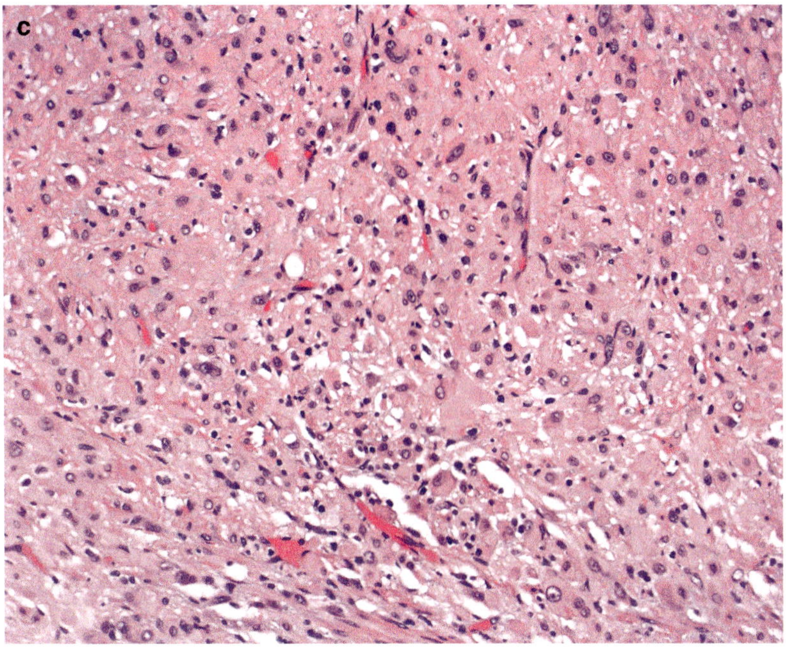

Fig. 7.50 (continued)

Table 7.28 Key pathologic features: Pseudomyogenic (epithelioid sarcoma-like) hemangioendothelioma

Often multifocal, more common in men
Spindled to epithelioid tumor cells with dense eosinophilic cytoplasm
Frequent admixed neutrophils
Immunophenotype
Positive for cytokeratin, ERG, FLI1, FOSB, variably positive for CD31, retained INI-1 expression
Negative for CD34
t(7;19) with *SERPINE-FOSB* fusion

Malignant Vascular Tumors

Epithelioid Hemangioendothelioma

Clinical Features

Epithelioid hemangioendothelioma (EHE) typically occurs in adult patients. In the skin it usually has a nondescript presentation as a skin-colored nodule and lacks the red to violaceous color of most cutaneous vascular tumors. Therefore, biopsies are often not submitted with the clinical suspicion of a vascular neoplasm. Epithelioid hemangioendothelioma recurs in about 10–15% of cases and metastasizes to regional lymph nodes or the lungs in 20–30% of cases. The overall mortality is about 10–20%. Given its relatively aggressive behavior, epithelioid hemangioendothelioma is now considered a fully malignant vascular tumor, rather than a tumor of intermediate malignancy. Surgery is the mainstay of treatment.

Pathologic Features

In deep-seated tumors, approximately half are associated with a pre-existing vessel and can be seen growing within the vessel and expanding the lumen. In such cases, constituent cells can be seen radiating out from the associated vessel. Intravascular growth is less common in cutaneous examples (Fig. 7.51a). The most important diagnostic feature is the cord-like to nested growth pattern of epithelioid endothelial cells embedded in a myxohyaline stroma. Well-formed multicellular vessels are not seen. However, the endothelial cells frequently show individual intracytoplasmic vacuoles (so-called blister cells) that may contain red blood cells (Fig. 7.51b). Generally, the nuclear features are relatively bland, but significant cytologic atypia may be

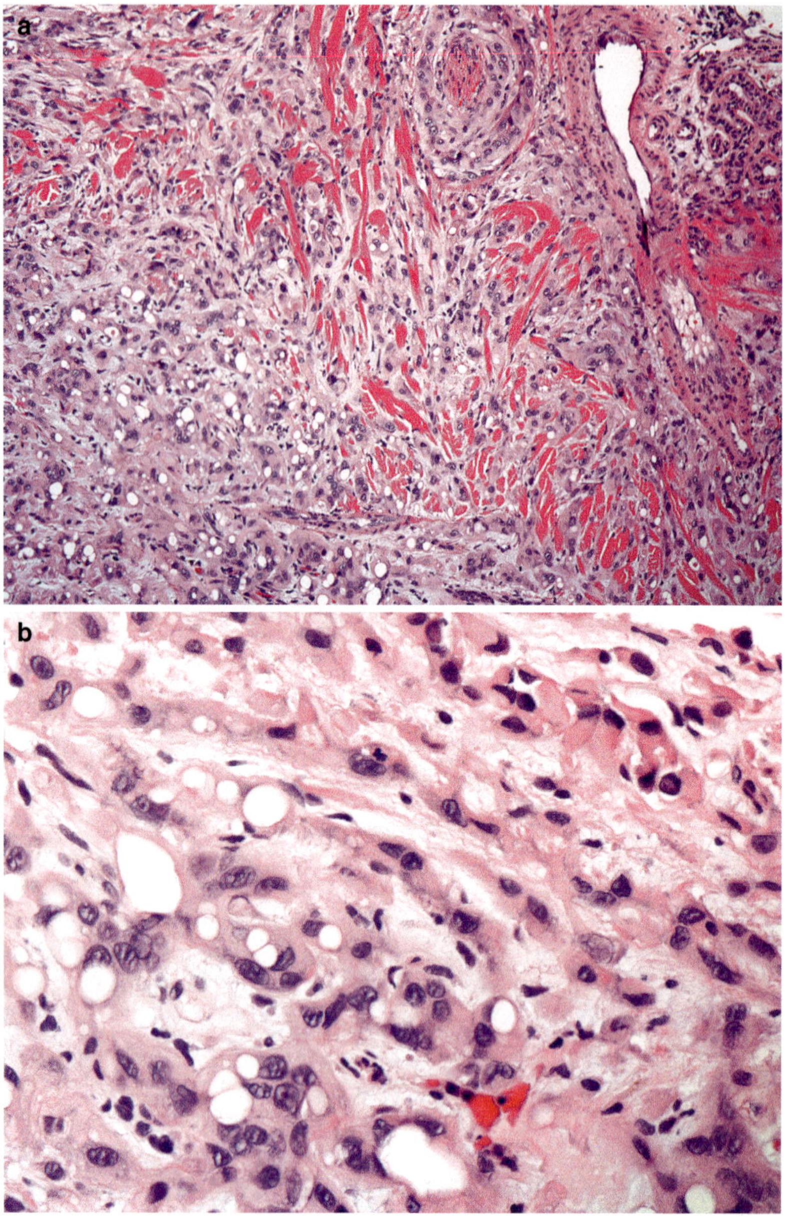

Fig. 7.51 Epithelioid hemangioendothelioma. (**a**) The tumor is composed of cords and nests of epithelioid tumor cells infiltrating the dermis. (**b**) Higher power image demonstrating cords of epithelioid endothelial cells, many with intracytoplasmic vacuoles

seen in up to 25% of cases. These lesions are immunoreactive for vascular markers CD31, CD34, and ERG. Rare cases may lose expression of CD34 or CD31. Importantly, approximately 25% of cases will also show immunoreactivity for cytokeratin, but it is typically less intense than the immunoreactivity seen for vascular markers.

There has been recent insight into the molecular pathogenesis of this entity. It is now known that this tumor has a consistent recurring t(1;3) resulting in a *WWTR1-CAMTA1* fusion transcript. *WWTR1* is a transcription factor highly expressed in endothelial cells, while *CAMTA1* is a transcription regulatory protein usually expressed in the brain. FISH to detect rearrangement of *CAMTA1* can be a useful ancillary diagnostic tool in difficult cases. Nuclear immunoreactivity for CAMTA1 by immunohis-

Table 7.29 Key pathologic features: epithelioid hemangioendothelioma

Cord-like growth pattern of small epithelioid endothelial cells
Intracytoplasmic vacuoles
Myxohyaline stroma
Immunophenotype
Positive for CD31, CD34, ERG, CAMTA1, 25% positive for cytokeratin
t(1;3) *WWTR1-CAMTA1* fusion

tochemistry is seen in over 90% of cases and represents an effective means of confirming the diagnosis, as other vascular tumors lack expression of this marker (Table 7.29).

Differential Diagnosis

The differential diagnosis of epithelioid hemangioendothelioma includes epithelioid sarcoma and pseudomyogenic (epithelioid sarcoma-like) hemangioendothelioma. These tumors have different growth patterns and immunophenotypes. Epithelioid sarcoma typically has a more solid, nodular proliferation of epithelioid cells, often with foci of central necrosis reminiscent of necrotizing granulomas. Epithelioid sarcoma demonstrates strong keratin and epithelial membrane antigen immunoreactivity, and approximately 50–60% of cases are positive for CD34; epithelioid sarcoma is negative for CD31 and shows loss of INI-1 (SMARCB1) expression. Pseudomyogenic (epithelioid sarcoma-like) hemangioendothelioma has a more solid, sheet-like growth pattern of epithelioid-to-spindled cells and is consistently negative for CD34 (see above). The growth pattern of epithelioid hemangioendothelioma can also cause confusion with metastatic carcinoma, especially metastatic breast or signet ring cell carcinomas of the GI tract which often have a cord-like arrangement of tumor cells. Cutaneous mixed tumors and related myoepitheliomas can also have a cord-like-to-nested growth pattern and have a similar appearing stroma. Evidence of true ductal lumen formation, when present, can aid in the distinction, as EHE does not demonstrate ductal differentiation. These tumors are negative for vascular markers.

Angiosarcoma

Clinical Features

Angiosarcoma may be primary cutaneous or secondary tumors related to radiation therapy or chronic lymphedema (see section below). Primary cutaneous angiosarcoma, with few exceptions, presents in the sun-damaged skin of the head and neck, implicating ultraviolet radiation as an etiological factor. Cutaneous angiosarcomas frequently begin as subtle bruise-like areas that subsequently progress to solitary or multiple violaceous nodules and/or plaques. All angiosarcomas are aggressive neoplasms. It is notoriously difficult to achieve negative surgical margins, and local recurrence is frequent, as is metastasis. Favored metastatic sites include the lungs and lymph nodes.

Pathologic Features

Angiosarcoma has a wide range of microscopic appearances. In most cases, there are complex vessels lined by atypical endothelial cells with enlarged hyperchromatic nuclei that dissect through the dermal collagen (Fig. 7.52a, b). Occasional cases can mimic intravascular papillary endothelial hyperplasia (Fig. 7.53). Multilayering of endothelial cells lining lumina and papillae formation are commonly seen (Fig. 7.54). In some cases, the individual tumor cells may not exhibit striking cytologic atypia, but the tumors' growth pattern demonstrates marked architectural complexity. Cases can also contain areas of solid growth (Fig. 7.55), as well as a mixture of solid sheet-like areas and vasoformative channels. In cases with a prominent solid growth pattern, vasoformative channels can usually be seen at the periphery of the tumor. Within solid areas, there usually is evidence of slit-like vascular spaces and intratumoral hemorrhage present. Cases may also have an epithelioid cytomorphology consisting of round cells with relatively abundant cytoplasm. Epithelioid angiosarcoma may have complex vascular channels (Fig. 7.56a) or present as solid sheets of cells (Fig. 7.56b). The tumor cells of epithelioid angiosarcoma often have amphophilic cytoplasm, which represents a clue to the diagnosis.

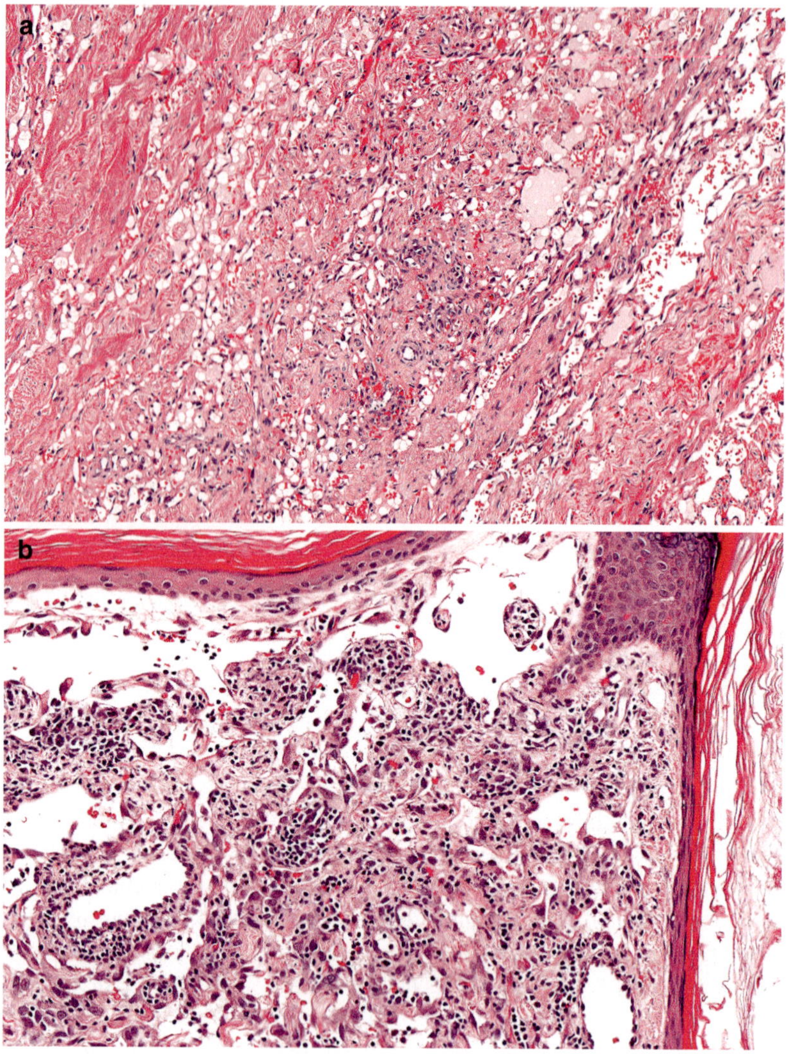

Fig. 7.52 Angiosarcoma. (**a**) Architecturally complex vessels lined by hyperchromatic endothelial cells dissecting through dermal collagen. (**b**) Higher power image demonstrating complex vessels lined by atypical endothelial cells in sun-damaged skin

Angiosarcomas are positive for vascular markers, with CD31 and ERG probably representing the best immunohistochemical markers to confirm endothelial differentiation, as long as one keeps in mind that histiocytes are also immunoreactive for CD31. In predominantly spindled angiosarcomas, CD34 is often a more effective marker than CD31. One should keep in mind the pitfall that epithelioid angiosarcomas can express keratins, EMA, and CD30, presenting potential sources of diagnostic confusion (Table 7.30). Unlike postradiation and lymphedema-associated angiosarcoma, primary cutaneous angiosarcoma is typically negative for MYC expression by immunohistochemistry and *MYC* amplification by FISH (see below).

Differential Diagnosis

The differential diagnosis with other vascular tumors has largely been discussed in previous sections. In summary, the presence of complex vessels lined by atypical endothelial cells in sun-damaged skin should prompt consideration of the diagnosis of angiosarcoma. In small biopsies of spindled forms of angiosarcoma, the differential diagnosis includes sarcomatoid squamous cell carcinoma, spindle cell melanoma, atypical fibroxanthoma, and pleomorphic dermal sarcoma. As

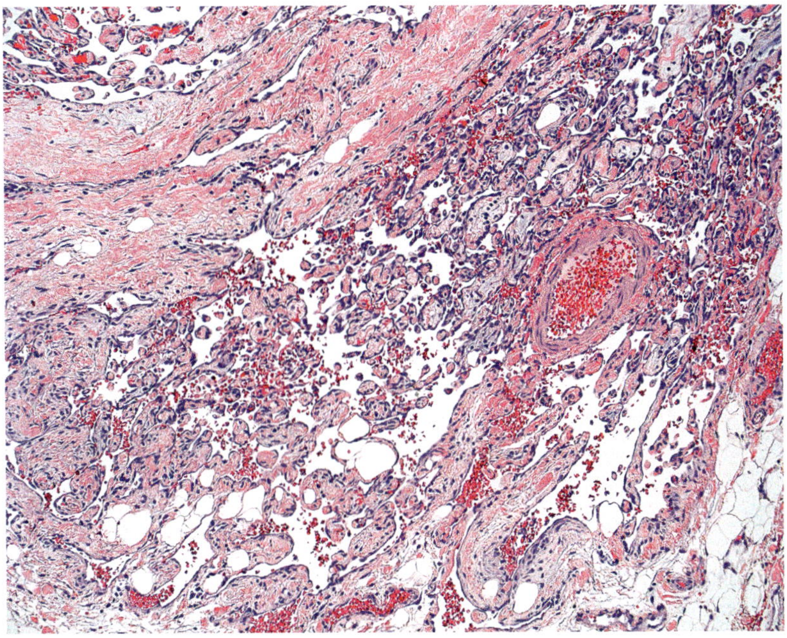

Fig. 7.53 Well-differentiated angiosarcoma mimicking intravascular papillary endothelial hyperplasia. The papillary structures extend outside of the confinements of the vessels and infiltrate adipose tissue

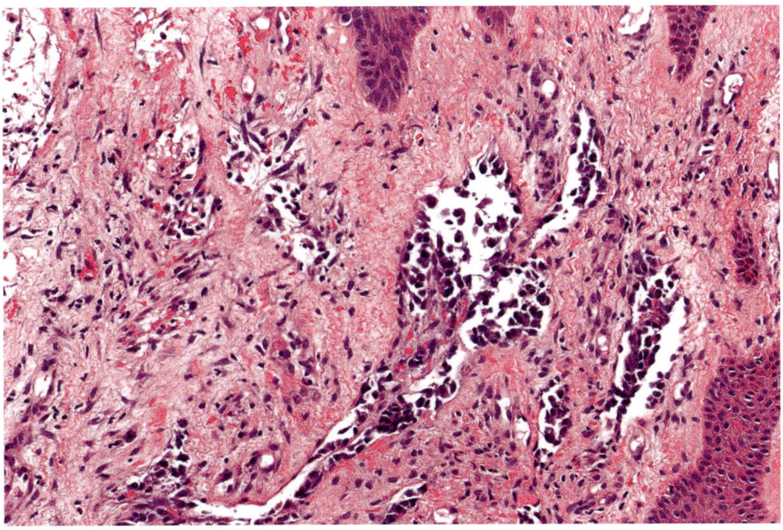

Fig. 7.54 Multilayering of atypical endothelial cells and intravascular papillae are common features of angiosarcoma

previously mentioned, examination of the periphery of spindled angiosarcoma often reveals atypical vascular channels seen in classic angiosarcoma, allowing for the diagnosis. In partially sampled lesions where the periphery is not available for examination, the presence of intratumoral hemorrhage should prompt consideration of angiosarcoma. In this setting, immunostains, especially ERG, should be used to exclude this possibility. In epithelioid angiosarcomas, the differential diagnosis usually includes a poorly differentiated carcinoma. The amphophilic cytoplasm and the presence of hemorrhage are clues to the diagnosis. In cases with CD30 expression, anaplastic large cell lymphoma is a potential consideration. Expression of vascular markers allows distinction from carcinoma and lymphoma.

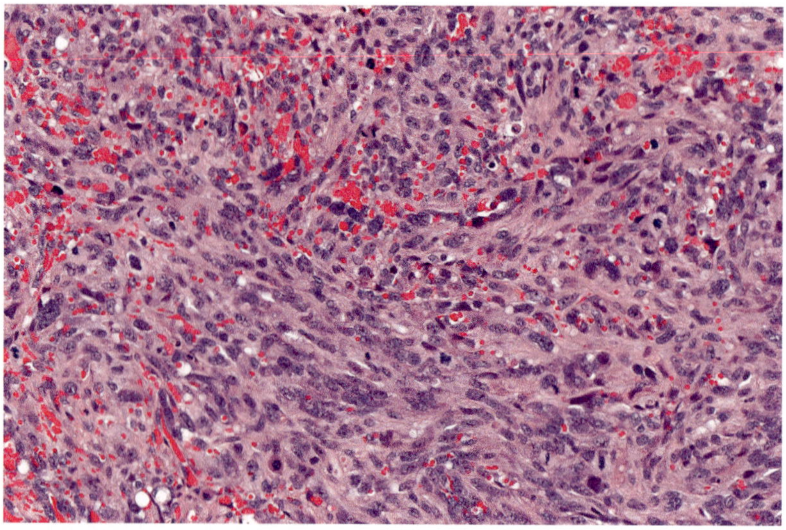

Fig. 7.55 Angiosarcoma with solid sheet-like proliferation of atypical, spindled endothelial cells. Note the intratumoral hemorrhage, a clue to the diagnosis

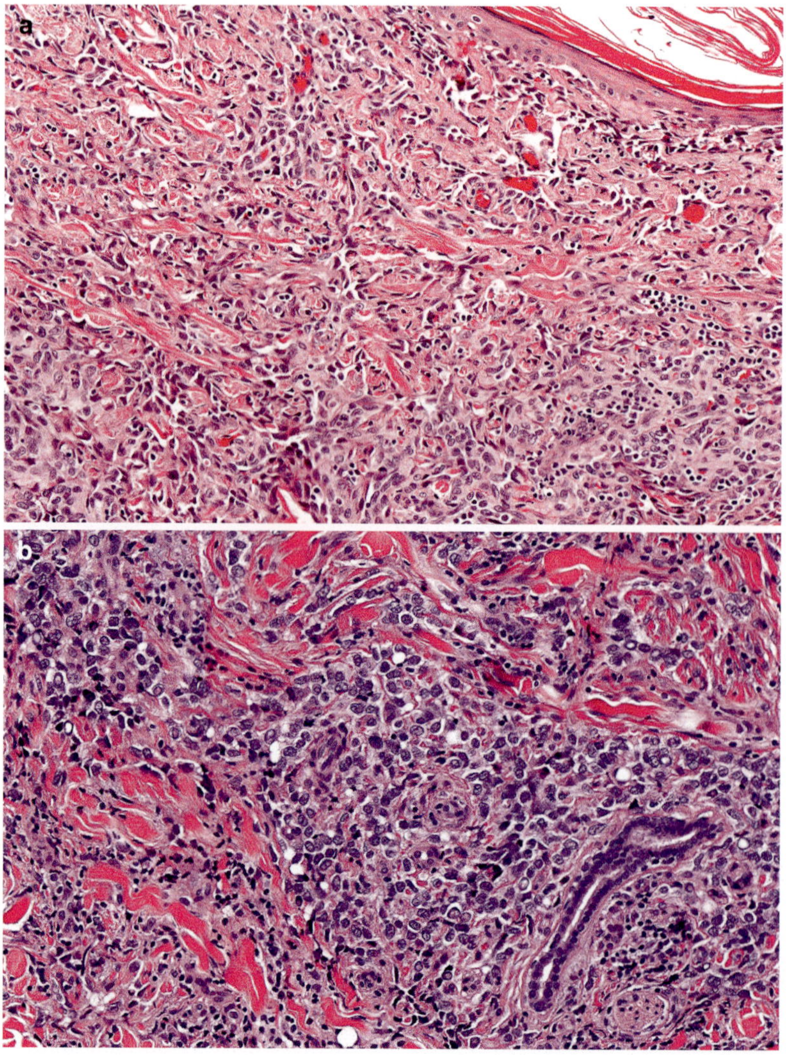

Fig. 7.56 Epithelioid angiosarcoma. (**a**) Architecturally complex vessels lined by combination of atypical hyperchromatic and epithelioid endothelial cells. (**b**) Epithelioid angiosarcoma with solid, sheet-like growth pattern

Table 7.30 Key pathologic features: angiosarcoma

Complex vascular channels to solid sheets
Cytologic atypia
Intratumoral hemorrhage
Immunophenotype
Positive for CD31, CD34, ERG
Pitfall: epithelioid angiosarcoma may be positive for cytokeratins

Radiation- and Lymphedema-Associated Vascular Tumors

Angiosarcoma

Clinical Features

Angiosarcoma can also arise secondary to radiation therapy and chronic lymphedema. Most postradiation angiosarcomas occur in the setting of breast cancer. They arise in the skin in the radiation field, with an average latency of 5 years. It should be noted that they can arise as soon as 1 year after radiation therapy. Radiation-induced angiosarcomas in other clinical settings typically have a latency of 10 years or more. Lymphedema-associated angiosarcoma historically was associated with radical mastectomy (Stewart-Treves syndrome), but with the move to more conservative surgical approaches, this is now uncommon. Lymphedema-associated angiosarcoma can be seen secondary to any cause of chronic lymphedema, such as morbid obesity or lymphedema secondary to filariasis. Lymphedema-associated angiosarcomas typically have a latency of 10 years or more. The clinical presentation of these lesions is similar to that of primary angiosarcoma, namely, expanding violaceous plaques, which may contain nodular areas.

Like primary cutaneous angiosarcoma, secondary angiosarcoma is an aggressive tumor with high rate of local recurrence and frequent metastasis to the lungs and lymph nodes. Interestingly, radiation-associated angiosarcomas arising in the skin of the breast may also metastasize to the contralateral breast. Surgery is the treatment of choice.

Pathologic Features

Secondary angiosarcomas have the same range of histologic features as conventional angiosarcoma. Two unusual histologic patterns have been described in cutaneous radiation-associated angiosarcoma of the breast: the capillary lobule pattern and the so-called radiation dermatitis-like pattern. In the capillary lobule pattern, there are distinct nodules of atypical vessels somewhat reminiscent of the cannonball pattern of tufted angioma (Fig. 7.57). In the radiation dermatitis-like pattern, there are individual atypical cells and noncomplex worm-like vessels lined by atypical endothelial cells (Fig. 7.58a, b). Radiation and lymphedema-associated angiosarcomas are positive for routine vascular markers. More than 90% of cases also have amplification of *MYC*, which can be detected by FISH. This group of angiosarcomas also has nuclear expression of MYC that can be demonstrated by immunohistochemistry (Table 7.31). Immunohistochemistry is an effective surrogate for FISH in most cases, but if there is any doubt with an individual case, FISH is the preferred technique.

Differential Diagnosis

Except in the case of well-differentiated angiosarcomas or cases with subtle histologic features, the differential diagnosis is rarely problematic. Radiation-induced atypical vascular lesion is the most problematic differential diagnosis. This is discussed in more detail below.

Radiation-Induced Atypical Vascular Lesion

Clinical Features

Postradiation atypical vascular lesions typically present in the radiation field on the skin of the breast in women with breast cancer treated conservatively with lumpectomy and adjuvant radiation therapy. On average, atypical vascular lesions present approximately 3 years after radiation therapy but can present in as little as 1 year to many years after radiation. They typically

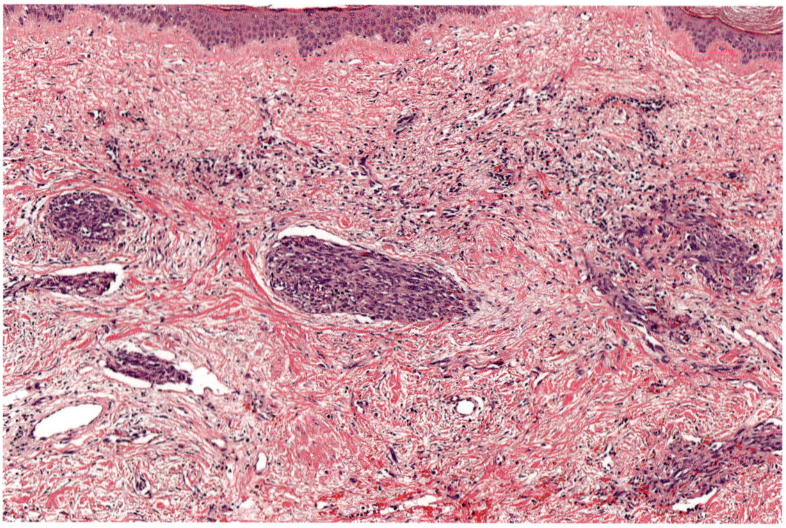

Fig. 7.57 Capillary lobule pattern of postradiation angiosarcoma characterized by discrete lobules of atypical endothelial cells

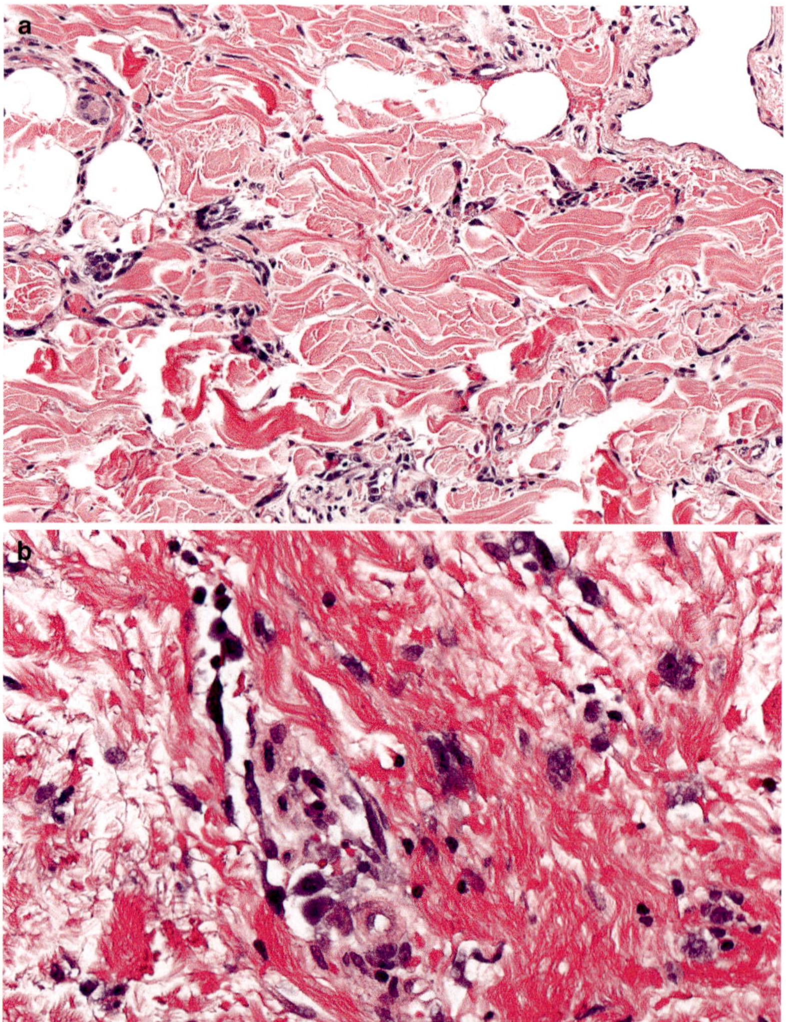

Fig. 7.58 Radiation dermatitis pattern of postradiation angiosarcoma. (**a**) Scattered atypical endothelial cells and focal vascular channel formation. (**b**) Note the associated hemorrhage and worm-like vascular channels lined by hyperchromatic endothelial cells

present as small solitary or multiple (0.1–6 cm) skin-colored to red papules or nodules within the radiation field. Sometimes they can be vesicular similar to cutaneous lymphatic malformations, and in the past, this variant has also been referred to as benign lymphangiomatous papule. Clinically, they pursue a benign clinical course, with only rare examples of angiosarcoma arising within AVLs. If completely excised, they do not recur, but new atypical vascular lesions can develop over time. If clinically feasible, conservative excision is recommended.

Pathologic Features

Microscopically, atypical vascular lesions are relatively well-circumscribed and symmetrical with a vaguely wedge-shaped silhouette. The well-formed vascular structures comprising the lesion are usually confined to the papillary and superficial-to-mid reticular dermis. In rare cases, the lesion may extend to the subcutis. The superficial portion typically contains more dilated vascular spaces than the deeper aspect. In the deeper component, the vessels are compressed and may show a dissecting pattern between collagen bundles. The vessels are lined by a single layer of endothelial cells. Some cases have papillary projections formed by the underlying stroma, but multilayering of endothelial cells and mitotic figures are not present. They have been divided into two histologic patterns: (1) lymphatic type and (2) vascular type. The former histologically mimics a cutaneous lymphatic malformation with ectatic vessels (Fig. 7.59), while the latter presents as well-formed small vessels lined by hobnail endothelial cells (Fig. 7.60), resembling hobnail lymphatic malformation (hobnail hemangioma) or acquired progressive lymphangioma. Both patterns tend to lack the multilayering of endothelial cells and show only mild, if any, cytologic atypia in the form of nuclear hyperchromasia and hobnailing (Table 7.32).

Table 7.31 Key pathologic features: radiation- and lymphedema-associated angiosarcoma

Most cases similar to conventional angiosarcoma
Rare deceptively bland cases
MYC amplification by FISH
Nuclear expression of MYC by immunohistochemistry

Differential Diagnosis

The primary differential diagnosis is with well-differentiated, postradiation angiosarcoma. The relative circumscription of atypical vascular lesions, bland cytology, and lack of multilayering typically allow distinction in most cases. However, sampling is critical, and the entire lesion needs to be visualized, particularly the base, before a diagnosis of atypical vascular lesion can be confidently rendered. Ancillary studies to detect *MYC*

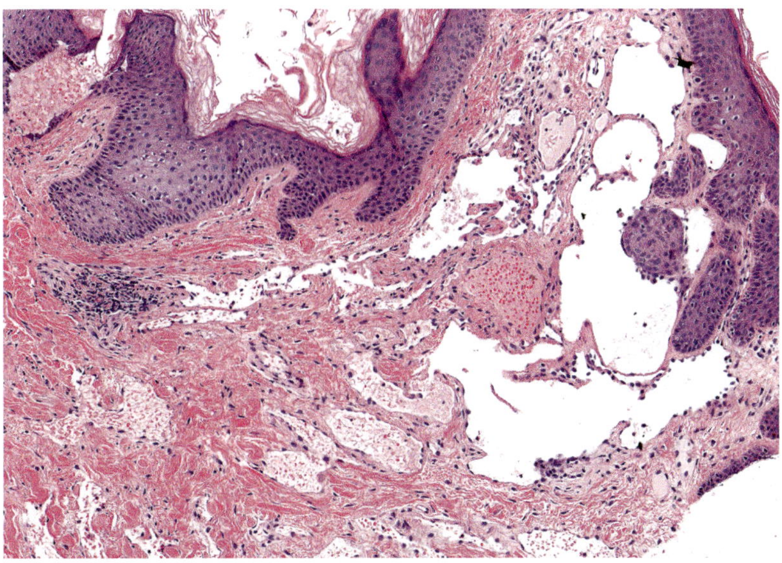

Fig. 7.59 Atypical vascular lesion, lymphatic type characterized by dilated vessels resembling cutaneous lymphatic malformation in the superficial dermis

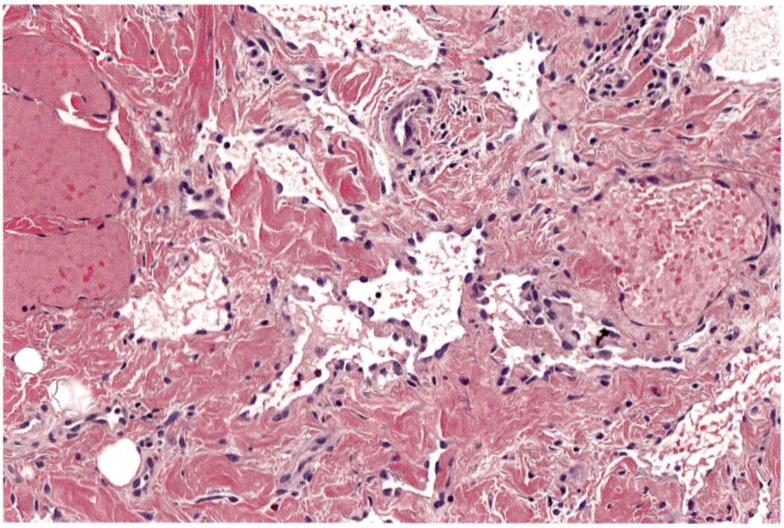

Fig. 7.60 Atypical vascular lesion, vascular type, characterized by vessels lined by hobnail endothelial cells resembling hobnail lymphatic malformation

Table 7.32 Key pathologic features: atypical vascular lesion

Small, circumscribed lesions
Generally confined to the dermis
Lymphatic type
Most common type
Ectatic vessels in dermis resembling lymphangioma
Hobnail endothelial cells
No overt nuclear cytologic atypia or mitotic activity
Vascular type
Capillary-like vessels
Hobnail endothelial cells
No overt nuclear cytologic atypia or mitotic activity
Negative for *MYC* amplification by FISH and MYC expression by immunohistochemistry

amplification or MYC expression are very useful. Unlike postradiation angiosarcoma, atypical vascular lesion lacks *MYC* amplification. It should be noted that focal MYC expression in atypical vascular lesions detected by immunohistochemistry has been reported, but they lack the diffuse strong nuclear expression of radiation-associated angiosarcoma.

Selected References

1. Antonescu CR, Le Loarer F, Mosquera JM, Sboner A, Zhang L, Chen CL, Chen HW, Pathan N, Krausz T, Dickson BC, Weinreb I, Rubin MA, Hameed M, Fletcher CD. Novel YAP1-TFE3 fusion defines a distinct subset of epithelioid hemangioendothelioma. Genes Chromosomes Cancer. 2013;52(8):775–84.
2. Ayturk UM, Couto JA, Hann S, Mulliken JB, Williams KL, Huang AY, Fishman SJ, Boyd TK, Kozakewich HP, Bischoff J, Greene AK, Warman ML. Somatic activating mutations in GNAQ and GNA11 are associated with congenital hemangioma. Am J Hum Genet. 2016;98(4):789–95.
3. Billings SD, Folpe AL, Weiss SW. Epithelioid sarcoma-like hemangioendothelioma. Am J Surg Pathol. 2003;27(1):48–57.
4. Billings SD, McKenney JK, Folpe AL, Hardacre MC, Weiss SW. Cutaneous angiosarcoma following breast-conserving surgery and radiation: an analysis of 27 cases. Am J Surg Pathol. 2004;28(6):781–8.
5. Brenn T, Fletcher CD. Cutaneous epithelioid angiomatous nodule: a distinct lesion in the morphologic spectrum of epithelioid vascular tumors. Am J Dermatopathol. 2004;26(1):14–21.
6. Brenn T, Fletcher CD. Radiation-associated cutaneous atypical vascular lesions and angiosarcoma: clinicopathologic analysis of 42 cases. Am J Surg Pathol. 2005;29(8):983–96.
7. Calonje E, Fletcher CD, Wilson-Jones E, Rosai J. Retiform hemangioendothelioma. A distinctive form of low-grade angiosarcoma delineated in a series of 15 cases. Am J Surg Pathol. 1994;18(2):115–25.
8. Couto JA, Vivero MP, Kozakewich HP, Taghinia AH, Mulliken JB, Warman ML, Greene AK. A somatic MAP3K3 mutation is associated with verrucous venous malformation. Am J Hum Genet. 2015;96(3):480–6.
9. Deyrup AT, Tighiouart M, Montag AG, Weiss SW. Epithelioid hemangioendothelioma of soft tissue: a proposal for risk stratification based on 49 cases. Am J Surg Pathol. 2008;32(6):924–7.
10. Doyle LA, Fletcher CD, Hornick JL. Nuclear expression of CAMTA1 distinguishes epithelioid Hemangioendothelioma from histologic mimics. Am J Surg Pathol. 2016;40(1):94–102.
11. Duprez R, Lacoste V, Brière J, Couppié P, Frances C, Sainte-Marie D, Kassa-Kelembho E, Lando

MJ, Essame Oyono JL, Nkegoum B, Hbid O, Mahé A, Lebbé C, Tortevoye P, Huerre M, Gessain A. Evidence for a multiclonal origin of multicentric advanced lesions of Kaposi sarcoma. J Natl Cancer Inst. 2007;99(14):1086–94.

12. Fanburg-Smith JC, Michal M, Partanen TA, Alitalo K, Miettinen M. Papillary intralymphatic angioendothelioma (PILA): a report of twelve cases of a distinctive vascular tumor with phenotypic features of lymphatic vessels. Am J Surg Pathol. 1999;23(9):1004–10.
13. Fernandez AP, Sun Y, Tubbs RR, Goldblum JR, Billings SD. FISH for MYC amplification and anti-MYC immunohistochemistry: useful diagnostic tools in the assessment of secondary angiosarcoma and atypical vascular proliferations. J Cutan Pathol. 2012;39(2):234–42.
14. Fineberg S, Rosen PP. Cutaneous angiosarcoma and atypical vascular lesions of the skin and breast after radiation therapy for breast carcinoma. Am J Clin Pathol. 1994;102(6):757–63.
15. Grayson W, Pantanowitz L. Histological variants of cutaneous Kaposi sarcoma. Diagn Pathol. 2008;3:31.
16. Gurbuz Y, Muezzinoglu B, Apaydin R, Yumbul AZ. Acral arteriovenous tumor (cirsoid aneurysm): clinical and histopathological analysis of 6 cases. Adv Clin Pathol. 2002;6(1):25–9.
17. Hornick JL, Fletcher CD. Pseudomyogenic hemangioendothelioma: a distinctive, often multicentric tumor with indolent behavior. Am J Surg Pathol. 2011;35(2):190–201.
18. Huang SC, Zhang L, Sung YS, Chen CL, Krausz T, Dickson BC, Kao YC, Agaram NP, Fletcher CD, Antonescu CR. Frequent FOS gene rearrangements in epithelioid hemangioma: a molecular study of 58 cases with morphologic reappraisal. Am J Surg Pathol. 2015;39(10):1313–21.
19. Hung YP, Fletcher CD, Hornick JL. FOSB is a useful diagnostic marker for pseudomyogenic hemangioendothelioma. Am J Surg Pathol. 2017;41(5):596–606.
20. ISSVA Classification of Vascular Anomalies ©2014 International Society for the Study of Vascular Anomalies. Available at issva.org/classification. Accessed 1 Nov 2017.
21. Ji Y, Chen S, Xiang B, Li K, Xu Z, Yao W, Lu G, Liu X, Xia C, Wang Q, Li Y, Wang C, Yang K, Yang G, Tang X, Xu T, Wu H. Sirolimus for the treatment of progressive kaposiform hemangioendothelioma: a multicenter retrospective study. Int J Cancer. 2017;141(4):848–55.
22. Joethy J, Al Jajeh I, Tay SC. Intravenous pyogenic granuloma of the hand – a case report. Hand Surg. 2011;16(1):87–9.
23. Ko JS, Billings SD. Diagnostically challenging epithelioid vascular tumors. Surg Pathol Clin. 2015;8(3):331–51.
24. Kurek KC, Pansuriya TC, van Ruler MA, van den Akker B, Luks VL, Verbeke SL, Kozakewich HP, Sciot R, Lev D, Lazar AJ, Fletcher CD, Bovée JV. R132C IDH1 mutations are found in spindle cell hemangiomas and not in other vascular tumors or malformations. Am J Pathol. 2013;182(5):1494–500.
25. Lawley LP, Cerimele F, Weiss SW, North P, Cohen C, Kozakewich HP, Mulliken JB, Arbiser JL. Expression of Wilms tumor 1 gene distinguishes vascular malformations from proliferative endothelial lesions. Arch Dermatol. 2005;141(10):1297–300.
26. Le Huu AR, Jokinen CH, Rubin BP, Mihm MC, Weiss SW, North PE, Dadras SS. Expression of prox1, lymphatic endothelial nuclear transcription factor, in Kaposiform hemangioendothelioma and tufted angioma. Am J Surg Pathol. 2010;34(11):1563–73.
27. Limaye N, Wouters V, Uebelhoer M, Tuominen M, Wirkkala R, Mulliken JB, Eklund L, Boon LM, Vikkula M. Somatic mutations in angiopoietin receptor gene TEK cause solitary and multiple sporadic venous malformations. Nat Genet. 2009;41(1):118–24.
28. Lyons LL, North PE, Mac-Moune Lai F, Stoler MH, Folpe AL, Weiss SW. Kaposiform hemangioendothelioma: a study of 33 cases emphasizing its pathologic, immunophenotypic, and biologic uniqueness from juvenile hemangioma. Am J Surg Pathol. 2004;28(5):559–68.
29. Martorell-Calatayud A, Balmer N, Sanmartín O, Díaz-Recuero JL, Sangueza OP. Definition of the features of acquired elastotic hemangioma reporting the clinical and histopathological characteristics of 14 patients. J Cutan Pathol. 2010;37(4):460–4.
30. Marušić Z, Billings SD. Histopathology of spindle cell vascular tumors. Surg Pathol Clin. 2017;10(2):345–66.
31. McMenamin ME, Fletcher CD. Reactive angioendotheliomatosis: a study of 15 cases demonstrating a wide clinicopathologic spectrum. Am J Surg Pathol. 2002;26(6):685–97.
32. Napekoski KM, Fernandez AP, Billings SD. Microvenular hemangioma: a clinicopathologic review of 13 cases. J Cutan Pathol. 2014;41(11):816–22.
33. Nätynki M, Kangas J, Miinalainen I, Sormunen R, Pietilä R, Soblet J, Boon LM, Vikkula M, Limaye N, Eklund L. Common and specific effects of TIE2 mutations causing venous malformations. Hum Mol Genet. 2015;24(22):6374–89.
34. Nayler SJ, Rubin BP, Calonje E, Chan JK, Fletcher CD. Composite hemangioendothelioma: a complex, low-grade vascular lesion mimicking angiosarcoma. Am J Surg Pathol. 2000;24(3):352–61.
35. North PE. Pediatric vascular tumors and malformations. Surg Pathol Clin. 2010;3(3):455–94.
36. North PE, Waner M, Mizeracki A, Mihm MC Jr. GLUT1: a newly discovered immunohistochemical marker for juvenile hemangiomas. Hum Pathol. 2000;31(1):11–22.
37. North PE, Waner M, Mizeracki A, Mrak RE, Nicholas R, Kincannon J, Suen JY, Mihm MC Jr. A unique microvascular phenotype shared by juvenile hemangiomas and human placenta. Arch Dermatol. 2001;137(5):559–70.
38. O'Donnell PJ, Pantanowitz L, Grayson W. Unique histologic variants of cutaneous Kaposi sarcoma. Am J Dermatopathol. 2010;32(3):244–50.
39. Parsons A, Sheehan DJ, Sangueza OP. Retiform hemangioendotheliomas usually do not express

D2-40 and VEGFR-3. Am J Dermatopathol. 2008;30(1):31–3.
40. Patton KT, Deyrup AT, Weiss SW. Atypical vascular lesions after surgery and radiation of the breast: a clinicopathologic study of 32 cases analyzing histologic heterogeneity and association with angiosarcoma. Am J Surg Pathol. 2008;32(6):943–50.
41. Perez MC, Padhya TA, Messina JL, Jackson RS, Gonzalez RJ, Bui MM, Letson GD, Cruse CW, Lavey RS, Cheong D, Forster MR, Fulp WJ, Sondak VK, Zager JS. Cutaneous angiosarcoma: a single-institution experience. Ann Surg Oncol. 2013;20(11):3391–7.
42. Perkins P, Weiss SW. Spindle cell hemangioendothelioma. An analysis of 78 cases with reassessment of its pathogenesis and biologic behavior. Am J Surg Pathol. 1996;20(10):1196–204.
43. Perry KD, Al-Lbraheemi A, Rubin BP, Jen J, Ren H, Jang JS, Nair A, Davila J, Pambuccian S, Horvai A, Sukov W, Tazelaar HD, Folpe AL. Composite hemangioendothelioma with neuroendocrine marker expression: an aggressive variant. Mod Pathol. 2017;30(11):1589–602.
44. Requena L, Kutzner H. Hemangioendothelioma. Semin Diagn Pathol. 2013;30(1):29–44.
45. Requena L, Sangueza OP. Cutaneous vascular anomalies. Part I. Hamartomas, malformations, and dilation of preexisting vessels. J Am Acad Dermatol. 1997a;37(4):523–49. quiz 549–52.
46. Requena L, Sangueza OP. Cutaneous vascular proliferation. Part II. Hyperplasias and benign neoplasms. J Am Acad Dermatol. 1997b;37(6):887–919. quiz 920–2.
47. Requena L, Sangueza OP. Cutaneous vascular proliferations. Part III. Malignant neoplasms, other cutaneous neoplasms with significant vascular component, and disorders erroneously considered as vascular neoplasms. J Am Acad Dermatol. 1998;38(2 Pt 1):143–75. quiz 176–8.
48. Sangüeza OP, Walsh SN, Sheehan DJ, Orland AF, Llombart B, Requena L. Cutaneous epithelioid angiomatous nodule: a case series and proposed classification. Am J Dermatopathol. 2008;30(1):16–20.
49. Shon W, Billings SD. Cutaneous malignant vascular neoplasms. Clin Lab Med. 2017;37(3):633–46.
50. Suurmeijer AJ, Fletcher CD. Papillary haemangioma. A distinctive cutaneous haemangioma of the head and neck area containing eosinophilic hyaline globules. Histopathology. 2007;51(5):638–48.
51. Tanas MR, Sboner A, Oliveira AM, Erickson-Johnson MR, Hespelt J, Hanwright PJ, Flanagan J, Luo Y, Fenwick K, Natrajan R, Mitsopoulos C, Zvelebil M, Hoch BL, Weiss SW, Debiec-Rychter M, Sciot R, West RB, Lazar AJ, Ashworth A, Reis-Filho JS, Lord CJ, Gerstein MB, Rubin MA, Rubin BP. Identification of a disease-defining gene fusion in epithelioid hemangioendothelioma. Sci Transl Med. 2011;3(98):98ra82.
52. Ten Broek RW, Bekers EM, de Leng WWJ, Strengman E, Tops BBJ, Kutzner H, Leeuwis JW, van Gorp JM, Creytens DH, Mentzel T, van Diest PJ, Eijkelenboom A, Flucke U. Mutational analysis using Sanger and next generation sequencing in sporadic spindle cell hemangiomas: a study of 19 cases. Genes Chromosomes Cancer. 2017;56(12):855–60.
53. Tennant LB, Mulliken JB, Perez-Atayde AR, Kozakewich HP. Verrucous hemangioma revisited. Pediatr Dermatol. 2006;23(3):208–15.
54. Tollefson MM, McEvoy MT, Torgerson RR, Bridges AG. Diffuse dermal angiomatosis of the breast: clinicopathologic study of 5 patients. J Am Acad Dermatol. 2014;71(6):1212–7.
55. Tong PL, Beer TW. Acquired elastotic hemangioma: ten cases with immunohistochemistry refuting a lymphatic origin in most lesions. J Cutan Pathol. 2010;37(12):1259–60.
56. Trindade F, Kutzner H, Tellechea Ó, Requena L, Colmenero I. Hobnail hemangioma reclassified as superficial lymphatic malformation: a study of 52 cases. J Am Acad Dermatol. 2012;66(1):112–5.
57. Tsang WY, Chan JK. Bacillary angiomatosis. A "new" disease with a broadening clinicopathologic spectrum. Histol Histopathol. 1992;7(1):143–52.
58. Verma SB, Vasani R. Stewart-Bluefarb syndrome revisited. Clin Exp Dermatol. 2016;41(5):522–5.
59. Wang L, Gao T, Wang G. Cutaneous lymphatic malformation characterized by swelling of digits: a report of six cases. J Cutan Pathol. 2014;41(5):451–6.
60. Yuri T, Yamazaki F, Takasu K, Shikata N, Tsubura A. Glomeruloid hemangioma. Pathol Int. 2008;58(6):390–5.

8 Perivascular Tumors

Steven D. Billings and Rajiv M. Patel

Abstract

This chapter focuses on a group of tumors that arise from perivascular "myoid" modified smooth muscle cells that invest blood vessels. This family of tumors includes angioleiomyoma, glomus tumor, glomuvenous malformation (glomangioma), glomangiomyoma, myopericytoma, myofibroma, glomus tumor of uncertain malignant potential, and malignant glomus tumor. This group of tumors, consisting of round to spindled cells that invest a proliferation of bland blood vessels, shows significant histologic and immunophenotypic overlap. Indeed, perivascular myoid cell tumors are often hybrid lesions that demonstrate a combination of histopathologic features of the aforementioned entities.

Angioleiomyoma

Clinical Features

Angioleiomyoma, also known as angiomyoma, is now considered to be part of the spectrum of pericytic tumors rather than smooth muscle neoplasms. They usually present on the extremities, especially the legs of middle-aged adults, as solitary nodules. The lesions are often painful, though not as commonly so as pilar leiomyomas. Women are more often affected than men (M:F, 1:2), except with respect to tumors arising in the head and neck, where men are more commonly affected. Rare acral cases have been described.

Pathologic Features

Angioleiomyomas are well-circumscribed tumors composed of interspersed vessels of varying thickness, which present in the subcutis or deep dermis. Classically, the vessels are relatively thick-walled (Fig. 8.1a), but this is not always the case. The tumor cells surrounding the vascular lumens often have a concentric pattern of growth that blends in with the surrounding smooth muscle (Fig. 8.1b), imparting substantial histologic overlap with myopericytoma. Myxoid change, thrombosis, and calcification are commonly seen. Rare cases have an epithelioid morphology or associated adipocytes. Degenerative atypia is rarely seen (so-called symplastic angioleiomyoma), and mitotic activity is typically absent. Nuclear palisading may rarely be present. Constituent tumor cells are positive for SMA, desmin, and H-caldesmon (Table 8.1).

S. D. Billings (✉)
Department of Pathology, Cleveland Clinic, Cleveland, OH, USA
e-mail: billins@ccf.org

R. M. Patel
Department of Pathology, University of Michigan Medical School, Ann Arbor, MI, USA

S. D. Billings et al. (eds.), *Soft Tissue Tumors of the Skin*,
https://doi.org/10.1007/978-1-4939-8812-9_8

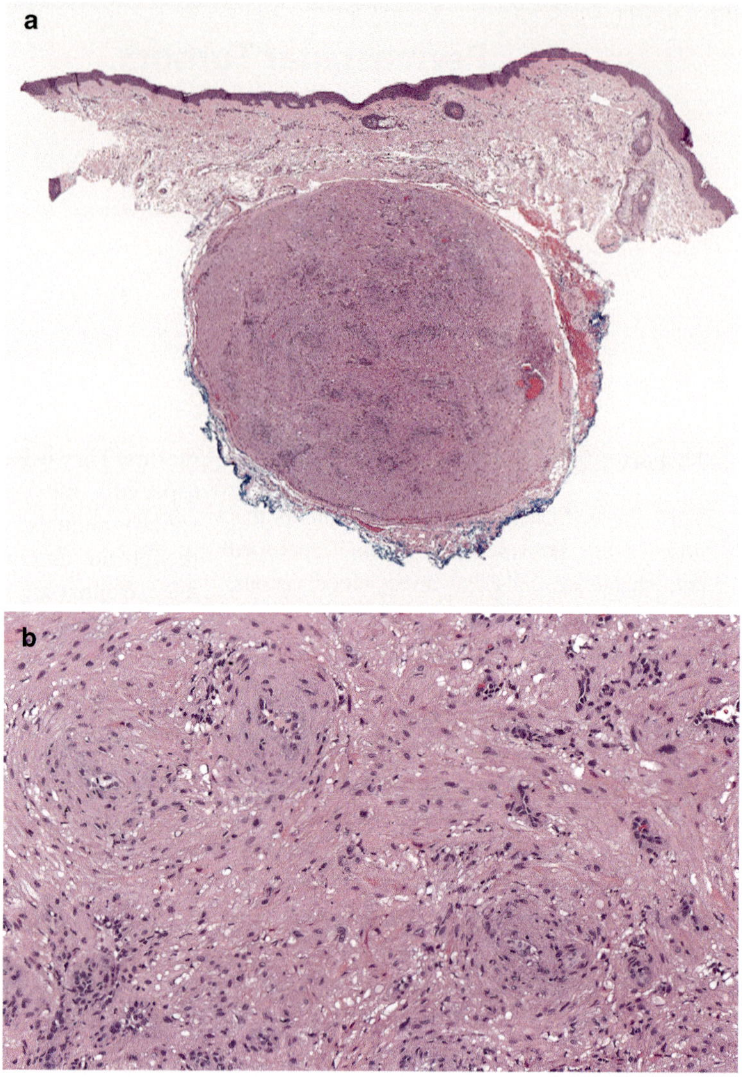

Fig. 8.1 Angioleiomyoma. (**a**) Low-power view of angioleiomyoma within the dermis. The lesion is composed of a well-circumscribed proliferation of blood vessels surrounded by smooth muscle, (**b**) high power view demonstrating concentric arrangement of smooth muscle around vessels

Table 8.1 Key pathologic features: angioleiomyoma

Well-circumscribed
Deep dermis and subcutis
Conspicuous vasculature, often thick-walled
Bland smooth muscle cells often concentrically arranged around vessels

Differential Diagnosis

Angioleiomyomas differ from cutaneous leiomyomas in their deeper location, prominent vascular component, and circumscribed nature. Like angioleiomyomas, leiomyosarcomas arising from vessels may be circumscribed, but they usually have some infiltration into surrounding soft tissue, more nuclear atypia and mitotic activity.

Glomus Tumor

Clinical Features

Glomus tumor is the most common member of this family of tumors. It typically presents in young adults in the distal extremities, especially the nail bed, as a small <1 cm painful nodule. Superficial tumors often have a red-blue appearance. Subungual tumors are somewhat more common in women. Glomus tumor is a benign lesion cured by simple excision.

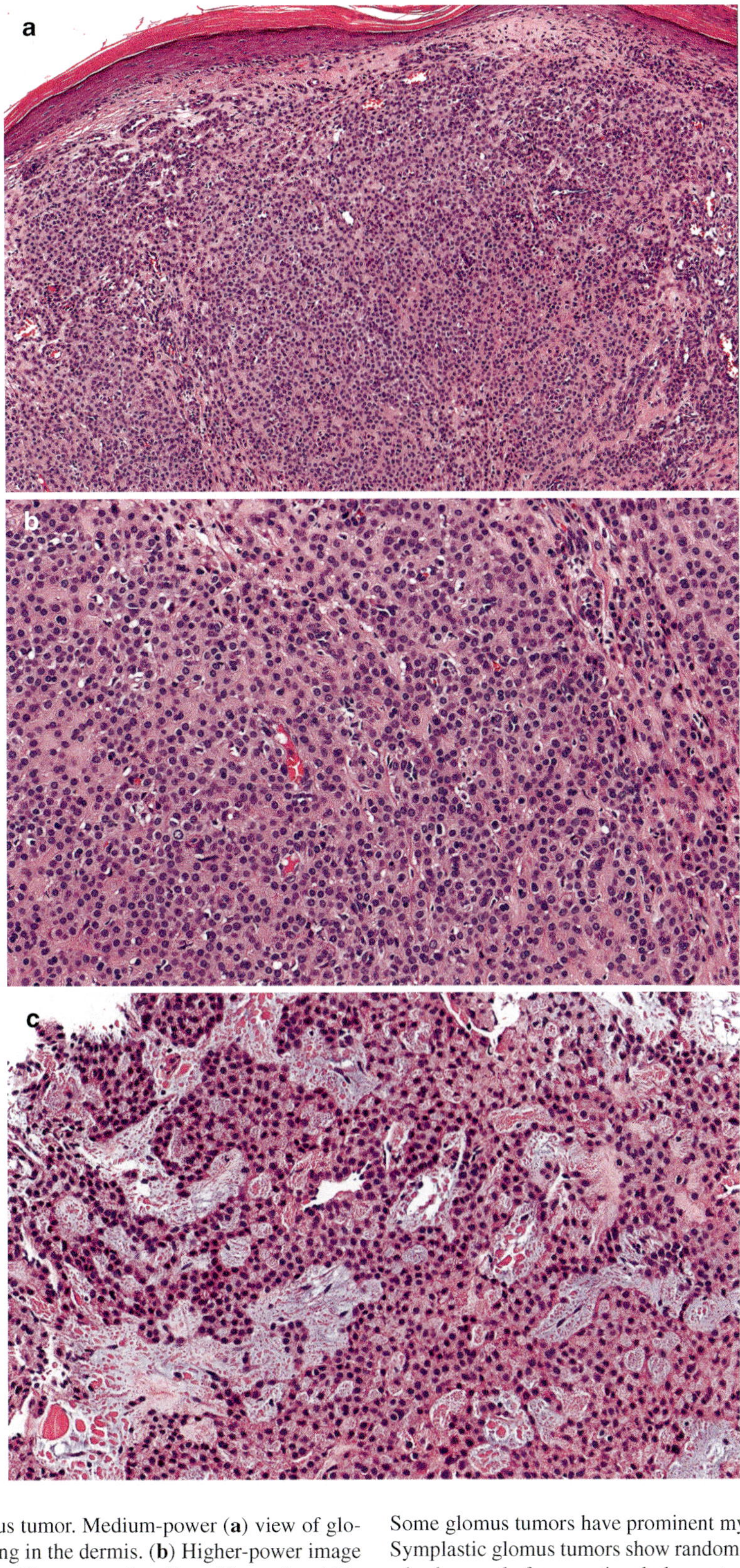

Fig. 8.2 Glomus tumor. Medium-power (**a**) view of glomus tumor arising in the dermis. (**b**) Higher-power image demonstrating uniform round cells with eosinophilic cytoplasm investing delicate capillary vasculature. (**c**) Some glomus tumors have prominent myxoid stroma. (**d**) Symplastic glomus tumors show random nuclear atypia in a background of conventional glomus tumor

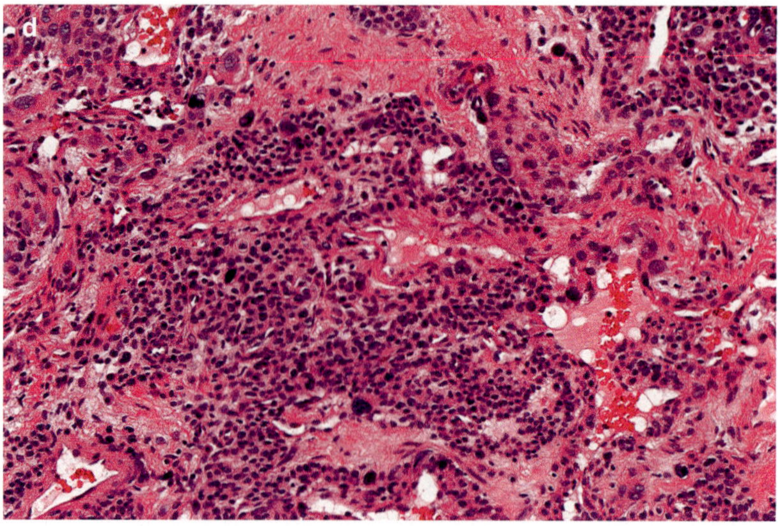

Fig. 8.2 (continued)

Table 8.2 Key pathologic features: glomus tumor

Uniform round to oval cells surrounding thin-walled vessels
SMA+, Type IV collagen+, desmin-
Symplastic glomus tumor: Scattered atypia without mitotic activity or necrosis

Pathologic Features

Glomus tumors typically consist of bland, uniform, round to oval cells arranged in solid nests or sheets that surround thin-walled blood vessels (Fig. 8.2a, b). The stroma investing constituent cells can vary from hyalinized to myxoid (Fig. 8.2c). Mitotic activity and necrosis are absent, though rare cases can show random nuclear atypia that is considered degenerative in nature, so-called symplastic glomus tumors (Fig. 8.2d). By immunohistochemistry, glomus tumors are positive for SMA and H-caldesmon but negative for desmin. Immunostains for type IV collagen highlight basement membrane material surrounding individual tumor cells. These lesions are negative for S100 protein, cytokeratin, and synaptophysin (Table 8.2).

Differential Diagnosis

The primary differential diagnosis is with other members of the perivascular myoid family of tumors detailed below. The closest histologic mimics are glomuvenous malformation and glomangiomyoma. The former has larger ectatic vessels and a thinner layer of surrounding glomus cells, while the latter resembles glomus tumor but with a transition from glomus cells to true smooth muscle. Symplastic glomus tumors need to be distinguished from malignant glomus tumor. The criteria for malignant glomus tumor are discussed below. Occasional cases may be confused with spiradenoma, but glomus tumors lack the two-cell population of that entity, have no ductal differentiation, and are negative for cytokeratins by immunohistochemistry. Similarly, glomus tumors can sometimes be mistaken for neuroendocrine tumors, but the absence of immunoreactivity for cytokeratins, synaptophysin, and chromogranin allows for their distinction. We have encountered rare cases with prominent myxoid stroma that resembled extraskeletal myxoid chondrosarcoma. Extraskeletal myxoid chondrosarcoma lacks the capillary vasculature of glomus tumor, is typically negative for SMA, and presents as a deep soft tissue mass.

Glomuvenous Malformation

Clinical Features

Glomuvenous malformation, formerly known as glomangioma, is typically an autosomal dominant familial tumor (~60%) that arises

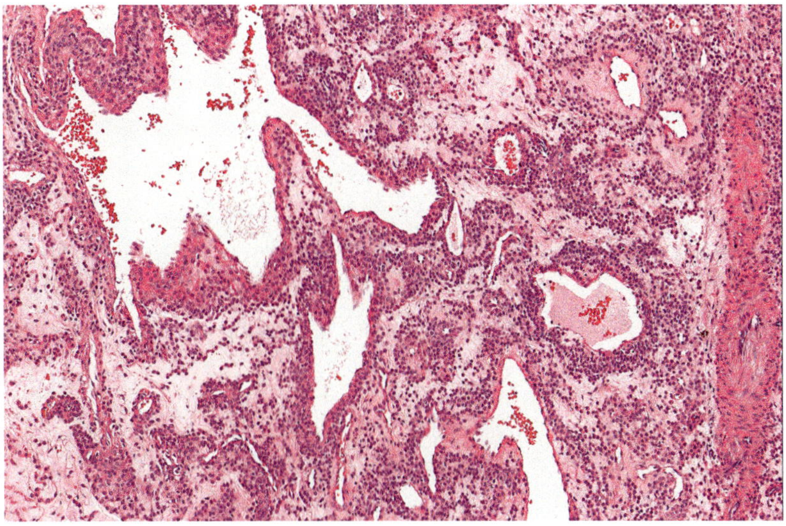

Fig. 8.3 Glomuvenous malformation with ectatic vessels lined by a thin layer of glomus cells

Table 8.3 Key pathologic features: glomuvenous malformation

Usually familial and often multifocal
Ectatic veins lined by clusters or thin layers of glomus cells

secondary to inherited loss of function mutations in *GLMN* (glomulin). Less commonly they are sporadic tumors. Clinically they are bluish-purple papulonodules or plaques with a cobblestone appearance. They can be relatively localized or multifocal, covering large areas of the skin. Most commonly they involve the extremities, but any location may be involved. Glomuvenous malformations tend to be less painful than conventional glomus tumor but are still typically painful upon palpation.

Pathologic Features

Glomuvenous malformations typically present as a large, poorly circumscribed proliferation of thin-walled ectatic vessels, lined by small clusters or thin layers of glomus cells (Fig. 8.3). Rare cases show close association with smooth muscle, hair follicles, and eccrine glands. Constituent cells have the same immunophenotype as conventional glomus tumors. (Table 8.3).

Differential Diagnosis

The ectatic vascular architecture of glomuvenous malformations allows their distinction from conventional glomus tumors. Glomangiomyomas often demonstrate some histologic overlap but also display transition from glomus cells to true smooth muscle. Venous malformations lack perivascular glomus cells.

Glomangiomyoma

Clinical Features

This is a rare subtype of glomus tumor that may have clinical overlap with glomus tumor and glomuvenous malformation. Rarely, it can be multifocal (glomangiomyomatosis).

Pathologic Features

Glomangiomyoma may largely resemble a glomus tumor or a glomuvenous malformation, and represents a defined phenotype along a histologic spectrum that includes these two tumors. In lesions resembling glomus tumor, there is a transition to spindled cells resembling true smooth muscle (Fig. 8.4). In those resembling glomuve-

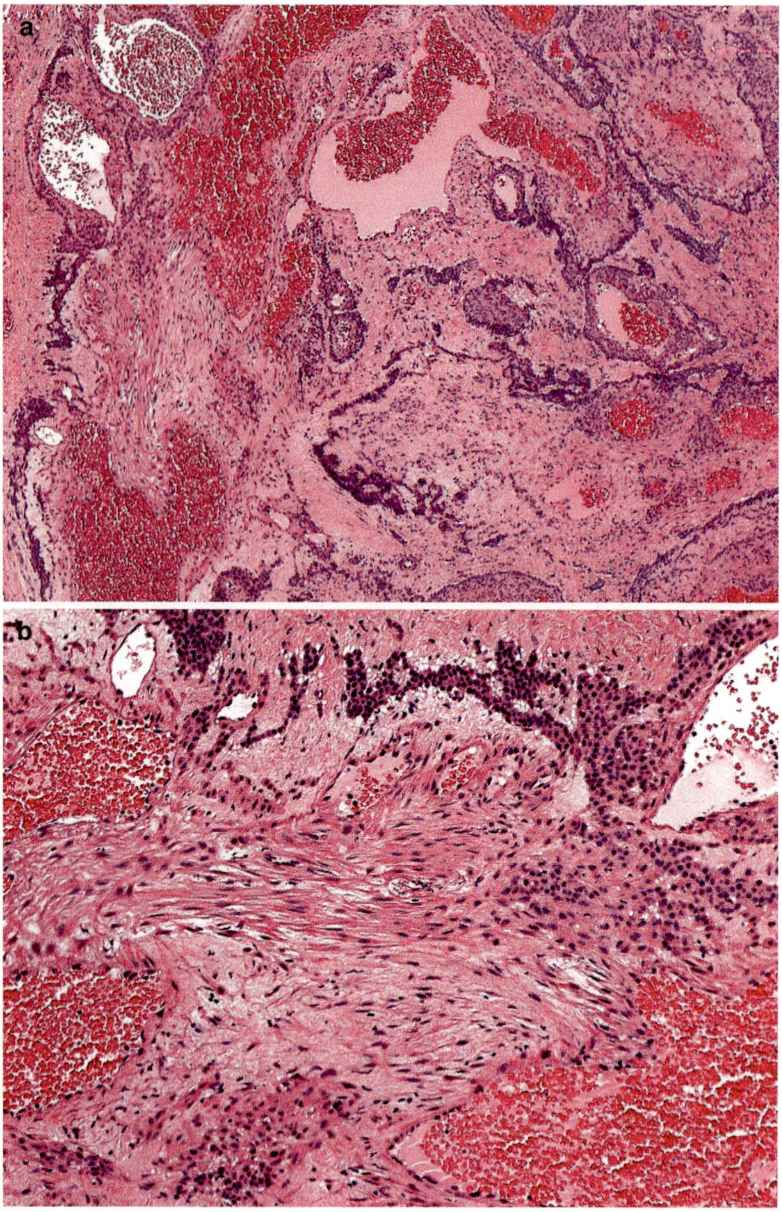

Fig. 8.4 Glomangiomyoma. (**a**). Low-power image demonstrating combination of round glomus cells and spindled cells in association with ectatic, thin-walled vessels. (**b**). Higher-power image demonstrating transition of glomus cells to smooth muscle cells. (Images courtesy of Dr. Thomas Brenn, University of Calgary)

nous malformation, the smooth muscle cells are admixed with the glomus cells.

Differential Diagnosis

The primary differential diagnosis is with glomus tumor and glomuvenous malformation. The distinction is largely academic. If there is evidence of transition from glomus cells to spindled smooth muscle cells, the diagnosis of glomangiomyoma is appropriate (Table 8.4).

Table 8.4 Key pathologic features: glomangiomyoma

Resembles either glomus tumor or glomuvenous malformation
Transition from round glomus cells to spindled smooth muscle cells

Myopericytoma

Clinical Features

Myopericytoma is a benign perivascular tumor that usually presents in middle-aged adults as a subcutaneous or dermal nodule of the distal extremities. Unlike glomus tumor and glomuvenous malformation, these lesions are usually asymptomatic. In the vast majority of cases, it is a benign tumor cured by simple excision. Rare patients present with multiple myopericytomas (myopericytomatosis).

Pathologic Features

Myopericytoma is usually a well-circumscribed tumor arising in the subcutis or dermis (Fig. 8.5a). The tumor is composed of plump

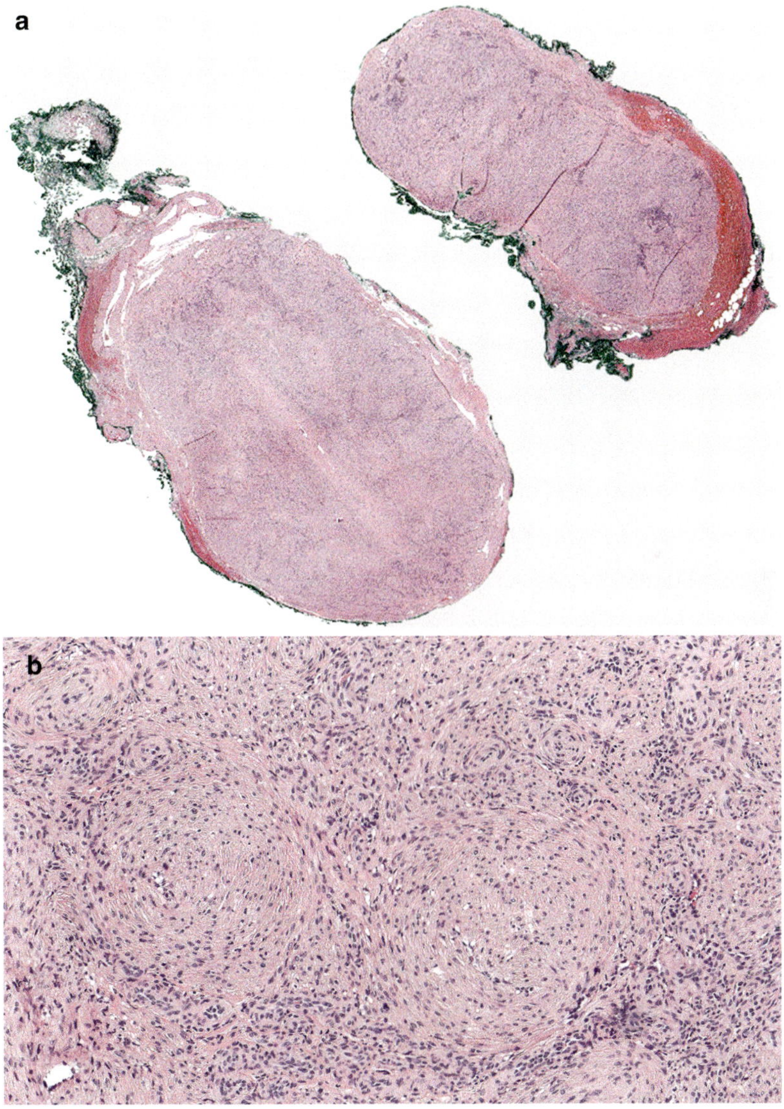

Fig. 8.5 Myopericytoma. (**a**) Myopericytoma is usually a well-circumscribed tumor arising in the subcutis or dermis. (**b**) Constituent tumor cells are spindled with eosinophilic cytoplasm, and in areas they condense around vessels in a concentric fashion. (**c**) Myopericytomas often have a hemangiopericytoma-like vasculature

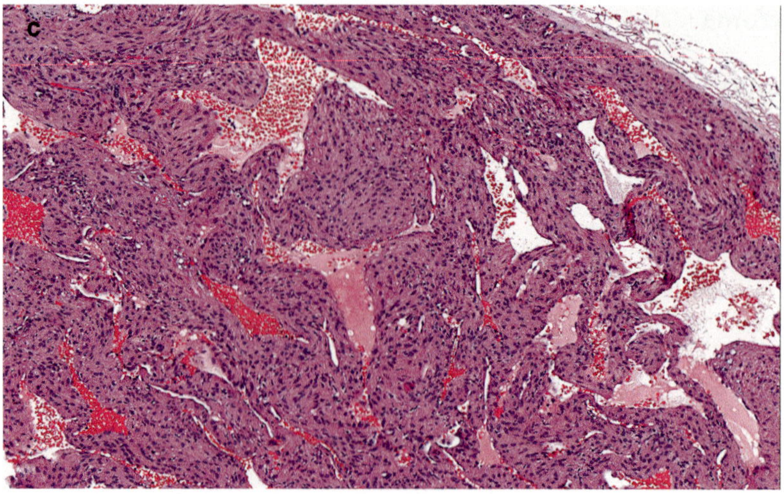

Fig. 8.5 (continued)

Fig. 8.6 Intravascular myopericytoma. A small percentage of cases are entirely intravascular. The native vascular wall is in the lower-left corner of the image

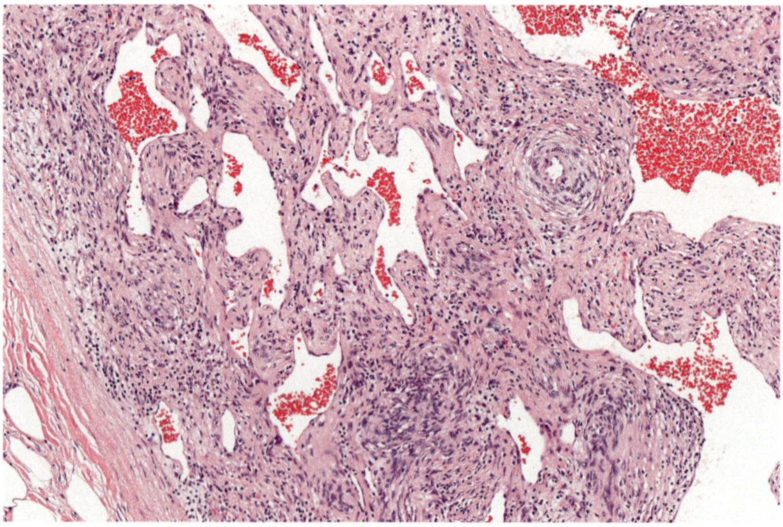

oval to spindled cells that surround the vessels, often in a concentric fashion (Fig. 8.5b). The vasculature varies from thin-walled compressed vessels to ectatic, branching hemangiopericytomatous vessels (Fig. 8.5c). A small subset presents as intravascular tumors (Fig. 8.6). Constituent tumor cells are usually positive for SMA and H-caldesmon but are typically negative for desmin and CD34. They are also negative for S100 protein, STAT6, and cytokeratins. Myopericytoma and myopericytomatosis have been linked to mutations in *PDGFRB*. A small subset has recurring *SRF-RELA* fusions and is more cellular and positive for desmin by immunohistochemistry (Table 8.5).

Rare malignant forms exist. Malignant examples have marked mitotic activity and often a fascicular growth pattern (Fig. 8.7). They maintain the perivascular growth pattern of conventional myopericytoma at least focally and are usually only partially SMA positive.

Differential Diagnosis

Myopericytoma differs from glomus tumors in having a predominantly spindled rather than round cell morphology. Angioleiomyomas have a similar concentric growth pattern of spindled cells around vessels, but the vessels have thicker walls and longer, more eosinophilic true smooth muscle cells that are positive for desmin. Myofibroma is a related tumor (see below) that has a biphasic pattern of myoid nodules and round to oval cells surrounding delicate, sometimes staghorn-like, vessels. Myopericytoma may have vessels that resemble those seen in solitary fibrous tumor, but solitary fibrous tumor does not have a concentric perivascular arrangement of tumor cells and is positive for CD34 and STAT6, unlike

Table 8.5 Key pathologic features: myopericytoma

Bland, short spindled cells arranged in concentric fashion around vessels
Vessels vary from thin and compressed to staghorn-like
Positive for SMA and H-caldesmon but usually negative for desmin
May be intravascular

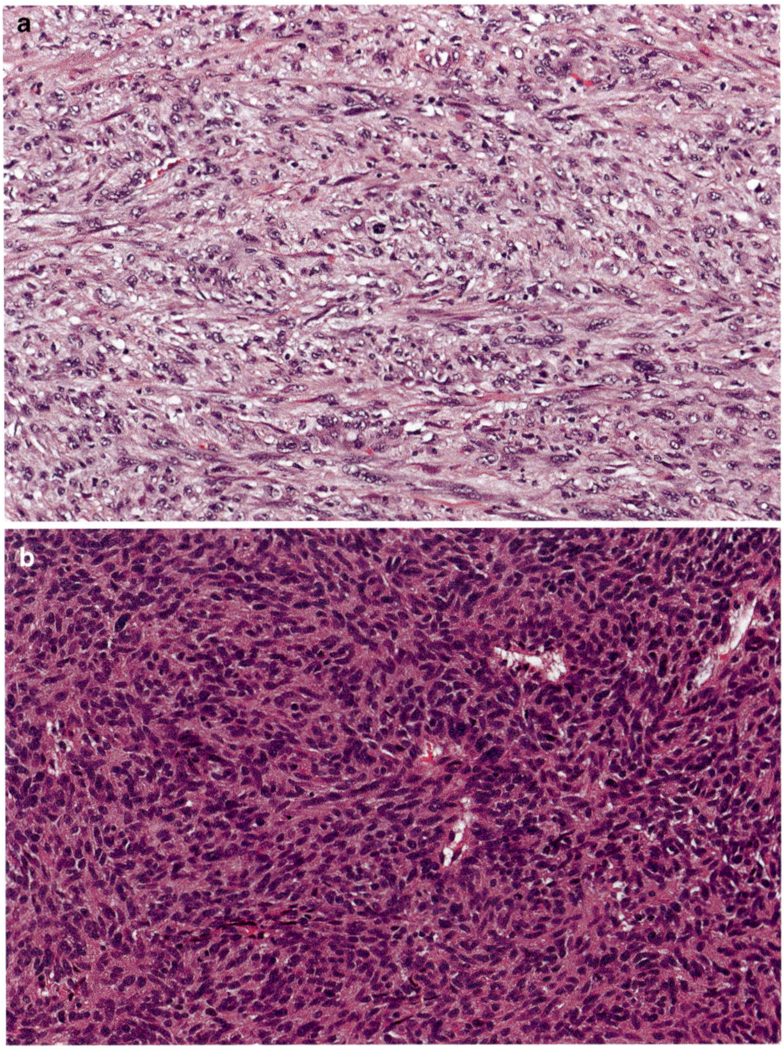

Fig. 8.7 Malignant myopericytoma. (**a**) Malignant myopericytoma with a fascicular growth pattern, atypia, and mitotic activity. (**b**) Malignant myopericytoma composed of a hypercellular proliferation of hyperchromatic oval tumor cells with condensation of tumor cells around capillary vasculature

myopericytoma. Based on the current WHO classification of soft tissue tumors, myopericytoma is often the best overall classification for hybrid tumors demonstrating features of more than one perivascular "myoid" tumor.

Myofibroma

Clinical Features

Once considered a fibroblastic tumor, myofibroma is now recognized as being part of the spectrum of perivascular "myoid" tumors and is related to myopericytoma and other tumors in this family. Myofibroma most commonly arises in young children but may also present in adult patients over a wide age range. Usually the tumor presents as a solitary mass but rarely can be multifocal (myofibromatosis). The head and neck region is the most commonly involved anatomic site, but the tumor can present in any location. Lesions typically are purplish cutaneous nodules. Myofibromatosis is associated with multifocal lesions involving deep soft tissue, bones, and viscera. Myofibroma is benign and cured by simple excision. Incompletely excised tumors may undergo spontaneous resolution.

Pathologic Features

Myofibroma is classically a biphasic tumor composed of pauci-cellular nodules of myoid spindled cells with eosinophilic cytoplasm embedded in a gray stroma and round cell areas associated with a distinct, often hemangiopericytoma-like, vasculature (Fig. 8.8a-c). Often, myoid nodules are present at the periphery of the lesion with the round cell component located more centrally, but the opposite pattern may also be seen. Occasional cases are relatively monophasic and composed predominantly of the pauci-cellular myoid component (Fig. 8.8d). Necrosis and vascular invasion may rarely be seen. More recently, myofibromas with atypical features have been described, including cases with hypercellular areas resembling fibrosarcoma, absent or diminished myoid nodules, infiltrative borders, and perineural invasion (Fig. 8.8e). These atypical features do not seem to adversely affect prognosis. By immunohistochemistry, myofibromas are typically positive for SMA and variably positive for desmin and H-caldesmon. They are negative for CD34, STAT6, S100 protein, and cytokeratin. Myofibromas have recently been associated with *PDGFRB* mutations (Table 8.6).

Differential Diagnosis

Myopericytoma lacks the biphasic morphology and gray stroma of the myoid nodules in myofibroma. Solitary fibrous tumor lacks myoid nodules and is positive for CD34 and STAT6. Leiomyomas have intersecting fascicles of smooth muscle and lack the round cell component.

Malignant Glomus Tumor and Glomus Tumor of Uncertain Malignant Potential

Clinical Features

While most glomus tumors in this category present as deep soft tissue masses, cutaneous forms do exist. Similar to other glomus tumors, cutaneous lesions present as purplish nodules, typically larger than 2 cm. Rare cases with a history of rapid growth arising in a longstanding lesion have been described, suggesting the possibility of malignant transformation of a precursor lesion. In the seminal study by Folpe and colleagues, malignant glomus tumors had a metastatic rate approaching 40%. Most of these lesions were deep soft tissue lesions, however. In our experience, similar to other sarcomas, superficial tumors in this category behave less aggressively, likely because they are more amenable to complete excision with tumor-free margins.

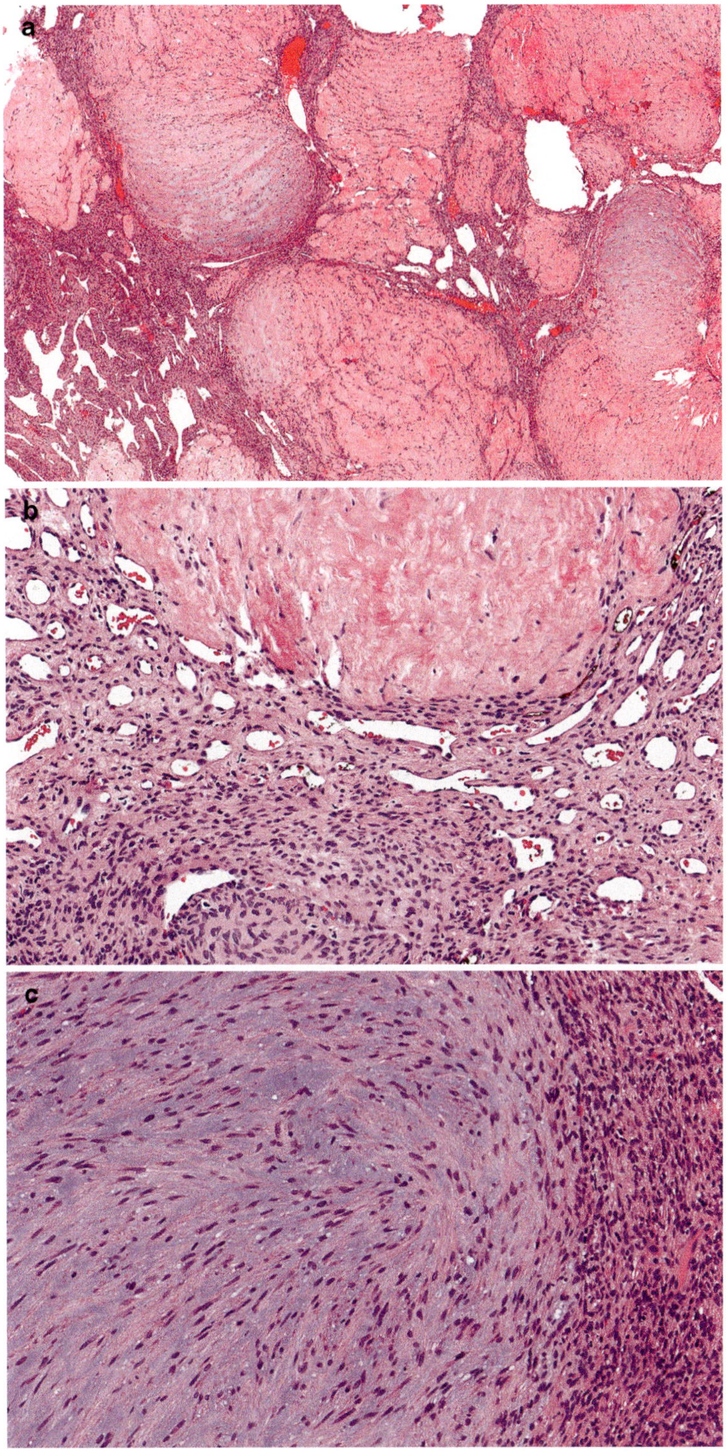

Fig. 8.8 Myofibroma. (**a**) Low-power image of myofibroma with biphasic morphology consisting of pauci-cellular myoid nodules surrounding cellular areas containing ovoid tumor cells and prominent capillary vasculature. (**b**) Higher-power image demonstrating the round to ovoid tumor cells and capillary vasculature. (**c**) Higher-power image of myoid nodule demonstrating eosinophilic myoid cells embedded in gray stroma. (**d**) Occasional cases are monophasic and composed almost exclusively of the myoid component. (**e**) Myofibromas with atypical features have been described, including cases with hypercellular areas resembling fibrosarcoma and absent or diminished myoid nodules

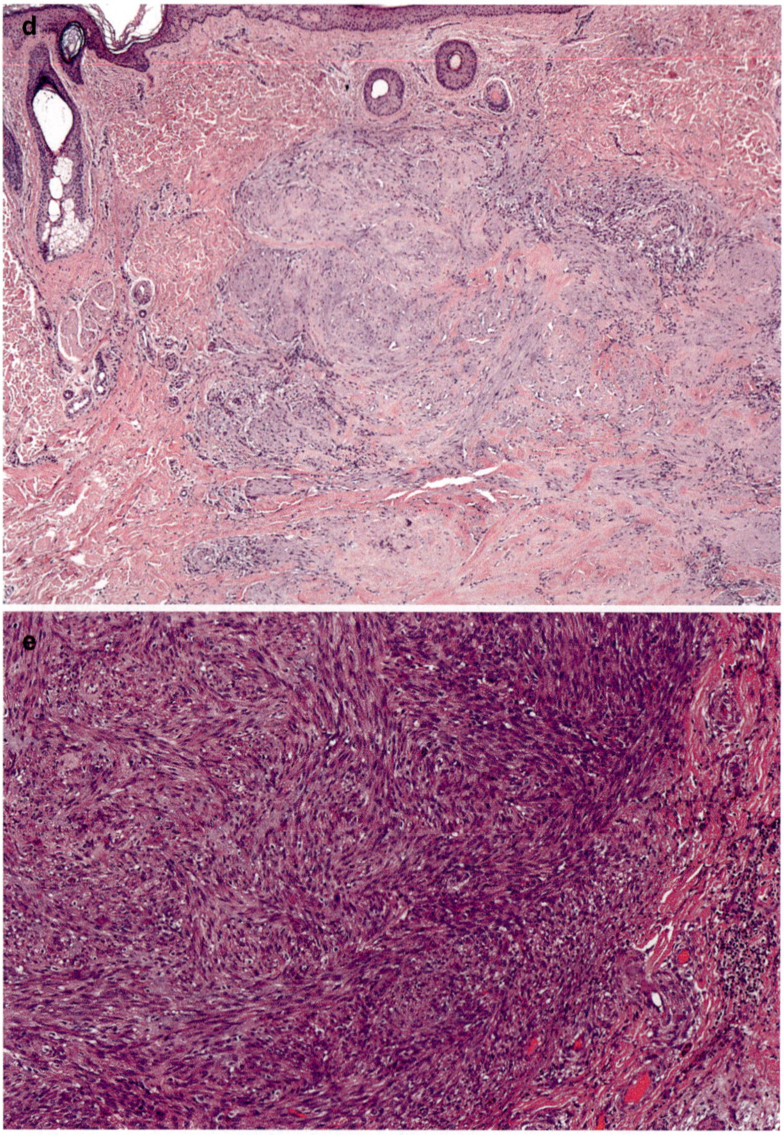

Fig 8.8 (continued)

Table 8.6 Key pathologic features: myofibroma

Biphasic tumor
Pauci-cellular myoid nodules of spindled cells with gray stroma
Round to ovoid cells arrayed around an associated capillary to hemangiopericytoma-like vasculature
SMA+, CD34-, STAT6-

Pathologic Features

Malignant glomus tumors typically have two morphologic patterns. The first resembles a conventional glomus tumor with sheets of round cells, though with nuclear atypia and mitotic activity (Fig. 8.9a). Alternately, they may resemble a spindle cell sarcoma like

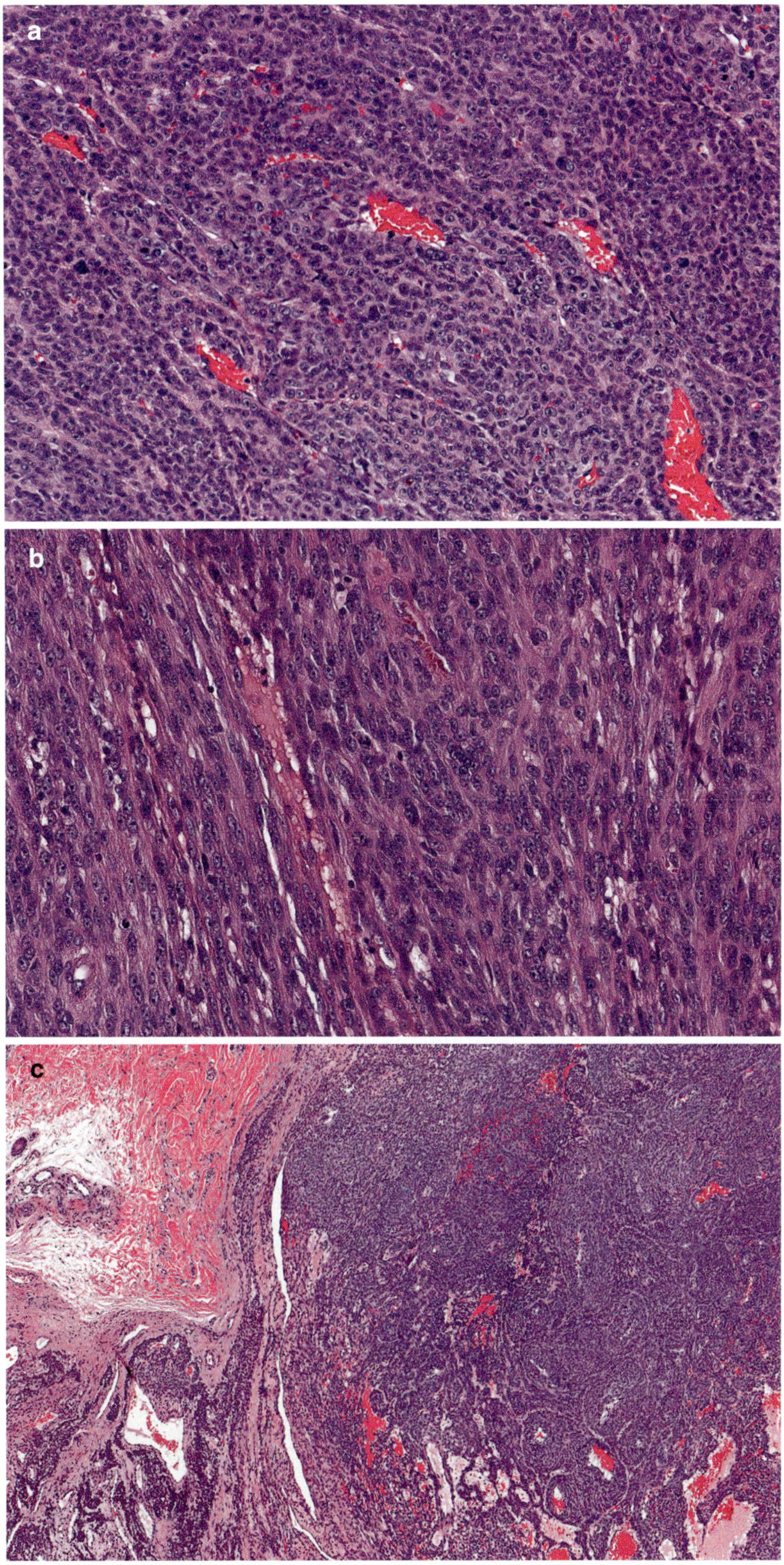

Fig. 8.9 Malignant glomus tumor. (**a**) Tumor composed of atypical round glomus cells with frequent mitotic figures. (**b**) Malignant glomus tumor with spindled morphology. (**c**) Transition from precursor glomus tumor (lower left) to hypercellular malignant glomus tumor (right)

fibrosarcoma or leiomyosarcoma (Fig. 8.9b). A rim of a precursor glomus tumor is sometimes evident (Fig. 8.9c). To be considered malignant, the tumor must have marked atypia and either mitotic activity >5/50 HPFs or atypical mitotic figures or large (size >2 cm) and deep location. Glomus tumors of uncertain malignant potential lack sufficient histologic features of malignancy, but are clearly not a conventional glomus tumor. Usually they lack atypia, but have mitotic activity, or are large or deeply located. As mentioned earlier, symplastic glomus tumors have atypia but no other features of malignancy. Like conventional glomus tumors, malignant ones are positive for SMA and will show, at least focally, a netlike pattern of basement membrane highlighted by type IV collagen stains (Table 8.7).

Differential Diagnosis

The differential diagnosis depends on the tumor morphology. Lesions with round cell features could be confused with rhabdomyosarcoma or Ewing sarcoma. The absence of immunoreactivity for desmin, myogenin, and MyoD1 can help distinguish malignant glomus tumor from rhabdomyosarcoma. For lesions with a spindled morphology, leiomyosarcoma enters the differential diagnosis. Leiomyosarcomas are typically positive for desmin. Positive immunoreactivity for type IV collagen also helps in the recognition of malignant glomus tumor.

Table 8.7 Key pathologic features: malignant glomus tumor and glomus tumor of uncertain malignant potential

Marked atypia and one of the following:
Mitotic activity >5/50 HPFs or
Atypical mitotic figures or
Size >2 cm and deep location
Tumors with no atypia but other features associated with malignancy = glomus tumor of uncertain malignant potential
Tumors with only atypia and no other features of malignancy = symplastic glomus tumor

Selected References

1. Agaimy A, Bieg M, Michal M, et al. Recurrent somatic PDGFRB mutations in sporadic infantile/solitary adult Myofibromas but not in Angioleiomyomas and Myopericytomas. Am J Surg Pathol. 2017;41(2):195–203.
2. Antonescu CR, Sung YS, Zhang L, Agaram NP, Fletcher CD. Recurrent SRF-RELA fusions define a novel subset of cellular Myofibroma/Myopericytoma: a potential diagnostic pitfall with sarcomas with myogenic differentiation. Am J Surg Pathol. 2017;41(5):677–84.
3. Boon LM, Mulliken JB, Enjolras O, Vikkula M. Glomuvenous malformation (glomangioma) and venous malformation: distinct clinicopathologic and genetic entities. Arch Dermatol. 2004;140(8):971–6.
4. Borroni RG, Grassi S, Concardi M, et al. Glomuvenous malformations with smooth muscle and eccrine glands: unusual histopathologic features in a familial setting. J Cutan Pathol. 2014;41(3):308–15.
5. Brouillard P, Ghassibé M, Penington A, et al. Four common glomulin mutations cause two thirds of glomuvenous malformations ("familial glomangiomas"): evidence for a founder effect. J Med Genet. 2005;42(2):e13.
6. Folpe AL, Fanburg-Smith JC, Miettinen M, Weiss SW. Atypical and malignant glomus tumors: analysis of 52 cases, with a proposal for the reclassification of glomus tumors. Am J Surg Pathol. 2001;25(1):1–12.
7. Granter SR, Badizadegan K, Fletcher CD. Myofibromatosis in adults, glomangiopericytoma, and myopericytoma: a spectrum of tumors showing perivascular myoid differentiation. Am J Surg Pathol. 1998;22(5):513–25.
8. Hung YP, Fletcher CDM. Myopericytomatosis: Clinicopathologic analysis of 11 cases with molecular identification of recurrent PDGFRB alterations in Myopericytomatosis and Myopericytoma. Am J Surg Pathol. 2017;41(8):1034–44.
9. LeBlanc RE, Taube J. Myofibroma, Myopericytoma, Myoepithelioma, and Myofibroblastoma of skin and soft tissue. Surg Pathol Clin. 2011;4(3):745–59.
10. Linos K, Carter JM, Gardner JM, Folpe AL, Weiss SW, Edgar MA. Myofibromas with atypical features: expanding the morphologic spectrum of a benign entity. Am J Surg Pathol. 2014;38(12):1649–54.
11. McMenamin ME, Fletcher CD. Malignant myopericytoma: expanding the spectrum of tumours with myopericytic differentiation. Histopathology. 2002;41(5):450–60.
12. Monteagudo C, Carda C, Llombart-Bosch A, Calduch L, Jordá E. Multiple glomangiomyoma versus glomangioma: conceptual and ultrastructural observations. Am J Dermatopathol. 2000;22(4):371–3.
13. Mravic M, LaChaud G, Nguyen A, Scott MA, Dry SM, James AW. Clinical and histopathological diagnosis of glomus tumor: an institutional experience of 138 cases. Int J Surg Pathol. 2015;23(3):181–8.

14. Oudijk L, den Bakker MA, Hop WC, et al. Solitary, multifocal and generalized myofibromas: clinicopathological and immunohistochemical features of 114 cases. Histopathology. 2012;60(6B):E1–11.
15. Yang JS, Ko JW, Suh KS, Kim ST. Congenital multiple plaque-like glomangiomyoma. Am J Dermatopathol. 1999;21(5):454–7.

9 Adipocytic Tumors

Steven D. Billings and Rajiv M. Patel

Abstract

Adipocytic tumors are commonly encountered in dermatopathology. Most are variants of lipomas, but rare cutaneous liposarcomas do occur. This chapter will cover the range of adipocytic tumors encountered in dermatopathology and discuss challenging variants and their differential diagnoses.

Lipoma

Clinical Features

Conventional lipomas typically present in middle-aged adults as painless masses most commonly involving the trunk but may be encountered at nearly any anatomic site. They are usually solitary but rarely may be multiple. Simple excision is curative. Local recurrence is exceptional.

S. D. Billings (✉)
Department of Pathology, Cleveland Clinic, Cleveland, OH, USA
e-mail: billins@ccf.org

R. M. Patel
Department of Pathology, University of Michigan Medical School, Ann Arbor, MI, USA

Pathologic Features

Lipomas are most commonly small subcutaneous masses composed of mature adipocytes and scattered collagen bundles (Fig. 9.1a). Mature adipose tissue often does not fix well on the short tissue processor runs used for dermatopathology specimens, causing the histotechnologist to cut thicker sections in order to produce an adequate tissue section. This may result in the appearance of Lochkern cells on the slide. Lochkern cells simply represent thickly sectioned adipocytes that have intranuclear vacuoles (Fig. 9.1b). The presence of ribbon-like cytoplasmic membranes in adipocytes is a clue that one is dealing with thickly sectioned adipose tissue. Lipomas may also be subject to trauma with attendant fat necrosis. Tissue macrophages with lipidized cytoplasm in foci of fat necrosis (Fig. 9.1c) should not be confused with lipoblasts or other sinister cells. Lipomas may also be extensively fibrotic, so-called fibrolipoma (Fig. 9.1d), or demonstrate myxoid change, designated as myxolipomas (Fig. 9.1e). The latter, less common finding can be seen in conventional lipomas and likely represents a degenerative phenomenon. Lipoma variants lack any significant cytologic atypia and mitotic activity.

Although conventional lipomas may have genetic alterations involving 12q13–12q15, most commonly by way of a t(3;12), there is no real

S. D. Billings et al. (eds.), *Soft Tissue Tumors of the Skin*,
https://doi.org/10.1007/978-1-4939-8812-9_9

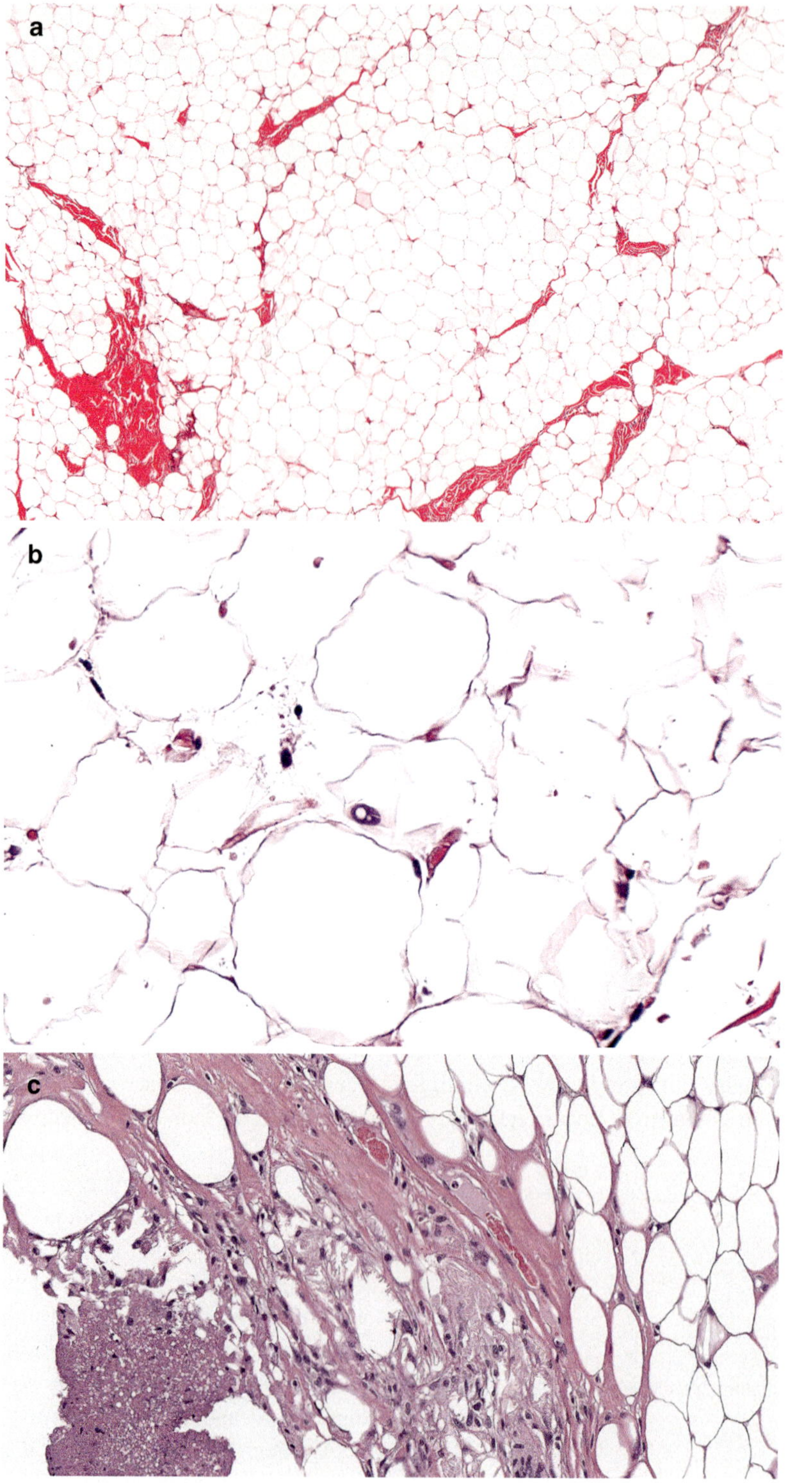

Fig. 9.1 Lipoma. (**a**) Lipomas are typically small subcutaneous masses composed of mature adipose and scattered collagen bundles. (**b**) Thickly sectioned adipose containing a Lochkern cell. These should not be confused with lipoblasts. (**c**) Lipoma with fat necrosis containing lipidized macrophages. (**d**) Extensively fibrotic lipomas are termed fibrolipomas. (**e**) Lipomas with extensive myxoid change are designated as myxolipomas

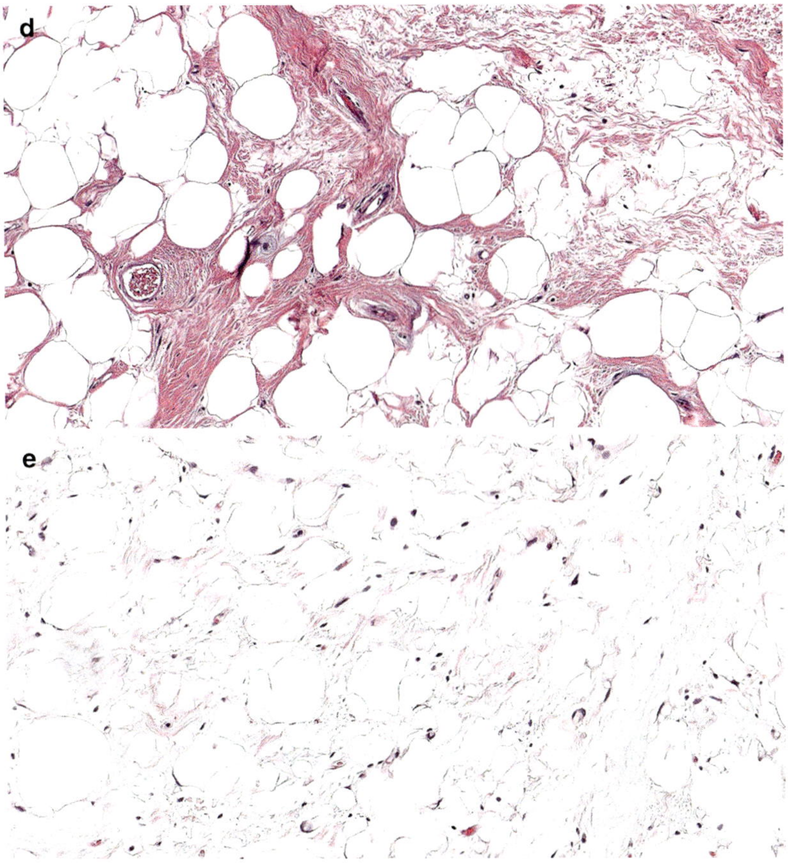

Fig. 9.1 (continued)

Table 9.1 Key pathologic features: lipoma

Composed of mature adipocytes
May have associated fibrous tissue (fibrolipoma)
May have myxoid change (myxoid lipoma)
Lochkern cells present in thick sections not to be confused with lipoblasts

role for ancillary molecular tests in the diagnosis of conventional lipomas. That being said, occasionally the need to exclude an atypical lipomatous tumor necessitates their use, particularly in limited biopsies. Conventional lipomas lack MDM2 expression by immunohistochemistry and show no evidence of *MDM2* amplification by FISH, while atypical lipomatous tumors/well-differentiated liposarcomas do demonstrate expression and amplification by these methods, respectively (Table 9.1).

Differential Diagnosis

Conventional lipomas are rarely diagnostically problematic. The primary differential diagnosis is normal mature adipose. Fibrolipomas and lipomas with fat necrosis need to be distinguished from atypical lipomatous tumor/well-differentiated liposarcoma. Lipomas lack the atypical, hyperchromatic spindle cells within expanded fibrous septa seen in atypical lipomatous tumor/well-differentiated liposarcoma. Nuclear immunohistochemical expression of MDM2 and *MDM2* gene amplification is also not seen in lipomas. As a caveat, histiocytes in fat necrosis can express MDM2 by immunohistochemistry, but they lack amplification of the gene. It is imperative not to overinterpret Lochkern cells and lipidized macrophages in lipomas with fat necrosis as lipoblasts. Lipoblasts are actually quite rare in atypical lipomatous tumor/well-differentiated liposarcoma and are not required to make the diagnosis. Myxolipoma can be confused with myxoid liposarcoma or lipoblastoma. Myxolipomas lack the delicate "chicken wire" capillary vasculature and true lipoblasts seen in those entities. Also, lipoblastomas are tumors of young children rather than adults.

Angiolipoma

Clinical Features

Angiolipomas usually occur in young adults, are more common in men, and frequently present as multiple painful subcutaneous nodules. The forearm is the most common location, but they can present in a wide variety of anatomic sites.

Pathologic Features

Histologically, these lesions are composed of mature adipose admixed with varying numbers of small arcades of capillaries (Fig. 9.2a). The vessels are often arrayed in clusters and associated with perivascular hyalinization and focal fibrin microthrombi formation (Fig. 9.2b). The number of vessels can be sparse, making it difficult to distinguish them from a conventional lipoma, or prominent where they obscure the adipocytic component leading to an appearance more akin to a vascular tumor (Fig. 9.2c).

Angiolipomas harbor low-level protein kinase D2 (*PRKD2*) mutations, with the highest level of mutations being in the adipocytes. It is postulated that this results in angiogenesis. Testing for this mutation is, however, of no diagnostic utility (Table 9.2).

Differential Diagnosis

Angiolipomas should be distinguished from conventional lipomas (in cases with relatively few characteristic vessels), hemangiomas and other vascular tumors (in cases with relatively little fat). The characteristic clusters of small capillaries containing fibrin microthrombi allow for their distinction from these lesions.

Spindle Cell Lipoma and Pleomorphic Lipoma

Clinical Features

Spindle cell lipoma and the related morphologic variant pleomorphic lipoma classically present on the upper back, posterior neck, or

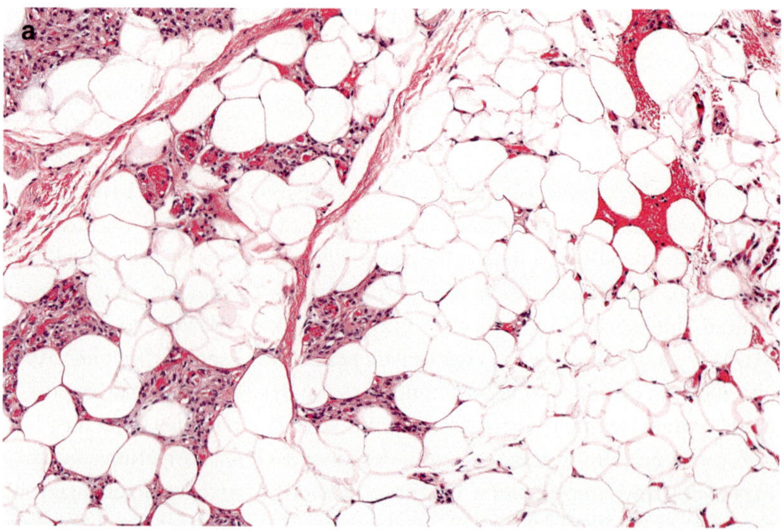

Fig. 9.2 Angiolipoma. (**a**) Angiolipomas are composed of a mixture of mature adipose and a varying number of small vessels. (**b**) Capillaries are arranged in clusters and associated with perivascular hyalinization and fibrin microthrombi formation. (**c**) In some cases vessels are so prominent as to obscure the adipocytic component leading to confusion with a vascular tumor

Fig. 9.2 (continued)

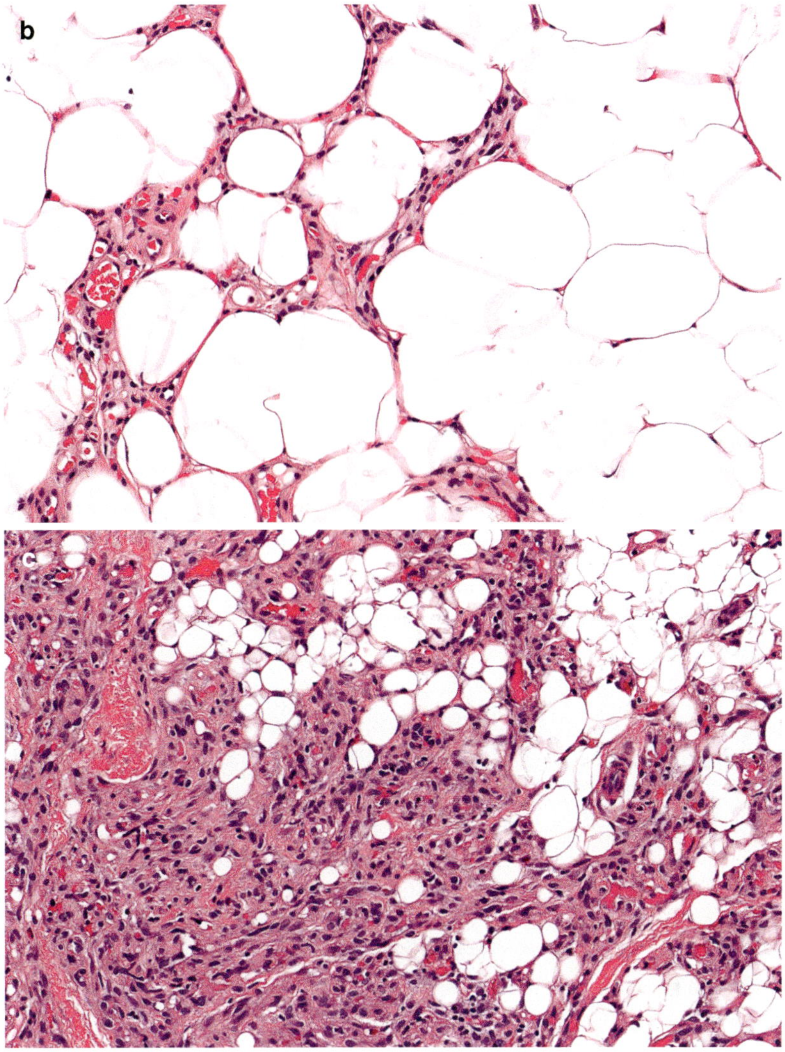

Table 9.2 Key pathologic features: angiolipoma

Usually multiple
Mature adipocytes with clusters of capillaries
Vessels contain frequent fibrin microthrombi
Rare cases have few mature adipocytes

scalp. However, they can also present on the face, in the oral cavity, and on the trunk and extremities; indeed they have been described in nearly every anatomic location imaginable. They are much more common in men (M:F, 10:1). In women, they have a different stereotypical location, with two-thirds of cases presenting outside the shawl distribution, most commonly the extremities. Spindle cell lipoma and pleomorphic lipoma are benign entities, cured by simple excision. Incompletely excised tumors may rarely recur.

Pathologic Features

Spindle cell lipoma is typically a circumscribed tumor arising in the subcutis composed of short fusiform-to-spindled cells, admixed with ropy collagen, varying amounts of myxoid stroma, mature adipocytes, and frequent mast cells (Fig. 9.3a). In more cellular examples, the spindled cells are often arranged in short fascicles

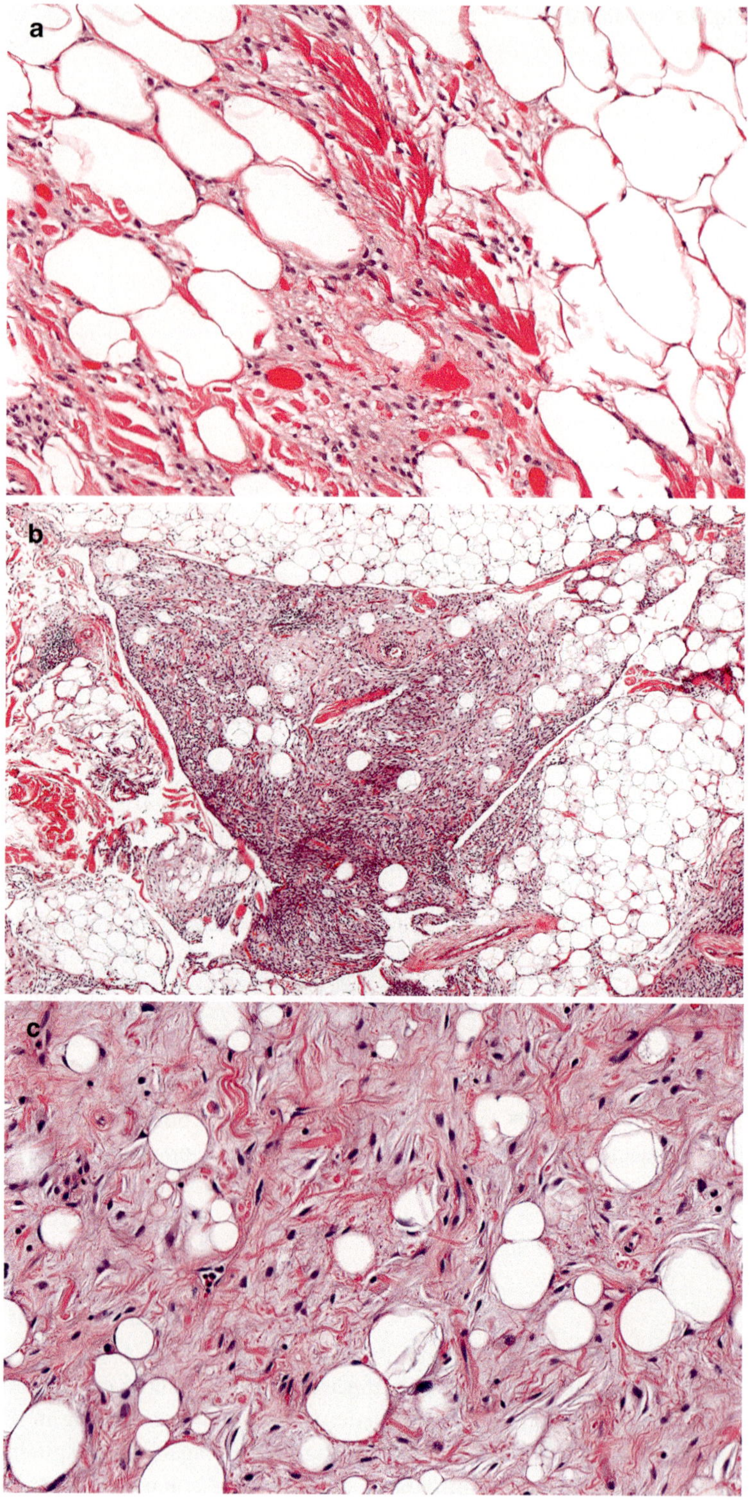

Fig. 9.3 Spindle cell lipoma. (**a**) Spindle cell lipoma is composed of short fusiform-to-spindled cells, admixed with ropy collagen, varying amounts of myxoid stroma, mature adipocytes, and frequent mast cells. (**b**) In cellular examples spindled cells are arranged in short fascicles that have been likened to a "school of fish." (**c**) Pauci-cellular examples have more abundant myxoid stroma. (**d**) In some cases there may be a pseudoangiomatous pattern with large irregular spaces mimicking ectatic vessels. (**e**) Examples with few to no mature adipocytes have been referred to as "fat-free or low-fat" spindle cell/pleomorphic lipomas. (**f**) Pleomorphic lipomas are identical to spindle cell lipomas in every aspect except for the presence of multinucleated floret-like giant cells with enlarged hyperchromatic nuclei

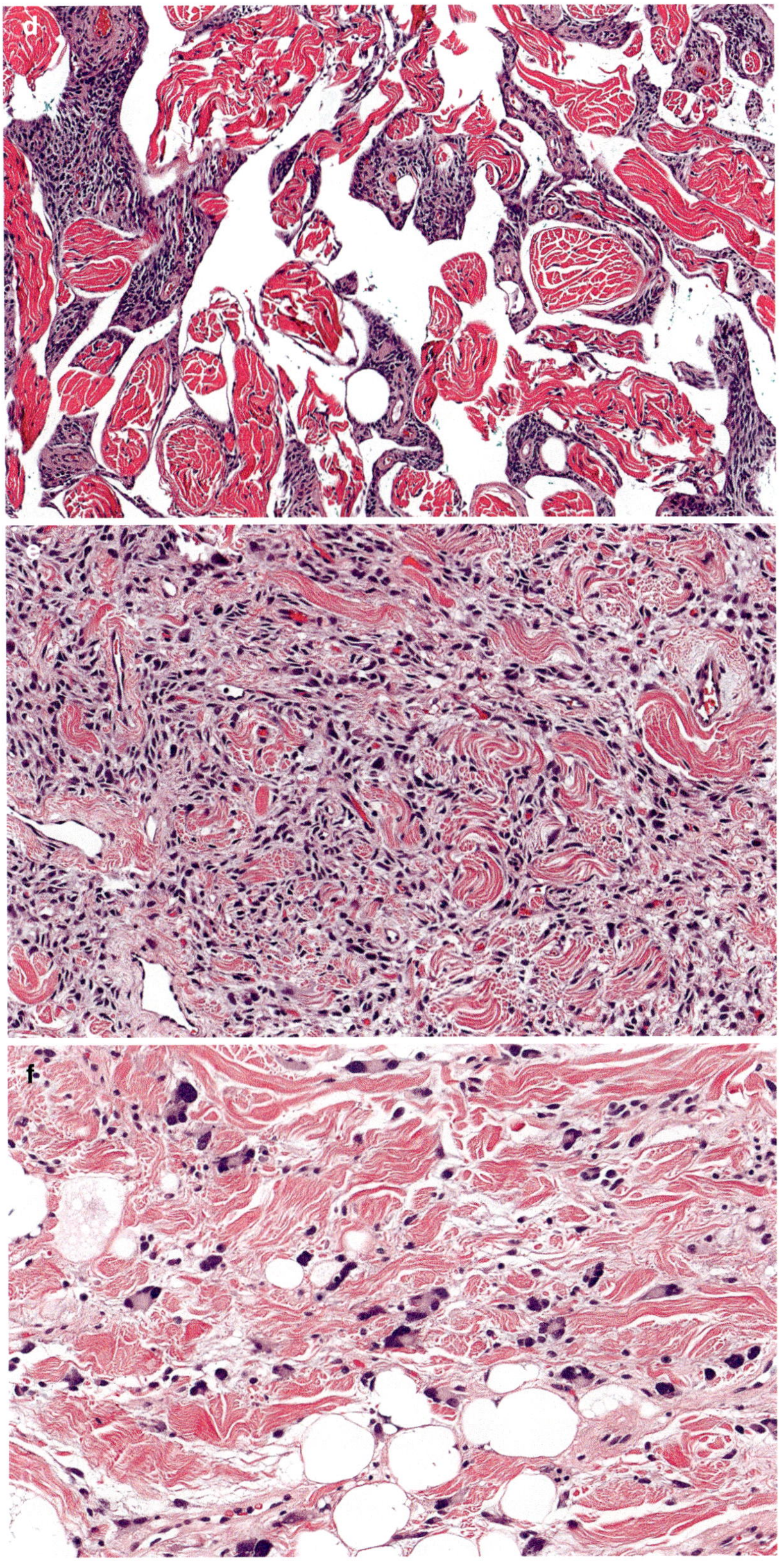

Fig. 9.3 (continued)

that have been likened to a "school of fish" (Fig. 9.3b). In less cellular examples, the fascicular pattern may be absent. Pauci-cellular examples often have more abundant myxoid stroma (Fig. 9.3c). In some cases there may be a pseudoangiomatous pattern with large irregular spaces mimicking ectatic vessels (Fig. 9.3d). Cases from the face typically arise in the dermis. Dermal spindle cell lipomas are not circumscribed, but instead have the same constituent components infiltrating between the reticular dermal collagen bundles. While in most cases adipose tissue is prominent, there are examples with few to no mature adipocytes (so-called "fat-free or low-fat" spindle cell/pleomorphic lipomas) (Fig. 9.3e). Spindle cell lipomas of the face often contain very little in the way of adipocytes. Pleomorphic lipomas are identical to spindle cell lipomas in every aspect except for the presence of multinucleated floret-like giant cells with enlarged hyperchromatic nuclei (Fig. 9.3f).

The spindle cell component in spindle cell lipoma and the pleomorphic cells in the pleomorphic lipoma are consistently positive for CD34. They are also typically positive for bcl-2. The constituent spindle cells are negative for S100 protein, though the adipocytes are positive. Spindle cell lipomas typically have losses of 13q14, the locus of the *RB1* gene. This can be demonstrated by FISH or by immunohistochemistry looking for loss of RB1 protein expression (Table 9.3).

Table 9.3 Key pathologic features: spindle cell and pleomorphic lipoma

Spindle cell lipoma and pleomorphic lipoma represent a histologic spectrum of the same tumor
In men most common on the upper back, posterior neck, and scalp
In women most common on the extremities
Spindle cell lipoma Bland spindle cells, ropy collagen, and mature adipocytes Myxoid stroma common Some cases with little to no adipose CD34+, RB1–, STAT6–
Pleomorphic lipoma Floret-like giant cells, bland spindle cells, ropy collagen, mature adipocytes Myxoid stroma common Some cases with little to no adipose CD34+, RB1–, STAT6–

Differential Diagnosis

The differential diagnosis of conventional spindle cell lipomas is rarely problematic. In cases with little to no fat, the diagnosis may be more difficult. Low-fat and fat-free examples can be confused with solitary fibrous tumor. Solitary fibrous tumor usually contains more mat-like rather than ropy collagen and often has a staghorn, hemangiopericytomatous vasculature, which is uncommon in spindle cell lipoma. Solitary fibrous tumors are positive for CD34 and STAT6, while spindle cell lipomas are positive for CD34 and negative for STAT6. Neurofibromas are distinguished by the random arrangement of their tumor cells and immunoreactivity for S100 protein and SOX10. Myxoid examples of spindle cell lipoma can be confused with myxoid dermatofibrosarcoma protuberans (DFSP), which is purely myxoid and lacks the ropy collagen that is invariably present in spindle cell lipoma. In addition, careful histologic examination often reveals areas of conventional DFSP in association with the more myxoid zones. Testing for the *PDGFB* gene rearrangement seen in DFSP can be helpful in problematic cases.

Pleomorphic lipomas need to be distinguished from undifferentiated pleomorphic sarcoma and pleomorphic liposarcoma. Pleomorphic lipomas still have the bland spindle cells and ropy collagen of conventional spindle cell lipomas, which are lacking in the latter two entities. Mitotic figures are also uncommon in pleomorphic lipoma and common in sarcomas. Pleomorphic lipomas with myxoid stroma similarly need to be distinguished from myxofibrosarcoma. Again the population of bland spindled cells and ropy collagen in the former aids in this distinction. It should be noted that CD34 is not helpful in the differential diagnoses outlined above, as any of the aforementioned neoplasms can be positive for this marker.

Chondroid Lipoma

Clinical Features

This is the least common lipoma subtype. It usually arises in the proximal extremities or limb girdles of adult women. It may be subcutaneous or arise in deep soft tissue.

Pathologic Features

Chondroid lipomas are well-circumscribed tumors composed of a lobular arrangement of cords and nests of tumor cells and adipocytes set within a myxochondroid-to-hyalinized stroma (Fig. 9.4a). Constituent cells have an epithelioid morphology with eosinophilic to vacuolated cytoplasm (Fig. 9.4b), and lipoblasts (Fig. 9.4c) are commonly present. There is a variable tumor vasculature composed of thin- and thick-walled vessels. Calcification and metaplastic bone may be present. Mitotic activity and pleomorphism are typically absent.

Lipoblasts are S100 protein positive. The tumor cells are negative for *MDM2* amplification. Chondroid lipoma has a recurring t(11;16)(q13;p12-13) resulting in a *C11* or *f95-MKL2* fusion (Table 9.4).

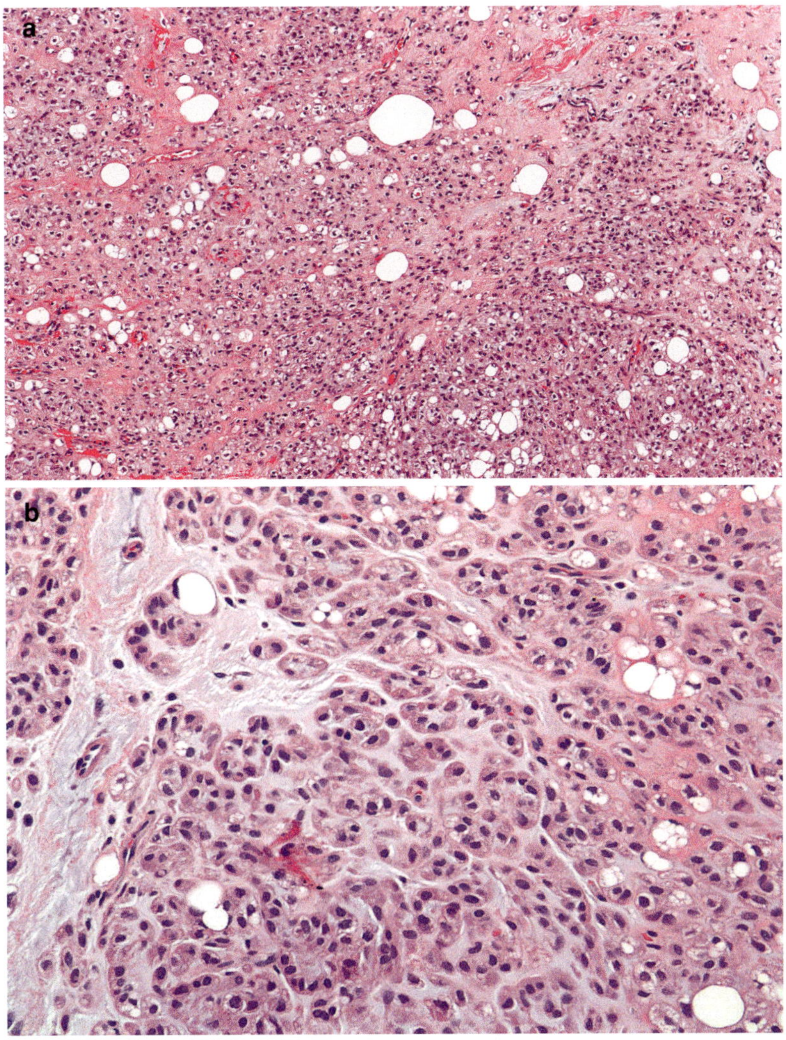

Fig. 9.4 Chondroid lipoma. (**a**) Chondroid lipomas are well-circumscribed tumors composed of a lobular arrangement of cords and nests of tumor cells and adipocytes set within a myxochondroid-to-hyalinized stroma. (**b**) Constituent cells have an epithelioid morphology with eosinophilic to vacuolated cytoplasm, and lipoblasts (**c**) are commonly present

Fig. 9.4 (continued)

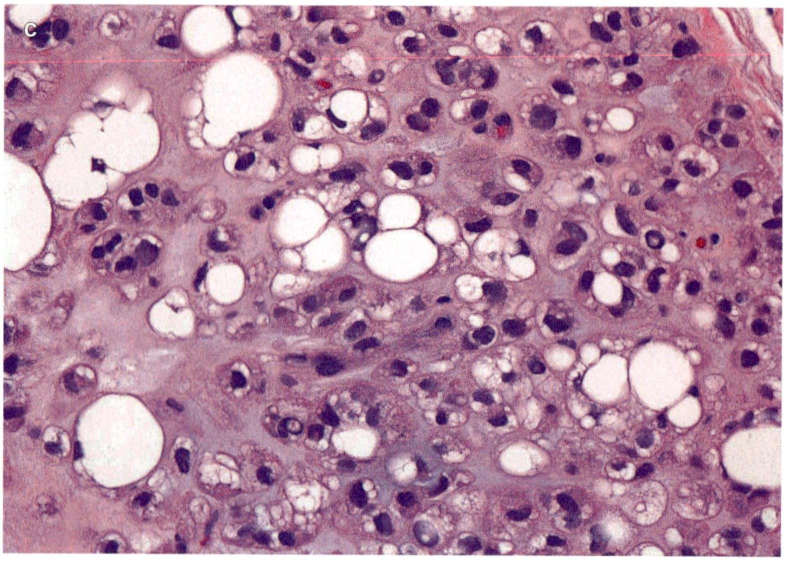

Table 9.4 Key pathologic features: chondroid lipoma

Lobular growth pattern
Cords and nests of epithelioid cells with vacuolated cytoplasm
Chondroid stroma
May have lipoblasts

Differential Diagnosis

Myxoid liposarcoma is a tumor of spindled cells rather than epithelioid cells and has a consistent plexiform capillary vasculature and a t(12;16) (see below). Soft tissue chondroma typically presents in the hands and feet and lacks adipocytic differentiation. Myoepithelioma lacks adipocytic differentiation and demonstrates immunoreactivity for at least some epithelial markers by immunohistochemistry. Extraskeletal myxoid chondrosarcoma has fibrous bands, often has hemorrhage, and the tumor cells, while epithelioid, are not vacuolated. Extraskeletal myxoid chondrosarcoma also has characteristic cytogenetic findings with either a t(9;17) or t(9;22) involving *NR4A3*.

Hibernoma

Clinical Features

Hibernoma is an uncommon neoplasm composed of brown fat. They are slightly more common in adult men with a wide age range. They are rare in children. The most common anatomic location is the thigh, followed by the shoulder, back, neck, chest, arm, and abdominal cavity or retroperitoneum. Hibernomas range from 1–24 cm, with an average size of 9 cm. Hibernoma is a benign tumor, which does not recur after complete excision.

Pathologic Features

Hibernomas are most often subcutaneous, mobile masses. Characteristically, their gross cut surface varies from tan to red brown. Histologically, tumors are composed, at least focally, of coarsely multivacuolated "mulberry-like" fat cells with small, central nuclei with no evidence of atypia or mitotic activity (Fig. 9.5). In general, hibernomas are more richly vascularized than typical lipomas. In addition to the classic morphology, myxoid, spindle cell, and lipoma-like variants have also been described. All are typically positive for S100 protein and rarely so for CD34. Hibernomas have characteristic rearrangements of 11q13–11q21 (Table 9.5).

Differential Diagnosis

Given the classic constellation of histologic features, one is unlikely to confuse hibernoma with

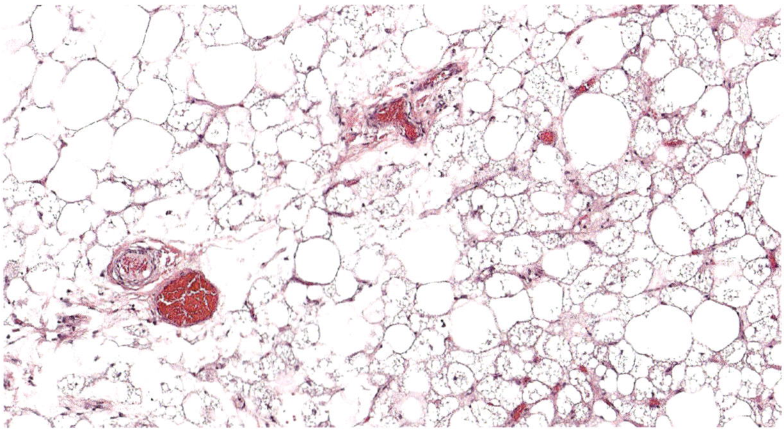

Fig. 9.5 Hibernoma. (**a**) Hibernomas are composed, at least focally, of coarsely multivacuolated "mulberry-like" fat cells with small, central nuclei with no evidence of atypia or mitotic activity

Table 9.5 Key pathologic features: hibernoma

Combination of brown fat and mature adipocytes
Brown fat Polygonal "mulberry-like" cells with eosinophilic, finely vacuolated cytoplasm and central bland nuclei
Typically S100 +, CD34–

other entities. The most important differential diagnosis is with atypical lipomatous tumor/well-differentiated liposarcoma, which demonstrates atypical, hyperchromatic stromal cells within expanded fibrous septa, not seen in hibernoma. Atypical lipomatous tumor is also *MDM2* amplified, unlike hibernoma.

Lipoblastoma

Clinical Features

Lipoblastoma is a rare tumor of infants that recapitulates fetal fat. It typically involves the extremities as a solitary mass, but may also present in the head and neck and deep soft tissues (e.g., retroperitoneum). Rarely, patients may have multiple lesions (lipoblastomatosis). It is more common in males than females (3:1, M/F). Lipoblastoma is a benign tumor treated with complete excision. Recurrences are common (13–46%) and likely the result of incomplete excision.

Pathologic Features

Lipoblastomas are well circumscribed, have a lobular growth pattern, and contain varying amounts of immature spindle cells, lipoblasts, and mature adipocytes delineated by fibrous septa (Fig. 9.6a). In areas containing immature spindle cells, myxoid stroma and a delicate plexiform capillary vasculature are often prominent and impart a histologic picture indistinguishable from myxoid liposarcoma (Fig. 9.6b). Over time the tumors may mature and contain an increased amount of mature fat compared with spindle cells and lipoblasts (Fig. 9.6c).

Approximately 70% of cases have abnormalities of *PLAG1*, found on 8q12.1, which is variably fused with *COL1A2* (7q21.3), *HAS2* (8q24.13), *RAD51B* (14q24.1), *COL3A1* (2q32.2), or *RAB2A* (8q12.1). Polysomy of chromosome 8 has also been described in tumors lacking rearrangements of *PLAG1*. Immunohistochemistry does not play a role in the diagnosis of lipoblastoma (Table 9.6).

Differential Diagnosis

The primary differential diagnosis is with myxoid liposarcoma. The clinical presentation allows distinction in most cases, as myxoid liposarcoma arising in an infant would be exceptional. Myxoid liposarcoma also has a t(12;16) resulting in a *FUS-DDIT3* fusion, unlike lipoblastoma. In a case with more mature adipose tissue, a conventional lipoma

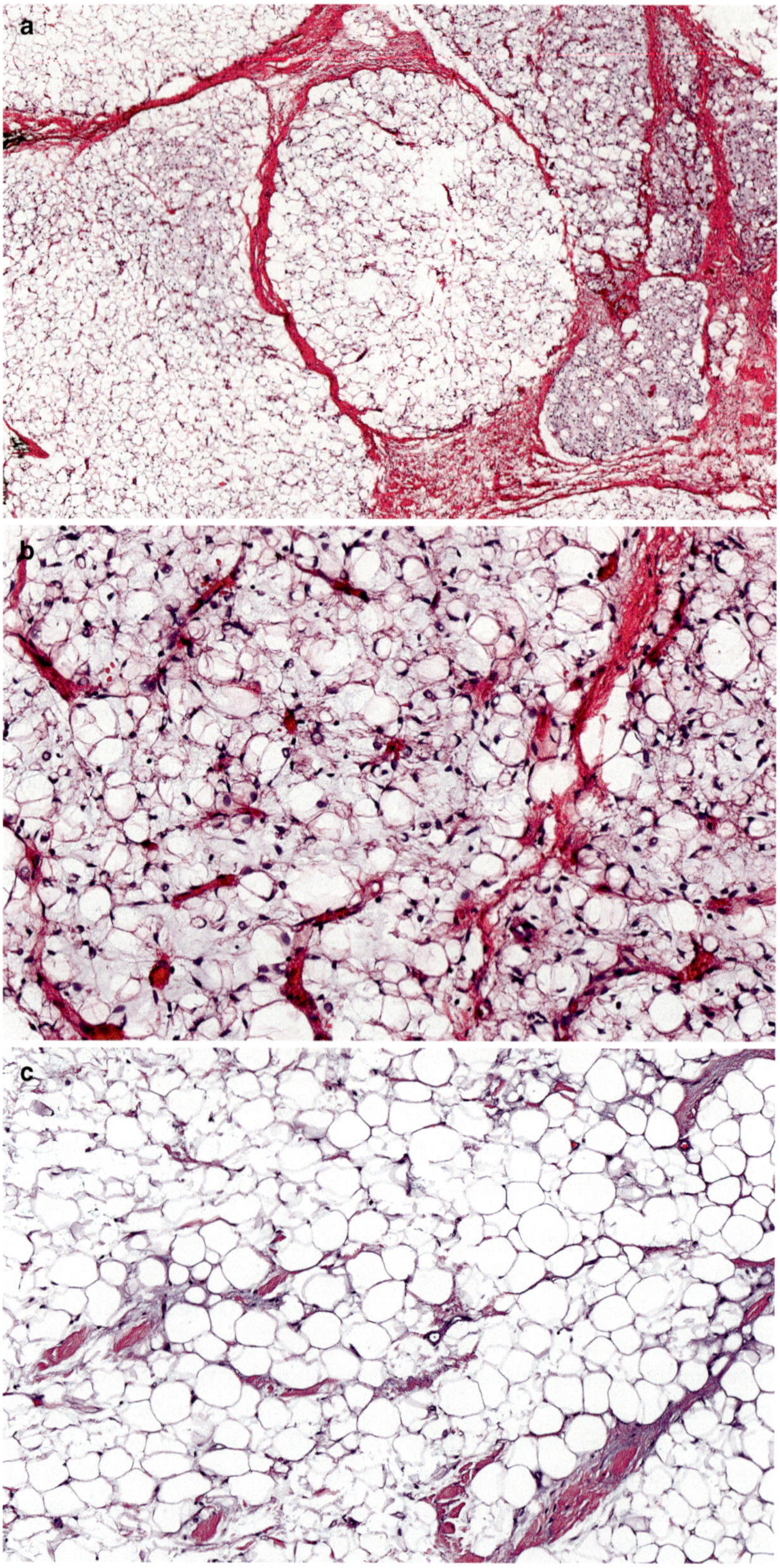

Fig. 9.6 Lipoblastoma. (**a**) Lipoblastomas are well circumscribed and have a lobular growth pattern with varying amounts of immature spindle cells, lipoblasts, and mature adipocytes delineated by fibrous septa. (**b**) In areas containing immature spindle cells, myxoid stroma and a delicate plexiform capillary vasculature are often prominent and histologically indistinguishable from myxoid liposarcoma. (**c**) Over time the tumors may mature and contain an increased amount of mature fat compared with spindle cells and lipoblasts

Table 9.6 Key pathologic features: lipoblastoma

Tumor of infants
Well circumscribed with lobular growth pattern
Spindle cells, lipoblasts, and mature adipocytes
Myxoid stroma with plexiform vasculature
Rearrangement of *PLAG1* common

could be considered in the differential. However, conventional lipomas are rare in children and typically lack the myxoid stroma and plexiform capillary vasculature of lipoblastoma.

Nevus Lipomatosus

Clinical Features

Nevus lipomatosus presents as solitary or grouped waxy, verrucous papules, or plaques on the buttocks, thigh, or lower back of children and young adults. This is a benign tumor cured by simple excision.

Pathologic Features

Lesions are comprised of mature adipocytes in the reticular dermis in association with overlying verrucous to papillomatous epidermal hyperplasia. Dermal adnexal structures are typically absent (Fig. 9.7) (Table 9.7).

Differential Diagnosis

The differential diagnosis is primarily with acrochordon (fibroepithelial polyp), which is essentially histologically identical except that it lacks mature adipocytes. Fibrolipoma could be considered in the differential, but that is a subcutaneous, rather than a dermal, lesion.

Pleomorphic Liposarcoma

Clinical Features

Unlike in the deep soft tissues where pleomorphic liposarcoma is the least common form of liposarcoma, it is the most common form in the skin and superficial soft tissue. It typically occurs in older patients, but children are rarely affected as well. The most common anatomic sites of involvement are the extremities followed by the trunk and head and neck. Lesions are typically small and superficial at presentation (~2 cm). Primary cutaneous pleomorphic liposarcoma may locally recur, particularly when incompletely excised, but distant metastasis has not been reported. Treatment is with wide excision. Adjuvant therapy is not typically necessary.

Pathologic Features

Superficial pleomorphic liposarcomas may be dermal and subcutaneous, purely subcutaneous, or purely dermal tumors. This neoplasm is usually composed of pleomorphic lipoblasts in association with hyperchromatic, pleomorphic spindled cells present in a fascicular-to-storiform growth pattern (Fig. 9.8a). A predominantly epithelioid proliferation of cells, in addition to the lipoblasts, is seen in roughly a quarter of cases (Fig. 9.8b). Pleomorphic lipoblasts are requisite for the diagnosis (Fig. 9.8c), but they are variably present, with some tumors containing only a few lipoblasts, while others have many. In rare cases the cellularity is relatively low, and the tumor can resemble a pleomorphic fibroma (Fig. 9.8d). In general, mitotic activity is typically conspicuous, and occasional cases will have necrosis.

Immunohistochemistry and molecular studies play little role in the diagnosis. The pleomorphic lipoblasts are variably positive for S100 protein, but the non-lipogenic component is typically negative. There may be variable immunoreactivity for SMA and CD34. Only rarely do they exhibit evidence of *MDM2* amplification (Table 9.8).

Differential Diagnosis

Recognition of pleomorphic lipoblasts allows the distinction of pleomorphic liposarcoma from undifferentiated pleomorphic sarcoma.

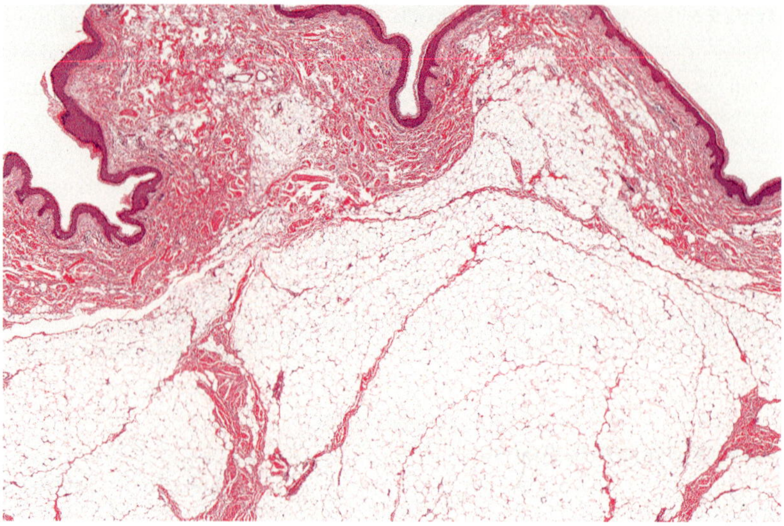

Fig. 9.7 Nevus lipomatosus. (**a**) Nevus lipomatosus is composed of mature adipocytes in the reticular dermis in association with overlying papillomatous epidermal hyperplasia. Dermal adnexal structures are typically absent

Table 9.7 Key pathologic features: nevus lipomatosus

Poorly circumscribed collections of mature adipocytes in reticular dermis
Lack of adnexal structures in dermis

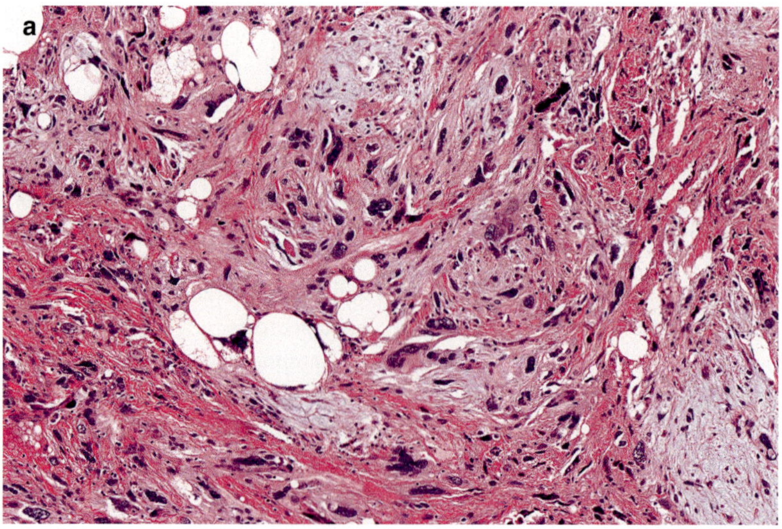

Fig. 9.8 Pleomorphic liposarcoma. (**a**) Pleomorphic liposarcoma is composed of pleomorphic lipoblasts in association with hyperchromatic, pleomorphic spindled cells present in a fascicular-to-storiform growth pattern. (**b**) A predominantly epithelioid proliferation of cells (left), in addition to the lipoblasts, is seen in roughly a quarter of cases. (**c**) Pleomorphic lipoblasts are requisite for the diagnosis. (**d**) In rare cases the cellularity is relatively low, and the tumor can resemble a pleomorphic fibroma

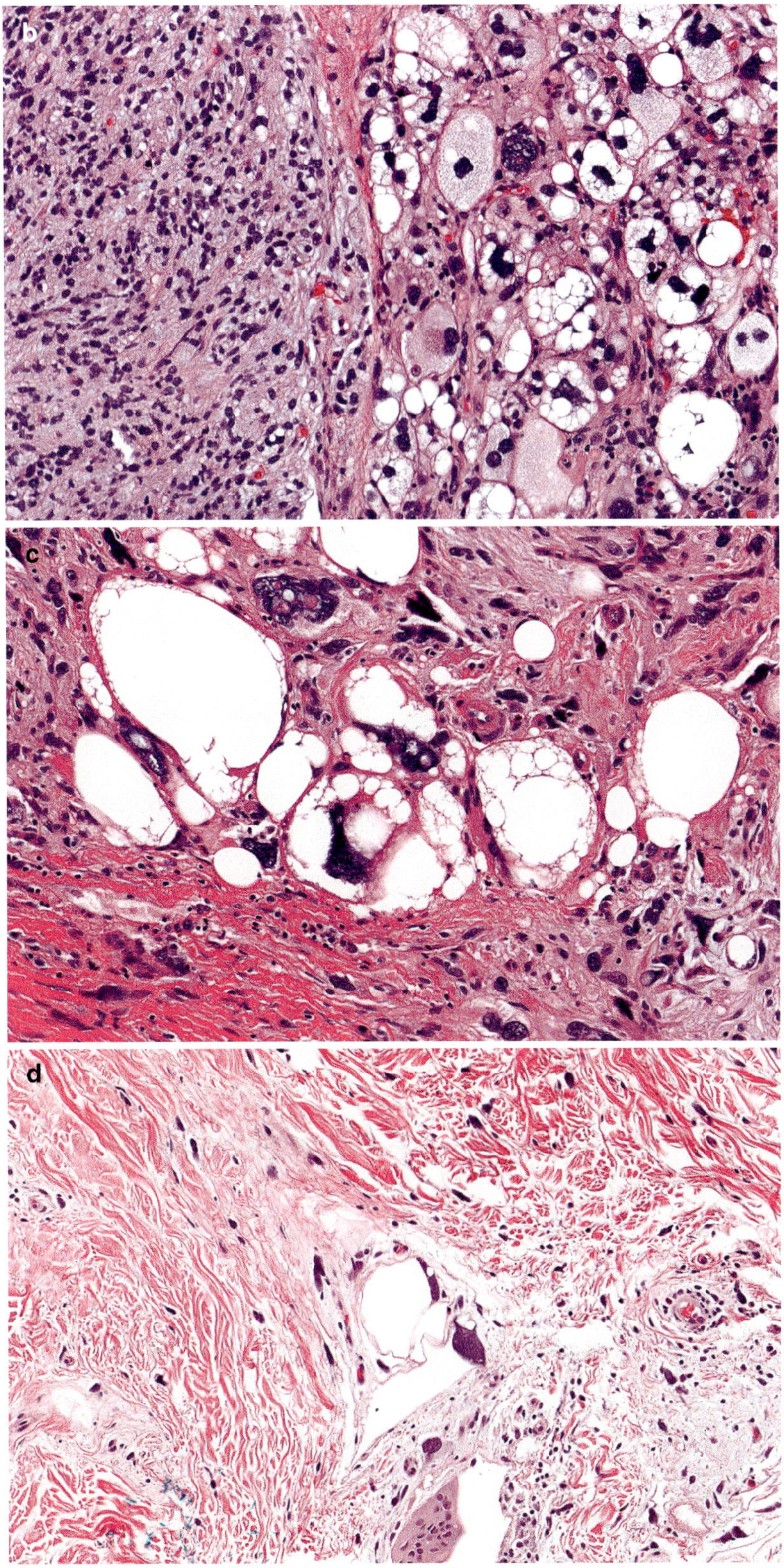

Fig. 9.8 (continued)

Table 9.8 Key pathologic features: pleomorphic liposarcoma

Pleomorphic tumor often resembling undifferentiated pleomorphic sarcoma
Variable number of pleomorphic lipoblasts
Rare hypocellular cases (pleomorphic fibroma-like)
A subset have cells with prominent epithelioid morphology

Pleomorphic lipoma has multinucleated floret-like giant cells, pleomorphic cells, and rarely lipoblasts, but the background bland spindled cells and ropy collagen are not seen in pleomorphic liposarcoma. Dedifferentiated liposarcoma has significant cytologic atypia, pleomorphism, and cellularity but does not typically contain pleomorphic lipoblasts, except in rare cases with "homologous" lipoblastic (pleomorphic liposarcoma-like) differentiation. The presence of a component of atypical lipomatous tumor/well-differentiated liposarcoma distinguishes dedifferentiated liposarcoma from pleomorphic liposarcoma. Demonstration of *MDM2* amplification by FISH also strongly favors a diagnosis of well-differentiated or dedifferentiated liposarcoma.

Atypical Lipomatous Tumor

Clinical Features

Atypical lipomatous tumor is the superficial equivalent of well-differentiated liposarcoma, the latter term being reserved for tumors arising in the deep soft tissues or retroperitoneum. It typically arises in adults in the extremities (or retroperitoneum in the case of well-differentiated liposarcoma). Atypical lipomatous tumor rarely occurs above the fascia as a mass of the subcutis. Local recurrence is frequent, owing to the difficulty of complete excision, particularly of deep-seated lesions. In the absence of dedifferentiation, there is no metastatic risk.

Pathologic Features

The tumor is composed predominantly of mature-appearing adipocytes delineated by fibrous bands containing scattered hyperchromatic, pleomorphic stromal spindle cells (Fig. 9.9a). Lipoblasts are almost never seen and are not required for the diagnosis. The atypical spindle cells often are first found to cluster around or be present within the walls of misshapen blood vessel present in the neoplasm (Fig. 9.9b). Some cases have a prominent inflammatory component or fibrous stroma in the background (Fig. 9.9c). However, these findings are less common in superficial examples. Overall, the cellularity of the lesion is low, and mitotic activity is absent to sparse. If present, these features should prompt consideration of the possibility of dedifferentiated liposarcoma.

Atypical lipomatous tumor has supernumerary ring and giant marker chromosomes that have amplified sequences of 12q14–12q15 that include *MDM2*, *CDK4*, *TSPAN31*, and *HMGA2*. Detection of amplification of *MDM2* by FISH is a reliable ancillary diagnostic test. Immunohistochemical stains for MDM2 and CDK4 can also be useful. In our experience stains for MDM2 are better than those for CDK4 (Fig. 9.9d). It should be pointed out that the immunostains work better on tumors that are more cellular and less lipogenic. FISH should be considered the gold standard ancillary diagnostic test (Table 9.9).

Differential Diagnosis

The primary differential diagnosis is with conventional lipoma, fibrolipoma, and pleomorphic lipoma. Neither conventional lipomas nor fibrolipomas have atypical stromal spindle cells. Pleomorphic lipoma may have atypical cells but also has the bland spindle cells and ropy collagen characteristic of conventional spindle cell lipoma. In contrast to atypical lipomatous tumor, amplification of *MDM2* is not seen in any of these lipoma subtypes.

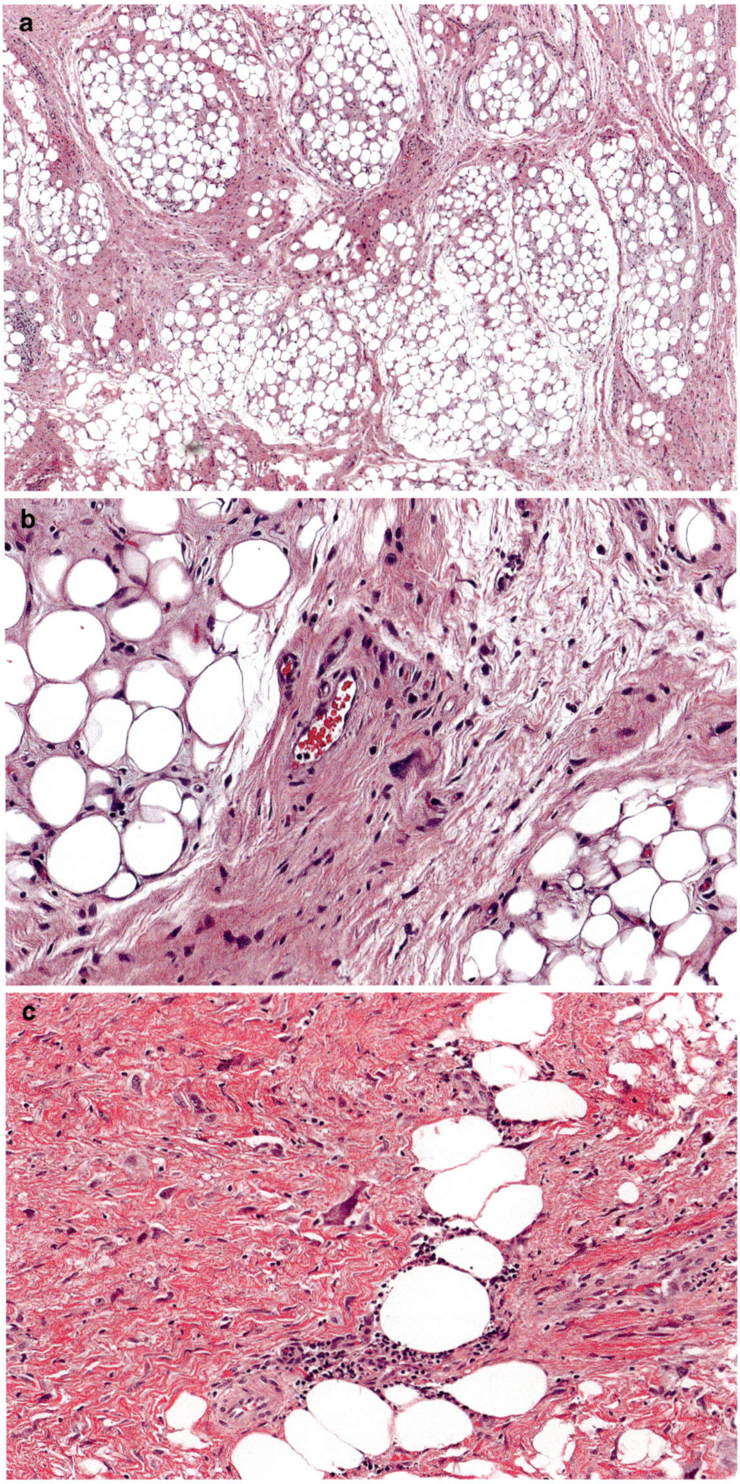

Fig. 9.9 Atypical lipomatous tumor. (**a**) The tumor is usually composed predominantly of mature-appearing adipocytes delineated by fibrous bands containing scattered hyperchromatic, pleomorphic stromal spindle cells. (**b**) The atypical spindle cells often are first found to cluster around or be present within the walls of misshapen blood vessels present in the neoplasm. (**c**) Some cases have a prominent inflammatory component or fibrous stroma in the background. (**d**) Immunohistochemical stains for MDM2 and CDK4 can be useful for diagnosis. In our experience stains for MDM2 (pictured) are better than CDK4

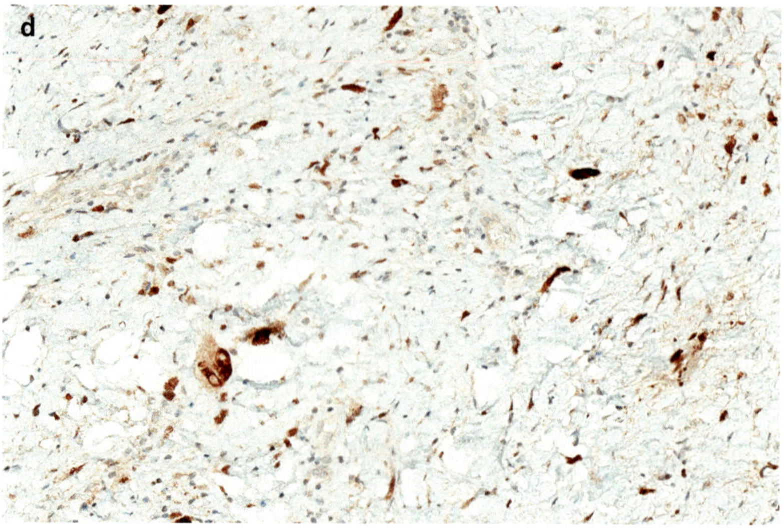

Fig. 9.9 (continued)

Table 9.9 Key pathologic features: atypical lipomatous tumor

Mature adipocytes delineated by fibrous bands
Pleomorphic stromal cells within expanded fibrous septa
Pleomorphic cells may cluster around abnormal blood vessels
Lipoblasts rare to absent
MDM2 amplified

Dedifferentiated Liposarcoma

Clinical Features

Dedifferentiated liposarcoma has the same general demographics as atypical lipomatous tumor. Similarly, cutaneous presentation is quite rare. Dedifferentiated liposarcoma has a risk of metastasis, but it is not certain if the risk presented by superficial tumors is the same as for deep-seated lesions. Similar to other superficial sarcomas, one would expect the risk of metastasis to be much lower for cutaneous dedifferentiated liposarcoma.

Pathologic Features

Classically, dedifferentiated liposarcoma is defined as a juxtaposition of a high-grade pleomorphic undifferentiated sarcoma adjacent to an atypical lipomatous tumor/well-differentiated liposarcoma (Fig. 9.10). Dedifferentiated liposarcoma with less pleomorphism and cellularity has also been described and termed so-called low-grade dedifferentiation. It has been suggested by Harry Evans that cases with increased cellularity, but with fewer than five mitotic figures per 10 HPF, be termed cellular atypical lipomatous tumors, as this subset of lesions appear to behave in a fashion similar to conventional atypical lipomatous tumors (Table 9.10).

Differential Diagnosis

Dedifferentiated liposarcoma is distinguished from pleomorphic undifferentiated sarcoma by the presence of a well-differentiated liposarcoma component.

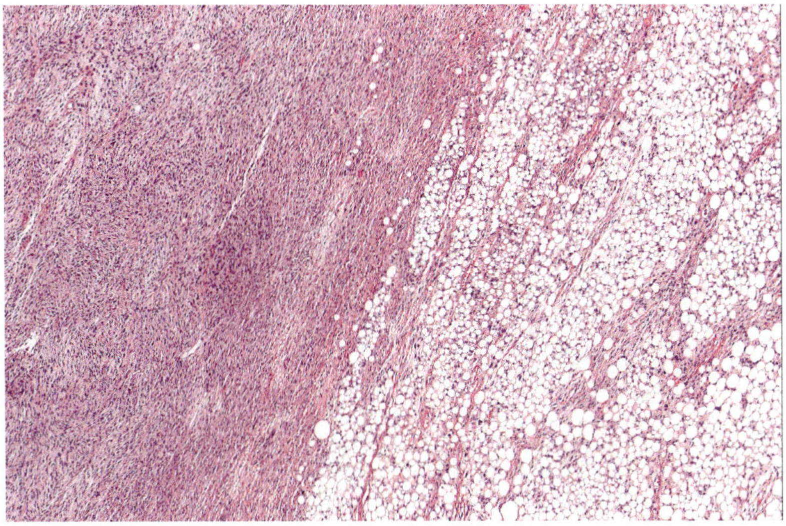

Fig. 9.10 Dedifferentiated liposarcoma. Dedifferentiated liposarcoma is defined as a juxtaposition of a high-grade pleomorphic undifferentiated sarcoma adjacent to an atypical lipomatous tumor/ well-differentiated liposarcoma

Table 9.10 Key pathologic features: dedifferentiated liposarcoma

Combination of atypical lipomatous tumor and component resembling undifferentiated pleomorphic sarcoma
Transition between components often abrupt
Mitotic rate >5/10 HPFs in dedifferentiated area
MDM2 amplification

Myxoid Liposarcoma

Clinical Features

This tumor typically presents in middle-aged adults. Myxoid liposarcoma is a deep-seated sarcoma of the extremities and only rarely presents as a superficial mass above the fascia. When arising in superficial locations, it may be more common in acral sites. Myxoid liposarcoma has a significant risk of metastasis, and this risk increases with an increased round cell component. This tumor has a propensity to metastasize to unusual locations, and the possibility of a metastasis should always be excluded when lesions present in the skin.

Pathologic Features

Grossly, myxoid liposarcoma has a gelatinous appearance on sectioning. Microscopically, it is usually composed of relatively bland oval to spindled cells in an abundant myxoid stroma in association with a delicate plexiform capillary vasculature (Fig. 9.11a). Univacuolated and multivacuolated, but not pleomorphic, lipoblasts are usually present (Fig. 9.11b). The myxoid stroma may contain acellular pools imparting a resemblance to a focus of pulmonary edema histologically (Fig. 9.11c). In some cases, the tumors are hypercellular, and the plexiform vasculature is obscured. The latter was previously termed round cell liposarcoma but is now designated as high-grade myxoid liposarcoma in the current WHO classification (Fig. 9.11d). Cases with as little as 5% round cell component may behave in a more aggressive fashion. Mitotic activity is typically low, especially at the pure myxoid liposarcoma end of the spectrum.

Immunohistochemistry plays no role in the diagnosis of myxoid liposarcoma. This tumor

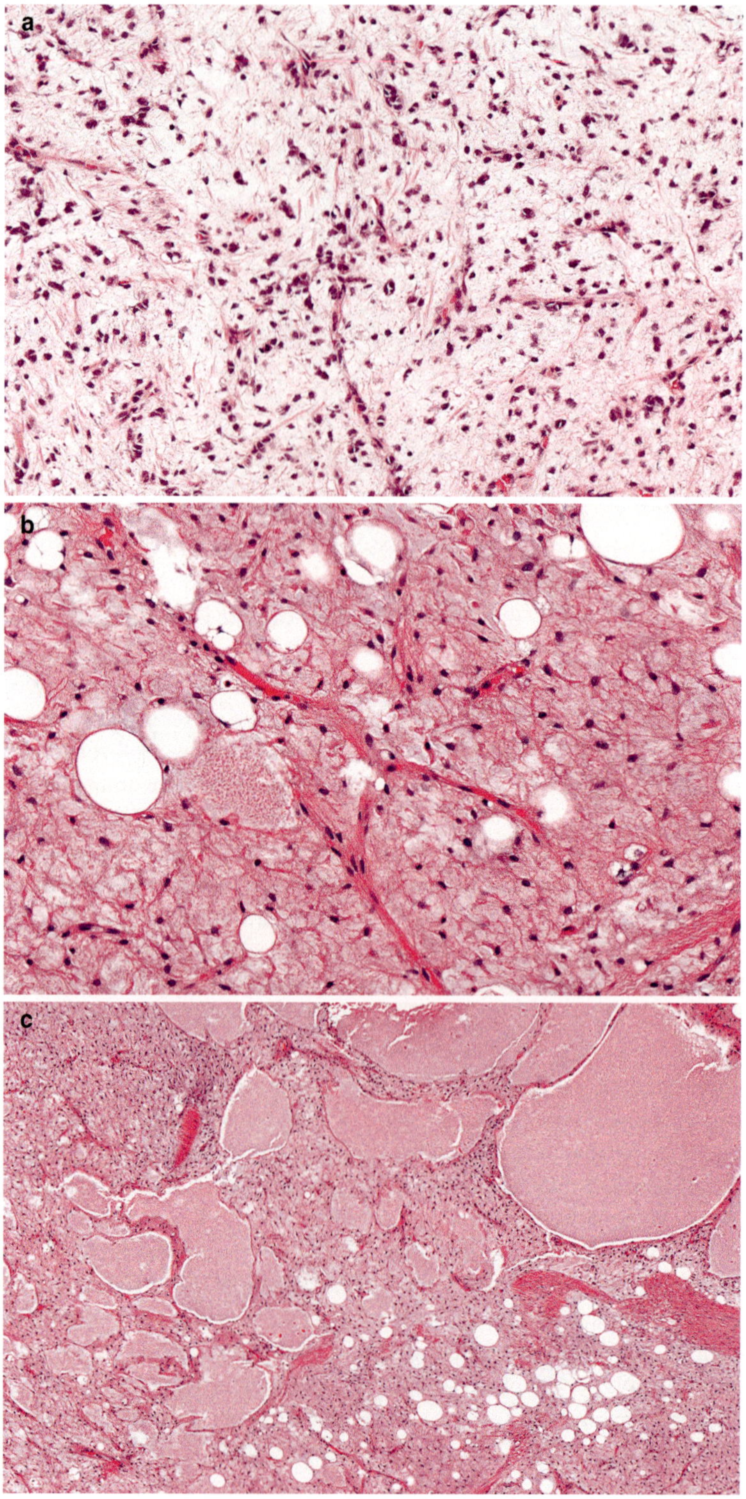

Fig. 9.11 Myxoid liposarcoma. (**a**) Myxoid liposarcoma is composed of relatively bland oval to spindled cells in an abundant myxoid stroma in association with a delicate plexiform capillary vasculature. (**b**) Univacuolated and multivacuolated, but not pleomorphic, lipoblasts are usually present. (**c**) The myxoid stroma may contain acellular pools resembling pulmonary edema histologically. (**d**) In some cases, the tumors are hypercellular, and the plexiform vasculature is obscured; this was previously termed round cell liposarcoma but is now designated as high-grade myxoid liposarcoma in the current WHO classification

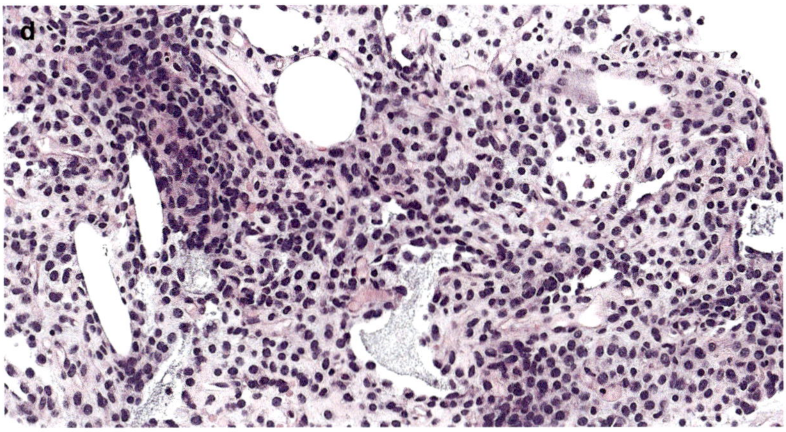

Fig. 9.11 (continued)

Table 9.11 Key pathologic features: myxoid liposarcoma

Bland oval to spindled cells in myxoid stroma
Variable numbers of lipoblasts
Plexiform capillary vasculature
t(12;16) *FUS-DDIT3* fusion

does have a t(12;16) *FUS-DDIT3* fusion. FISH to detect either *FUS* or *DDIT3* rearrangements are commonly used ancillary diagnostic tests to confirm the diagnosis (Table 9.11).

Differential Diagnosis

Lipoblastoma can have areas indistinguishable from myxoid liposarcoma, but lipoblastoma is a tumor of infants and young children. It also does not have the same cytogenetic abnormality. Myxoid DFSP has a more uniform distribution of spindled to stellate cells without the evenly distributed plexiform vessels. It should be pointed out that myxoid DFSP can have vessels that resemble those of myxoid liposarcomas in areas, but this is usually a focal finding. FISH for *PDGFB* rearrangement can be used to confirm the diagnosis of DFSP in difficult cases. Myxofibrosarcoma has more nuclear atypia and coarser curvilinear vessels than myxoid liposarcoma. Neither DFSP nor myxofibrosarcoma has true lipoblasts. FISH to detect *FUS* or *DDIT3* rearrangement will easily identify myxoid liposarcoma in problematic cases.

Selected References

1. Billings SD, Folpe AL. Diagnostically challenging spindle cell lipomas: a report of 34 "low-fat" and "fat-free" variants. Am J Dermatopathol. 2007;29(5):437–42.
2. Buehler D, Marburger TB, Billings SD. Primary subcutaneous myxoid liposarcoma: a clinicopathologic review of three cases with molecular confirmation and discussion of the differential diagnosis. J Cutan Pathol. 2014;41(12):907–15.
3. Byun JY, Choi YW, Choi HY, Myung KB. A case of dedifferentiated Liposarcoma that developed in the dermis. Ann Dermatol. 2008;20(4):204–8.
4. Carvalho GS, Cavalcanti SM, Herênio AS, Teixeira MA, Alencar ER, Gonçalves SP. Nevus lipomatosus cutaneous superficialis. An Bras Dermatol. 2016;91(5 suppl 1):114–5.
5. Chen BJ, Mariño-Enríquez A, Fletcher CD, Hornick JL. Loss of retinoblastoma protein expression in spindle cell/pleomorphic lipomas and cytogenetically related tumors: an immunohistochemical study with diagnostic implications. Am J Surg Pathol. 2012;36(8):1119–28.
6. Coffin CM. Lipoblastoma: an embryonal tumor of soft tissue related to organogenesis. Semin Diagn Pathol. 1994;11(2):98–103.
7. Collins MH, Chatten J. Lipoblastoma/lipoblastomatosis: a clinicopathologic study of 25 tumors. Am J Surg Pathol. 1997;21(10):1131–7.
8. Dadone B, Refae S, Lemarié-Delaunay C, Bianchini L, Pedeutour F. Molecular cytogenetics of pediatric adipocytic tumors. Cancer Genet. 2015;208(10):469–81.
9. Dei Tos AP, Mentzel T, Fletcher CD. Primary liposarcoma of the skin: a rare neoplasm with unusual high grade features. Am J Dermatopathol. 1998;20(4):332–8.
10. Enzinger FM, Harvey DA. Spindle cell lipoma. Cancer. 1975;36(5):1852–9.

11. Evans HL. Atypical lipomatous tumor, its variants, and its combined forms: a study of 61 cases, with a minimum follow-up of 10 years. Am J Surg Pathol. 2007;31(1):1–14.
12. Furlong MA, Fanburg-Smith JC, Miettinen M. The morphologic spectrum of hibernoma: a clinicopathologic study of 170 cases. Am J Surg Pathol. 2001;25(6):809–14.
13. Gardner JM, Dandekar M, Thomas D, Goldblum JR, Weiss SW, Billings SD, Lucas DR, McHugh JB, Patel RM. Cutaneous and subcutaneous pleomorphic liposarcoma: a clinicopathologic study of 29 cases with evaluation of MDM2 gene amplification in 26. Am J Surg Pathol. 2012;36(7):1047–51.
14. Hofvander J, Arbajian E, Stenkula KG, Lindkvist-Petersson K, Larsson M, Nilsson J, Magnusson L, von Steyern FV, Rissler P, Hornick JL, Mertens F. Frequent low-level mutations of protein kinase D2 in angiolipoma. J Pathol. 2017;241(5):578–82.
15. Ko JS, Daniels B, Emanuel PO, Elson P, Khachaturov V, McKenney JK, Goldblum JR, Billings SD. Spindle cell lipomas in women: a report of 53 cases. Am J Surg Pathol. 2017;41(9):1267–74.
16. Mehregan AH, Tavafoghi V, Ghandchi A. Nevus lipomatosus cutaneous superficialis (Hoffmann-Zurhelle). J Cutan Pathol. 1975;2(6):307–13.
17. Meis JM, Enzinger FM. Chondroid lipoma. A unique tumor simulating liposarcoma and myxoid chondrosarcoma. Am J Surg Pathol. 1993;17(11):1103–12.
18. Paredes BE, Mentzel T. Atypical lipomatous tumor/"well-differentiated liposarcoma" of the skin clinically presenting as a skin tag: clinicopathologic, immunohistochemical, and molecular analysis of 2 cases. Am J Dermatopathol. 2011;33(6):603–7.
19. Roh HS, Lee HE, Park MH, Ko JY, Ro YS. Subcutaneous myxoid and round cell liposarcoma. Ann Dermatol. 2011;23(3):338–41.
20. Sheng W, Lu L, Wang J. Cellular angiolipoma: a clinicopathological and immunohistochemical study of 12 cases. Am J Dermatopathol. 2013;35(2):220–5.
21. Shmookler BM, Enzinger FM. Pleomorphic lipoma: a benign tumor simulating liposarcoma. A clinicopathologic analysis of 48 cases. Cancer. 1981;47(1):126–33.
22. Thomson TA, Horsman D, Bainbridge TC. Cytogenetic and cytologic features of chondroid lipoma of soft tissue. Mod Pathol. 1999;12(1):88–91.
23. Thway K, Flora RS, Fisher C. Chondroid lipoma: an update and review. Ann Diagn Pathol. 2012;16(3):230–4.
24. Weiss SW. Lipomatous tumors. Monogr Pathol. 1996;38:207–39.

Nerve Sheath and Related Tumors

10

Steven D. Billings

Abstract

This chapter reviews the wide spectrum of cutaneous nerve sheath tumors. The vast majority are benign tumors, including neurofibromas, schwannomas, perineuriomas, granular cell tumors, and various neuroma subtypes. Malignant granular cell tumor, malignant peripheral nerve sheath tumor, and Ewing sarcoma, a malignant neuroectodermal tumor, are also rarely encountered in the skin. Diagnostic criteria and practical considerations are emphasized.

Neurofibroma

Clinical Features

There are three histologic subtypes of neurofibroma: localized (conventional), diffuse, and plexiform neurofibroma. Localized neurofibroma is the most common cutaneous nerve sheath tumor encountered in dermatopathology practice. It usually presents in young adults, but can be seen at any age. Men and women are affected equally. Clinically, lesions can be polypoid and resemble intradermal nevi or acrochordons or present as deeper dermal papulonodules.

Diffuse neurofibromas are an uncommon variant that usually present in the head and neck of children and young adults. Most patients do not have neurofibromatosis, but a subset may have this condition. Clinically, the lesions are ill-defined, infiltrative tumors of the dermis and subcutis. Rare cases can be quite large.

Plexiform neurofibroma is pathognomonic for neurofibromatosis type 1 (NF1). They typically develop early in life, are diagnosed macroscopically based on imaging or gross pathologic features, and present as large plexiform soft tissue masses with a characteristic "bag of worms" appearance. These lesions must be distinguished from neurofibromas with merely a microscopic plexiform growth pattern, which are not necessarily associated with NF1.

Neurofibromas are benign tumors, usually cured by simple excision. True plexiform neurofibromas have a significant risk of malignant transformation to malignant peripheral nerve sheath tumor.

Pathologic Features

Localized neurofibroma is typically a circumscribed but unencapsulated tumor composed of haphazardly arranged bland spindled to comma-shaped cells set in a collagenous, variably myxoid, stroma (Fig. 10.1). The stroma has a light pink hue and is finer than reticular dermal colla-

S. D. Billings (✉)
Department of Pathology, Cleveland Clinic, Cleveland, OH, USA
e-mail: billins@ccf.org

S. D. Billings et al. (eds.), *Soft Tissue Tumors of the Skin*,
https://doi.org/10.1007/978-1-4939-8812-9_10

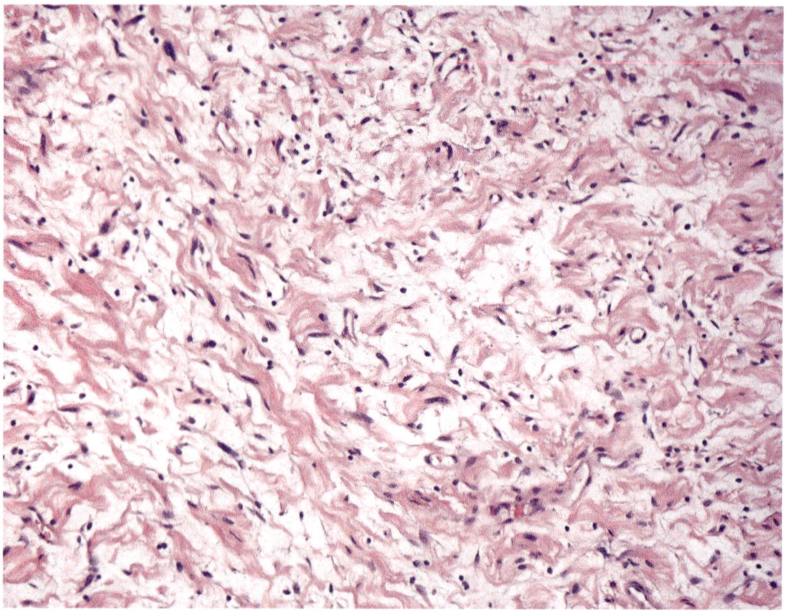

Fig. 10.1 Neurofibroma with bland spindled cells with wavy nuclei embedded in a variably collagenous and myxoid stroma

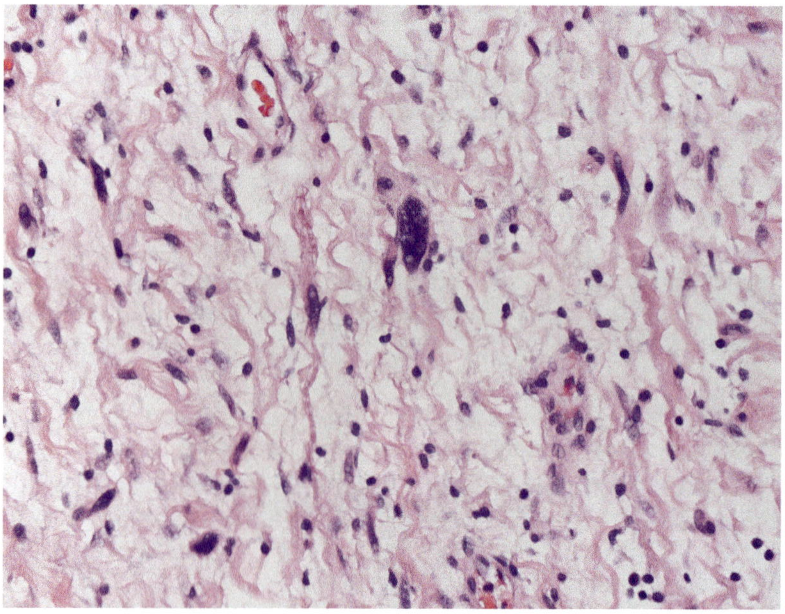

Fig. 10.2 Neurofibroma with degenerative atypia consisting of scattered cells with enlarged pleomorphic nuclei

gen bundles. Scattered mast cells are present, but this is not a specific feature. Occasional cases will demonstrate cytologic atypia consisting of scattered spindle cells with enlarged hyperchromatic and pleomorphic nuclei with smudgy chromatin (Fig. 10.2). This atypia is considered degenerative in nature and is not indicative of malignant transformation, unless the changes are diffuse and associated with increased cellularity and mitotic activity (see malignant peripheral nerve sheath tumor below). By immunohistochemistry, neurofibromas are variably positive for S100 protein, EMA, and CD34, recapitulating the different constituents of normal nerves: Schwann cells, perineurial cells, and perineurial fibroblasts, respectively.

In diffuse neurofibroma, the cellular components are the same as in localized neurofibroma.

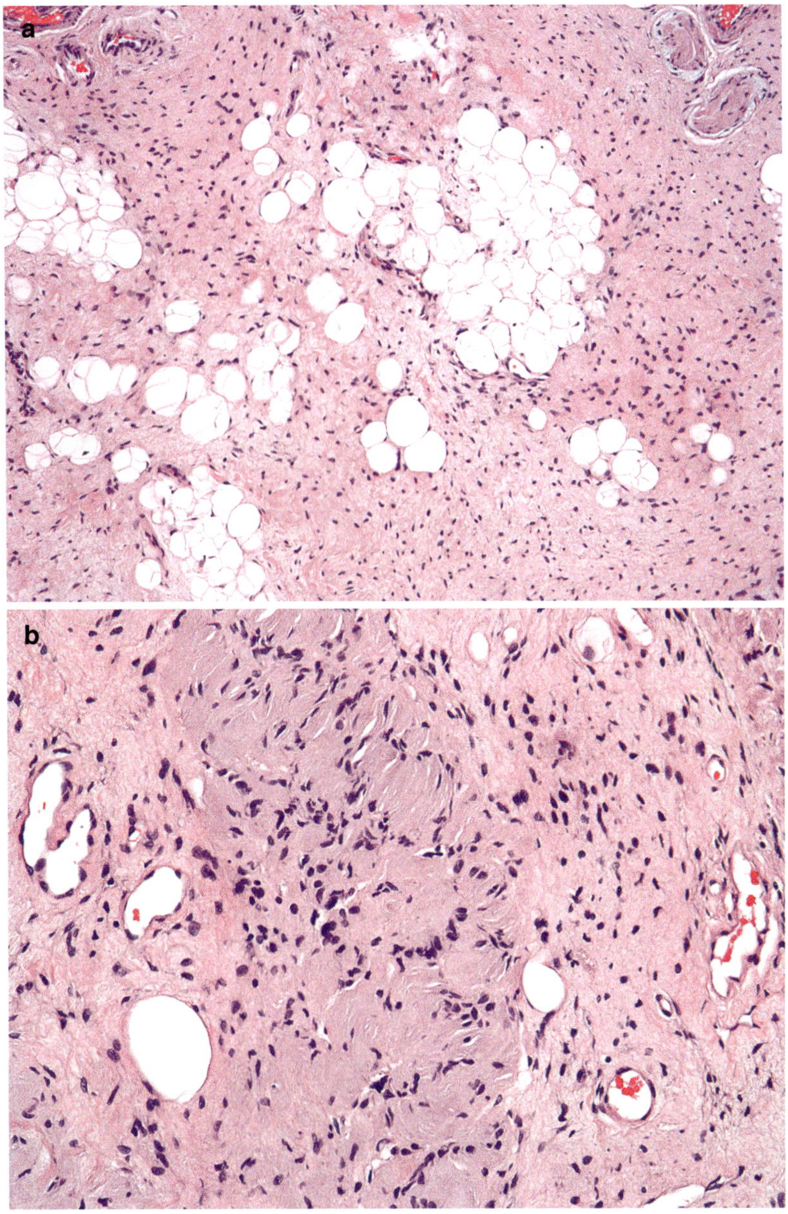

Fig. 10.3 (**a**) Diffuse neurofibroma infiltrating through adipose tissue of the subcutis. (**b**) Meissner body formation seen in the center of the picture is typical of diffuse neurofibroma

In contradistinction to the latter, the tumor is poorly circumscribed and infiltrates around preexisting dermal structures, extending into the subcutis (Fig. 10.3a). The tumor cells are more evenly distributed in the stroma compared with conventional neurofibromas. Diffuse neurofibromas often exhibit structures that resemble Meissner corpuscles (Fig. 10.3b).

Neurofibromas with a plexiform growth pattern consist of tangled, markedly expanded nerve fibers composed of spindled to comma-shaped nuclei that resemble the tumor cells of conventional neurofibroma (Fig. 10.4). They may also have areas resembling diffuse neurofibroma (Table 10.1).

Differential Diagnosis

For localized neurofibroma, the differential diagnosis includes schwannoma, perineurioma,

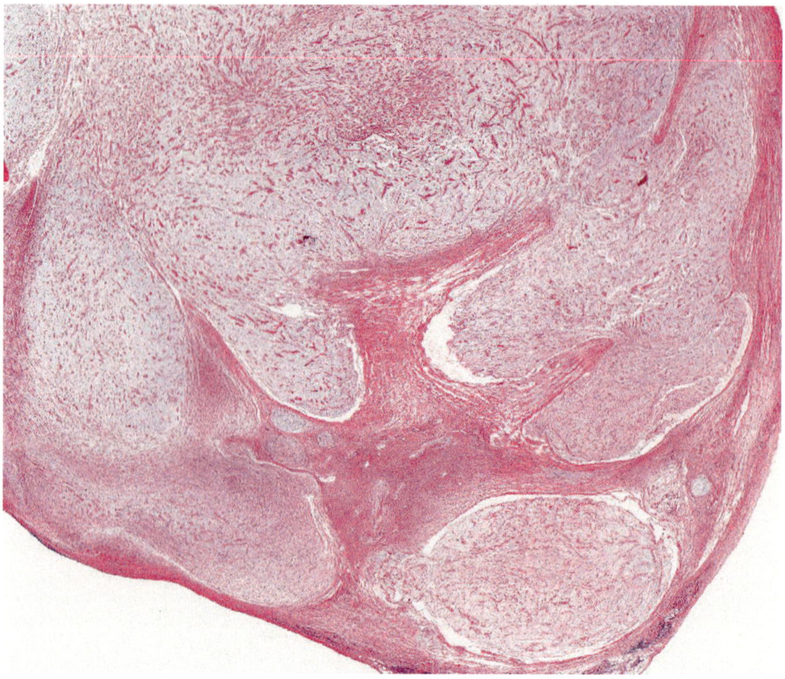

Fig. 10.4 Plexiform neurofibroma with expanded nerve fibers in a distinctly plexiform pattern

Table 10.1 Key pathologic features: neurofibroma

Bland spindled cells with wavy nuclei in collagenous to myxoid stroma
May have focal atypia
Variably positive for S100, EMA, CD34
Diffuse neurofibroma
Infiltrative growth pattern
Meissner corpuscle-like bodies
Plexiform neurofibroma
Plexiform growth pattern
Associated with neurofibromatosis

neurotized intradermal nevus, and dermatofibroma. Schwannoma has distinct hypo- and hypercellular areas, typically has a fibrous capsule, and is diffusely positive for S100 protein, rather than the more patchy positivity seen in neurofibroma. Perineurioma has a more swirling arrangement of tumor cells with elongated cytoplasmic processes and is positive for EMA and often CD34, but is negative for S100 protein. Less common but also useful stains include claudin-1 and GLUT-1, which are typically positive in perineuriomas. Some intradermal nevi will undergo neurotization, a process by which deep dermal melanocytes become more spindled and resemble the constituent cells of neurofibromas. However, there are usually conventional nested melanocytes in the superficial dermis that facilitate recognition of a melanocytic lesion. Neurotized nevi also do not have the same tumor formed stroma as neurofibromas. Dermatofibromas may be confused with neurofibromas at low magnification. However the spindled cells of dermatofibromas intercalate around preexisting collagen bundles of the reticular dermis in a characteristic fashion (collagen trapping), and secondary elements such as multinucleated giant cells, foamy histiocytes and hemosiderin-laden macrophages are typically present at least focally. Dermatofibromas are also negative for S100 protein.

Diffuse neurofibromas need to be distinguished from dermatofibrosarcoma protuberans, especially the myxoid variant. Diffuse neurofibromas and dermatofibrosarcoma protuberans can both infiltrate into the fat and are immunoreactive for CD34, but dermatofibrosarcoma protuberans lacks Meissner bodies and is negative for S100 protein. In difficult cases, molecular studies such as FISH or PCR can be utilized to look for the characteristic t(17;22) translocation of dermatofibrosarcoma protuberans.

The primary differential diagnosis is with other forms of neurofibroma. One should keep in mind that it is often difficult, if not impossible, to make a diagnosis of plexiform neurofibroma on small skin biopsies. The diagnosis is best reserved for large tumors that are suspected to be plexiform neurofibromas clinically or by imaging studies. It should be remembered that NF1 patients also often have numerous localized neurofibromas and sometimes diffuse neurofibromas. Plexiform schwannoma also enters the differential diagnosis. Plexiform schwannomas tend to be much smaller than plexiform neurofibromas and have distinct Antoni A and Antoni B areas, which are not found in plexiform neurofibromas.

Schwannoma

Clinical Features

Schwannoma (neurilemoma) is a benign nerve sheath tumor composed almost entirely of neoplastic Schwann cells. The age range at presentation is wide and no gender or ethnic predisposition has been identified. In cutaneous lesions, the dermis and subcutis of the head and neck region and flexor surfaces of extremities are most commonly involved, but they may arise in almost any superficial location. The presentation is usually that of a solitary, slow-growing, asymptomatic mass, sometimes with a duration of a few years. Occasionally, patients may experience pain or paresthesia.

Most schwannomas are sporadic and solitary. Multiple schwannomas should prompt evaluation for familial or syndromic causes. Bilateral vestibular nerve schwannoma is a well-known pathognomonic feature of neurofibromatosis type 2, in addition to schwannomas at other sites, congenital cataract, meningioma, and glioma. Schwannomatosis is the other syndrome that may cause multiple non-intradermal schwannomas (excluding bilateral vestibular nerve involvement), which are usually of late onset (30s) with accompanying cutaneous pain. Approximately 10% of schwannomatosis cases are familial/hereditary; the remainder are sporadic.

Schwannomas are benign tumors with simple enucleation being curative in most cases. Large deeper-seated lesions may require surgical resection. Recurrence of classic schwannoma is very rare, but cellular schwannoma has a higher risk of local recurrence. Plexiform schwannoma can recur and may be locally infiltrative in some cases. However, distant metastasis does not occur. Malignant transformation, as discussed below, is exceptionally rare.

Pathologic Features

Grossly, schwannomas are encapsulated and tan-yellow in color. They may be fusiform or globular and are usually eccentric to an associated nerve. Superficial cases are usually smaller than 5 cm, whereas deep tumors may grow to a considerable size. Large schwannomas are also prone to develop secondary changes including cystic degeneration and hemorrhage.

Microscopically schwannomas are well-circumscribed and encapsulated. Lymphoid aggregates are often appreciated at the periphery at low magnification. The classical image of a schwannoma consists of a biphasic pattern: cellular "Antoni A" and less cellular, loose or sometimes myxoid "Antoni B" areas (Fig. 10.5). The well-known Verocay body represents a structure formed by two parallel rows of tumor cells vaguely palisading around a central zone rich in eosinophilic fibrillary processes (Fig. 10.6). Constituent tumor cells are mostly spindled and arranged in short fascicles or vague whorls and have fusiform nuclei with inconspicuous nucleoli and lightly eosinophilic cytoplasm with indistinct cell borders. Nuclear pseudoinclusions can be seen occasionally. Rare examples with adipocytic/lipoblastic differentiation mimicking signet ring cells have been reported. Degenerative changes are quite common, including hyalinized/thrombosed vessels, hemorrhage, cystic change, xanthomatous histiocytes, and stromal hyalinization (Fig. 10.7a). Hyperchromatic, bizarre nuclei with "smudged" chromatin can often be noticed even at low to intermediate magnification, but the mitotic count is low and atypical mitotic figures are absent (Fig. 10.7b). The term "ancient schwannoma" refers to tumors with low mitotic rate and significant degenerative nuclear atypia. Several important variants merit additional attention and are discussed individually below (Table 10.2).

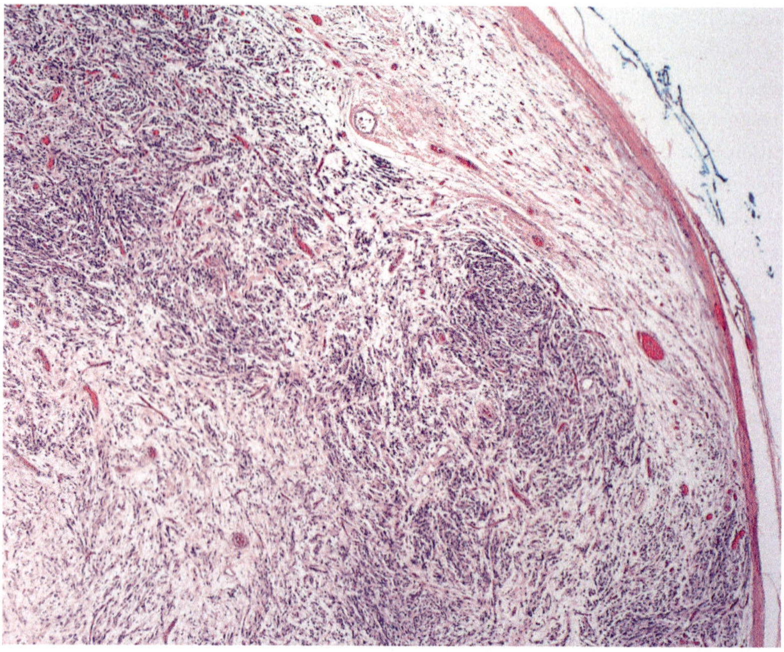

Fig. 10.5 A. Schwannoma with true capsule and cellular Antoni A areas and hypocellular Antoni B areas

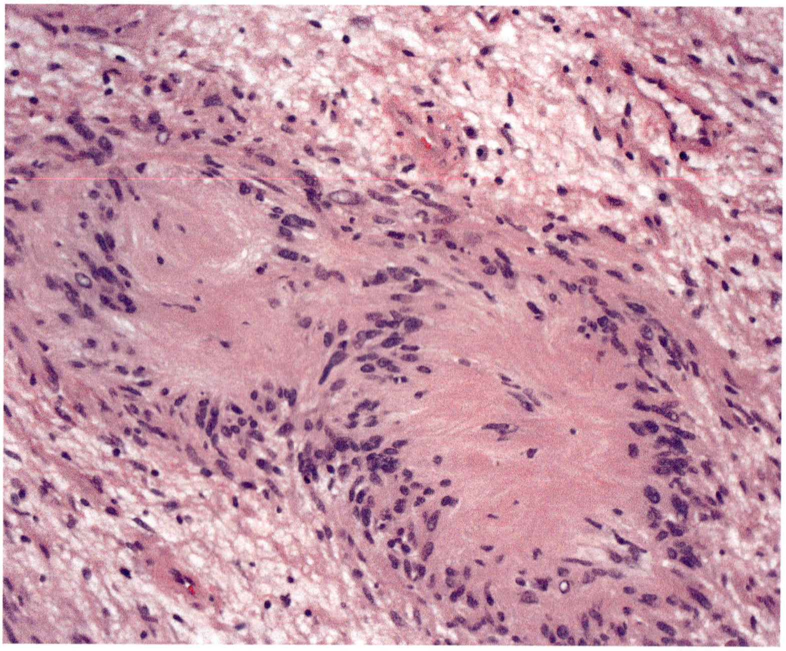

Fig. 10.6 Verocay body characterized by distinct palisading of tumor nuclei

Cellular Schwannoma

Cellular schwannoma is a distinct variant in that it is composed almost exclusively of cellular "Antoni A" areas without Verocay body formation or nuclear palisading (Fig. 10.8). In extreme cases, the spindle cells may be arranged in long fascicles similar to the herringbone pattern seen in fibrosarcoma. Loose or cystic areas account for no more than 10% of the entire tumor. Mitotic figures are more common compared to conventional schwannoma and range from 0 to 4/10 per high-power fields (HPFs). Atypical mitotic

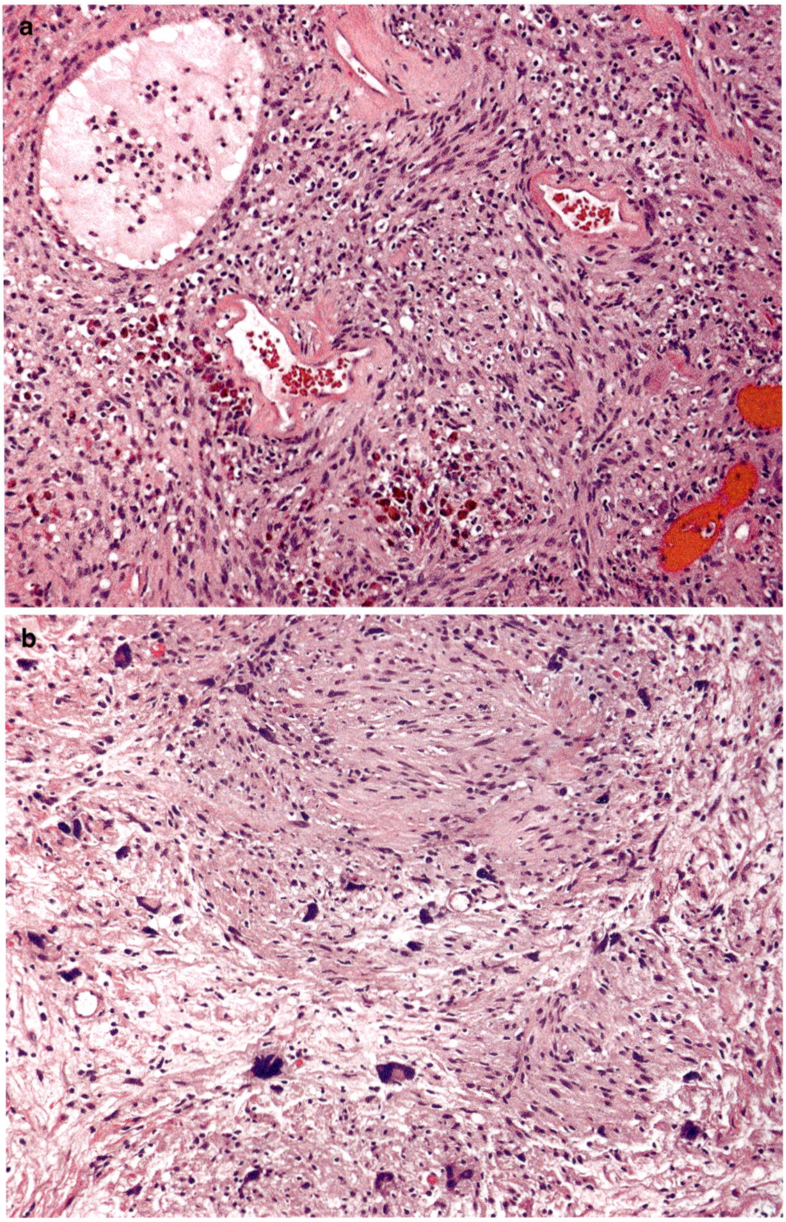

Fig. 10.7 (**a**) Schwannoma with hyalinized vasculature. (**b**) Degenerative atypia in a schwannoma

figures are absent. Most cases are deeply located, but subcutaneous cases are occasionally seen.

Plexiform Schwannoma

Plexiform schwannoma occurs in the dermis or subcutaneous tissue. As the name suggests, the tumors have a multinodular growth pattern with individual thin fibrous capsules (Fig. 10.9). Interconnection of nodules can be appreciated on serial sections. The cytomorphology of the nodules is similar to the "Antoni A" areas seen in classic schwannomas, though the cellularity is usually higher and Verocay bodies are seen less frequently. "Antoni B" areas with hyalinized vessels and foci of cystic change may be seen in some of the nodules. Mitotic activity is typically inconspicuous, but cases with as many as 8/10 HPFs have been reported. In some cases,

Table 10.2 Key pathologic features: schwannoma

Fibrous capsule
Hypercellular and hypocellular areas composed of bland spindled cells
Hyalinized vessels often present
May have degenerative atypia
Spindled cells strongly positive for S100, but negative for CD34
Cellular schwannoma
Lacks hypocellular areas
May have mitotic figures up to 4/10 HPFs
Plexiform schwannoma
Multinodular growth pattern
Microcystic/reticular schwannoma
Rare
Reticulated, cord-like growth pattern
Epithelioid schwannoma
Predominantly composed of epithelioid Schwann cells
25% multinodular
Mitotic rate low
Neuroblastoma-like schwannoma
Collagenous nodules surrounded by tumor cells
Still has features of conventional schwannoma

significant nuclear atypia is also present. Melanin pigment has been reported in rare cases. Plexiform schwannoma in infants can be congenital and present extremely worrisome features including infiltrative growth in the form of small peripheral nodules, high cellularity, high mitotic counts (up to 31/10 HPFs), and lack of some important characteristics of conventional schwannomas, such as lymphoid aggregates, "Antoni B" areas, and hyalinized thick-walled vessels. Indeed, such lesions were originally described as plexiform malignant peripheral nerve sheath tumor in the earlier literature. Although there are occasional cases of plexiform schwannoma in patients with NF1 or NF2, this association is weak at best in contrast to the association of plexiform neurofibromas with NF1.

Microcystic/Reticular Schwannoma

Microcystic/reticular schwannoma has a predilection for the gastrointestinal tract, but dermal and subcutaneous cases have been described.

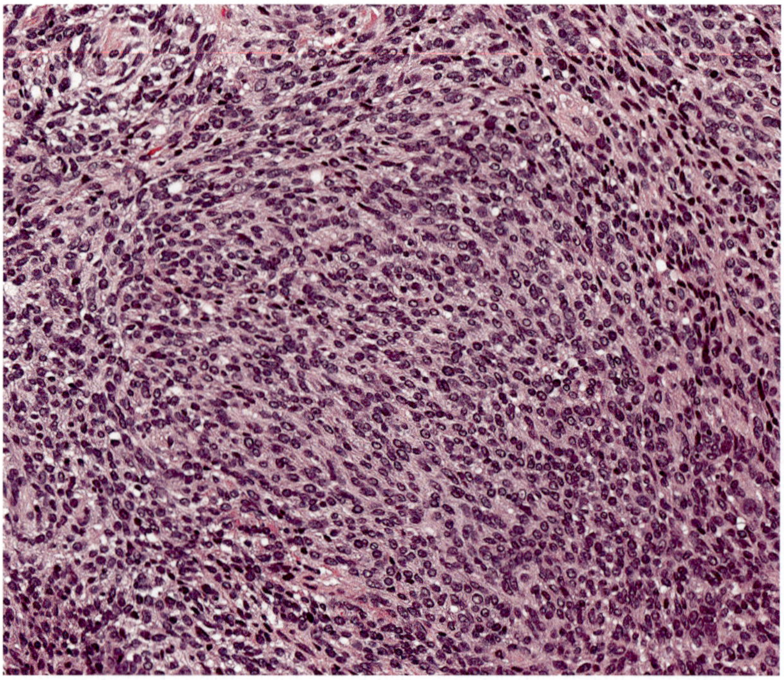

Fig. 10.8 Cellular schwannoma with fascicles of uniform spindled cells and no hypocellular areas

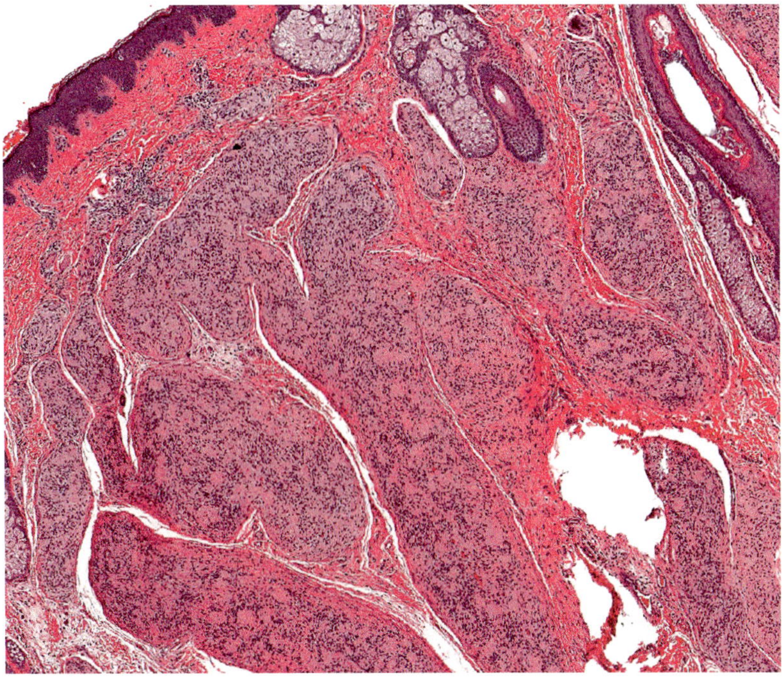

Fig. 10.9 Plexiform schwannoma demonstrating interconnecting nodules in the dermis surrounded by thin capsule

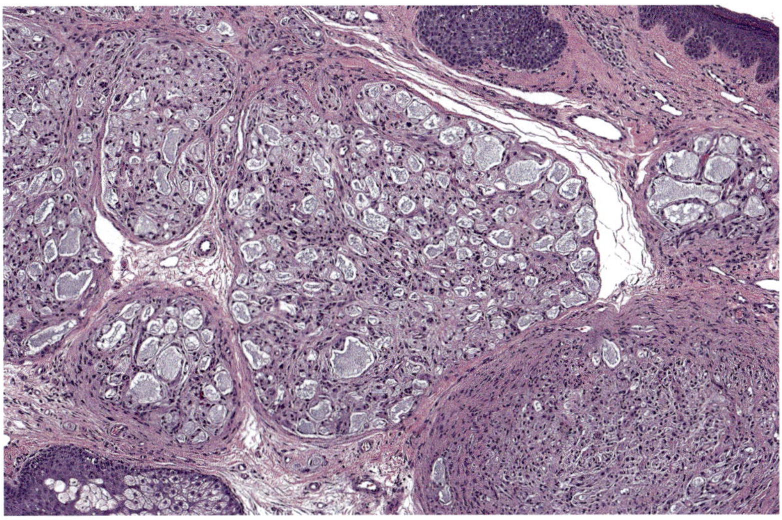

Fig. 10.10 Reticular schwannoma characterized by cords and strands of tumor cells in a myxoid stroma

These lesions are usually well-circumscribed or multilobular and may not be entirely encapsulated. It is characterized by the presence of microcystic and reticular areas composed of anastomosing cords and strands of tumor cells embedded in a variably myxoid to collagenous stroma (Fig. 10.10). Individual cells are spindled to ovoid and may be signet-like in some cases. Areas of conventional schwannoma, seen in some cases, can be a helpful diagnostic clue to the schwannoma diagnosis.

Epithelioid Schwannoma

Epithelioid schwannoma is predominantly composed of epithelioid cells (>50%). The dermis and subcutis of the extremities are the most

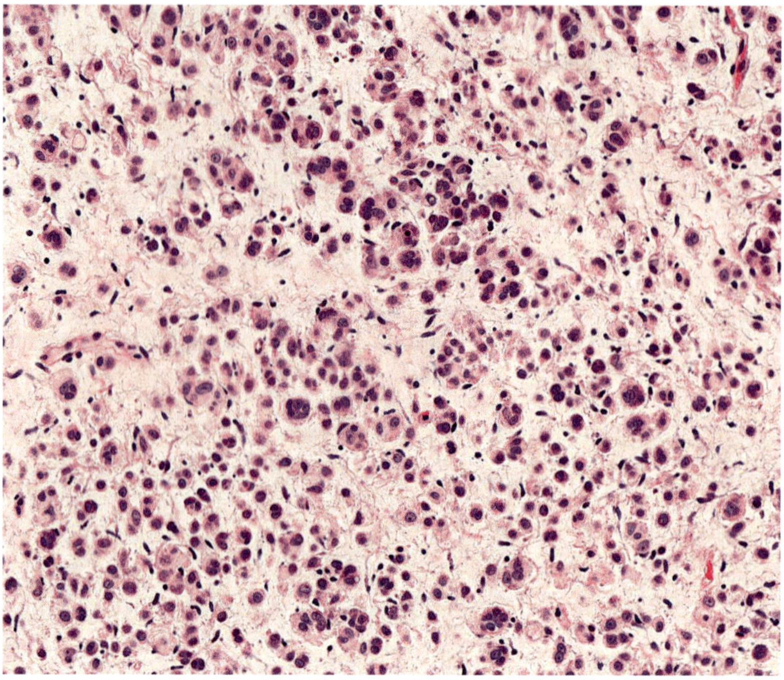

Fig. 10.11 Epithelioid schwannoma is predominantly composed of epithelioid rather than spindled Schwann cells

common sites of involvement. Most lesions are less than 5 cm, well-circumscribed, and ensheathed by a layer of perineurium. About a quarter of cases are multinodular. The tumors are composed of tight clusters, cords, or individual epithelioid cells (Fig. 10.11). Hyalinized vessels are present in the majority of cases (95%). Giant collagen rosette-like structures are seen occasionally. Cases with significant nuclear atypia (nuclear to cytoplasmic size ratio > 3:1) and mitotic index >3/10 HPFs, which fall short of criteria for a diagnosis of epithelioid malignant peripheral nerve sheath tumor, have been designated as "atypical variants," although the prognosis for these lesions is no different from typical schwannomas.

Neuroblastoma-Like Schwannoma

This is an unusual schwannoma variant in which tumor cells palisade around central collagenous cores mimicking the rosettes of a neuroblastoma (Fig. 10.12). They still have a capsule and the typical immunophenotype of a conventional schwannoma.

Pseudoglandular Schwannoma and Schwannomas with True Glands

Schwannomas with glandular structures are rare. Most of the cases represent schwannomas with central degeneration resulting in pseudoglandular structures that appear to be lined by epithelioid Schwann cells. Schwannomas with "true glands" are exceedingly rare with only a dozen reported cases. In addition to the rarity of such tumors, one has to exclude the possibility of entrapped dermal appendages. Hence, although it is difficult to draw firm conclusions, suffice it to say that the presence of glands or gland-like structures does not appear to have an adverse effect on the benign nature of schwannomas with these features in the very limited number of reported cases.

Schwannoma with Secondary Malignancy

Malignant change in neurofibromas, especially in the setting of neurofibromatosis 1, is well-recognized and not infrequent. In comparison, secondary malignancy developing in schwannomas is much rarer and typically seen in deep soft

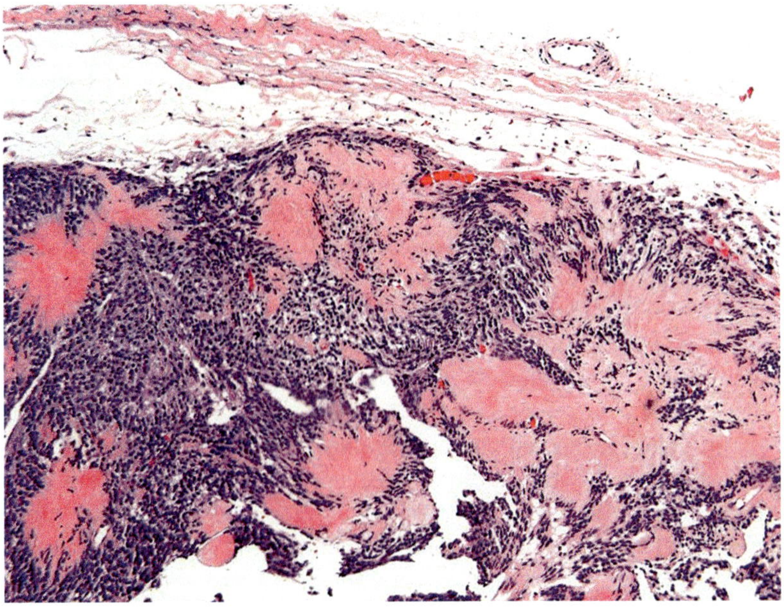

Fig. 10.12 Neuroblastoma-like schwannoma characterized by palisading arrangement of tumor cells around central zone of collagen that mimics the rosettes seen in neuroblastoma

tissue tumors rather than cutaneous ones. Cases with malignant change have been reported in the literature under the terms epithelioid malignant change, epithelioid malignant peripheral nerve sheath tumor, and even epithelioid angiosarcoma. Epithelioid malignant change is defined by scattered large epithelioid tumor cells with vesicular chromatin and prominent nucleoli, which are distinct from the hyperchromatic nuclei of degenerative or "ancient" schwannomas.

Immunohistochemical stains for S100 protein are diffusely and strongly positive in almost all constituent cells, which is a diagnostic feature different from the patchy weak to moderate staining seen in neurofibromas. Immunohistochemical stains for SOX10 are similarly diffusely positive, but have a nuclear staining pattern. Collagen IV or laminin shows diffuse pericellular staining. Neurofilament protein stains may help identify axons of preexisting nerves at the periphery of the tumor, in contrast to axon entrapment in the midst of neurofibromas. GFAP can be positive in some cases, and cross reactivity with cytokeratins leading to positive staining has been reported in rare cases. EMA highlights the perineurium/capsule. Synaptophysin, HMB45, and Melan-A stains are typically negative in schwannomas.

Electron microscopy is rarely needed or used nowadays but shows the diagnostic abundant reduplicated basal lamina.

Germline *SMARCB1* (INI1, hBAF47) mutation has been identified in 30–60% of familial and 10% of sporadic cases of schwannomatosis. Most of these are missense mutations in contrast to the deletion and truncation seen in hereditary rhabdoid tumor syndrome, although rare overlapping cases do exist. A recent study demonstrated *LZTR1* germline missense mutations in 80% of a strictly defined subset of schwannomatosis cases (loss of portion of 22q and mutated NF2 in the remaining allele, but lacking germline *SMARCB1* mutation). The molecular abnormalities underlying schwannomatosis appear to be heterogeneous with many different molecular subsets likely awaiting discovery by future studies.

Differential Diagnosis

The picture of a classical schwannoma with its biphasic patterns is distinct and has a limited differential diagnosis. Solitary circumscribed neuroma (palisaded encapsulated neuroma) has morphologic overlap, but the clefting artifact characteristic of solitary circumscribed neuroma allows distinction (see below). Distinction from neurofibroma is usually quite straightforward. Neurofibroma is usually circumscribed but not encapsulated. A blue-grayish mucinous matrix is often evident with the characteristic "shredded carrot" collagen. The biphasic pattern of schwannoma is absent. Immunohistochemical stains for S100 protein highlight some of the cells rather than the diffuse, strong immunoreactivity of schwannoma. Neurofilament also labels the axons within neurofibromas. Hybrid nerve sheath tumors composed of neurofibroma and schwannoma may take the form of background neurofibroma with scattered nodules of schwannoma, simulating "Antoni B" and "Antoni A" patterns.

The morphologic variants of schwannoma may pose some diagnostic difficulty and have a longer list of differential diagnoses. Cellular schwannoma can be easily misdiagnosed as a spindle cell sarcoma due to its hypercellularity and sometimes high mitotic rate. However, its circumscription and encapsulation are crucial hints to its benign nature. Careful sampling and searching for the paucicellular "Antoni B" areas of conventional schwannoma can be helpful if present. Diffuse and intense S100 positivity is not a feature of typical malignant peripheral nerve sheath tumors, and if this is seen in a biopsy of a cellular spindle cell neoplasm, it strongly suggests a cellular schwannoma. There are exceptions to this rule however, so one must proceed with caution and consider all of the histopathologic and clinical features that are presented in a given case. Cutaneous malignant peripheral nerve sheath tumors are also exceedingly rare, and most have areas of typical precursor neurofibroma. Spindle cell/desmoplastic melanoma is frequently amelanotic, with only S100 protein or SOX10 positivity, and therefore may mimic cellular schwannoma. However, spindle cell/desmoplastic melanoma is often associated with a junctional melanocytic component, infiltrative borders, cellular atypia, mitotic activity, and lymphoid aggregates.

Plexiform schwannoma must be distinguished from plexiform neurofibroma, which is diagnostic of neurofibromatosis 1 (NF1) and carries risk of malignant transformation to malignant peripheral nerve sheath tumor. By definition, plexiform neurofibroma must be able to be diagnosed grossly or on imaging studies to be pathognomonic of NF1. A microscopically apparent plexiform growth pattern, in and of itself, is insufficient for a diagnosis of NF1. In additional to the morphologic differences between schwannoma and neurofibroma, the pattern of S100 protein immunoreactivity is also very helpful since it is strongly and diffusely positive in plexiform schwannoma, whereas the stain only highlights a subset of cells in plexiform neurofibroma.

The microcystic/reticular growth pattern is not limited to schwannoma but can be seen in perineurioma, myoepithelial neoplasms, dermal nerve sheath myxoma and ossifying fibromyxoid tumor (OFMT). A panel of immunostains including S100 protein, EMA, and cytokeratin can easily exclude reticulated/microcystic perineurioma and myoepithelial neoplasms given the former is EMA positive and S100 protein negative and the latter is cytokeratin/EMA and S100 protein positive. Dermal nerve sheath myxoma has a distinct predilection to arise in the fingers and is distinctly myxoid in appearance, unlike schwannomas. This tumor is also diffusely positive for S100 protein and may have focal CD34 positivity, but unlike schwannomas, they are typically positive for GFAP and may be positive for neuron-specific enolase and CD57. Ossifying fibromyxoid tumor (OFMT) has a characteristic peripheral bony shell in 80% of cases. S100 protein is positive in most cases but is less intense and diffuse than the staining pattern seen in a typical schwannoma. In addition, SOX10 is almost always negative in OFMT but is consistently positive in schwannoma.

A list of epithelioid neoplasms comes into the differential diagnosis of epithelioid schwannoma, with nodular or metastatic melanoma and epithelioid malignant peripheral nerve sheath tumor being the most important ones to recognize given their aggressive clinical behavior. Nodular melanomas typically have a junctional component and are not encapsulated. Metastatic melanomas may be circumscribed, but still lack a capsule. Melanomas have more cytologic atypia and mitotic activity as well. Immunoreactivity for melanocyte-specific markers (e.g., Melan-A, HMB45, MiTF) easily allows their distinction from schwannoma. Epithelioid malignant peripheral nerve sheath tumor grows in a multinodular fashion with a predilection for superficial locations. Epithelioid malignant peripheral nerve sheath tumors have more significant nuclear atypia, vesicular chromatin, higher mitotic rate, atypical mitoses, necrosis, and usually a focally myxoid stroma. Identification of a conventional schwannoma component and associated classic secondary elements such as thick-walled vessels, hemosiderin deposition, and foamy macrophages can be of tremendous help. INI1 loss by immunohistochemistry is seen in half of epithelioid malignant peripheral nerve sheath tumors and can be helpful if present. Careful histomorphologic and immunohistochemical evaluation is essential to reaching the correct diagnosis.

Neuroblastoma-like schwannoma needs to be distinguished from true neuroblastoma. The clinical presentation of these two entities is quite different and very helpful for making the diagnosis. Neuroblastoma arises in deep soft tissue, is often associated with the adrenal gland, and is a neoplasm of infants. Neuroblastoma-like schwannoma can be confused with the hyalinizing spindle cell tumor with giant collagen rosettes variant of low-grade fibromyxoid sarcoma. Low-grade fibromyxoid sarcoma lacks the distinct capsule of schwannoma and by immunohistochemistry is positive for MUC4 and negative for S100 protein.

Perineurioma

Clinical Features

Perineurioma is an uncommon benign peripheral nerve sheath tumor composed of cells with perineurial differentiation. In comparison to neurofibroma and schwannoma, perineurioma was recognized as a distinct entity only fairly recently. It has no association with neurofibromatosis. Perineuriomas can be divided into intraneural perineurioma, extraneural or soft tissue perineurioma, sclerosing perineurioma, and mucosal perineurioma, based on their distinct clinicopathologic features.

Intraneural perineurioma was previously classified under terms such as localized hypertrophic neuropathy and hypertrophic interstitial neuritis, which actually are lesions that represent Schwann cell proliferations with a true "onion bulb" appearance (see below). Intraneural perineurioma most commonly presents in young people under the age of 40, with a slight female predominance. The ulnar, radial, median, peroneal, and sciatic nerves are the most common nerves affected, but involvement of other nerves has been reported, including those in the head and neck. These lesions are usually associated with a long history of progressive neural deficit. Imaging demonstrates segmental enlargement of the involved nerve.

Extraneural or soft tissue perineurioma, the most common form, occurs in a wide age range with an equal sex distribution. The extremities and trunk are the most common locations, with fewer cases described in the head and neck region. About 10% are limited to the dermis and half are subcutaneous, while a third occur in the deep soft tissues. Most cases present as a painless mass, although associated pain is present in a subset of cases.

Sclerosing perineurioma is a distinct variant of perineurioma in that it almost exclusively occurs in the dermis and/or subcutis of acral sites of young people with a male predominance. Although distinctly uncommon, non-acral examples have been described.

Mucosal perineuriomas present as colon polyps in middle age adults and will not be discussed further here.

Perineuriomas are benign tumors with very low risk of local recurrence. Intraneural perineurioma may be associated with neural deficits if involving major nerves.

Pathologic Features

Intraneural perineuriomas present as fusiform segmental enlargement of involved nerves. On histologic examination, there is a diffuse perineurial spindle cell proliferation ensheathing individual nerve fibers and their associated Schwann cells in a multilayered, concentric fashion, creating the characteristic "pseudo-onion bulb" appearance (Fig. 10.13). Despite this highly characteristic histologic feature on cross-sections, it is less straightforward to recognize on longitudinal sections. The latter demonstrate abundant perineurial cells arranged in parallel within thickened nerve bundles. The constituent perineurial cells are cytologically bland with oval to fusiform nuclei, homogeneous chromatin, and scant eosinophilic cytoplasm. Mitotic activity is minimal. Occasional large, degenerate, hyperchromatic nuclei similar to those seen in ancient schwannoma or neurofibroma can be seen; this change has no clinical significance.

Soft tissue perineuriomas have a mean size of 4 cm but occasionally can be much larger. Cutaneous examples tend to be smaller at presentation. They are non-encapsulated but well-circumscribed tumors. Plexiform or multinodular growth patterns have been reported. Microscopically, infiltrative growth is seen in a small subset of cases. Cellularity varies, but hypocellular lesions are the most common. Soft tissue perineurioma has a swirling to fascicular arrangement of bland spindled cells with elongated slender cytoplasmic processes in a variably myxoid and collagenous stroma (Fig. 10.14). Some cases have laminated, long fascicles with frequent clefting (Fig. 10.15). Areas with tumor cells intercalating between collagen bundles, reminiscent of collagen trapping seen in dermatofibromas, may be present. The tumor cells are embedded in a variably collagenous to myxoid stroma. If the background stroma is predominantly myxoid, the tumor may have a reticular or microcystic appearance. Most tumor cells are spindled with wavy, buckled nuclei with homogeneous chromatin, no nucleoli and long thin cytoplasmic processes with indistinct cell boundaries. In some cases, the cells may be plumper with more cytoplasm. Mitotic activity is minimal. Large hyperchromatic nuclei may be seen rarely, analogous to degenerative ancient change in schwannomas or neurofibromas.

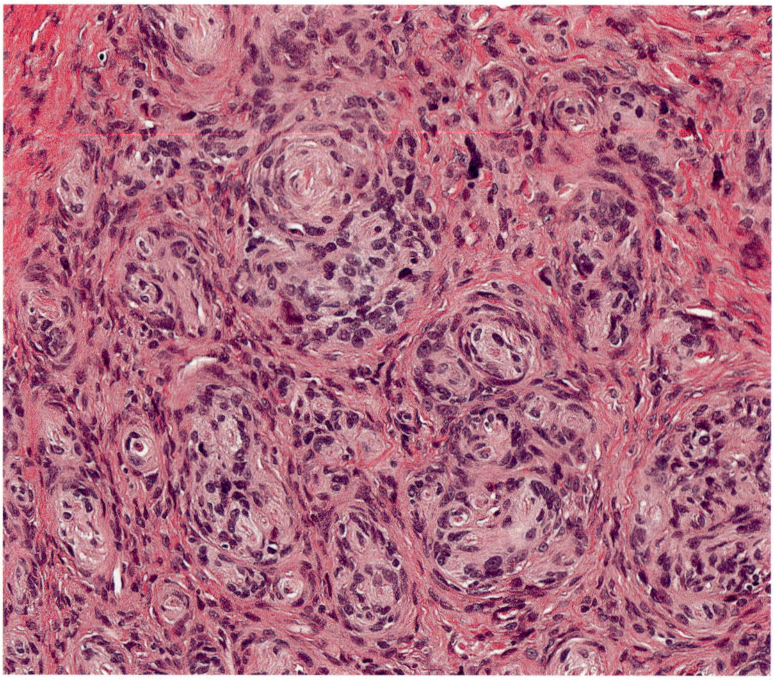

Fig. 10.13 Intraneural perineurioma with concentric proliferation of perineurial cells surrounding nerve fibers

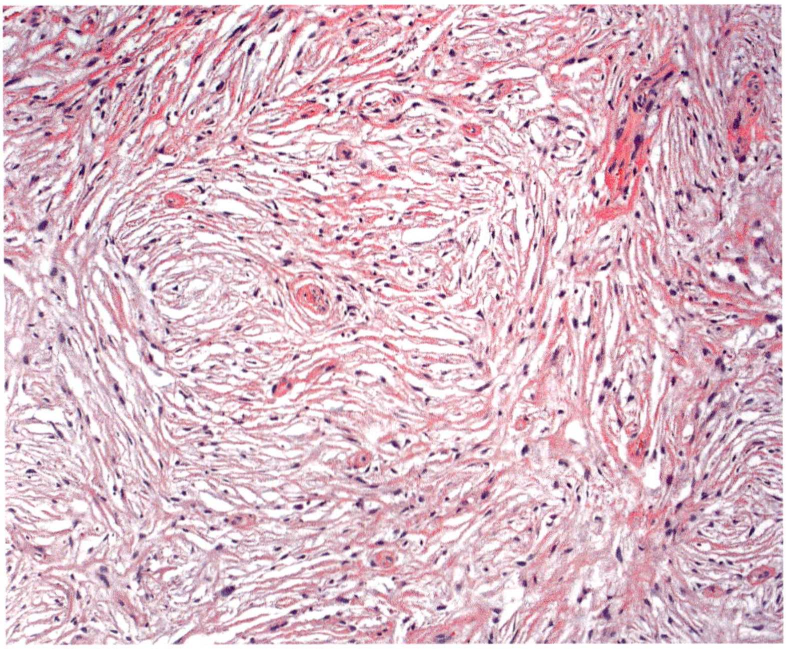

Fig. 10.14 Perineuriomas typically have a swirling pattern of bland spindled cells with elongated, delicate cytoplasmic processes in a variably myxoid and collagenous stroma

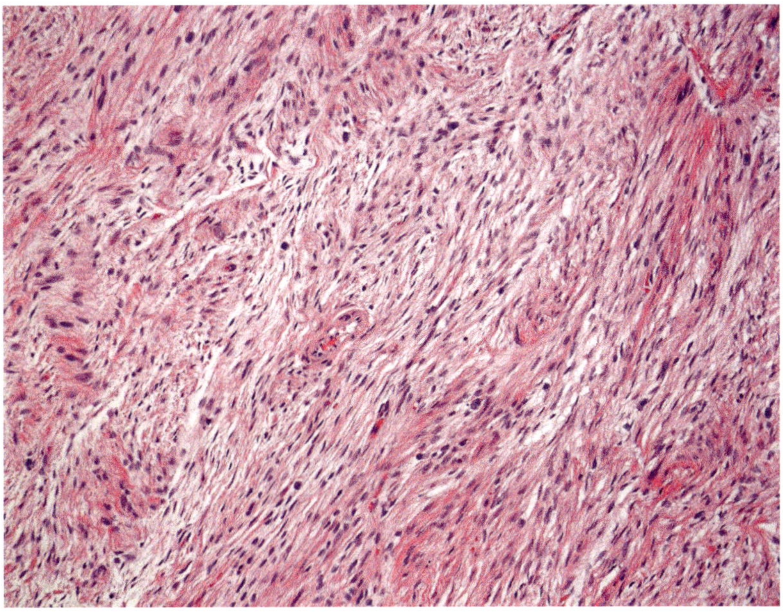

Fig. 10.15 Perineurioma with predominantly fascicular pattern

Sclerosing perineurioma has a mean size of 1.5 cm, well-circumscribed borders, and a firm, rubbery consistency grossly. Microscopically all cases have a densely collagenous or hyalinized stroma with intervening variably spindled to epithelioid tumor cells, with fine chromatin and small nucleoli. The cells have a cord-like to trabecular growth pattern (Fig. 10.16). Mitotic activity is very low and cytologic atypia is minimal (Table 10.3). Perineuriomas are positive for EMA, GLUT1, and claudin-1. Immunoreactivity for EMA is almost definitional for the diagnosis, but it can be very weak and focal, typically requiring examination at high magnification to

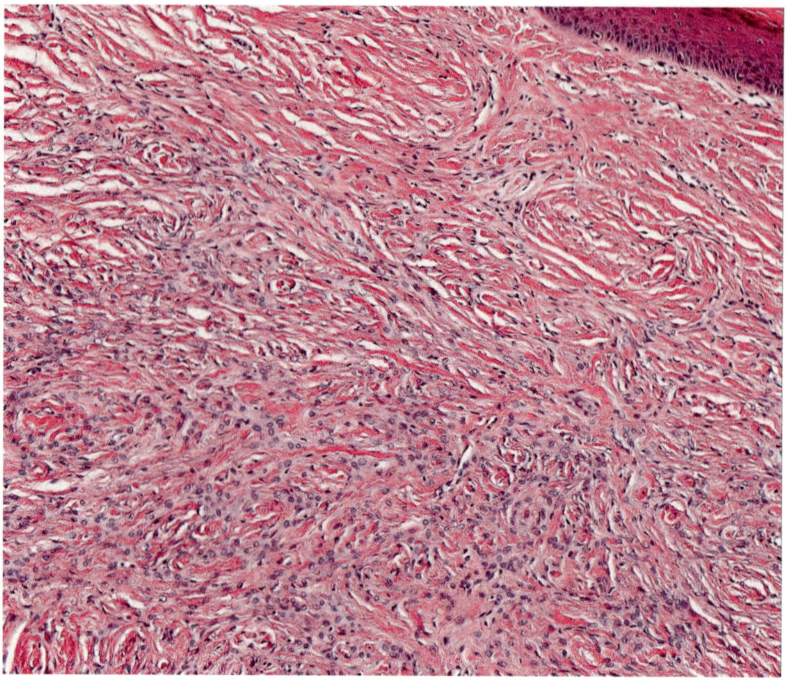

Fig. 10.16 Sclerosing perineurioma has a cord-like to reticular pattern of more epithelioid cells in a collagenous stroma

Table 10.3 Key pathologic features: perineurioma

Positive for EMA, variably positive for CD34, negative for S100
Intraneural perineurioma
Concentric proliferation of perineurial cells around nerves imparting "onion bulb" appearance
Soft tissue perineurioma
Swirling to fascicular growth pattern
Myxoid to collagenous stroma
Bland spindled cells with elongated cytoplasmic processes
Sclerosing perineurioma
Usually acral location
Spindled to epithelioid cells in cord-like pattern
Dense collagenous stroma

recognize positive cells (Fig. 10.17). The long, tapered cytoplasmic processes are typically the portion of the cell that stain the strongest, but they can be difficult to detect due to their delicate, slender appearance. Immunoreactivity for claudin-1 is stronger but only positive in about 30% of cases of soft tissue perineurioma. Immunoreactivity for claudin-1 is more frequent in sclerosing perineurioma. Perineuriomas are usually immunoreactive for CD34 and can sometimes have a "fingerprint" pattern of CD34 immunoreactivity. The tumor cells are negative for S100 protein, desmin, cytokeratin, and MUC4. Laminin and collagen IV highlight the surroundings of tumor cells. Loss of chromosome 22q has been reported.

Differential Diagnosis

The differential diagnosis for perineurioma is very broad given its diverse histologic features. Intraneural perineurioma needs to be distinguished from hypertrophic neuropathy, as seen in Charcot-Marie-Tooth disease, a disorder in which the peri-axonal sheath is composed of Schwann cells rather than normal perineurial cells. S100 protein and EMA stains are helpful in this differential, as Schwann cells are S100 positive, while perineurial cells are EMA positive. Superficial soft tissue-type perineurioma may be confused with dermatofibrosarcoma protuberans due to the sometimes shared storiform growth pattern, but perineurioma is much less cellular than conventional dermatofibrosarcoma protuberans. Myxoid dermatofibrosarcoma protuberans has a purely myxoid stroma rather than a

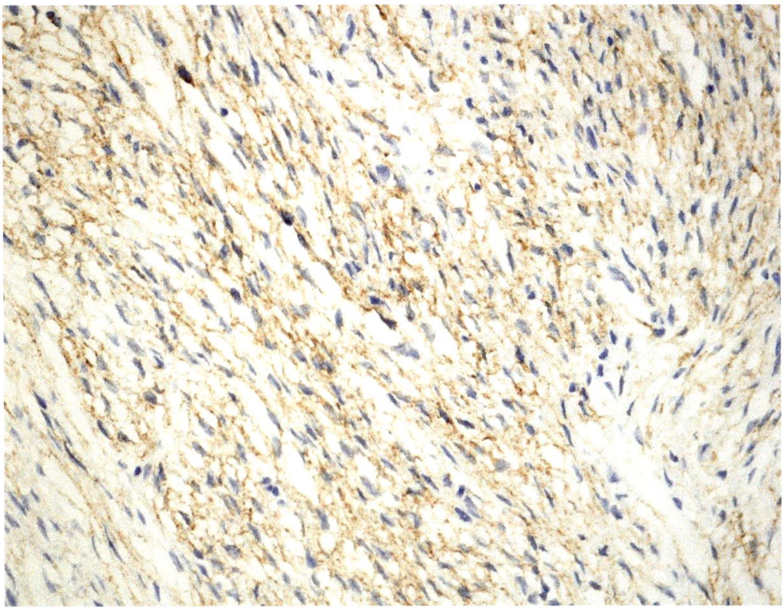

Fig. 10.17 EMA stain in perineurioma highlighting delicate cytoplasmic processes

collagenous and myxoid stroma of soft tissue perineurioma. Immunoreactivity for EMA and claudin-1 is not typically seen in dermatofibrosarcoma protuberans. Neurofibromas can be mistaken for perineurioma, but the tumor cells in neurofibroma have a random growth pattern and do not have the elongated cytoplasmic processes of perineurial cells. Neurofibromas are positive for S100 protein, unlike perineurioma. It should be pointed out that neurofibromas typically have some admixed perineurial cells. Finally, low-grade fibromyxoid sarcoma can have areas that very closely resemble perineurioma. Indeed, this is the most important and difficult malignant neoplasm to differentiate from perineurioma in our experience. Low-grade fibromyxoid sarcoma can be positive for EMA but, in contrast to perineurioma, is consistently positive for MUC4 by immunohistochemistry. The reticulated/microcystic pattern seen in some perineuriomas may be seen in schwannoma, myoepithelial tumors, ossifying fibromyxoid tumor, and extraskeletal myxoid chondrosarcoma. Identification of more conventional components of these neoplasms in conjunction with reticular foci is the most effective way to distinguish these entities from perineurioma. In addition, a limited panel of immunohistochemical stains including S100 protein, EMA, and/or claudin-1 and cytokeratins can be very helpful in excluding schwannoma, myoepithelial tumors, and ossifying fibromyxoid tumor.

Sclerosing perineurioma occurs almost exclusively in the digits; therefore other acral tumors, including fibroma of tendon sheath and superficial acral fibromyxoma, figure into the differential diagnosis. Fibroma of tendon sheath, which one can essentially consider as a variant of nodular fasciitis, is associated with a tendon sheath, lacks the cord-like growth pattern of sclerosing perineurioma, and is negative for EMA. Superficial acral fibromyxoma is composed of spindled to stellate cells rather than epithelioid cells and has a random to fascicular growth pattern. Superficial acral fibromyxoma is positive for CD34 and variably positive for EMA but is negative for claudin-1.

Hybrid Schwannoma/Perineurioma

Clinical Features

Tumors having both features of schwannoma and perineuriomas have recently been described. They typically occur in young to middle-aged adults, affecting men and women equally, and present as painless masses of the subcutis and/or dermis with a wide anatomic distribution. This is a benign tumor with rare local recurrence after excision.

Pathologic Features

Tumors are circumscribed but unencapsulated. Constituent cells are spindled with long cytoplasmic processes and are variably arranged in storiform to whorled to lamellar growth patterns (Fig. 10.18). Distinct areas of schwannoma and perineurioma are usually identifiable. Degenerative atypia can rarely be present, as can mitotic activity. Hybrid lesions are immunoreactive for S100 protein, EMA, and CD34. Most tumors also express claudin-1. The S100 protein-positive cells and EMA-positive cells are arranged in parallel layers in a laminated fashion (Fig. 10.19) (Table 10.4).

Differential Diagnosis

The tumor can closely resemble a soft tissue perineurioma, but soft tissue perineurioma lacks immunoreactivity for S100 protein. Neurofibroma can be a consideration, but the Schwann cells in neurofibroma tend to be shorter, and perineurial cells in neurofibroma are more scattered without the lamellar pattern of hybrid schwannoma-perineurioma. Low-grade fibromyxoid sarcoma resembles the perineurial component of these lesions but can be distinguished by its MUC4 positivity. The characteristic t(7;16) translocation of LGFMS can be identified by FISH or PCR in problematic cases.

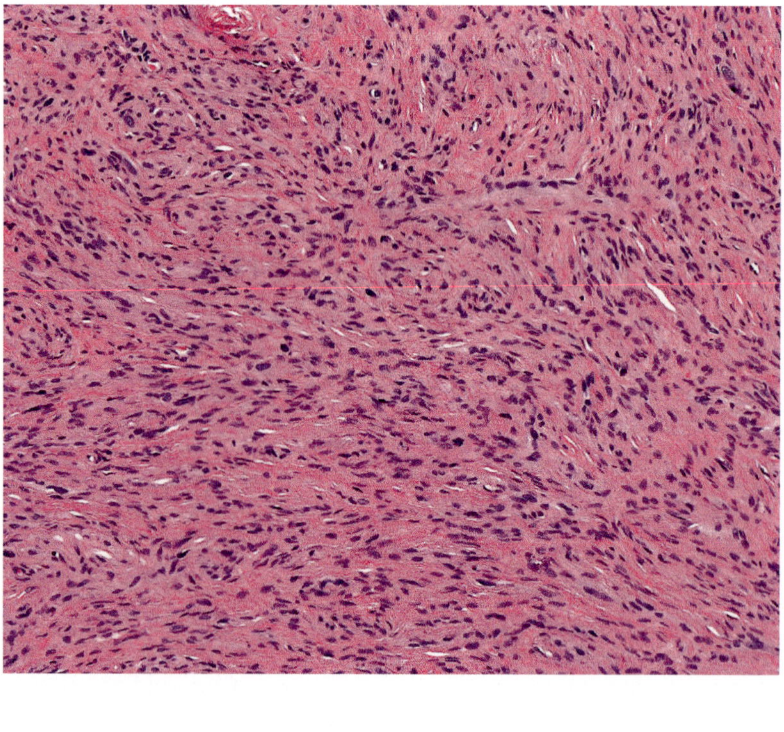

Fig. 10.18 Hybrid schwannoma/perineurioma with spindled cells arranged in lamellar growth pattern

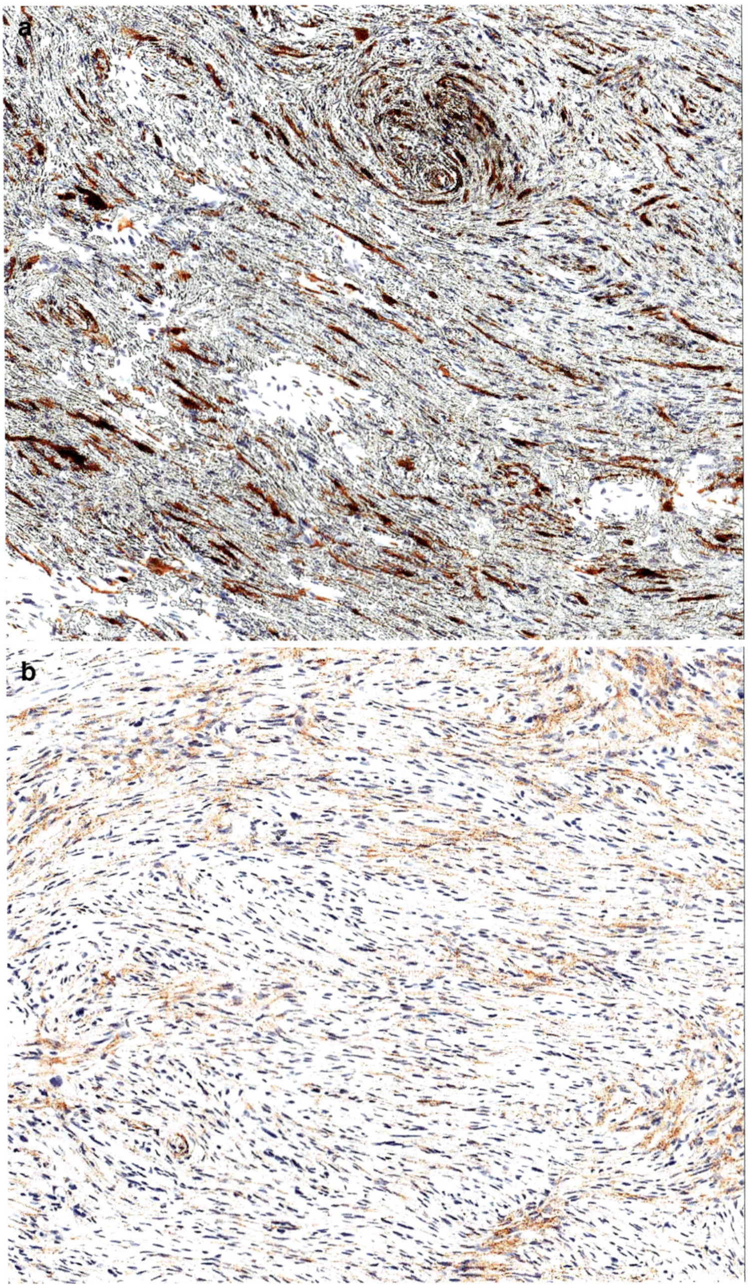

Fig. 10.19 (**a** and **b**) Immunohistochemical stains for S100 protein (**a**) and EMA (**b**) highlighting alternating arrangement of Schwann cells and perineurial cells, respectively

Table 10.4 Key pathologic features: hybrid schwannoma/perineurioma

Circumscribed but unencapsulated
Variably storiform, swirling to lamellar growth pattern
Distinct schwannoma and perineurioma areas often present
S100 positive Schwann cells alternate in a parallel arrays with EMA positive perineurial cells

Granular Cell Tumor

Clinical Features

Granular cell tumor, described in 1926 by Abrikossoff, is a benign tumor with nerve sheath differentiation that has highly characteristic cells with eosinophilic granular cytoplasm.

Although it usually occurs in adults in the third and fourth decades, all age groups are affected and the male to female ratio is approximately equal. There is a predilection for people of African descent. The tongue is considered one of the most common sites, but a significant portion occur in the skin. In 5–10% of cases, there may be multiple lesions present. An association between Noonan syndrome with multiple lentigines and multiple granular cell tumors has been reported. Granular cell tumors can be asymptomatic or pruritic and typically present as a small cutaneous nodule averaging just over 1 cm in size.

Granular cell tumors are benign in the vast majority of cases, although rare malignant forms exist (see below). Conservative resection is sufficient in most cases. Recurrence is rare.

Pathologic Features

Grossly, granular cell tumor appears as firm nodules in the dermis or subcutis. Microscopically, it is unencapsulated and poorly circumscribed with a gray-pink tinge at low magnification. The large, polygonal cells are arranged in vague nests or trabeculae with a syncytial appearance due to the presence of indistinct cell borders (Fig. 10.20). Focal spindling of cells may be present in some cases. The cytoplasm is granular and eosinophilic (Fig. 10.21) due to the accumulation of phagolysosomes, which are PAS positive and diastase resistant. Pustulo-ovoid bodies of Milian, large eosinophilic granules surrounded by a clear halo, have been reported to be present in almost all cases. The nuclei range from small and hyperchromatic to vesicular with distinct nucleoli. Scattered nuclear degenerative atypia can be identified in some cases but, in itself, is not diagnostic of malignancy. A few additional features of granular cell tumor are worth noting. In squamous epithelium-lined areas such as the skin, tongue, and esophagus, granular cell tumor is often associated with overlying pseudoepitheliomatous hyperplasia (Fig. 10.22), which is a classical pitfall for a misdiagnosis as squamous cell carcinoma in superficial biopsies. Another feature that may be alarming to the unwary is the presence of dense collagen fibrosis in some cases, potentially mimicking the desmoplasia seen in some malignancies. Finally, the intimate associa-

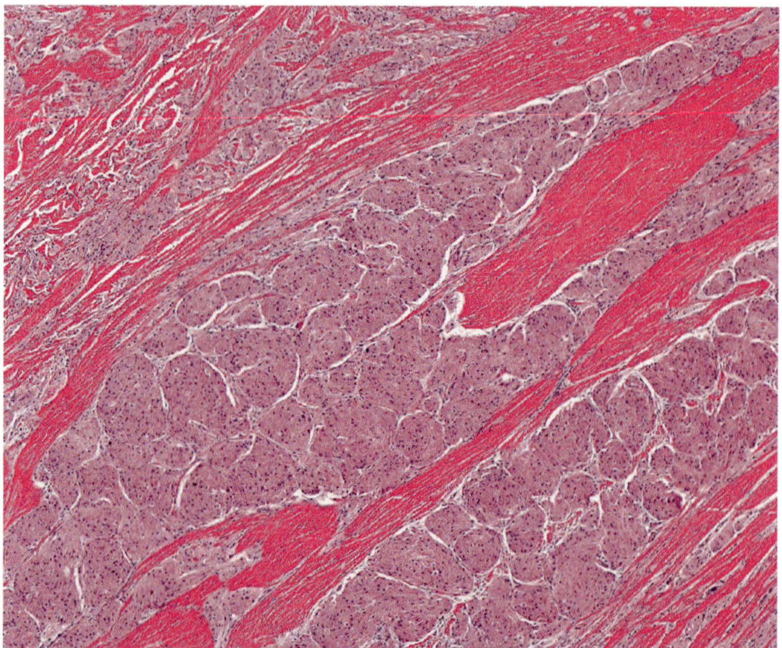

Fig. 10.20 Granular cell tumor with nested growth pattern

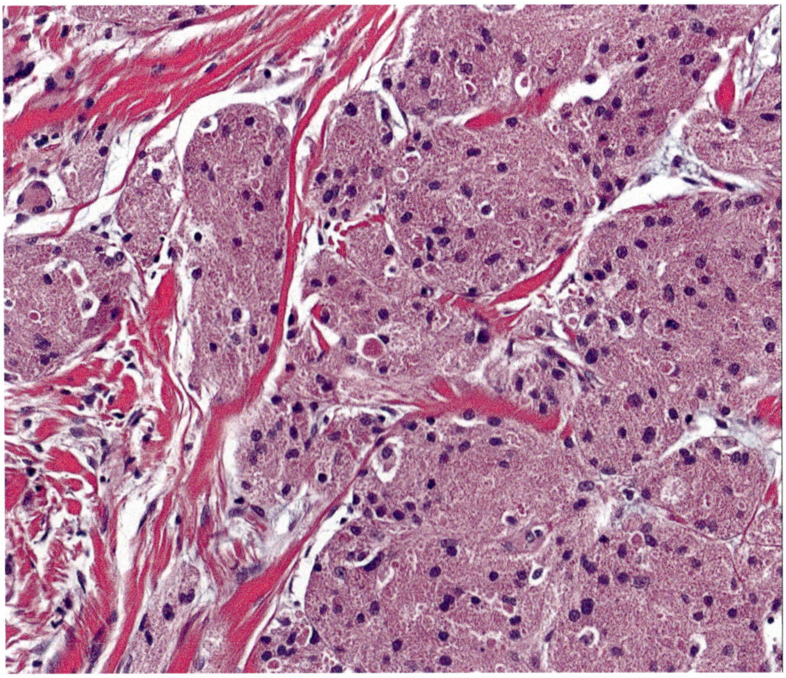

Fig. 10.21 The tumor cells of granular cell tumor have abundant eosinophilic granular cytoplasm. Pustulo-ovoid bodies of Milian, large eosinophilic granules surrounded by a clear halo, are also present

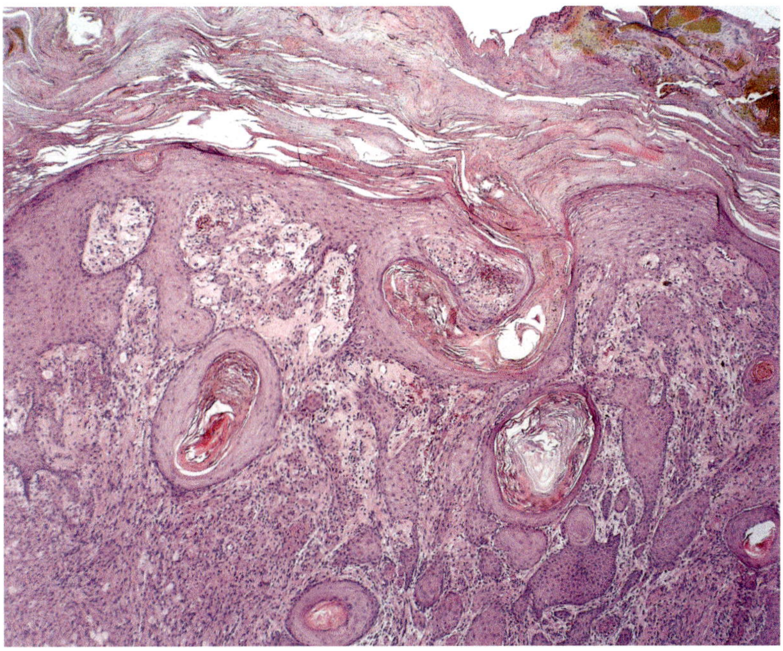

Fig. 10.22 Pseudoepitheliomatous hyperplasia overlying a dermal granular cell tumor

tion of some GCT with small nerves can be misinterpreted as perineural invasion (Fig. 10.23). Rare cases with unusual features, such as a plexiform growth pattern, clear cytoplasm, and epidermal involvement, have been reported (Table 10.5).

Granular cell tumors are usually strongly and diffusely positive for S100 protein, SOX10, TFE3, calretinin, and inhibin. CD68, CD163, NKI-C3, and MiTF may also be positive but are nonspecific. They are typically negative for

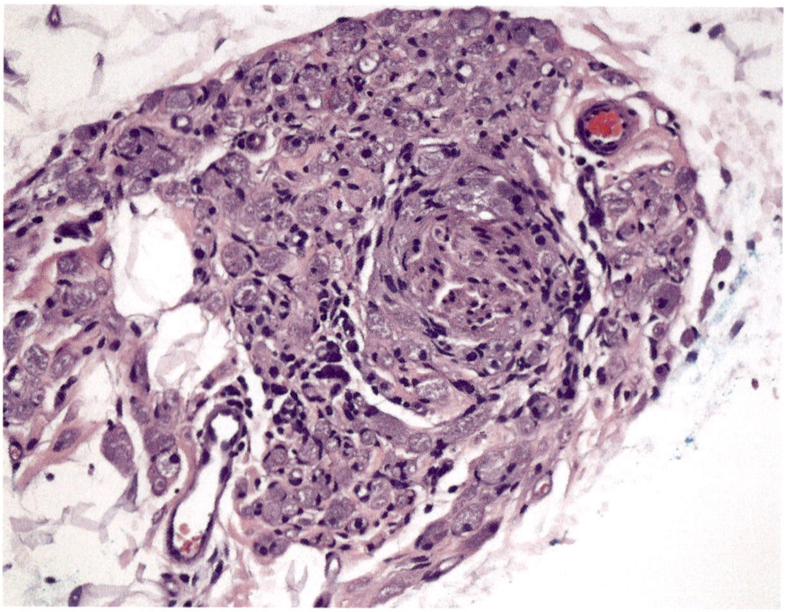

Fig. 10.23 Granular cell tumor surrounding nerve fiber

Table 10.5 Key pathologic features: granular cell tumor

Large polygonal cells with abundant eosinophilic granular cytoplasm
Usually bland nuclear features
May have overlying pseudoepitheliomatous hyperplasia
S100+, SOX10+, TFE3+, calretinin+, inhibin+, PAS+

desmin, cytokeratin, GFAP, Melan-A (may rarely be positive), and HMB45.

Differential Diagnosis

Adult-type rhabdomyoma frequently occurs in the mucosa and soft tissues of the head and neck region, which overlaps with the site propensity of granular cell tumor. Microscopically adult rhabdomyoma consists of cells with eosinophilic cytoplasm and scattered vacuolated "spider cells." Cell borders are well defined, unlike in granular cell tumor. Positivity for desmin in a tumor with these features is diagnostic. Hibernoma is usually a subcutaneous lesion with distinct multi-vacuolated "mulberry cells" recapitulating those seen in brown fat. A subset of hibernomas are composed of cells with predominantly eosinophilic cytoplasm. S100 protein stains are not helpful in this differential diagnosis, since both neoplasms are positive with this antibody. The distinction between these lesions relies on careful examination of H&E stained sections and the identification of the conventional components of hibernoma. Alveolar soft part sarcoma (ASPS) usually occurs in the deep soft tissue, but cases arising in the tongue or orbit have been reported, especially in children. ASPS is usually composed of well-formed nests separated by delicate vascular channels, in contrast to the vague nests of granular cell tumor. S100 protein, SOX10, and inhibin stains are negative in ASPS. TFE3 staining is positive in a subset of ASPS as a result of the presence of the protein product of the *ASPL-TFE3* gene fusion, which is not seen in granular cell tumor. Characteristic rhomboid crystals are present. The crystals are PAS-positive, diastase resistant. The crystals may vary in number from sparse to numerous.

Polypoid granular cell tumor/primitive non-neural granular cell tumors and congenital granular cell tumors merit a short discussion here since, although their names are similar, they represent different entities. Polypoid granular cell tumor/primitive nonneural granular cell tumor is a rare neoplasm, with relatively few series and case reports in the literature. Most cases present as a polypoid mass centered in the dermis surrounded by an epidermal collarette. The tumors have more cytologic atypia and mitotic activity than classic granular cell tumors. Neural markers such as S100 protein are consistently negative. Only rare cases of local recurrence or lymph node metastasis have been reported. Even in these cases, the biologic behavior appears to be indolent and the prognosis favorable. Congenital granular cell tumor, or congenital epulis, occurs mostly as an anterior maxillary alveolar ridge mass in female infants. This stereotypic presentation, together with the lack of S100 protein immunoreactivity, enables distinction from conventional granular cell tumor.

Atypical and Malignant Granular Cell Tumor

Clinical Features

Malignant granular cell tumor is very rare and, by definition, the malignant counterpart of conventional benign granular cell tumors. Since its original description in 1945, many cases have been reported, most in the form of single case reports. A commonly used, although not universally embraced, classification system was developed by Fanburg-Smith and colleagues in 1998 to delineate benign from malignant and atypical granular cell tumors. Most malignant granular cell tumors show a female predominance, typically in the fourth to fifth decade, and involvement of various anatomic locations, particularly the trunk and extremities.

In the largest series, 39% of patients with malignant granular cell tumors with available follow-up information succumbed to disease with a median interval of 3 years. Unfavorable prognostic indicators include older age, large tumor size, local recurrence, metastasis, a Ki-67 labeling index greater than 10%, and p53 immunoreactivity. Wide local excision is the primary treatment. In contrast, the behavior of atypical granular cell tumor appears to be in line with conventional granular cell tumor. None of the atypical cases in this series developed metastasis. That being said, it is usually our recommendation to conservatively but completely excise atypical granular cell tumors given the limited experience with this entity in published series.

Pathologic Features

Grossly, malignant granular cell tumors tend to be large (median size 4 cm), in comparison to atypical and benign granular cell tumors. Most are subcutaneous with poor circumscription and infiltrative borders. All tumors share the common feature of granular eosinophilic cytoplasm. Malignant granular cell tumor is defined by the presence of three or more of the following histologic features: (1) necrosis, (2) spindling, (3) pleomorphism, (4) high nuclear to cytoplasmic (N:C) ratio, (5) vesicular nuclei with large nucleoli, and (6) increased mitotic activity (>2 mitoses/10 high-power fields at 200× magnification) (Fig. 10.24). Those having only one or two features are designated as atypical granular cell tumors (Table 10.6).

Malignant and atypical granular cell tumors have the same immunophenotype as conventional granular cell tumors. They are positive for S100 protein, SOX10, neuron-specific enolase, and CD57. Many are positive (>50% cells) for p53. They are negative for desmin, cytokeratin, GFAP, Melan-A, and HMB45. Cytogenetic studies have not demonstrated specific, recurring abnormalities.

Differential Diagnosis

The differential diagnosis of malignant granular cell tumor includes other tumors with eosinophilic cytoplasm and significant atypia. Melanomas may have abundant eosinophilic

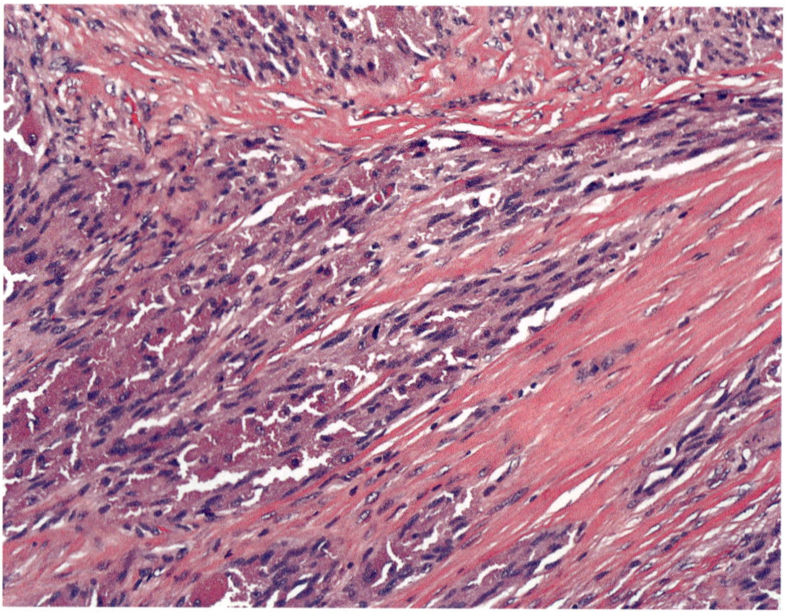

Fig. 10.24 Malignant granular cell tumor demonstrating spindling of tumor cells and mitotic activity (Courtesy of Dr. Karen Fritchie, Mayo Clinic, Rochester, MN)

Table 10.6 Key pathologic features: malignant granular cell tumor

Similar to conventional granular cell tumor
Must have three of the following six features
Necrosis, spindling, high N:C ratio, vesicular nuclei with large nucleoli, increased mitotic activity (>2/10 200× fields)

cytoplasm but are positive for melanocyte-specific markers such as HMB45, Melan-A, and MiTF. Other S100 protein-positive neoplasms with eosinophilic cytoplasm that are negative for melanocyte-specific markers may enter the differential diagnosis, including myoepithelial carcinoma and epithelioid malignant nerve sheath tumor. Some myoepithelial carcinomas have eosinophilic cytoplasm, but they usually demonstrate variable positivity for cytokeratins, EMA, p63, calponin, and smooth muscle actin. Epithelioid malignant nerve sheath tumor has a lobulated growth pattern and usually lacks granular eosinophilic cytoplasm. Loss of INI1 staining, if present (seen in 50% of cases), is helpful in confirming the diagnosis.

Dermal Nerve Sheath Myxoma

Clinical Features

Dermal nerve sheath myxoma is a benign nerve sheath tumor previously reported under the term myxoid neurothekeoma. Immunohistochemical and ultrastructural studies have confirmed the schwannian nature of dermal nerve sheath myxoma, but not cellular neurothekeoma, which led to their separation into distinct entities (cellular neurothekeoma is discussed in the fibrohistiocytic chapter). Dermal nerve sheath myxoma usually presents in the third to fifth decades with no gender predilection. It presents most commonly in the skin or subcutaneous tissue of the extremities, especially the fingers, as painless slow-growing nodules. Dermal nerve sheath myxoma has a local recurrence rate approaching 40–50%, a relative high rate compared to other benign tumors. Multiple recurrences have been reported, but not metastasis. Complete excision is preferable given the potential for recurrence.

Pathologic Features

Most dermal nerve sheath myxomas are small (<2.5 cm) and located in the dermis or superficial subcutaneous tissue. Grossly they are well-demarcated nodules with a mucoid or gelatinous appearance. Microscopically, they have a characteristic tightly arranged multinodular growth pattern with intervening thin fibrous septa (Fig. 10.25). The individual nodules of tumor have a uniformly myxoid matrix in which spindled to stellate Schwann cells with a reticulated/microcystic growth pattern are embedded (Fig. 10.26) (Table 10.7). Some of the cells have a distinct ringlike morphology, resembling monovacuolated lipoblasts or signet ring cells. Nuclear pseudoinclusions can be seen occasionally, as in other schwannian tumors, but true nuclear palisading and Verocay body formation is rare. The complex vasculature commonly seen in other myxoid tumors is absent. Cytologic atypia and mitotic activity is usually minimal. Immunostains for S100 protein are positive in the tumor cells, supporting their schwannian differentiation. GFAP and CD57 stains are often positive as well. EMA stains usually highlight the perineurial cells encircling individual tumor nodules; the latter finding is not required for the diagnosis.

Differential Diagnosis

The differential diagnosis of dermal nerve sheath myxoma includes other myxoid tumors that often involve the extremities, including myxofibrosarcoma, acral fibromyxoma, and plexiform neurofibroma with myxoid change. Myxofibrosarcoma often occurs in the subcutaneous tissues of the more proximal extremities of elderly patients. The clinical features as well as scattered cytologic atypia and a characteristic curvilinear vasculature allow its distinction from dermal nerve sheath myxoma. Myxofibrosarcoma is negative for S100 protein. Acral fibromyxoma is CD34 positive and lacks the multinodular growth pattern as well as

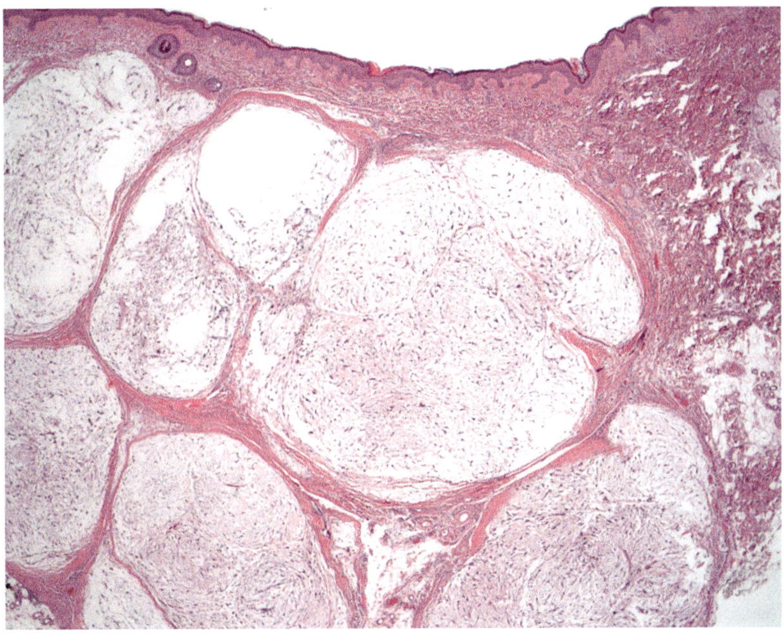

Fig. 10.25 Low-power image of dermal nerve sheath myxoma demonstrating discrete myxoid nodules separated by thin fibrous septa

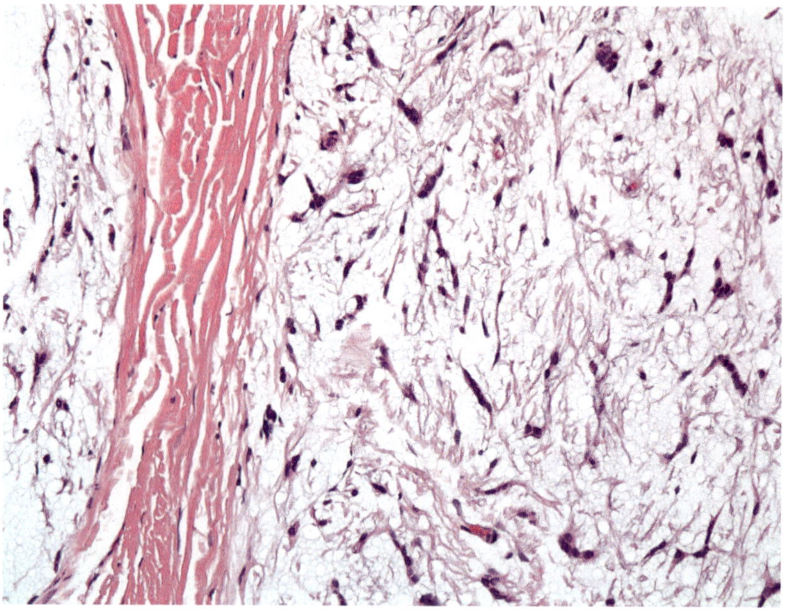

Fig. 10.26 Higher-power image of dermal nerve sheath myxoma

Table 10.7 Key pathologic features: dermal nerve sheath myxoma

Myxoid nodules separated by fibrous septa
Spindled to stellate cells in myxoid stroma
S100+
Benign, but local recurrence rate ~40–50%

S100 protein positivity. Plexiform neurofibroma is an important entity to recognize due to its association with neurofibromatosis type 1. The tumor nodules of plexiform neurofibroma are usually less compact than those seen in dermal nerve sheath myxoma, and the individual tumor nodules are composed of mixed wavy schwannian cells with buckled or comma-shaped nuclei and spindled fibroblasts. Neurofibromas also have more conspicuous collagen in the stroma. Immunoreactivity for S100 protein is not as diffuse and uniform as in dermal nerve sheath myxoma and GFAP is negative.

Dermal nerve sheath myxoma also needs to be differentiated from cellular neurothekeoma. Cellular neurothekeoma also has a nodular to nested appearance, but is less compact, less myxoid, and not separated by the distinct fibrous septations in most cases. Cellular neurothekeomas are composed of epithelioid to spindled cells with more abundant eosinophilic cytoplasm. Cellular neurothekeomas are variably positive for nonspecific markers NKI/C3, PGP9.5, CD68, MiTF, and SMA and negative for S100 protein and GFAP, unlike dermal nerve sheath myxoma.

Solitary Circumscribed Neuroma (Palisaded Encapsulated Neuroma)

Clinical Features

Originally described as palisaded encapsulated neuroma by Reed and colleagues, solitary circumscribed neuroma has become the preferred terminology for this lesion, as many cases have less than perfect palisading and encapsulation. Most patients are in their 40s–60s with equal sex distribution. The head and neck region, especially the face, is most commonly involved. Rare cases may be mucosa-based. The typical presentation is that of a solitary, painless dome-shaped papule or polypoid nodule measuring several millimeters.

Pathologic Features

Most are located in the dermis. Microscopically, the tumor is well-circumscribed but with an incomplete perineurium/fibrous capsule in most cases (Fig. 10.27). A small subset of cases can be multinodular or plexiform. An association with a small nerve may be seen at the base of the lesion. The spindled Schwann cells are arranged in fascicles or small nodules. Whorling and palisading are inconspicuous. Artificial cracks and clefts between the fascicles and nodules are often appreciable at low magnification and serve as a useful diagnostic clue (Fig. 10.28). There are

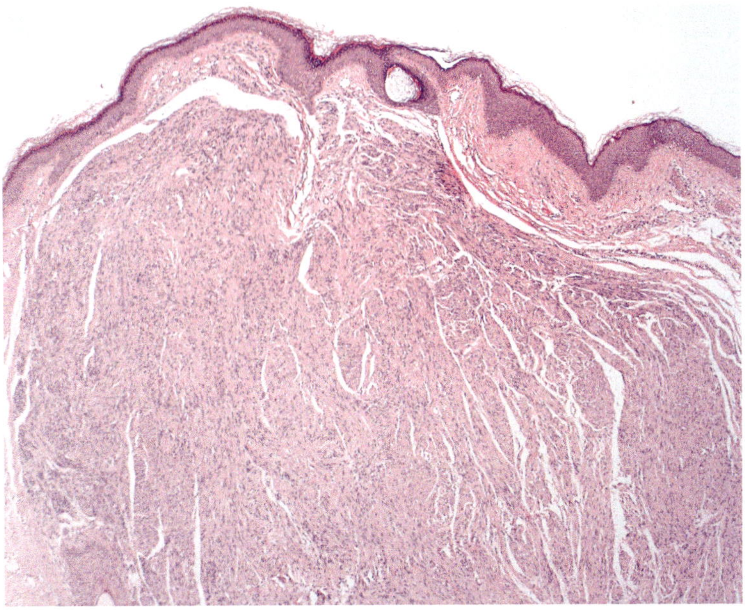

Fig. 10.27 Low-power image of solitary circumscribed neuroma

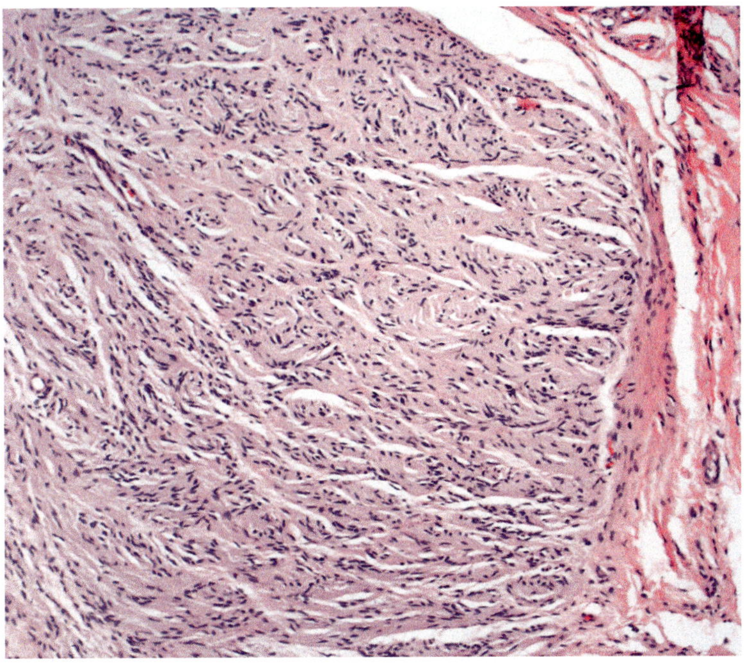

Fig. 10.28 Characteristic clefting between spindled cells of solitary circumscribed neuroma

Table 10.8 Key pathologic features: solitary circumscribed neuroma

Also known as palisaded encapsulated neuroma
Usually present on head and neck, especially face
Well circumscribed with thin capsule
Fascicles of spindled cells with clefting
S100+

admixed axons, but their visualization requires silver stains or neurofilament immunohistochemistry. S100 protein stains the Schwann cells. EMA is positive only in the perineurium (Table 10.8).

Differential Diagnosis

Solitary circumscribed neuroma is highly characteristic and the diagnosis is usually straightforward. The primary differential diagnosis is schwannoma. Schwannomas have a more developed capsule, as well as distinct cellular "Antoni A" and less cellular, loose "Antoni B" areas. Schwannomas lack the clefting artifact of solitary circumscribed neuroma. Verocay bodies are not seen in solitary circumscribed neuroma. It was originally thought that the presence of axons within the tumor allowed distinction from schwannoma, but schwannomas may also contain axons. Neurofibromas have a more heterogeneous appearance due to their mixed composition of Schwann cells, fibroblasts, and loose collagen fibers. When a solitary circumscribed neuroma demonstrates a plexiform growth pattern, it is important not to mistake it for a plexiform neurofibroma given this lesion's clinical implication. Mucosal neuromas may have a very similar histologic appearance, but most cases are multiple and associated with multiple endocrine neoplasia type 2b. They represent hyperplastic nerves with individual perineurium. Due to the fascicular growth of spindle cells, cutaneous leiomyoma may enter the differential, although the wavy buckled schwannian nuclei instead of cigar-shaped smooth muscle cell nuclei, as well as the cracking artifact, are distinct to solitary circumscribed neuroma. A simple panel of stains including S100 protein and desmin are sufficient to separate these two lesions from one another.

Other Neuromas

Neuromas are a group of entities that microscopically share similar histologic features. They resemble disorganized but otherwise relatively normal nerve fibers.

Traumatic Neuroma

Traumatic neuromas are seen in sites of previous injury or trauma prone areas. They resemble disorganized, but relatively normal nerve twigs. Nerves are often present in a fibrotic stroma related to the prior injury (Fig. 10.29).

Morton Neuroma

This is a variant of traumatic neuroma that typically arises between the 2nd and 3rd toes. Microscopically it resembles a normal nerve that has been expanded with some degenerative changes including an increase in myoid stroma; this lesion is typically very painful.

Pacinian Neuroma

Pacinian neuromas usually occur on the digits at sites of trauma. Morphologically they resemble clusters of enlarged Pacinian corpuscles (Fig. 10.30). This lesion is quite rare.

Rudimentary Polydactyly (Supernumerary Digit)

Although it likely represents a developmental abnormality, it is considered in the group of

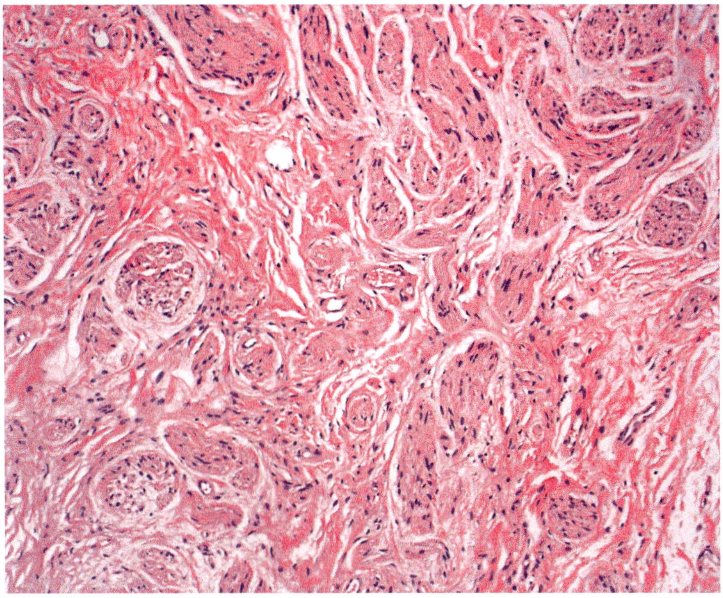

Fig. 10.29 Disorganized nerve fibers of traumatic neuroma

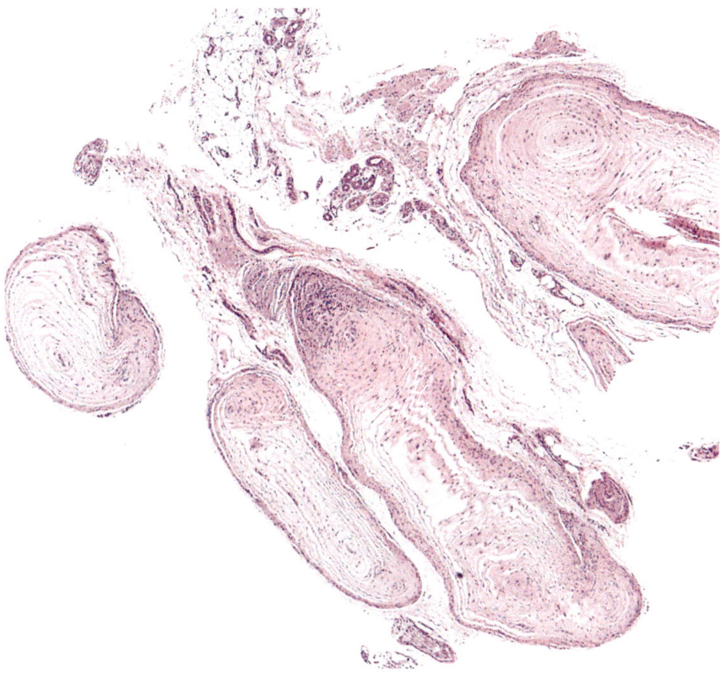

Fig. 10.30 Pacinian neuroma characterized by abnormal, enlarged Pacinian corpuscles

neuromas owing to its morphologic overlap with these lesions. This unusual lesion occurs at the base of the fifth finger. It is almost always present at birth. Microscopically, it is a polypoid soft tissue lesion that contains tangled, but otherwise normal, nerves (Fig. 10.31).

The neuroma group is summarized in Table 10.9.

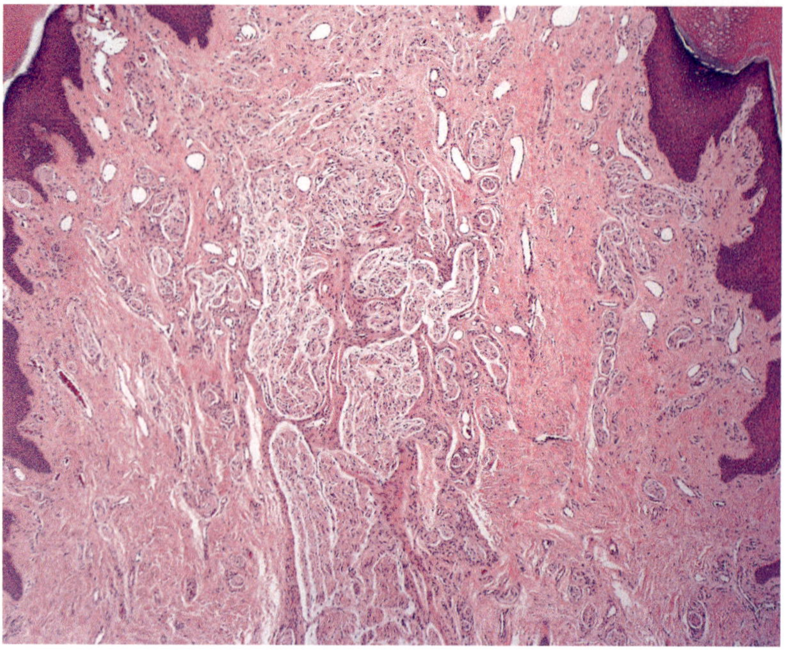

Fig. 10.31 Rudimentary polydactyly is composed of tangled nerves in the dermis of a polypoid lesion that presents on the base of the fifth digit

Table 10.9 Key pathologic features: neuromas

Disorganized but relatively normal nerves or neural structures
Some degenerative changes common
Rudimentary polydactyly: polypoid lesion at base of 5th finger

Meningioma

Clinical Features

There are three subtypes of meningiomas of the skin. Type I lesions present as congenital lesions derived from ectopic arachnoid cells. Type II and III meningiomas present in adults, usually in middle age. Type II lesions occur around sensory organs and are derived from arachnoid cells surrounding nerve bundles. Type III lesions are most common in the scalp and are direct extensions or, less commonly, metastases from dural-based tumors. With the exception of malignant meningiomas that have metastasized to the skin, meningiomas are benign tumors cured by simple excision.

Pathologic Features

Type I meningiomas are composed of pseudovascular spaces lined by meningothelial cells (Fig. 10.32). Types II and III are characterized by more discrete nests/nodules of meningothelial cells in a swirling arrangement (Fig. 10.33). Psammoma bodies, when present, can be a helpful clue to the diagnosis. Type III meningiomas tend to have a more diffuse growth pattern (Table 10.10). Meningiomas are positive for EMA and negative for cytokeratins, S100 protein, and CD34. Type II and III meningiomas are also positive for p63.

Differential Diagnosis

Type I lesions may be confused with angiosarcoma or lymphangioma, but presentation in children and absence of immunoreactivity for vascular markers aid in this distinction. Type II lesions can be confused with cellular neurothekeoma. Cellular neurothekeoma is nega-

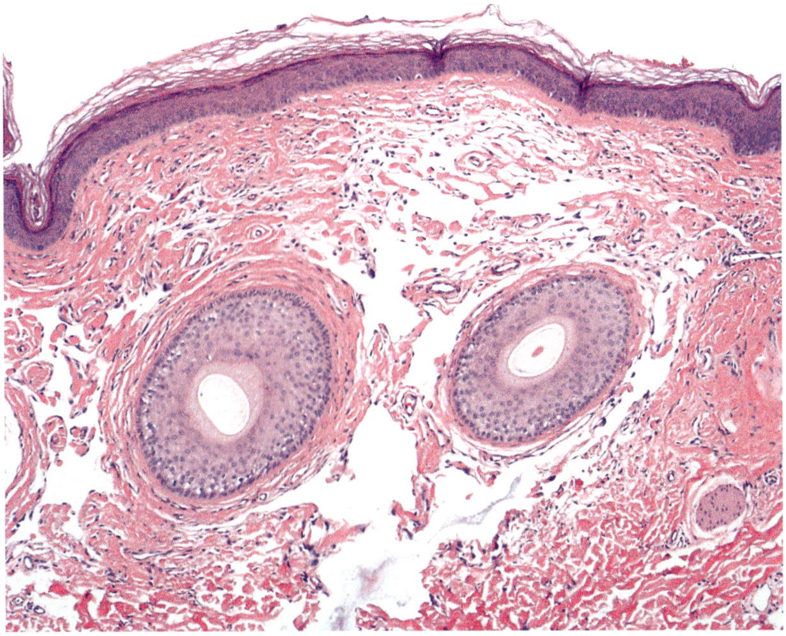

Fig. 10.32 Type I meningioma consisting of dilated pseudovascular spaces lined by meningothelial cells (Courtesy of Dr. Karen Fritchie, Mayo Clinic, Rochester, MN)

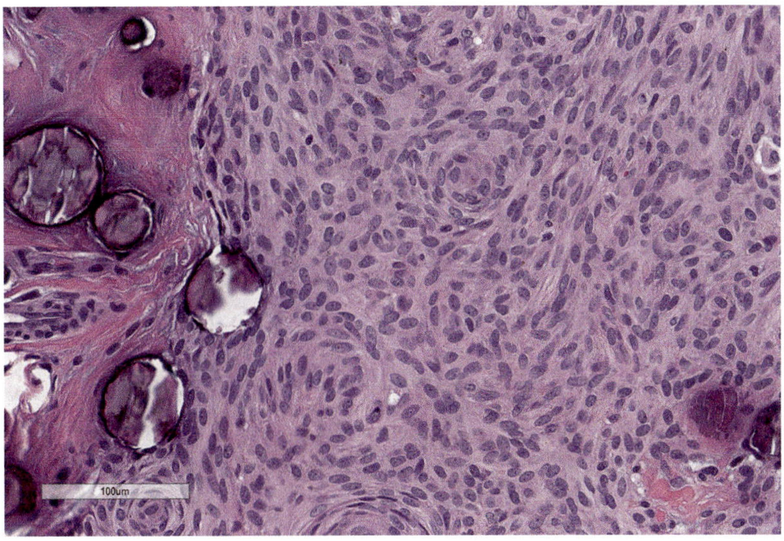

Fig. 10.33 Type III meningioma characterized by swirling arrangement of meningothelial cells and scattered psammoma bodies

tive for EMA and variably positive for NKI/C3, PGP9.5, MiTF, SMA, and CD68. Type III lesions can be confused with dermatofibromas and DFSP. The growth pattern of meningiomas is whirling and focally nested and meningiomas are negative for CD34. Dermatofibromas are more heterogeneous tumors and lack immunoreactivity for EMA.

Malignant Peripheral Nerve Sheath Tumor (MPNST)

Clinical Features

Approximately 25–50% of MPNSTs occur in the setting of neurofibromatosis. The remaining are sporadic tumors that occur in young to

Table 10.10 Key pathologic features: meningioma

EMA positive; negative for cytokeratin, S100, and CD34
Type I
Congenital lesions
Pseudovascular growth pattern
Type II
Present around sensory organs
Discrete nodules of meningothelial cells
Psammoma bodies common
Type III
Scalp
Whorled to syncytial growth pattern
Psammoma bodies common

middle-aged adults. They typically arise in deep soft tissue, but presentation in the skin does rarely occur. In the setting of cutaneous MPNST, the tumors are usually smaller than their deep soft tissue counterparts, with most cases <5 cm in size. Most present on the head and neck and men are slightly more commonly affected than women. Cutaneous MPNSTs are associated with NF-1 in close to half of reported cases.

In contrast to most superficial sarcomas, cutaneous MPNST is still associated with aggressive behavior with a similar rate of progression as their deep soft tissue counterparts. In one series of four patients, three developed metastases and died from their disease.

Pathologic Features

MPNSTs usually are composed of fascicles of hyperchromatic spindled cells and can have a herringbone pattern reminiscent of fibrosarcoma (Fig. 10.34). The fascicles often vary in cellularity imparting a marbled appearance to the tumor. A swirling pattern is sometimes seen. Nuclear palisading is uncommon and is present in less than 10% of cases. The individual tumor cells are usually spindled and sometimes have wavy nuclei. There is often increased cellularity around vessels and the tumor cells often push into the walls of the vessels. Heterologous elements are seen in about 10% of cases in deep soft tissue including cartilage, bone, glandular epithelium, rhabdomyoblasts, and angiosarcoma. When rhabdomyoblasts are present, the tumor may be classified as a malignant triton tumor. An epithelioid variant consisting predominantly of round to polygonal tumor cells with abundant eosinophilic cytoplasm also exists (Fig. 10.35). In cutaneous cases, the tumor is almost always associated with a precursor neurofibroma, usually of the sporadic rather than plexiform type (Table 10.11).

MPNSTs demonstrate immunoreactivity for S100 protein in about 50% of cases overall and is typically, but not always, focal. Immunoreactivity for S100 protein seems to be somewhat more common in cutaneous MPNST and can be strong and diffuse, but the positivity is often less in the malignant cells than that seen in the precursor neurofibroma or nerve. Epithelioid MPNST is often strongly positive for S100 protein, often more so than the precursor neurofibroma. Immunoreactivity for SOX10 is seen in about two-thirds of MPNSTs, and it may be a better marker than S100 protein. More recently, it has been shown that MPNSTs lose histone H3K27 methylation in about 50% of cases of spindled MPNST. Immunostains for this marker appear to be relatively specific but suffer from a relative lack of sensitivity.

Differential Diagnosis

The differential diagnosis includes other spindle cell sarcomas, such as synovial sarcoma, leiomyosarcoma, fibrosarcomatous dermatofibrosarcoma protuberans (DFSP), and malignant solitary fibrous tumor. Synovial sarcoma may express S100 protein in up to 30% of cases but is also positive for cytokeratin and TLE-1. Synovial sarcoma also has a characteristic t(X;18) involving *SSX* and *SS18* genes that can be detected by FISH or PCR. Leiomyosarcoma is usually more eosinophilic and will be positive for SMA and desmin. Fibrosarcomatous DFSP typically has evidence of a precursor DFSP component, rather than a neurofibroma component, and is usually CD34 positive and negative for S100 protein. FISH or PCR to demonstrate the t(17;22) with

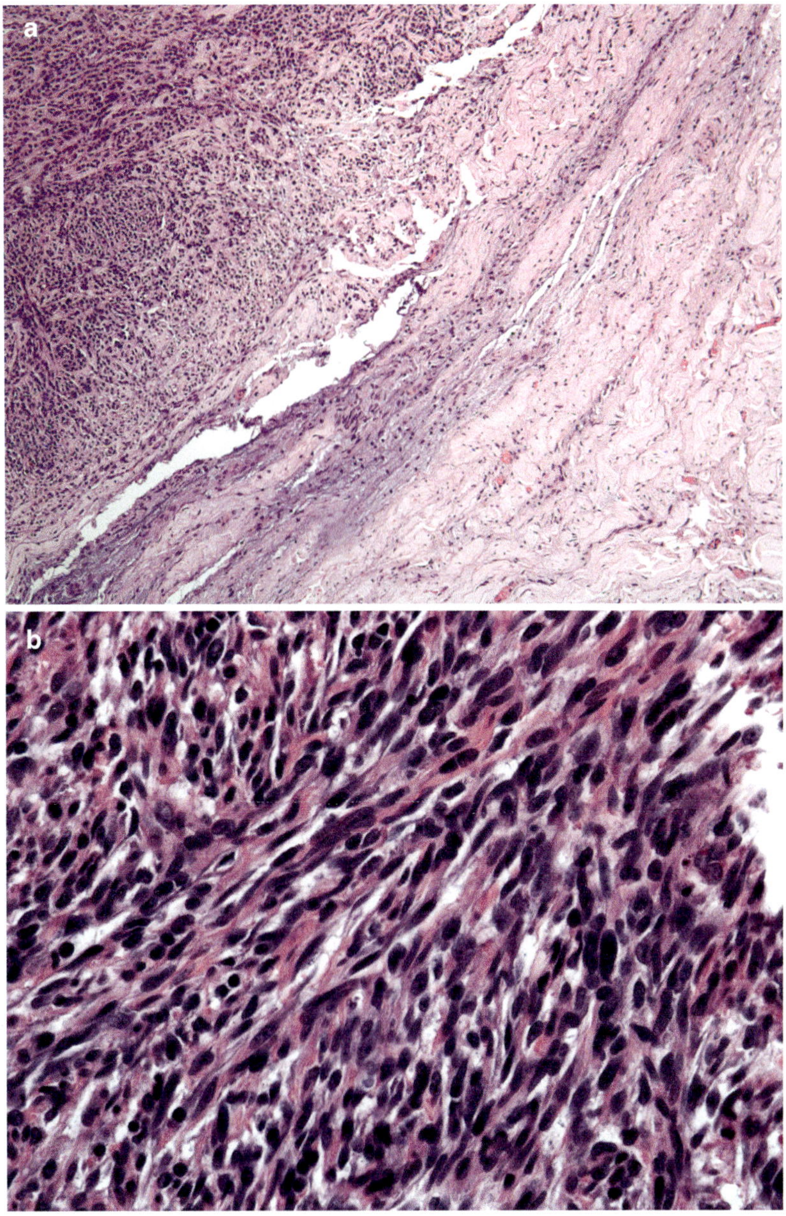

Fig. 10.34 (**a**) Malignant peripheral nerve sheath tumor with abrupt transition from precursor neurofibroma to malignant peripheral nerve sheath tumor component. (**b**) Higher-power image of malignant peripheral nerve sheath tumor demonstrating fascicles of atypical, hyperchromatic spindled cells

rearrangement of *PDGFB* of DFSP can be helpful in problematic cases. Malignant solitary fibrous tumor has shorter fascicles and a prominent vasculature and is positive for CD34 and STAT6. Epithelioid MPNST needs to be distinguished from metastatic carcinoma and melanoma. Epithelioid MPNST usually does not express keratin and are negative for melanocytic markers such as HMB45.

Ewing Sarcoma

Clinical Features

Although not a true nerve sheath tumor, Ewing sarcoma is a neuroectodermal tumor and thus discussed in this chapter. Cutaneous Ewing sarcoma is rare, with most reports in the literature representing single case reports or small series.

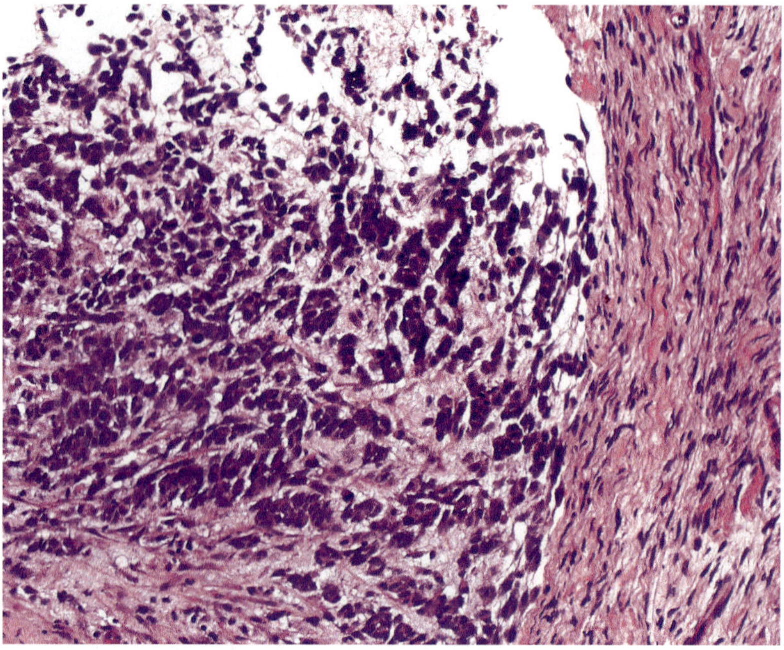

Fig. 10.35 Epithelioid malignant peripheral nerve sheath tumor composed of atypical epithelioid cells with eosinophilic cytoplasm arising in precursor neurofibroma

Table 10.11 Key pathologic features: malignant peripheral nerve sheath tumor (MPNST)

Rare
Often arise in association with precursor neurofibroma
Conventional MPNST
Fascicles of atypical hyperchromatic spindled cells
Variably positive for S100
Frequent loss of histone H3K27 methylation
Epithelioid MPNST
Sheets of atypical epithelioid cells
Strongly positive for S100

Similar to conventional Ewing sarcoma, most patients are young adults, with rare cases presenting in elderly patients. No site predilection is noted. For some unknown reason, Ewing sarcoma is much more common in patients of European descent compared with patients with Asian or African ancestry. Clinically, the lesions can be nondescript cutaneous nodules or have an epidermal collarette with clinical resemblance to pyogenic granuloma.

Although there is little collective experience with cutaneous Ewing sarcoma, presentation in the skin appears to be associated with a better overall prognosis compared to deeply situated tumors. That being said, metastasis has developed from cutaneous tumors. At the very least, patients need to have the tumor completely excised, and patients treated with surgery alone have done well. Many have also been treated with adjuvant chemotherapy.

Pathologic Features

The tumors typically arise in the dermis and are composed of sheets of undifferentiated round cells with little cytoplasm and uniform nuclei that have a somewhat stippled chromatin pattern and small nucleoli (Fig. 10.36a, b). Mitotic activity and apoptosis are typically, but not invariably, conspicuous.

Immunohistochemical stains for CD99 are very sensitive for Ewing sarcoma and show strong membranous immunoreactivity (Fig. 10.36c), though it should be noted that CD99 is not a very specific marker. Cases may have nuclear immunoreactivity for FLI1 or ERG. These stains are more useful in tumors with translocations involving those genes (see below). Other markers such as CD57, NSE, S100

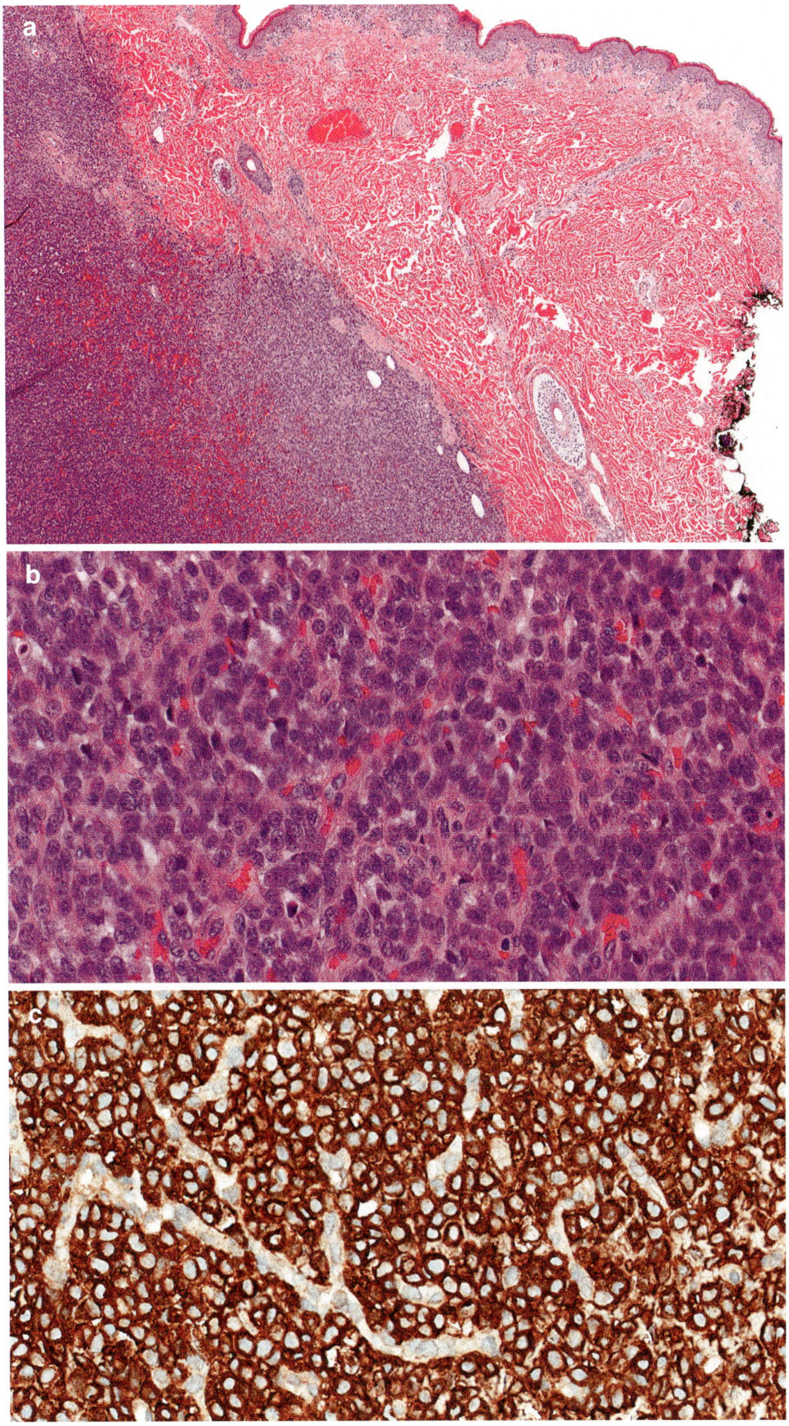

Fig. 10.36 (**a**) Low-power image demonstrating Ewing sarcoma arising in the dermis. (**b**) Ewing sarcoma is composed of sheets of uniform, atypical round cells with stippled chromatin. (**c**) Ewing sarcoma with strong membranous immunoreactivity for CD99

Table 10.12 Key pathologic features: cutaneous Ewing sarcoma

Sheets of uniform round cells with scant cytoplasm and stippled chromatin
Positive for CD99 with strong membranous pattern
t(11;22)*EWSR1-FLI1* >90% of cases

protein, and synaptophysin may be positive but are of limited diagnostic utility. Pitfalls include immunoreactivity for AE1/3 and CD117 in about 25% of cases and desmin in rare cases. Ewing sarcoma is negative for SMA, melanocyte-specific markers, TdT, and myogenin.

Molecular methods are invaluable for confirming the diagnosis, especially in difficult cases. About 90% of cases have a recurrent t(11;22) involving *EWSR1* from chromosome 22q12 and *FLI1* from 11q24. Detecting this rearrangement by PCR or break-apart FISH probes are effective means for reaching the diagnosis, with FISH techniques being more sensitive (91% for FISH and 59% for PCR). If FISH is employed, it should be remembered that a variety of tumors may have *EWSR1* rearrangements. In addition to the common *EWRS1-FLI1* fusion, alternate fusion partners for *EWSR1* include *ERG*, *ETV-1*, *E1AF*, as well as other rarer partners. As *EWSR1* is the most consistent partner, it is the most logical first choice for FISH probes, although rare cases have *FUS-ERG* or *FUS-FEV* fusions (Table 10.12).

Differential Diagnosis

The differential diagnosis of cutaneous cases includes rhabdomyosarcoma, Merkel cell carcinoma, lymphoblastic lymphoma, poorly differentiated synovial sarcoma, malignant glomus tumor, and in rare cases angiomatoid fibrous histiocytoma. Merkel cell carcinoma has more irregular nuclear contours, often with nuclear molding and neuroendocrine stippled chromatin. Merkel cell carcinoma can be immunoreactive for CD99, and this represents a diagnostic pitfall in older patients. Merkel cell carcinoma is positive for CK20 (in a perinuclear dot pattern) in contrast to Ewing sarcoma. Lymphoblastic lymphoma is positive for CD99 and can be positive for FLI1, but also expresses TdT, unlike Ewing sarcoma. Synovial sarcoma is usually a spindle cell tumor, but poorly differentiated round cell forms exist. Synovial sarcoma may express CD99 but also is immunoreactive for TLE1 and has a t(X;18) involving *SS18-SSX*. Malignant glomus tumor can histologically resemble Ewing sarcoma but is positive for SMA. Rare cases of angiomatoid fibrous histiocytoma can have round cell morphology, but angiomatoid fibrous histiocytoma consistently has a fibrous pseudocapsule and peripheral lymphoid cuff. It should be noted that angiomatoid fibrous histiocytoma can be positive for CD99 (50%) and has an *EWSR1* rearrangement in the majority of cases.

Selected References

1. Abbas O, Bhawan J. Cutaneous plexiform lesions. J Cutan Pathol. 2010;37(6):613–23.
2. Allison KH, Patel RM, Goldblum JR, Rubin BP. Superficial malignant peripheral nerve sheath tumor: a rare and challenging diagnosis. Am J Clin Pathol. 2005;124(5):685–92.
3. Avninder S, Ramesh V, Vermani S. Benign nerve sheath myxoma (myxoid neurothekeoma) in the leg. Dermatol Online J. 2007;13(2):14.
4. Erstine EM, Ko JS, Rubin BP, McKenney JK, Goldblum JR, Billings SD. Broadening the anatomic landscape of sclerosing perineurioma: A series of 5 cases in nonacral sites. Am J Dermatopathol. 2016 Nov 11. [Epub ahead of print] PubMed.
5. Evans HL. Sporadic superficial diffuse neurofibromas with repeated local recurrence over many years and a tendency toward malignant change: a report of 3 cases. Am J Surg Pathol. 2013;37(7):987–94.
6. Fanburg-Smith JC, Meis-Kindblom JM, Fante R, Kindblom LG. Malignant granular cell tumor of soft tissue: diagnostic criteria and clinicopathologic correlation. Am J Surg Pathol. 1998;22(7):779–94.
7. Fletcher CD, Theaker JM. Digital pacinian neuroma: a distinctive hyperplastic lesion. Histopathology. 1989;15(3):249–56.
8. Fletcher CD, Davies SE, McKee PH. Cellular schwannoma: a distinct pseudosarcomatous entity. Histopathology. 1987;11(1):21–35.
9. Fox MD, Billings SD, Gleason BC, Thomas AB, Cibull TL. Cutaneous meningioma: a potential diagnostic pitfall in p63 positive cutaneous neoplasms. J Cutan Pathol. 2013;40(10):891–5.
10. Goldblum JR, Beals TF, Weiss SW. Neuroblastoma-like neurilemoma. Am J Surg Pathol. 1994;18(3):266–73.

11. Hart J, Gardner JM, Edgar M, Weiss SW. Epithelioid schwannomas: an analysis of 58 cases including atypical variants. Am J Surg Pathol. 2016;40(5):704–13.
12. Hornick JL, Fletcher CD. Soft tissue perineurioma: clinicopathologic analysis of 81 cases including those with atypical histologic features. Am J Surg Pathol. 2005;29(7):845–58.
13. Hornick JL, Bundock EA, Fletcher CD. Hybrid schwannoma/perineurioma: clinicopathologic analysis of 42 distinctive benign nerve sheath tumors. Am J Surg Pathol. 2009;33(10):1554–61.
14. Kacerovska D, Michal M, Kazakov DV. Hybrid Epithelioid Schwannoma/Perineurioma. Am J Dermatopathol. 2016;38(7):e90–2.
15. Kaku Y, Fukumoto T, Louise Opada G, Anan T, Kimura T. A clinicopathologic and immunohistochemical study of 7 cases of sclerosing perineurioma. Am J Dermatopathol. 2015;37(2):122–8.
16. Kao GF, Laskin WB, Olsen TG. Solitary cutaneous plexiform neurilemmoma (schwannoma): a clinicopathologic, immunohistochemical, and ultrastructural study of 11 cases. Mod Pathol. 1989;2(1):20–6.
17. Koutlas IG, Scheithauer BW. Palisaded encapsulated ("solitary circumscribed") neuroma of the oral cavity: a review of 55 cases. Head Neck Pathol. 2010;4(1):15–26.
18. Lisle A, Jokinen C, Argenyi Z. Cutaneous pseudoglandular schwannoma: a case report of an unusual histopathologic variant. Am J Dermatopathol. 2011;33(5):e63–5.
19. Lupton JR, Epps RE, Figueroa P, Kupiec A, Sulica VI. Plexiform neurofibroma with massive hand involvement. J Am Acad Dermatol. 2000;43(6):1136–7.
20. Luzar B, Falconieri G. Cutaneous malignant peripheral nerve sheath tumor. Surg Pathol Clin. 2017;10(2):337–43.
21. Luzar B, Tanaka M, Schneider J, Calonje E. Cutaneous microcystic/reticular schwannoma: a poorly recognized entity. J Cutan Pathol. 2016;43(2):93–100.
22. Macarenco RS, Ellinger F, Oliveira AM. Perineurioma: a distinctive and underrecognized peripheral nerve sheath neoplasm. Arch Pathol Lab Med. 2007;131(4):625–36.
23. Machado I, Cruz J, Lavernia J, Llombart-Bosch A. Solitary, multiple, benign, atypical, or malignant: the "Granular Cell Tumor" puzzle. Virchows Arch. 2016;468(5):527–38.
24. Miedema JR, Zedek D. Cutaneous meningioma. Arch Pathol Lab Med. 2012;136(2):208–11.
25. Noonan VL, Greene DJ, Brodsky G, Kabani SP. Extraneural sclerosing perineurioma of the buccal mucosa: a case report and clinicopathologic review. Head Neck Pathol. 2010;4(2):169–73.
26. Pérez-González YC, Pagura L, Llamas-Velasco M, Cortes-Lambea L, Kutzner H, Requena L. Primary cutaneous malignant granular cell tumor: an immunohistochemical study and review of the literature. Am J Dermatopathol. 2015;37(4):334–40.
27. Robson AM, Calonje E. Cutaneous perineurioma: a poorly recognized tumour often misdiagnosed as epithelioid histiocytoma. Histopathology. 2000;37(4):332–9.
28. Rodríguez-Peralto JL, Riveiro-Falkenbach E, Carrillo R. Benign cutaneous neural tumors. Semin Diagn Pathol. 2013;30(1):45–57.
29. Rubin AI, Yassaee M, Johnson W, Elenitsas R, Zaladonis J Jr, Seykora JT. Multiple cutaneous sclerosing perineuriomas: an extensive presentation with involvement of the bilateral upper extremities. J Cutan Pathol. 2009;36(Suppl 1):60–5.
30. Sheth S, Li X, Binder S, Dry SM. Differential gene expression profiles of neurothekeomas and nerve sheath myxomas by microarray analysis. Mod Pathol. 2011;24(3):343–54.
31. Suchak R, Luzar B, Bacchi CE, Maguire B, Calonje E. Cutaneous neuroblastoma-like schwannoma: a report of two cases, one with a plexiform pattern, and a review of the literature. J Cutan Pathol. 2010;37(9):997–1001.
32. Sundarkrishnan L, Bradish JR, Oliai BR, Hosler GA. Cutaneous cellular pseudoglandular schwannoma: an unusual histopathologic variant. Am J Dermatopathol. 2016;38(4):315–8.
33. Thomas C, Somani N, Owen LG, Malone JC, Billings SD. Cutaneous malignant peripheral nerve sheath tumors. J Cutan Pathol. 2009;36(8):896–900.

Genital Mesenchymal Tumors

11

Karen J. Fritchie

Abstract

A variety of mesenchymal tumors can arise in the cervix, vulvovaginal, and inguinoscrotal regions including lipomatous neoplasms, peripheral nerve sheath tumors, and sarcomas such as rhabdomyosarcoma. Consequently, this chapter will focus on lesions that solely or predominantly affect the soft tissues of the distal genital tract, beginning with the genital stromal tumors. This group includes fibroepithelial stromal polyp, cellular angiofibroma, mammary-type myofibroblastoma, angiomyofibroblastoma, and aggressive angiomyxoma. As genital stromal tumors are notorious for significant morphologic and immunophenotypic overlap, key histologic features of each entity will be emphasized. Two rare lesions involving the vulva, prepubertal vulval fibroma and massive vulval edema, will also be reviewed. Finally, the chapter ends with a discussion of smooth muscle tumors of the external genitalia. Even though the morphology of smooth muscle tumors of the vulva, vagina, and scrotum is similar to those at other sites, each of these locations has unique criteria for distinguishing leiomyomas from leiomyosarcomas.

K. J. Fritchie (✉)
Mayo Clinic, Department of Laboratory Medicine and Pathology, Division of Anatomic Pathology, Rochester, MN, USA
e-mail: Fritchie.Karen@mayo.edu

Genital Stromal Tumors

The genital stromal tumors are a family of mesenchymal lesions that predominantly occur in the skin and soft tissue of the vulvovaginal, cervical, inguinoscrotal, and pelvic regions and include fibroepithelial stromal polyp, cellular angiofibroma, mammary-type myofibroblastoma, angiomyofibroblastoma, and aggressive angiomyxoma. These tumors are thought to originate from cells within the hormonally responsive specialized stroma of the distal genital tract. Thus, they exhibit a tremendous amount of morphologic, immunophenotypic, and genetic overlap, oftentimes resulting in diagnostic challenges. Fortunately, most genital stromal tumors are benign requiring only simple excision.

Fibroepithelial Stromal Polyp

Clinical Features

Fibroepithelial stromal polyps, first described by Norris and Taylor in 1965, characteristically present as single or multiple polypoid or pedunculated

Table 11.1 Key pathologic features: fibroepithelial stromal polyp

Spindle to stellate fibroblasts in fibrous or myxoid stroma. Polypoid appearance with multinucleated stromal cells adjacent to epithelial-stromal interface

S. D. Billings et al. (eds.), *Soft Tissue Tumors of the Skin*,
https://doi.org/10.1007/978-1-4939-8812-9_11

masses in the vagina and vulva but may occur in the cervix or arise from anal mucosa. These polyps show convincing similarities with superficial cervicovaginal myofibroblastoma, indicating that both likely represent the same entity. The majority of fibroepithelial stromal polyps harbor a stalk, a helpful diagnostic clue, while the remaining cases are sessile or show a frond-like papillary configuration. Fibroepithelial stromal polyps range from less than 1 cm in diameter to greater than 18 cm, although most are less than 4 cm. They are hormonally responsive and, consequently, are noted most frequently in reproductive-aged females or during pregnancy. However, the age distribution of these lesions is broad, and they have been reported from infancy to postmenopausal females. This is a benign tumor cured by simple excision.

Pathologic Features

Histologic examination reveals a variably cellular polypoid proliferation of spindled to stellate-shaped cells in a fibrotic, myxomatous, or edematous background (Fig. 11.1a–c). One of the key histologic features of fibroepithelial stromal polyp is its superficial location. Lesional cells approach and abut the overlying squamous epithelium with characteristic multinucleated stromal cells present near the stromal-epithelial interface (Fig. 11.1c, Table 11.1). Pseudosarcomatous features including hypercellularity (typically centrally located), cytologic atypia, increased mitotic activity (greater than 10 mitotic figures/10 high-power fields), and atypical mitoses are well documented in fibroepithelial stromal polyps and seem to have no effect on clinical behavior (Fig. 11.1e, f).

Differential Diagnosis

The main differential diagnosis of fibroepithelial stromal polyp includes other genital stromal tumors and embryonal rhabdomyosarcoma. The superficial location of fibroepithelial stromal polyp, lack of distinct border, polypoid appearance, and presence of multinucleated stromal cells help to differentiate it from other members of the genital stromal tumor family. Embryonal rhabdomyosarcoma overwhelmingly affects children less than 10 years and shows increased cellularity toward the surface of the lesion (cambium layer) (Fig. 11.1g) rather than near the center of the mass. While both fibroepithelial stromal polyp and embryonal rhabdomyosarcoma exhibit desmin reactivity, the latter will also express the skeletal muscle-specific markers myogenin and myoD1 (Fig. 11.1h).

Cellular Angiofibroma (Angiomyofibroblastoma-Like Tumor of the Male Genital Tract)

Clinical Features

In 1997 Nucci and colleagues described a series of four vulvar tumors with prominent blood vessels and a distinct spindle cell component, introducing the term "cellular angiofibroma." Over the next several years, tumors with similar morphology were reported in the inguinoscrotal region of male patients under the designation of "angiomyofibroblastoma-like tumor of the male genital tract." Cellular angiofibroma most commonly affects middle-aged females in the fifth decade of life (range 20–78 years). The vast majority of these tumors present as a slowly enlarging superficial mass (median size 6 cm, range 0.6–25 cm) in vulvovaginal or inguinoscrotal soft tissue. Less common locations include the perineum, periurethral soft tissue, anus, and retroperitoneum. Cellular angiofibroma is a benign tumor cured by simple excision. Rare cases of cellular angiofibroma and angiomyofibroblastoma with malignant transformation have been reported, but there is no evidence to date that these cases behave more aggressively than tumors with conventional features.

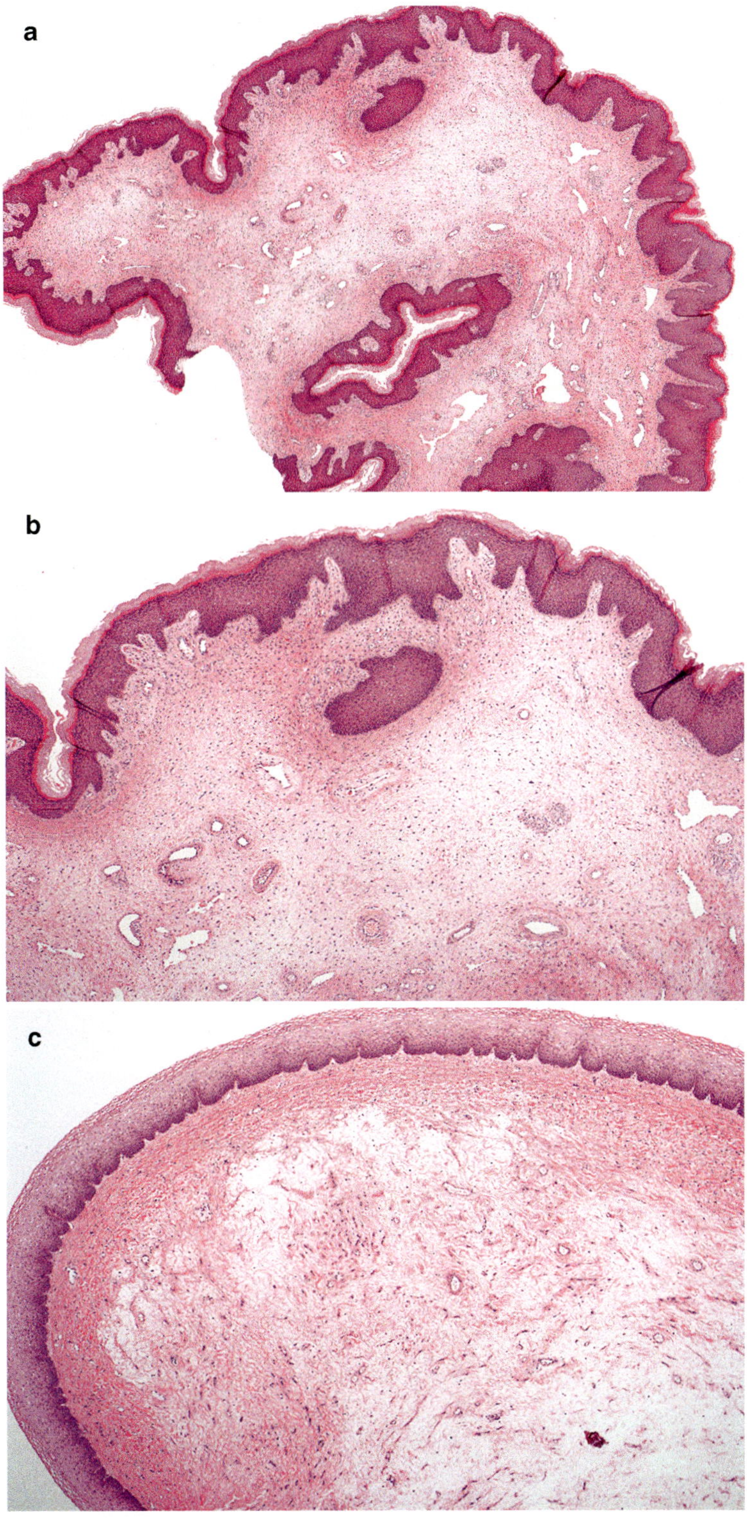

Fig. 11.1 Low-power examination (**a**) of a fibroepithelial stromal polyp shows distinct polypoid architecture. The stroma may be hyalinized (**b**) or myxomatous (**c**). Characteristic multinucleated stromal cells (**d**) are identified at the epithelial interface. Pseudosarcomatous change may manifest as hypercellularity (**e**) or cytologic atypia (**f**) with increased mitotic activity. In contrast to fibroepithelial stromal polyps, embryonal rhabdomyosarcoma shows increased cellularity at the stromal-epithelial interface (cambium layer) (**g**) and immunoreactivity for myogenin (**h**) and myoD1. (Photo credit for g and h to Dr. Alyaa Al-Ibraheemi, Boston Children's Hospital, Boston, MA)

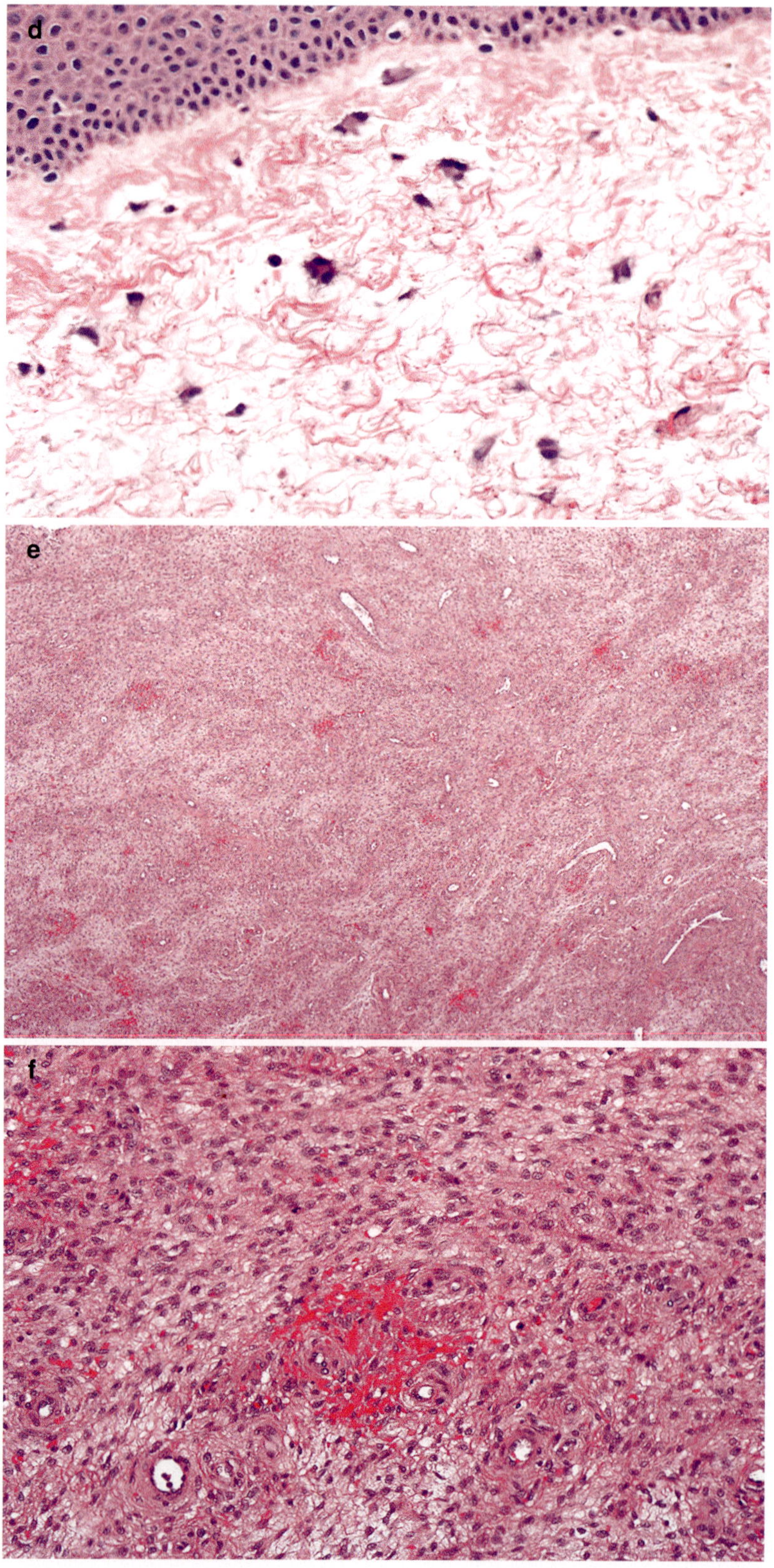

Fig. 11.1 (continued)

Fig. 11.1 (continued)

g

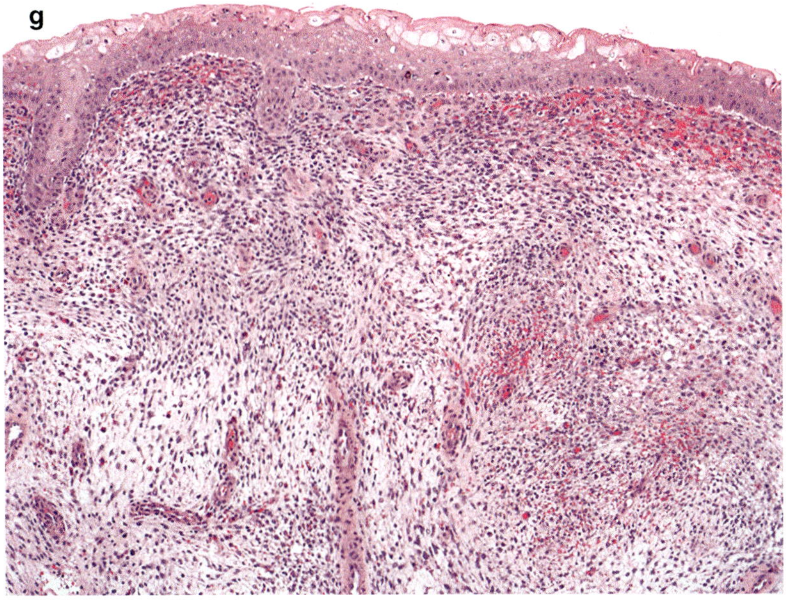

h

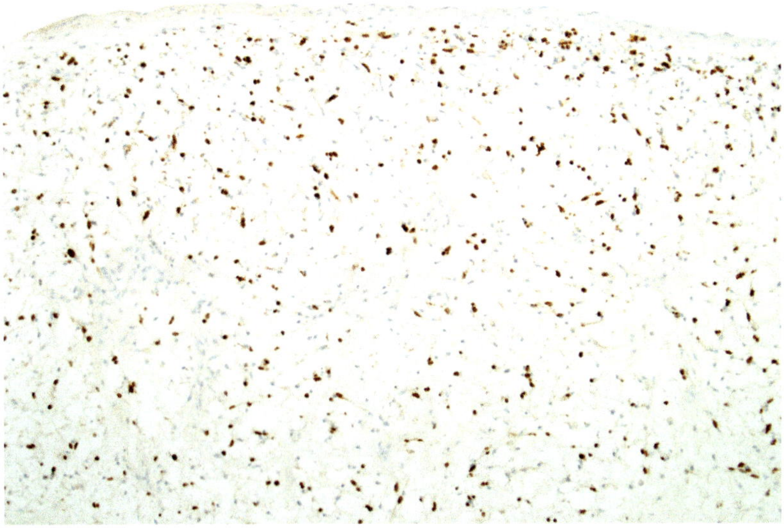

Pathologic Features

Cellular angiofibromas are well-circumscribed tumors composed of uniform ovoid to spindle-shaped cells with wavy or plump nuclei in a fibrous, collagenous, or edematous background (Fig. 11.2a). The stroma contains numerous obvious small- to medium-sized blood vessels and wispy collagen bundles (Fig. 11.2b). A subset of cases harbors a component of mature adipose tissue (Fig. 11.2c). While the majority of cellular angiofibromas have indolent morphologic features lacking significant atypia or mitotic activity, sarcomatous transformation has been reported. The sarcomatous component manifests as discrete foci resembling pleomorphic liposarcoma or undifferentiated pleomorphic sarcoma (Fig. 11.2d and Table 11.2).

Differential Diagnosis

The main differential diagnosis of cellular angiofibroma is mammary-type myofibroblastoma. As both entities share overlapping morphologic and immunophenotypic features, show monoallelic loss of *RB1*, and have similar clinical behavior, the distinction is academic. However, the recognition of a prominent vascular component with conspicuous hyalinization of the blood vessel walls is more in keeping with the diagnosis of cellular angiofibroma.

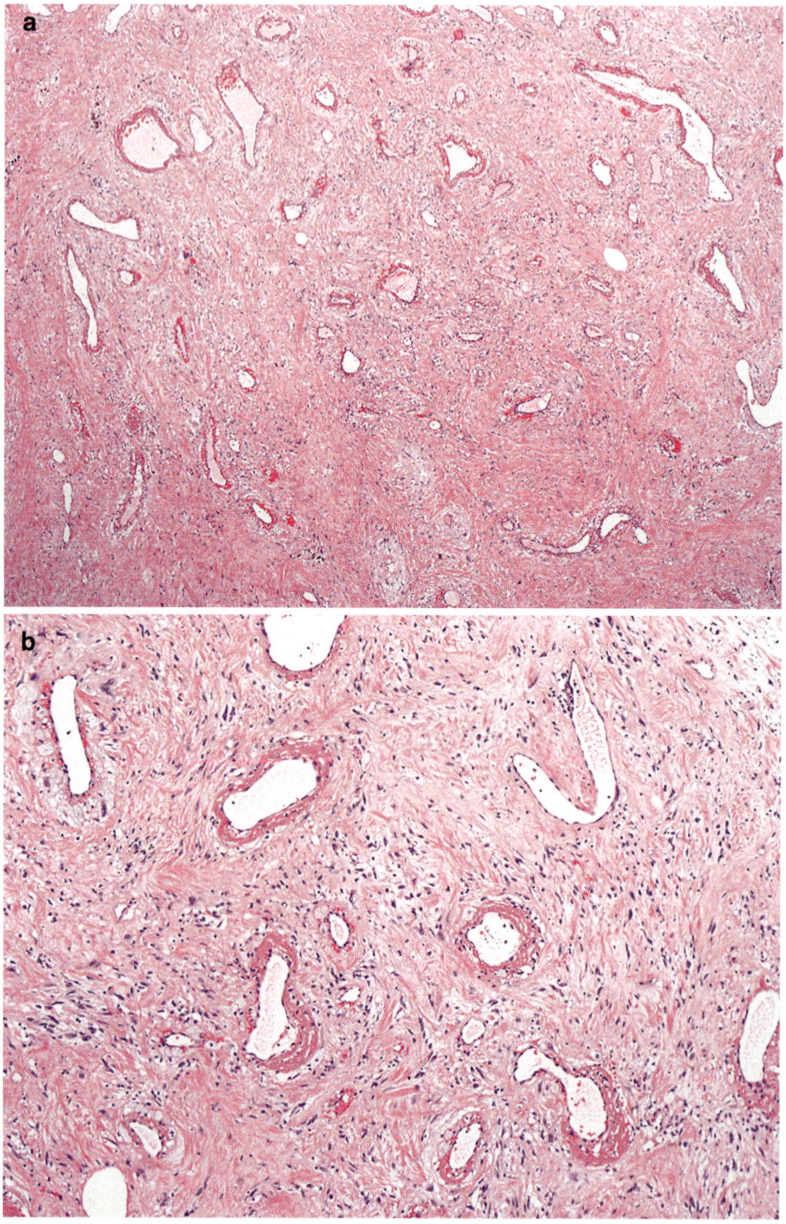

Fig. 11.2 A distinctive feature of cellular angiofibroma is prominent small- and medium-sized blood vessels (**a**) admixed with spindled cells in a collagenous background. Higher-power examination shows variable hyalinization of the vessel walls (**b**). Wispy collagen bundles are also appreciated in the stroma. A subset of cellular angiofibromas contain mature fat (**c**). A rare example of sarcomatous transformation with foci of pleomorphic liposarcoma (**d**)

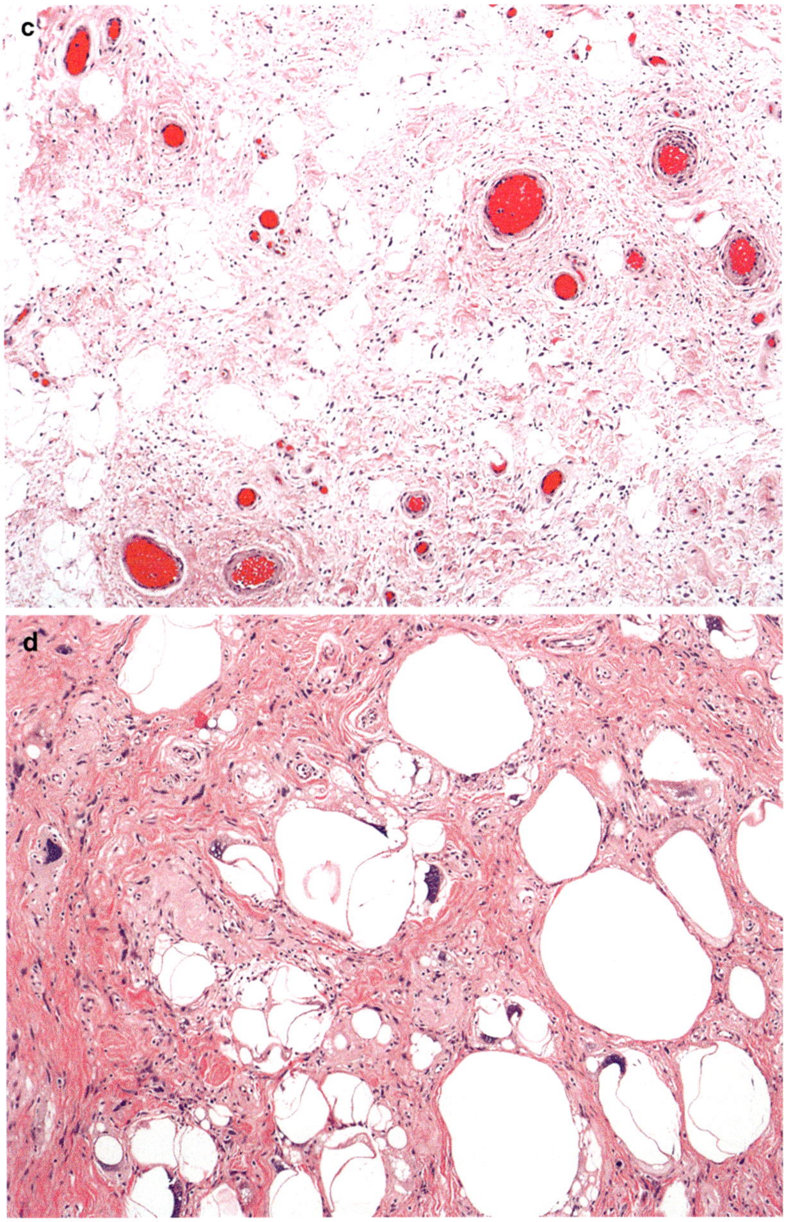

Fig. 11.2 (continued)

Table 11.2 Key pathologic features: cellular angiofibroma

Prominent small- to medium-sized hyalinized blood vessels
RB1 loss

Mammary-Type Myofibroblastoma

Clinical Features

Myofibroblastoma was initially described as a distinct stromal neoplasm arising in breast parenchyma with a predilection for elderly males, but the clinical spectrum was eventually expanded to include extra-mammary sites. In a series of 143 cases of mammary-type myofibroblastoma by Howitt and Fletcher, nearly half of the lesions arose in vulvar, groin, or inguinal regions. The male:female was approximately 2:1 with a mean age at presentation of 54 years (range 4–96 years). Tumors are well-circumscribed (Fig. 11.3a) and generally range from less than 1 cm to greater than 10 cm (median 5.5 cm).

Pathologic Features

Microscopic sections of mammary-type myofibroblastoma reveal bland spindled cells with short stubby nuclei deposited in a variably hyalinized or collagenous stroma (Fig. 11.3b, c). Thick collagen bundles may be conspicuous. Some tumors show foci of adipocytic differentiation (Fig. 11.3d), while others may exhibit epithelioid morphology (Fig. 11.3e). Cytologic atypia and mitotic activity are infrequent (Table 11.3).

Differential Diagnosis

As mentioned in the preceding section, the main differential diagnosis of mammary-type myofibroblastoma is cellular angiofibroma. The most helpful diagnostic clue favoring cellular angiofibroma

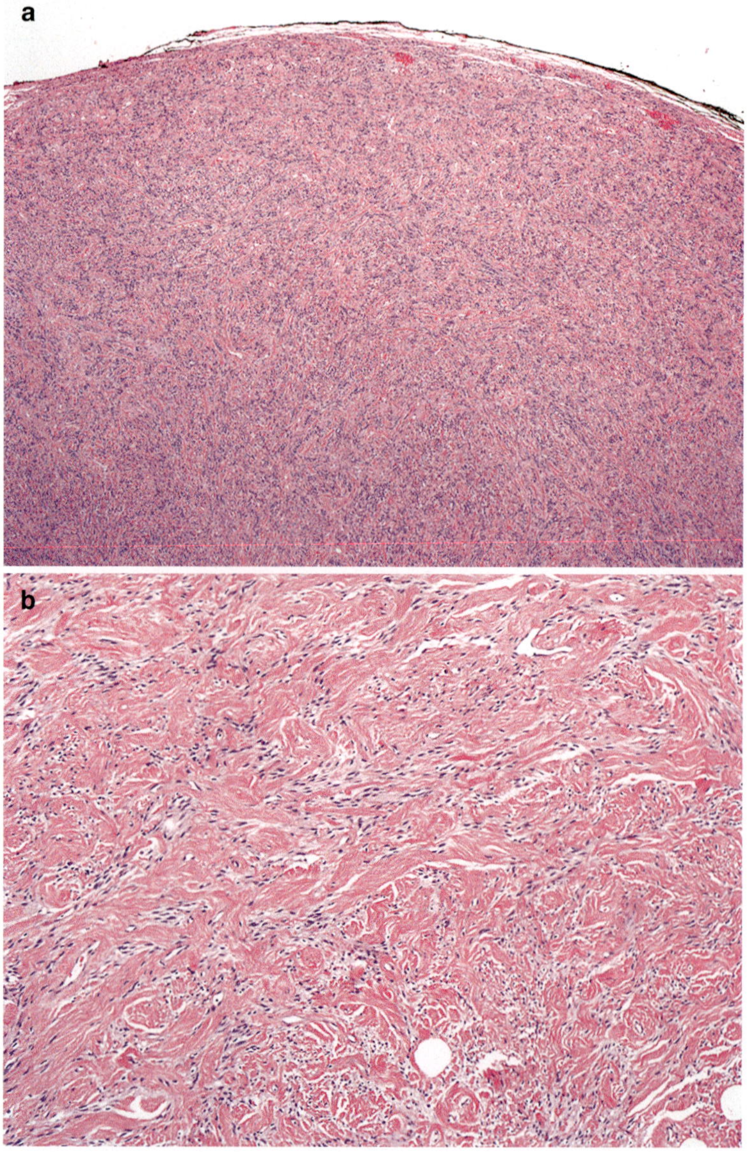

Fig. 11.3 Mammary-type myofibroblastoma is a well-circumscribed mesenchymal tumor (**a**) characterized by bland spindled to ovoid-shaped cells in a hyalinized background (**b**). A helpful diagnostic clue is the presence of thick collagen bundles (**c**). Similar to other genital stromal tumors, mammary-type myofibroblastoma may also harbor a well-differentiated adipocytic component (**d**). Occasionally, mammary-type myofibroblastoma is composed of predominantly of cells with epithelioid morphology (**e**)

Fig. 11.3 (continued)

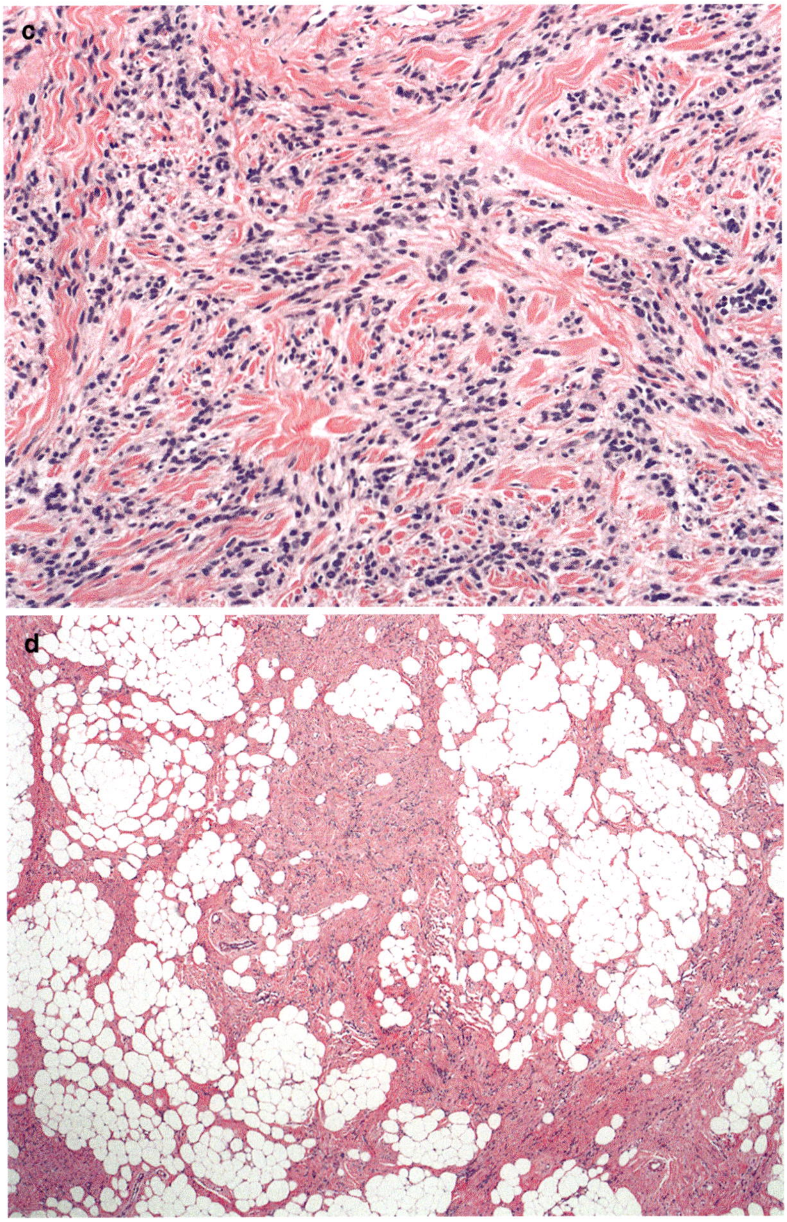

Table 11.3 Key pathologic features: mammary-type myofibroblastoma

Conspicuous broad bands of eosinophilic collagen
RB1 loss

over mammary-type myofibroblastoma is a prominent vascular component, which is generally absent in the latter. Occasionally, mammary-type myofibroblastoma may be mistaken for a smooth muscle neoplasm or solitary fibrous tumor. Even though mammary-type myofibroblastoma and smooth muscle tumors can express actin and desmin, the former contains broad eosinophilic collagen bundles lacking in smooth muscle neoplasms. The presence of CD34 immunoreactivity also supports the diagnosis of mammary-type myofibro-

Fig. 11.3 (continued)

e

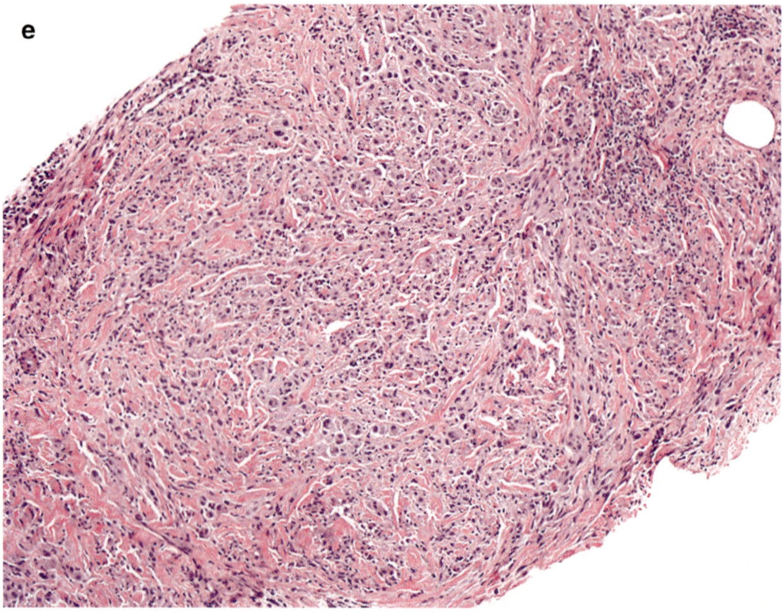

blastoma over leiomyoma or leiomyosarcoma. While not specific, the presence of hyalinized and staghorn-shaped blood vessels suggests solitary fibrous tumor. Additionally, as solitary fibrous tumors harbor *NAB2-STAT6* fusions, they show nuclear expression of STAT6.

Angiomyofibroblastoma

Clinical Features

Angiomyofibroblastoma occurs in the vulva and vagina of reproductive-aged females. Most tumors are well-circumscribed masses ranging from 1 to 12 cm, and many are present for several years before coming to clinical attention. This is a benign tumor, but a case with histologic features of malignancy has been reported. It is not certain how this impacts behavior, as experience is still too limited to be definitive at this point.

Pathologic Features

These tumors are characterized by ovoid to spindled cells in a myxoid or edematous matrix. The cellularity of angiomyofibroblastoma varies with alternating hypocellular and hypercellular zones. The lesional cells often aggregate around delicate small capillary-sized blood vessels where they show a plump, plasmacytoid, or occasionally multinucleated appearance (Fig. 11.4a, b and Table 11.4). Rare cases harbor mature adipose tissue (Fig. 11.4c). A single case of angiomyofibroblastoma with sarcomatous transformation has been described, but the vast majority of these tumors have banal histologic findings.

Differential Diagnosis

The differential diagnosis of angiomyofibroblastoma primarily includes other members of the genital stromal tumor family. The presence of plasmacytoid mononuclear cells "spinning" off from delicate blood vessels is the most important clue in the diagnosis of this entity.

Deep Angiomyxoma

Clinical Features

Deep (aggressive) angiomyxoma is a rare myxoid mesenchymal neoplasm that predominantly occurs in vulvovaginal, pelvic, and perineal regions of females. Cases involving the perineum and inguinoscrotal soft tissue in men have also been reported. Tumors are slow-growing gelatinous cyst-like masses, often thought clinically to represent a Bartholin gland cyst, and may measure up to 60 cm. Most deep angiomyxomas present in the third decade of life, but the age range is broad. This tumor is locally aggressive but without risk of metastasis; local recurrence occurs in approximately 30–40% of cases. Wide local excision with negative margins is advocated to minimize this risk. There is also evidence to suggest that gonadotropin-releasing hormone (GnRH) agonists may be helpful in recurrences or cases not amenable to surgical management.

Pathologic Features

Microscopic examination shows a poorly circumscribed proliferation of sparsely spaced spindled to stellate-shaped cells in a myxoid stroma (Fig. 11.5a). Significant cytologic atypia is absent (Fig. 11.5b), and mitotic figures are difficult to identify. Mast cells are often prominent. These tumors harbor a conspicuous vasculature comprised of variably ectatic and hyalinized small- and large-sized blood vessels (Table 11.5)

Differential Diagnosis

While all members of the genital stromal tumor family may exhibit myxoid features, deep angiomyxoma can be distinguished from other genital stromal tumors by a uniformly hypocellular

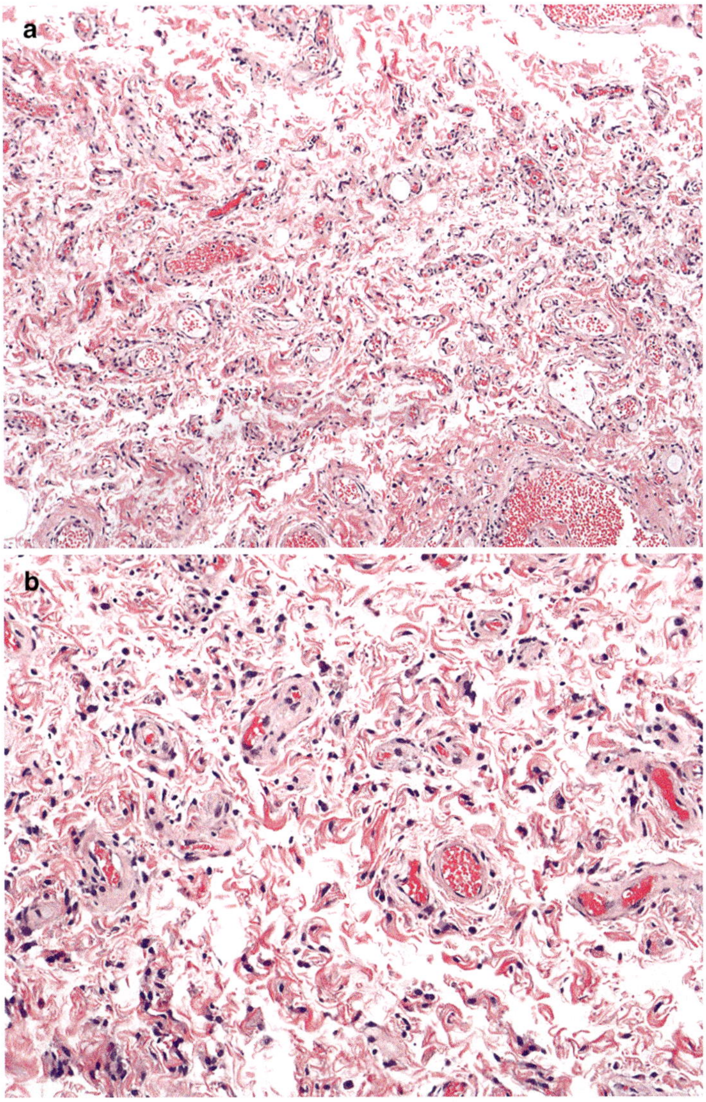

Fig. 11.4 Angiomyofibroblastoma is composed of predominantly delicate, small capillary-sized blood vessels (**a**) in myxoid stroma. The lesional cells are epithelioid or plasmacytoid as they appear to "spin" off from the blood vessels (**b**). Mature fat may be present (**c**)

Fig. 11.4 (continued)

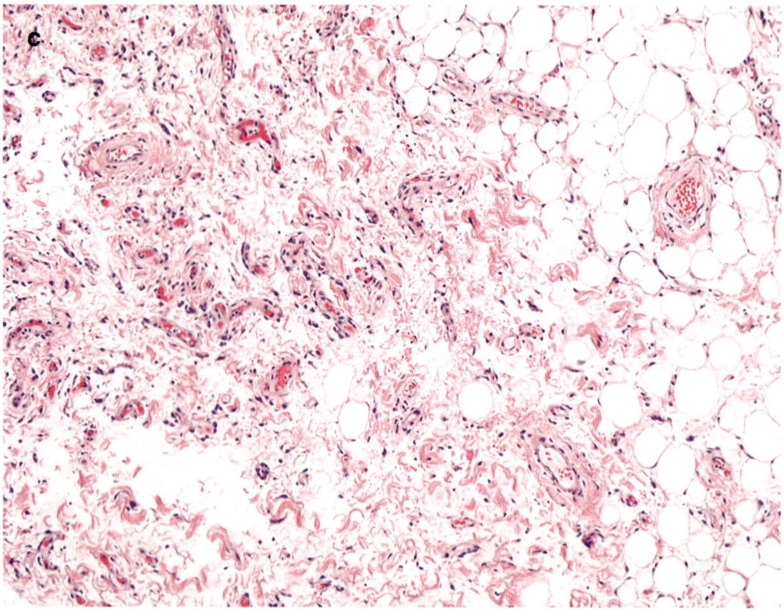

Table 11.4 Key pathologic features: angiomyofibroblastoma

Myxoid stroma with alternating hypocellular and hypercellular zones. Plasmacytoid cells spinning off from blood vessels

appearance and infiltrative growth pattern. Furthermore, as its name implies, this tumor typically involves deep soft tissue, whereas the remainder of lesions in this group are usually superficially situated. Well-differentiated liposarcoma may also arise in the pelvis/groin and show myxoid morphology; however well-differentiated liposarcoma is characterized by atypical spindle cells with enlarged hyperchromatic nuclei and *MDM2* amplification, which are absent in deep angiomyxoma.

Ancillary Studies for Genital Stromal Tumors

Immunohistochemistry

Virtually all genital stromal tumors express a combination of desmin, actin, CD34, and estrogen and progesterone receptors. Consequently, this panel is of limited value in rendering a specific diagnosis. Loss of RB expression is expected in cellular angiofibroma and mammary-type myofibroblastoma but not in the other members of this group, making this marker helpful if available. Importantly, stains for S100 protein and skeletal muscle markers (myogenin, myoD1) are negative in genital stromal tumors.

Genetics

RB1/13q14

Mammary-type myofibroblastoma and cellular angiofibroma are genetically linked by monoallelic or biallelic loss of *RB1*/13q14 (Fig. 11.6). The *RB1* locus encodes the retinoblastoma (RB) protein, a tumor suppressor protein important in cell cycle progression. As a result, these tumors show loss of RB immunoexpression by immunohistochemistry. A limited number of angiomyofibroblastomas, fibroepithelial stromal polyps, and aggressive angiomyxomas evaluated for deletion of *RB1*/13q14 by fluorescence in situ hybridization and/or RB by immunohistochemistry have failed to show loss of this locus.

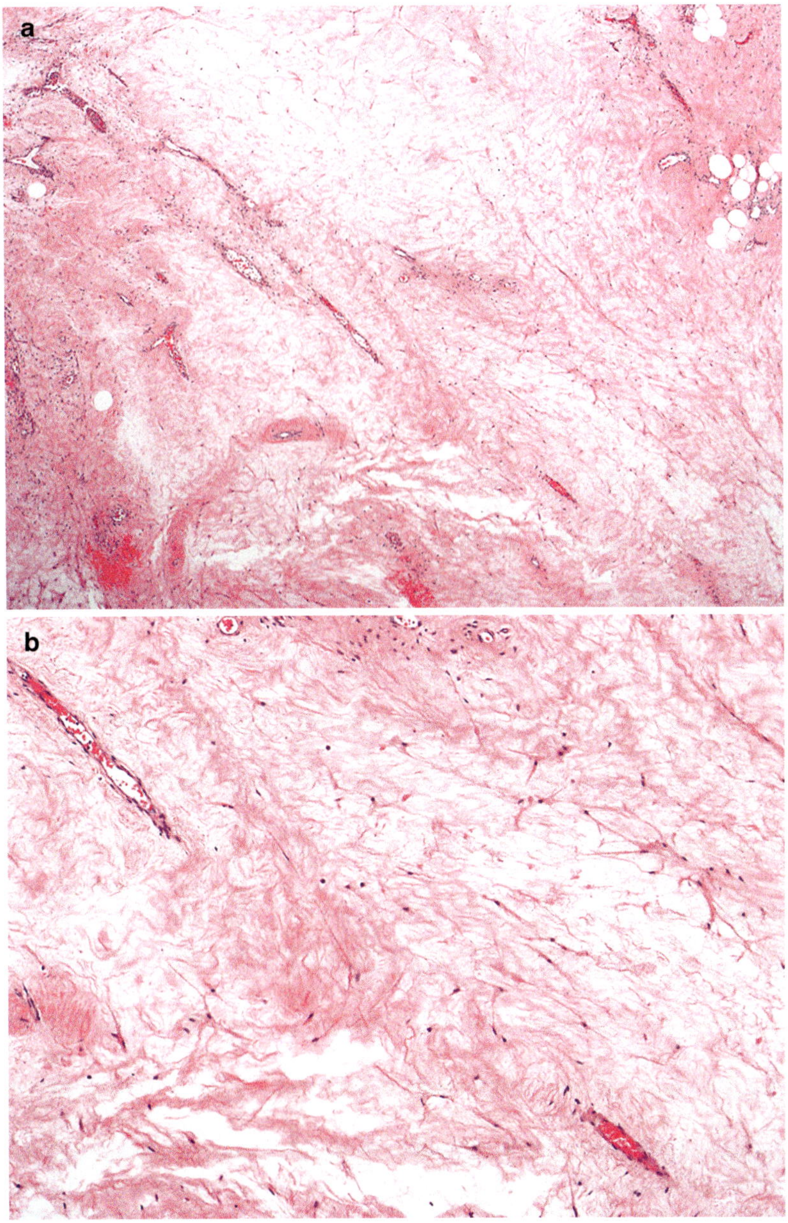

Fig. 11.5 Histologic examination of an deep angiomyxoma shows a uniformly hypocellular proliferation of spindle- to stellate-shaped cells in a myxoid stroma (**a**). High-power examination shows absence of cytologic atypia (**b**)

Table 11.5 Key pathologic features: aggressive angiomyxoma

Deep-seated and large (generally greater than 10 cm)
Infiltrative growth pattern
Uniformly hypocellular without cytologic atypia

HMGA2/12q14.3

Karotypic and interphase fluorescence in situ hybridization studies have shown genetic rearrangements of the high-mobility group A gene (*HMGA2*/12q14.3) in approximately one-third of deep angiomyxomas, while up to 90% of these tumors show expression of HMGA2 by immunohistochemistry. *HMGA2* encodes a protein involved in chromatin architecture and gene expression. However, the utility of this marker as a diagnostic tool is unclear as *HMGA2* rearrangements/HMGA2 expression have also been identi-

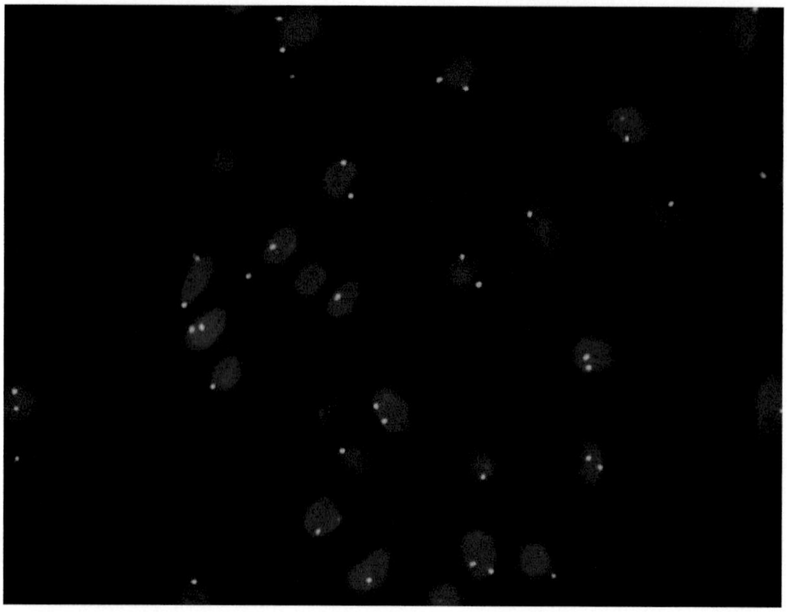

Fig. 11.6 Fluorescence in situ hybridization of mammary-type myofibroblastoma and cellular angiofibroma shows loss of *RB1*

fied in fibroepithelial stromal polyps, smooth muscle tumors, and a variety of other mesenchymal neoplasms.

Prepubertal Vulval Fibroma

Clinical Features

Prepubertal vulval fibroma is a rare mesenchymal tumor that presents in young females. In the largest series to date, Iwasa and Fletcher described 11 cases in patients ranging from 4 to 12 years. Two-thirds of cases in this report involved the labia majora, and sizes ranged from 2 to 8 cm. Similar lesions including "childhood asymmetric labium majus enlargement" (CALME) and "prepubertal labial fibrous hyperplasia" are thought to represent a physiologic response to hormones and may be related to prepubertal vulval fibroma. Prepubertal vulval fibroma is benign but may recur, especially if incompletely excised (Fig. 11.7).

Pathologic Features

Microscopically, prepubertal vulval fibroma is poorly circumscribed, involves submucosal or subcutaneous tissue, and consists of uniform spindled cells deposited in a collagenous or edematous stroma. Intralesional small- or medium-sized blood vessels, mature fat, and bundles of nerves are a common finding. Extensive myxoid change may be appreciated, but atypia and significant mitotic activity are not a feature of this entity (Table 11.6). The lesional cells are positive for CD34; immunoreactivity for actins, desmin, S100 protein, and estrogen/progesterone receptor is absent.

Differential Diagnosis

The differential diagnosis of prepubertal vulval fibroma includes fibroepithelial stromal polyp and deep angiomyxoma. While fibroepithelial stromal polyps may arise in the pediatric age group, they predominantly affect females of reproductive age. Histologically, fibroepithelial stromal polyps are distinctly polypoid in appearance and contain multinucleated stromal cells at the epithelial interface. Deep angiomyxoma arises in deep soft tissues of the lower genital tract and pelvis and contains myxoid rather than edematous or collagenous stroma. It is exceedingly uncommon in children. Finally, both fibroepithelial stromal polyps and deep angiomyxomas generally express desmin and estrogen/progesterone receptor, which are lacking in prepubertal vulval fibroma.

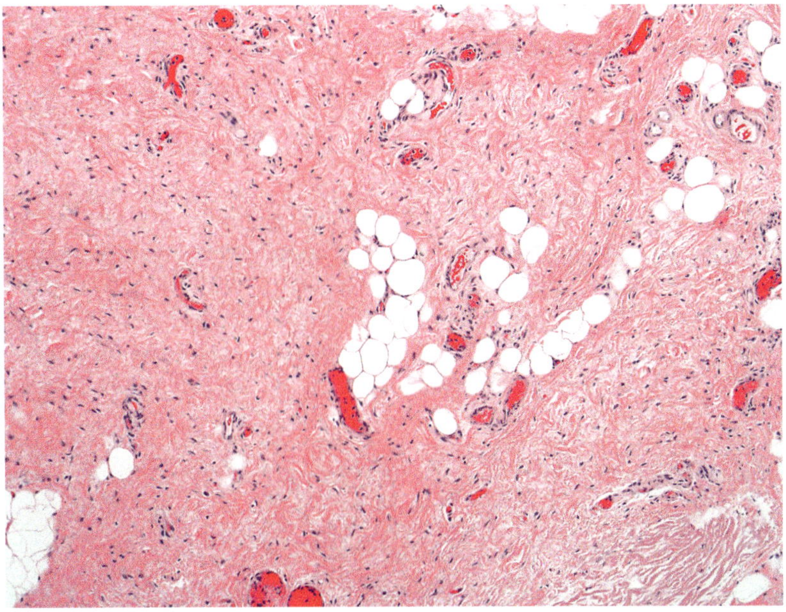

Fig. 11.7 Prepubertal vulval fibroma consists of uniform spindled cells within a collagenous stroma. (Photo credit to Dr. Alyaa Al-Ibraheemi, Boston Children's Hospital, Boston, MA)

Table 11.6 Key pathologic features: prepubertal vulval fibroma

Poorly circumscribed
Uniform spindled cells deposited in a collagenous or edematous stroma
May seen entrapped nerves or fat

Massive Vulval Edema

Clinical Features

Massive vulval edema is a site-specific variant of massive localized lymphedema. This pseudoneoplastic condition is likely related to chronic lymphatic obstruction. While this process most commonly affects morbidly obese or immobilized patients, similar lesions have been described during pregnancy and even as unilateral vulvar masses in competitive female cyclists. In a review of 17 cases by Fadare and colleagues, patients ranged in age from 19 to 59 years (median 39 years), and the lesions measured up to 45 cm (mean 6.1 cm). Massive vulval edema may recur after resection, especially if the predisposing factors (obesity, immobilization) persist.

Pathologic Features

Histologic examination of massive vulval edema shows markedly edematous subcutaneous adipose tissue underlying a sclerotic dermis (Fig. 11.8a, b). Adipocytes are arranged in a lobular configuration separated by fluid and hypocellular fibrous septa. The fibrous septa contain occasional multinucleated cells and fibroblasts (Fig. 11.8c), a subset of which may show mild reactive atypia. Perivascular chronic inflammation is a consistent finding and often a helpful clue as to the diagnosis (Table 11.7).

Differential Diagnosis

Massive vulval edema is commonly confused with deep angiomyxoma as both are characterized by a relatively hypocellular proliferation of bland spindle cells. However, aggressive angiomyxoma is deep-seated unlike massive vulval edema, which affects subcutaneous tissue. Additionally, the stroma of massive vulval edema is edematous rather than myxoid and contains prominent lymphocytic infiltrates around vascular channels. Finally, correlation with clinical presentation is often helpful as a history of morbid obesity or immobilization should raise suspicion for massive vulval edema.

Smooth Muscle Tumors of the External Genitalia

Clinical Features

Smooth muscle tumors of the external genitalia (vulva, vagina, and scrotum) are uncommon, but their gross and microscopic appearance is comparable to tumors arising at nongenital sites. Leiomyomas outnumber leiomyosarcomas in the vulva and vagina, while most smooth muscle tumors in the scrotum are malignant.

Pathologic Features

Gross examination of smooth muscle tumors of the vulva and vagina reveals well-circumscribed masses with a solid whorled cut surface. Those arising in the scrotum are more likely exhibit an infiltrative growth pattern. Histologic review shows plump spindle cells with brightly eosinophilic cytoplasm and blunt-ended nuclei arranged in interlacing fascicles. Variants include epithelioid morphology and myxoid change (Fig. 11.9). Unfortunately, given the rarity of these tumors,

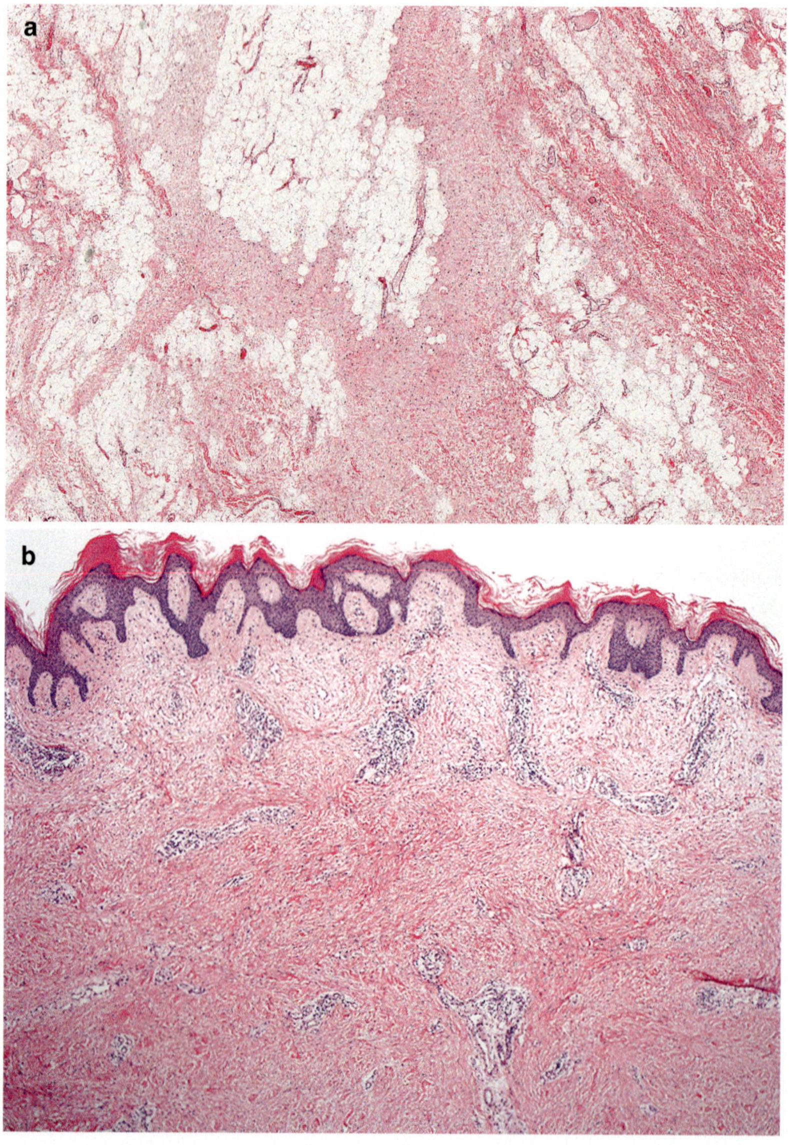

Fig. 11.8 Massive vulval edema is characterized by lobules of mature fat separated by edematous and fibrous septa (**a**). The overlying epidermis is often sclerotic with lymphoid aggregates surrounding lymphovascular spaces (**b**). Closer inspection of the fibrous septa reveals bland fibroblasts with a reactive appearance (**c**)

Fig. 11.8 (continued)

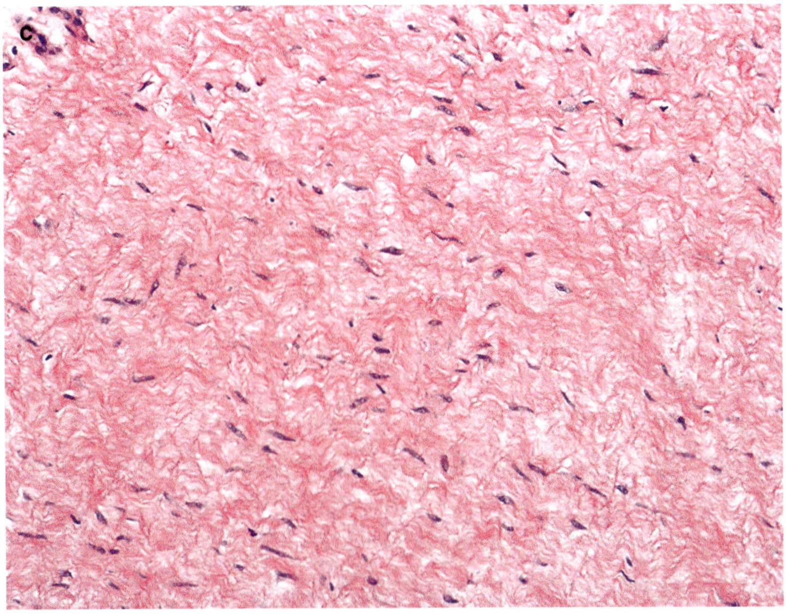

Table 11.7 Key pathologic features: massive vulval edema

Markedly edematous subcutaneous adipose tissue underlying a sclerotic dermis
Hypocellular fibrous septa with reactive fibroblasts and myofibroblasts

studies defining criteria for differentiating leiomyoma and leiomyosarcoma at these sites are limited. Distinguishing benign from malignant smooth muscle tumors of the vulva, vagina, and scrotum involves evaluating a combination of size, infiltrative growth, cytologic atypia, and mitotic rate (Tables 11.8 and 11.9). As expected, the lesional cells are immunoreactive for actin, desmin, and h-caldesmon.

Table 11.8 Key pathologic features: genital smooth muscle tumors

Vulvar leiomyoma
Well-circumscribed
Usually small
Lacks atypia
Low mitotic rate
Vulvar leiomyosarcoma
Often large (>5 cm)
Infiltrative
Cytologic atypia
Mitotic activity
Scrotal leiomyoma
Poorly circumscribed
No atypia or mitotic activity
Scrotal leiomyosarcoma
Any mitotic activity
Often cytologic atypia

Differential Diagnosis

Smooth muscle tumors with conventional features may be confused with mammary-type myofibroblastoma, while those with marked myxoid change can lead to the erroneous diagnosis of deep angiomyxoma. The lesional cells of mammary-type myofibroblastoma typically lack the bright eosinophilic color of cells of smooth muscle derivation. Additionally, mammary-type myofibroblastomas are CD34-positive. A misdiagnosis of deep angiomyxoma can be avoided by thorough sampling of the tumor as even myxoid smooth muscle tumors will generally show foci with traditional histology.

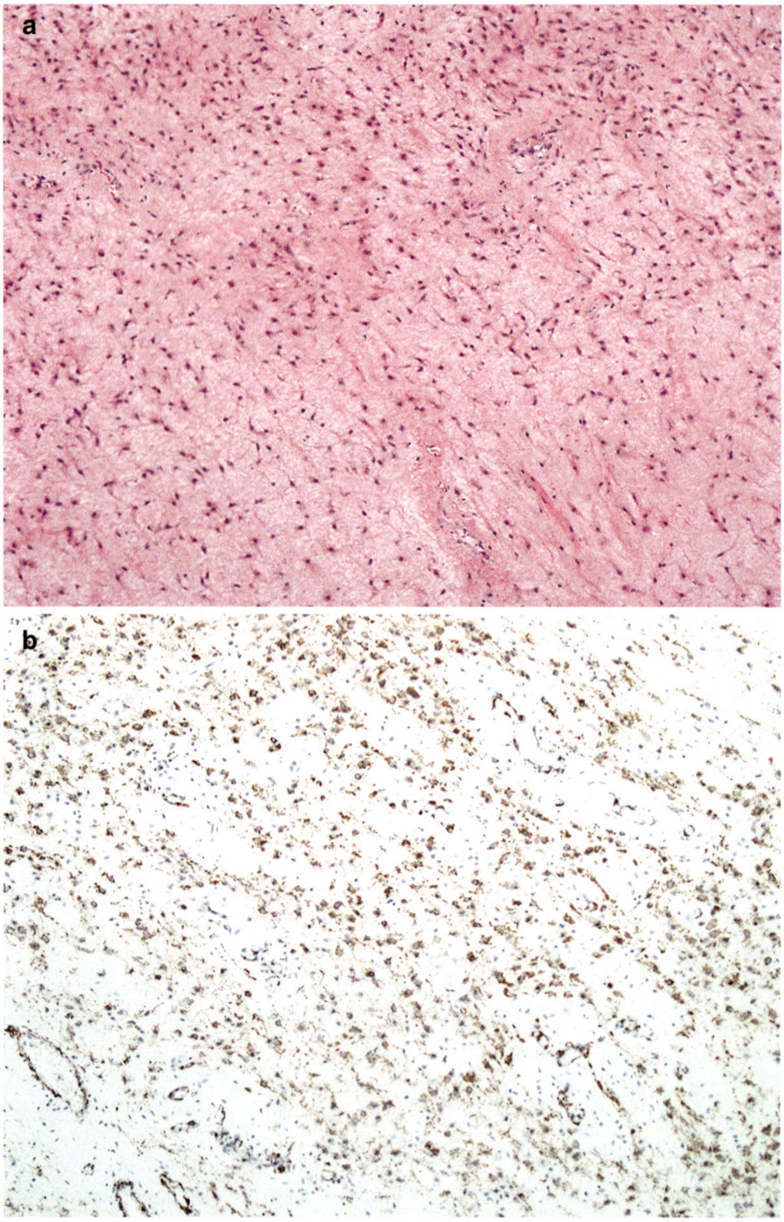

Fig. 11.9 Leiomyoma of the vulvar with significant myxoid change (**a**). Like conventional smooth muscle tumors, the lesional cells are positive for smooth muscle actin (**b**) and desmin (**c**). Smooth muscle tumors of the external genitalia may occasionally exhibit epithelioid morphology (**d**)

Fig. 11.9 (continued)

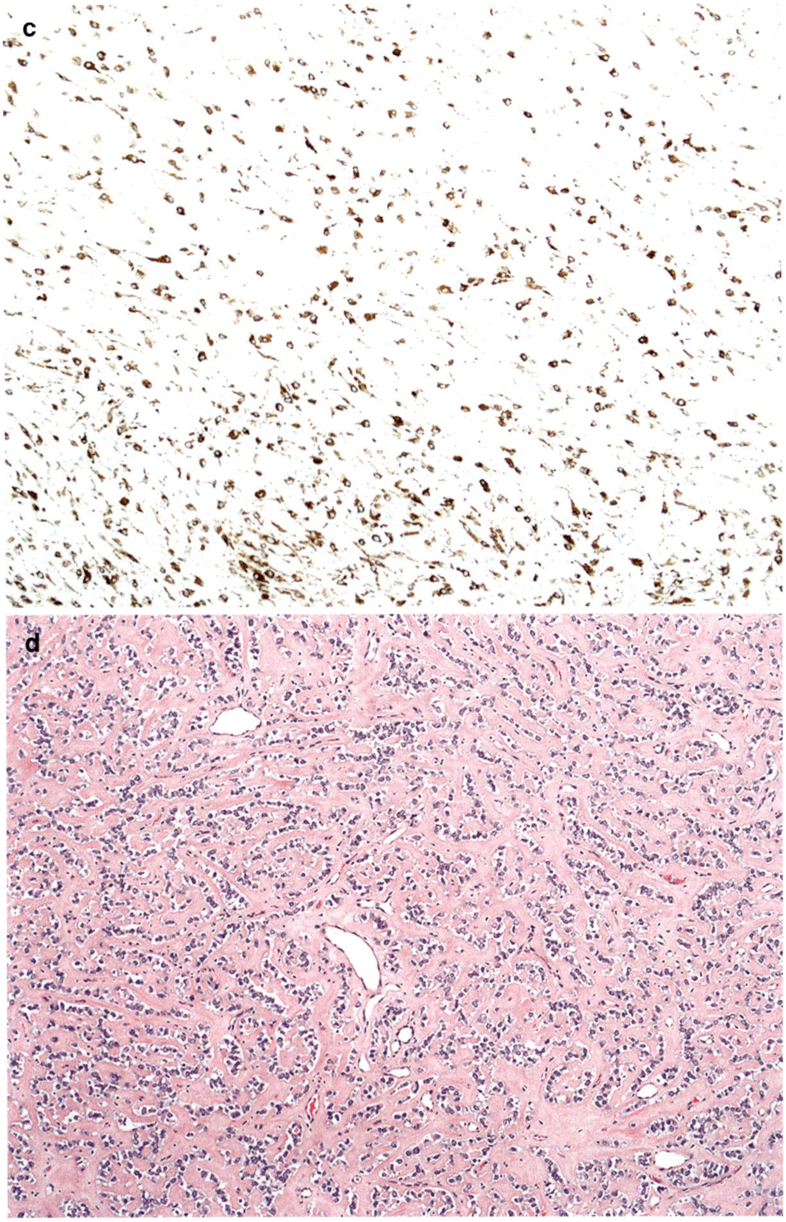

Table 11.9 Classification criteria for smooth muscle tumors of external genitalia

	Criteria for classification	Classification
Vulva	Gross size ≥ 5 cm Infiltrative margin Moderate-marked cytologic atypia Mitotic rate ≥ 5/10 HPFs	0 or 1 feature: leiomyoma 2 features: atypical leiomyoma 3 or 4 features: leiomyosarcoma
Vagina	Significant cytologic atypia Mitotic rate ≥ 5/10 HPFs Infiltrative margin	Significant cytologic atypia and mitotic rate ≥ 5/10 HPFs: leiomyosarcoma Infiltrative margin: leiomyosarcoma
Scrotum	Cytologic atypia Mitotic rate	No cytologic atypia or mitotic activity: leiomyoma (complete excision and clinical follow-up recommended) Cytologic atypia without mitotic activity: atypical smooth muscle tumor of uncertain biologic potential Any mitotic activity: leiomyosarcoma

HPF high-power fields

Selected References

1. Sayeed S, Xing D, Jenkins SM, et al. Criteria for risk stratification of vulvar and vaginal smooth muscle tumors: an evaluation of 71 cases comparing proposed classification systems. Am J Surg Pathol. 2018;42:84–94.
2. Chen E, Fletcher CD. Cellular angiofibroma with atypia or sarcomatous transformation: clinicopathologic analysis of 13 cases. Am J Surg Pathol. 2010;34:707–14.
3. Chen BJ, Marino-Enriquez A, Fletcher CD, et al. Loss of retinoblastoma protein expression in spindle cell/pleomorphic lipomas and cytogenetically related tumors: an immunohistochemical study with diagnostic implications. Am J Surg Pathol. 2012;36:1119–28.
4. Dreux N, Marty M, Chibon F, et al. Value and limitation of immunohistochemical expression of HMGA2 in mesenchymal tumors: about a series of 1052 cases. Mod Pathol. 2010;23:1657–66.
5. Fletcher CD, Tsang WY, Fisher C, et al. Angiomyofibroblastoma of the vulva. A benign neoplasm distinct from aggressive angiomyxoma. Am J Surg Pathol. 1992;16:373–82.
6. Flucke U, van Krieken JH, Mentzel T. Cellular angiofibroma: analysis of 25 cases emphasizing its relationship to spindle cell lipoma and mammary-type myofibroblastoma. Mod Pathol. 2011;24:82–9.
7. Howitt BE, Fletcher CD. Mammary-type myofibroblastoma: clinicopathologic characterization in a series of 143 cases. Am J Surg Pathol. 2016;40:361–7.
8. Iwasa Y, Fletcher CD. Cellular angiofibroma: clinicopathologic and immunohistochemical analysis of 51 cases. Am J Surg Pathol. 2004a;28:1426–35.
9. Iwasa Y, Fletcher CD. Distinctive prepubertal vulval fibroma: a hitherto unrecognized mesenchymal tumor of prepubertal girls: analysis of 11 cases. Am J Surg Pathol. 2004b;28:1601–8.
10. Laskin WB, Fetsch JF, Mostofi FK. Angiomyofibroblastoma like tumor of the male genital tract: analysis of 11 cases with comparison to female angiomyofibroblastoma and spindle cell lipoma. Am J Surg Pathol. 1998;22:6–16.
11. Matoso A, Chen S, Plaza JA, et al. Symplastic leiomyomas of the scrotum: a comparative study to usual leiomyomas and leiomyosarcomas. Am J Surg Pathol. 2014;38:1410–7.
12. McMenamin ME, Fletcher CD. Mammary-type myofibroblastoma of soft tissue: a tumor closely related to spindle cell lipoma. Am J Surg Pathol. 2001;25:1022–9.
13. Medeiros F, Erickson-Johnson MR, Keeney GL, et al. Frequency and characterization of HMGA2 and HMGA1 rearrangements in mesenchymal tumors of the lower genital tract. Genes Chromosomes Cancer. 2007;46:981–90.
14. Miettinen M, Fetsch JF. Evaluation of biological potential of smooth muscle tumours. Histopathology. 2006;48:97–105.
15. Miettinen M, Wahlstrom T, Vesterinen E, et al. Vaginal polyps with pseudosarcomatous features. A clinicopathologic study of seven cases. Cancer. 1983;51:1148–51.
16. Newman PL, Fletcher CD. Smooth muscle tumours of the external genitalia: clinicopathological analysis of a series. Histopathology. 1991;18:523–9.
17. Nielsen GP, Rosenberg AE, Koerner FC, et al. Smooth-muscle tumors of the vulva. A clinicopathological study of 25 cases and review of the literature. Am J Surg Pathol. 1996;20:779–93.
18. Nielsen GP, Young RH, Dickersin GR, et al. Angiomyofibroblastoma of the vulva with sarcomatous transformation ("angiomyofibrosarcoma"). Am J Surg Pathol. 1997;21:1104–8.
19. Norris HJ, Taylor HB. Polyps of the vagina. A benign lesion resembling sarcoma botryoides. Cancer. 1966;19:227–32.
20. Nucci MR, Granter SR, Fletcher CD. Cellular angiofibroma: a benign neoplasm distinct from angiomyofibroblastoma and spindle cell lipoma. Am J Surg Pathol. 1997;21:636–44.

21. Nucci MR, Young RH, Fletcher CD. Cellular pseudosarcomatous fibroepithelial stromal polyps of the lower female genital tract: an underrecognized lesion often misdiagnosed as sarcoma. Am J Surg Pathol. 2000;24:231–40.
22. Steeper TA, Rosai J. Aggressive angiomyxoma of the female pelvis and perineum. Report of nine cases of a distinctive type of gynecologic soft-tissue neoplasm. Am J Surg Pathol. 1983;7:463–75.
23. Tavassoli FA, Norris HJ. Smooth muscle tumors of the vagina. Obstet Gynecol. 1979a;53:689–93.
24. Tavassoli FA, Norris HJ. Smooth muscle tumors of the vulva. Obstet Gynecol. 1979b;53:213–7.
25. Vang R, Connelly JH, Hammill HA, et al. Vulvar hypertrophy with lymphedema. A mimicker of aggressive angiomyxoma. Arch Pathol Lab Med. 2000;124:1697–9.
26. Wargotz ES, Weiss SW, Norris HJ. Myofibroblastoma of the breast. Sixteen cases of a distinctive benign mesenchymal tumor. Am J Surg Pathol. 1987;11:493–502.

12 Soft Tissue Tumors of Uncertain Histogenesis

Darya Buehler

Abstract

The mesenchymal tumors discussed in this chapter represent a diverse group with distinctive morphologic, immunophenotypic, and molecular genetic features. Many of these tumors arise in the dermis or subcutis and can closely mimic cases routinely encountered in dermatopathology practice such as melanoma, carcinoma, dermatofibroma (fibrous histiocytoma), nerve sheath tumors, or granulomatous inflammation. Others occupy deep and visceral locations and cause diagnostic difficulties when encountered in an unusual site, such as the dermis or subcutis. Reviewed herein are epithelioid sarcoma (ES), clear cell sarcoma (CCS), perivascular epithelioid cell tumor (PEComa), ossifying fibromyxoid tumor (OFMT), pleomorphic hyalinizing angiectatic tumor (PHAT), hemosiderotic fibrolipomatous tumor (HFLT), Rosai-Dorfman disease (RDD), solitary fibrous tumor (SFT), synovial sarcoma (SS), alveolar soft part sarcoma (ASPS), and cutaneous myoepithelial tumors. The discussion emphasizes the clinicopathologic features, differential diagnosis, and important diagnostic pitfalls encountered with these neoplasms, as well as diagnostically useful immunohistochemical and molecular genetic findings.

Epithelioid Sarcoma

Clinical Features

Epithelioid sarcoma (ES) is a distinctive malignant neoplasm with predominantly epithelioid cytomorphology. There are two types of ES: the conventional, or distal-type, and the proximal-type, which has a predilection for proximal or axial locations, rhabdoid morphology, and more aggressive behavior. Both types are characterized by mutations in the *SMARCB1/hSNF5/INI1* gene on chromosome 22q11.

Distal-type ES presents over a wide age range, with a peak incidence in the second to third decades, and may occur in young children as well. Distal-type ES usually manifests as a firm, slowly growing subcutaneous nodule, plaque, or nonhealing ulcer in the distal extremities, especially the fingers, hands, and forearms, though more proximal locations may be affected. The patients often present with a long-standing history of recurrent "inflammation," "warts," or "ulcers" on the fingers. Distal-type ES tends to grow along nerve trunks, fascial planes, and tendons, accounting for the very high rate of local recurrence (80–90%). The clinical course is pro-

D. Buehler (✉)
Pathology and Laboratory Medicine, University of Wisconsin School of Medicine and Public Health, Madison, WI, USA
e-mail: buehler2@wisc.edu

S. D. Billings et al. (eds.), *Soft Tissue Tumors of the Skin*,
https://doi.org/10.1007/978-1-4939-8812-9_12

tracted, with late metastases in up to 50% of patients, most commonly involving the lymph nodes and lung and, less often, bones and skin (especially the scalp). The 5-year overall survival is 65–78% and up to 92% in children.

Proximal-type ES typically occurs as a deep-seated mass in a relatively older population, usually in the fourth decade and above. Common sites include the proximal limbs and limb girdles, as well as the pelvis, perineum, genital areas, head and neck, and mediastinum. In contrast to the slow, indolent course of distal-type ES, proximal-type ES behaves aggressively with rapid progression and early systemic metastases in up to 75% of patients. The treatment of choice for both distal and proximal-type ES is radical excision; adjuvant radiotherapy and chemotherapy have been used with some success. Although sometimes performed, the benefit of lymph node dissection or sentinel lymph node biopsy and completion lymph node dissection in epithelioid sarcoma remains uncertain.

Pathologic Features

Distal-type ES usually presents as an infiltrative dermal or subcutaneous nodule or nodules with ill-defined margins. There is often a zone of central geographic necrosis or fibrosis around which tumor cells show a palisaded arrangement, resembling granuloma annulare or an infectious granuloma (Fig. 12.1a, b). Cytologically, distal-type ES is composed of relatively uniform epithelioid or spindle cells arranged in nests or cords. The cells have round to oval nuclei, vesicular chromatin, inconspicuous nucleoli, and abundant eosinophilic cytoplasm and may resemble histiocytes (Fig. 12.1c). Nuclear atypia ranges from mild to severe, but many examples of this lesion demonstrate deceptively bland cytology (Fig. 12.2a), and mitotic activity is usually relatively low (<5/10 HPF). Perineural and vascular invasion, when present, are helpful in establishing the diagnosis in cytologically bland cases (Fig. 12.2b). Variable amounts of chronic inflammation and fibrosis are present and can cause distal-type ES to be mistaken for an inflammatory process (Fig. 12.3a), while spindle cell areas can mimic a fibroblastic or fibrohistiocytic lesion (Fig. 12.3b). Other reported morphologic features include hemorrhage, necrosis, angiomatoid change, calcifications, and osseous or cartilaginous metaplasia.

Proximal-type ES is a large, subcutaneous, or deep-seated mass composed of sheets of large, overtly atypical, and mitotically active epithelioid cells with round nuclei, prominent nucleoli, and dense abundant eosinophilic cytoplasm (Fig. 12.4a, b). A frequent finding is the presence of perinuclear hyaline eosinophilic rhabdoid inclusions (Fig. 12.4c). Ultrastructurally, these inclusions are composed of whorls of cytokeratin intermediate filaments.

By immunohistochemistry (IHC), most distal- and proximal-type ES express cytokeratins and EMA, but immunoreactivity for cytokeratin 5/6 is usually absent. Approximately 60% of all cases are positive for CD34. Occasionally, SMA and S100 protein may be focally positive as well. Factor XIIIa may occasionally be positive in spindle ES, which may lead to diagnostic confusion with fibrous histiocytomas (dermatofibromas). Both types of ES are characterized by the inactivation of *SMARCB1/hSNF5/INI1* gene on chromosome 22q11, which encodes a subunit of the SWI/SNF chromatin remodeling complex. This results in loss of nuclear expression of INI1 in greater than 90% of all cases. Because INI1 is ubiquitously expressed in normal tissues and most neoplasms, immunohistochemical staining to detect loss of INI1 expression is a very useful diagnostic tool (Fig. 12.5 and Table 12.1).

Differential Diagnosis

The most important mimickers of distal-type ES are granulomatous inflammatory processes (e.g., granuloma annulare, rheumatoid nodule, and necrobiosis lipoidica), infectious granulomas, and benign fibrohistiocytic tumors. The benign histiocytes and fibroblasts in these entities lack cytologic atypia, which is usually at least focally present in distal-type ES. The histiocytes in the nonneoplastic granulomatous proliferations and fibrous histiocytomas express CD68 and CD163, lack cytokeratin and EMA immunoreactivity, and retain nuclear INI1 expression. A high index of suspicion for distal-type ES should be maintained in any distal extremity lesion from a young patient, especially if the clinical history suggests a long-standing, recurrent, or otherwise unusual process. A low threshold for the application of cytokeratin immunostaining should be maintained in such circumstances.

Distal-type ES with more overt cytologic atypia can resemble cutaneous adnexal carcinoma or squamous cell carcinoma, which have substantial immunohistochemical overlap with distal-type ES. However, it is very unusual for a

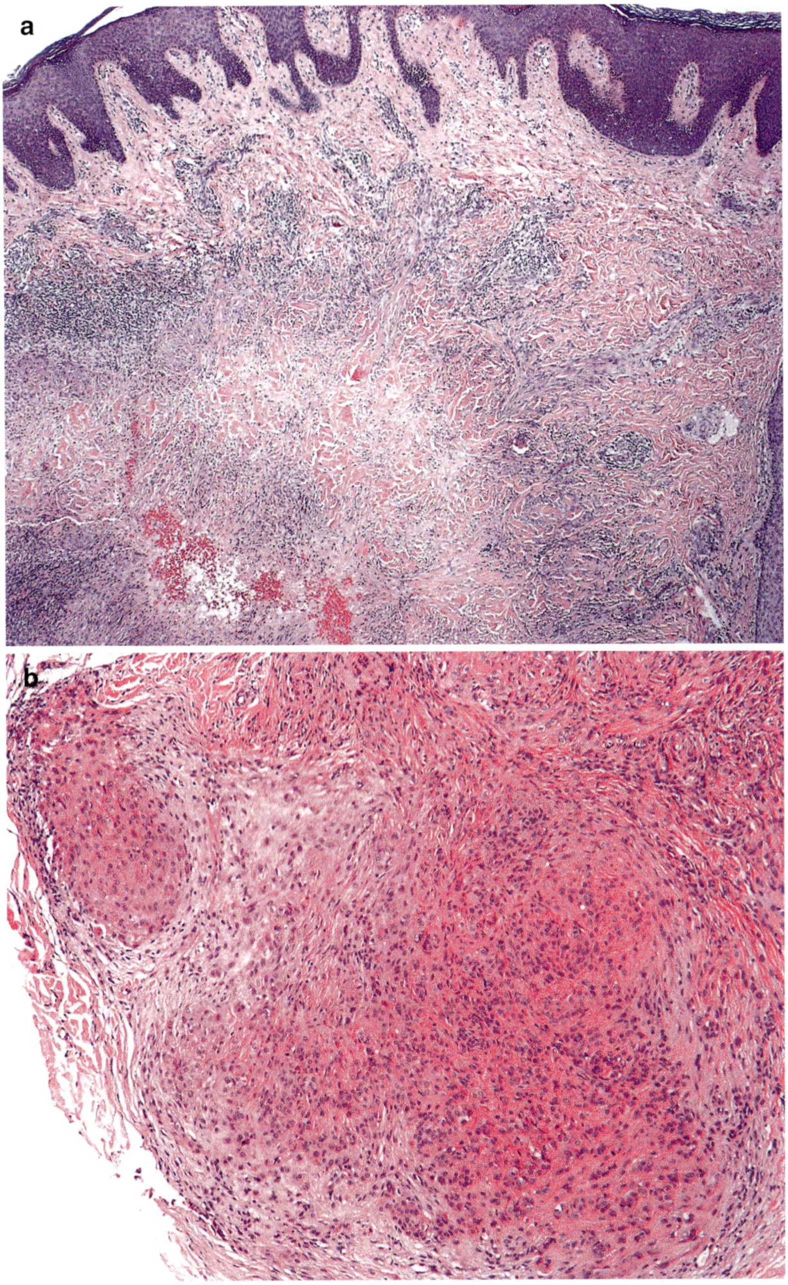

Fig. 12.1 Distal-type epithelioid sarcoma. (**a**) The tumors cells have a palisading granuloma-like growth pattern resembling granuloma annulare. (**b**) Solid nodule of epithelioid tumor cells resembling an infectious granuloma. (**c**) Uniform epithelioid to spindle cells with mild nuclear atypia and occasional mitoses

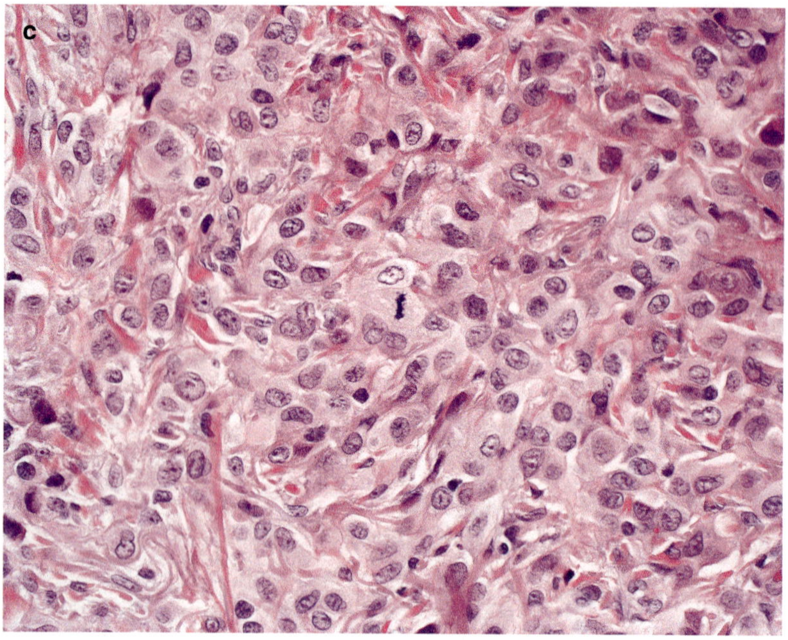

Fig. 12.1 (continued)

carcinoma to form a zone of geographic necrosis with peripheral palisading. By IHC, adnexal and squamous cell carcinomas are negative for CD34 and retain nuclear expression of INI1. Squamous cell carcinomas typically express CK5/6, unlike distal-type ES.

Pseudomyogenic hemangioendothelioma, originally described as epithelioid sarcoma-like hemangioendothelioma, is a distinctive epithelioid vascular neoplasm of intermediate malignancy that also may arise in the distal extremities of young adults and present as multifocal disease. The aptly named tumor is composed of sheets or fascicles of plump, cytokeratin-positive epithelioid, or spindle cell with abundant eosinophilic cytoplasm, mild nuclear atypia, and low mitotic activity, all of which may be seen in distal-type ES. It differs from ES by its prominent fascicular myoid component and lack of a nodular growth pattern and geographic necrosis with peripheral palisading. Both tumors express cytokeratins, but unlike ES, pseudomyogenic hemangioendothelioma is also positive for vascular markers ERG and CD31 (50–80%), is negative for CD34 and EMA, has retained INI1 expression, and shows nuclear expression of FOSB, a product of pathognomonic *SERPINE1/FOSB* rearrangement. See Chap. 7 for a detailed discussion of pseudomyogenic hemangioendothelioma.

Proximal-type ES is readily recognizable as a high-grade malignancy, but it can closely mimic other malignant cutaneous tumors with epithelioid morphology. Amelanotic melanoma can be distinguished from proximal-type ES by expression of melanocytic markers, lack of cytokeratin and CD34 expression, and retained INI1 expression. Epithelioid angiosarcoma often has a solid growth pattern like proximal-type ES and may express cytokeratins and CD34. However, epithelioid angiosarcoma consistently expresses additional vascular markers (particularly ERG and CD31) and retains nuclear INI1 expression. Epithelioid malignant peripheral nerve sheath tumor (MPNST) may arise from a nerve and is strongly and diffusely positive for S100 protein and usually negative for cytokeratins. INI1 IHC is less helpful in this context, as approximately 70% of epithelioid MPNSTs have loss of INI1 expression. Perhaps the most difficult tumor in the differential diagnosis is myoepithelial carcinoma (malignant

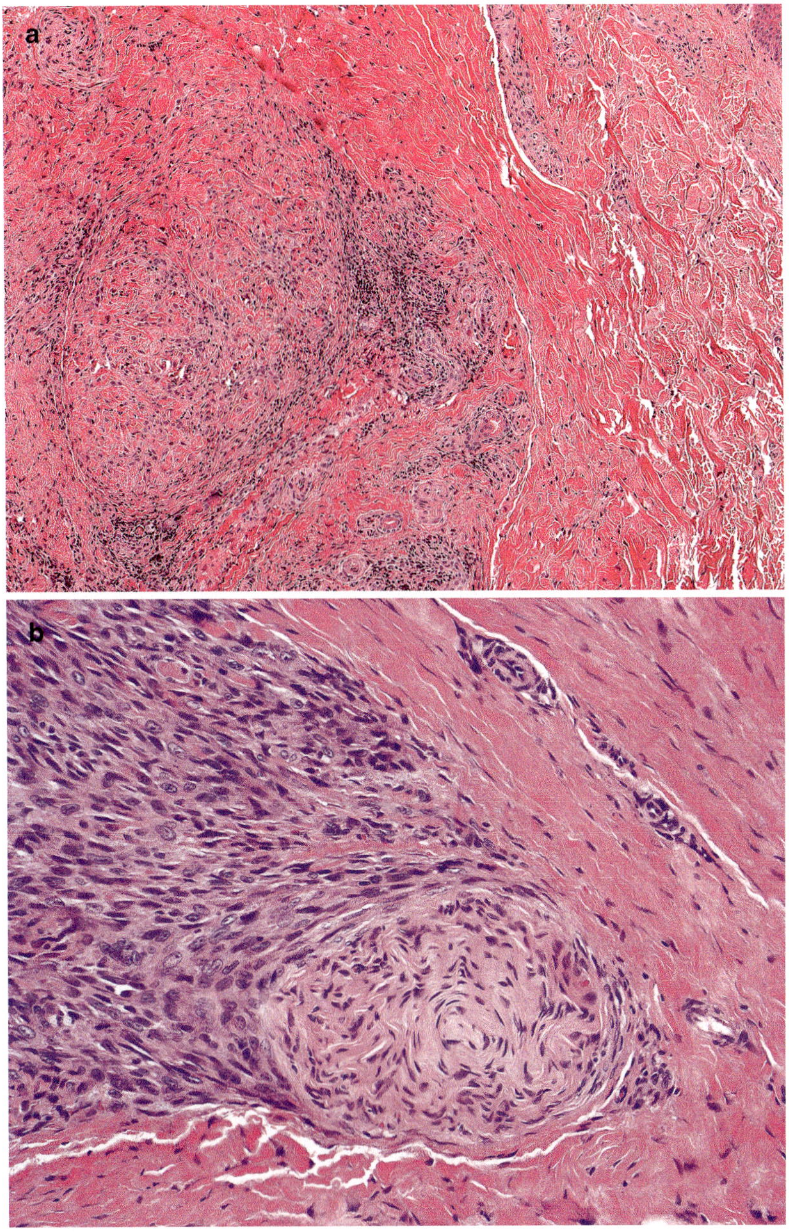

Fig. 12.2 (**a**) A subtle example of distal-type epithelioid sarcoma with minimal cytologic atypia involving the dermis. (**b**) Perineural invasion in epithelioid sarcoma

myoepithelioma). Myoepithelial carcinoma is a more morphologically heterogeneous tumor that typically co-expresses cytokeratins and markers of myoepithelial differentiation such as p63, SMA, GFAP, and/or S100 and is negative for CD34. Approximately 50% of cases show rearrangement of *EWSR1*. A potential pitfall is that myoepithelial carcinoma shows loss of INI1 expression in approximately 50% of cases.

Clear Cell Sarcoma

Clinical Features

Clear cell sarcoma (CCS) is a rare soft tissue sarcoma with bona fide melanocytic differentiation, reflected in its former name "malignant melanoma of soft parts." CCS usually presents in young adults in the second to fourth decades,

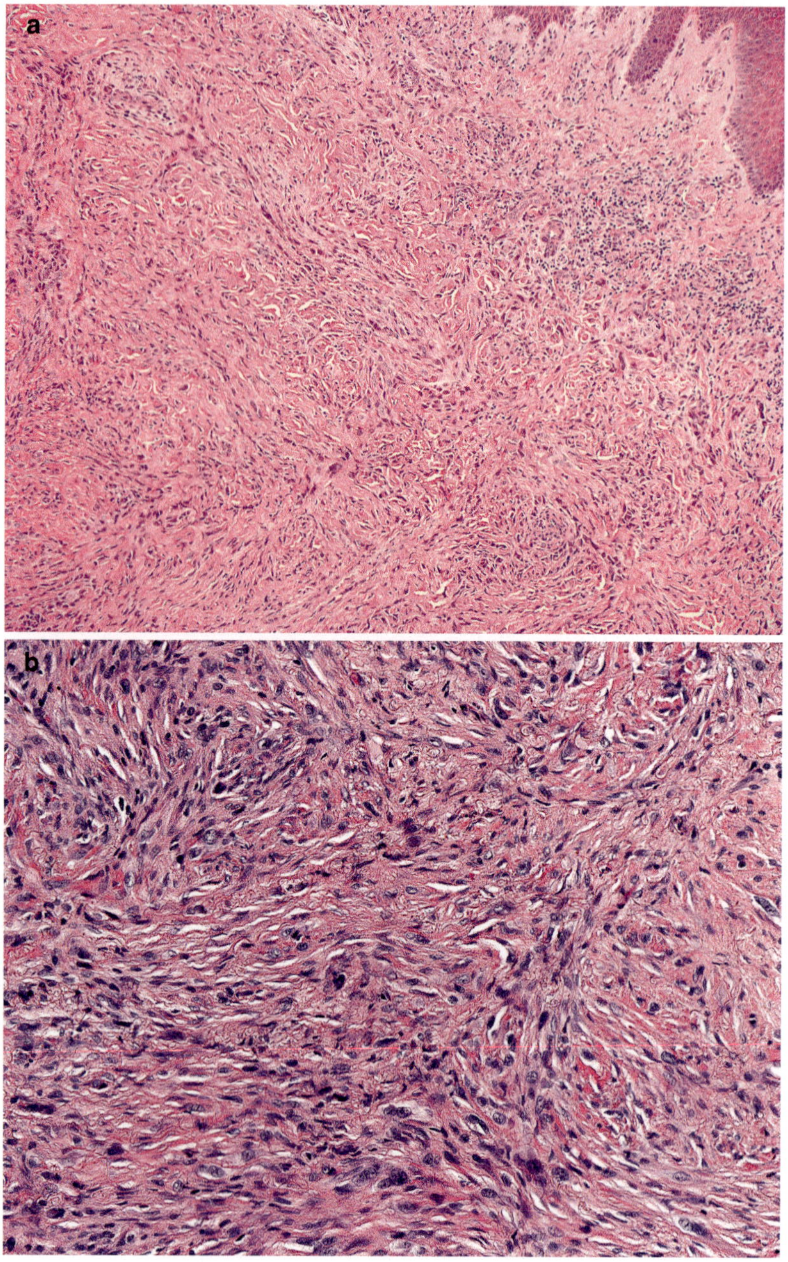

Fig. 12.3 Distal-type epithelioid sarcoma. (**a**) Prominent fibrosis and chronic inflammation that can be misinterpreted as an inflammatory process. (**b**) Spindle cell areas can be mistaken for a fibroblastic or a fibrohistiocytic lesion

although a wide age range may be affected. The tumors show a predilection for the distal limbs, especially the ankle and foot, and present as a slowly growing, deep soft tissue mass with an attachment to tendons, aponeuroses, or fasciae. Occasionally, they may present as a superficial primary cutaneous lesion arising in the dermis (Fig. 12.6). Cutaneous CCS also tends to occur in the distal extremities and less frequently on the trunk, proximal limbs, or head and neck and is usually small, <2 cm in size. CCS has a protracted clinical course but ultimately behaves aggressively, with a propensity for local recurrence in up to 40% of patients and a high rate of lymph

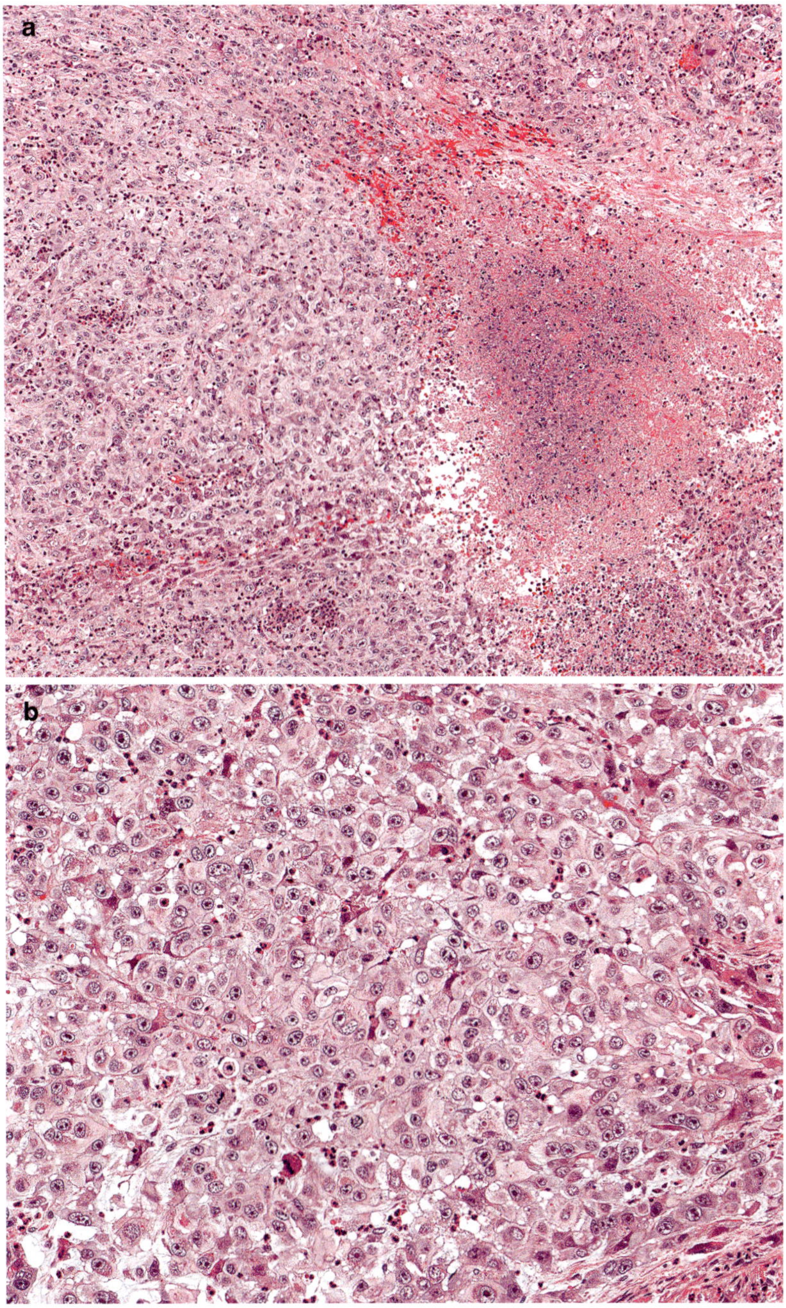

Fig. 12.4 Proximal-type ES. (**a**) Large subcutaneous overtly malignant mass with necrosis. (**b**) Sheets of large epithelioid cells with eccentric nuclei, prominent nucleoli, and abundant eosinophilic cytoplasm. (**c**) Perinuclear hyaline eosinophilic rhabdoid inclusion in proximal-type epithelioid sarcoma (arrow)

Fig. 12.4 (continued)

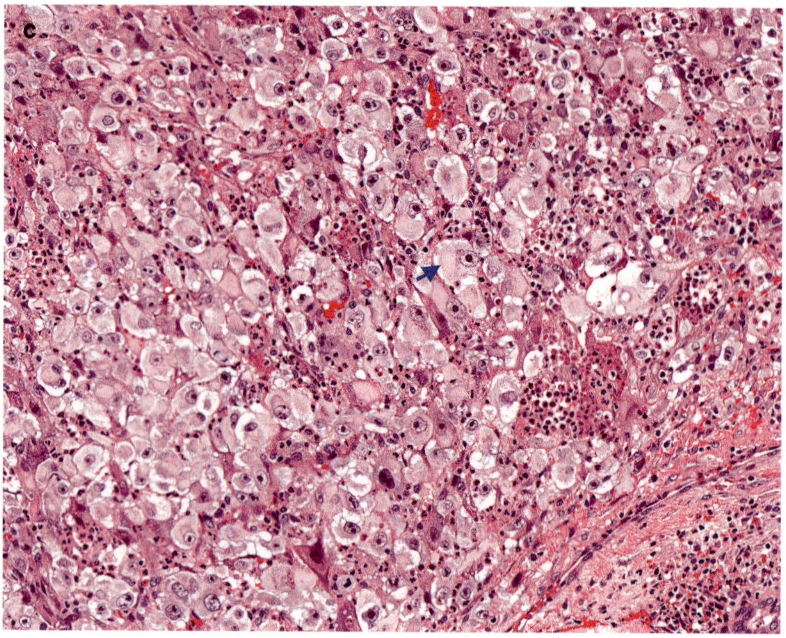

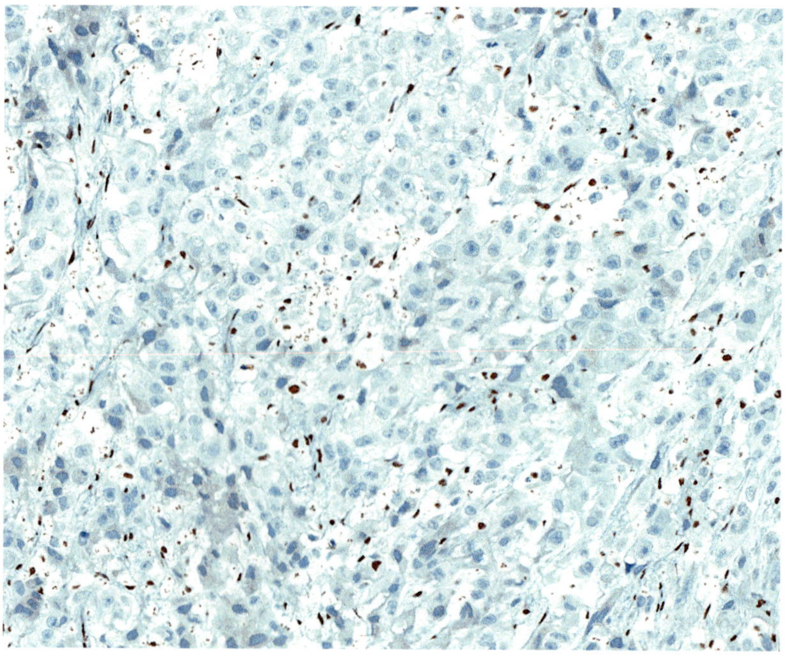

Fig. 12.5 Loss of expression of INI1 in epithelioid sarcoma (background stromal fibroblasts and lymphocytes retain nuclear expression)

node and systemic metastases, most often to the lungs and bones. The 5-year overall survival is 40–60%. Adverse prognostic features include large size, necrosis, local recurrence, and, in some reports, lymph node metastasis. The behavior of cutaneous CCS appears to be similar to its deep-seated counterpart, although the number of reported cases with available follow-up is small.

Table 12.1 Key pathologic features: epithelioid sarcoma

Distal-type ES
- Nodular growth often surrounding a geographic zone of necrosis with peripheral palisading - Uniform epithelioid to spindle cells that can resemble histiocytes - Nuclear atypia can be very mild, especially in cases with predominantly spindle cell morphology; mitotic activity is usually low (<5/10 HPF) - Perineural and vascular invasion are common
Proximal-type ES
- Sheets of large epithelioid cells with round nuclei, prominent nucleoli, and dense eosinophilic cytoplasm - Marked nuclear atypia and mitotic activity, necrosis - Perinuclear hyaline "rhabdoid" inclusions
Both types of ES express cytokeratins, EMA, and CD34 (60%) and demonstrate loss of SMARCB1/INI1 nuclear expression (90%)

Radical excision remains the treatment of choice. There are no uniform guidelines regarding lymph node dissection or sentinel lymph node biopsy in CCS. Conventional chemotherapy is of little benefit, but candidate therapeutic targets have been proposed, including c-Met.

Pathologic Features

CCS is composed of nests and fascicles of uniform spindle to fusiform cells separated by fibrous septa (Fig. 12.7a). The overlying dermis is usually uninvolved, and the epidermis is intact, but in cutaneous CCS, the epidermis may be ulcerated. Most cutaneous CCS are dermal-based tumors. However, nests of tumor cells at the dermal-epidermal junction mimicking the junctional component of a malignant melanoma as well as intraepidermal pagetoid spread may occur (Fig. 12.7b). The cytoplasmic clearing in constituent tumor cells occurs due to the accumulation of glycogen, but truly optically clear cytoplasm is uncommon in CCS; more often, the cytoplasm is palely eosinophilic and finely granular, resembling that of a cellular blue

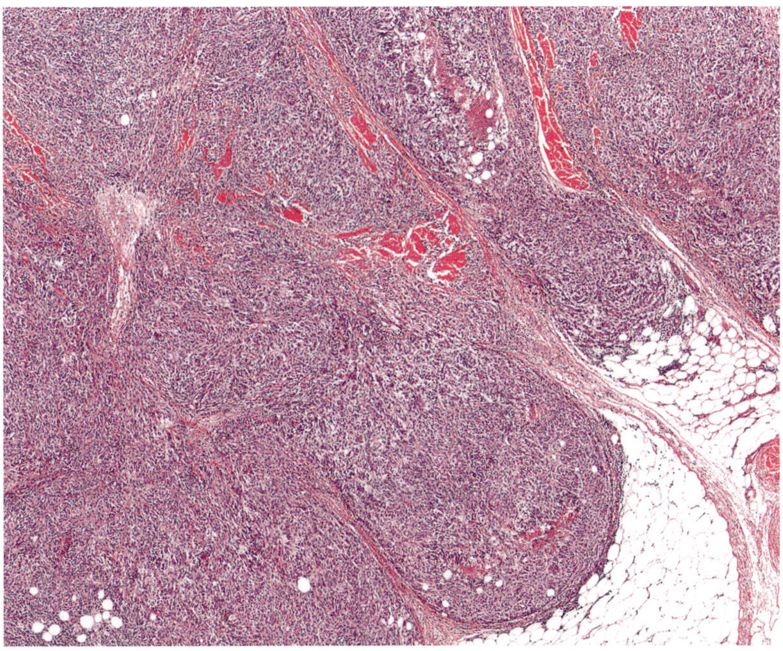

Fig. 12.6 Primary cutaneous clear cell sarcoma involving the dermis and superficial subcutis

nevus or melanoma (Fig. 12.8a). In most cases, the cells are overtly atypical with large vesicular nuclei and prominent nucleoli, but marked nuclear pleomorphism is not a characteristic feature. The mitotic rate is highly variable, and the stroma is usually sclerotic. Multinucleated wreath-like tumor giant cells, when present, are a very helpful diagnostic feature (Fig. 12.8b). Melanin pigment is seen in a minority of cases. Less common morphologic variations include rhabdoid features, bizarre pleomorphic cells, alveolar architecture due to cellular dyshesion, and a seminoma-like pattern. Metastatic CCS may acquire a more epithelioid or pleomorphic appearance reminiscent of conventional malignant melanoma or carcinoma.

Clear cell sarcomas diffusely express S100 protein and, in most cases, co-express the mela-

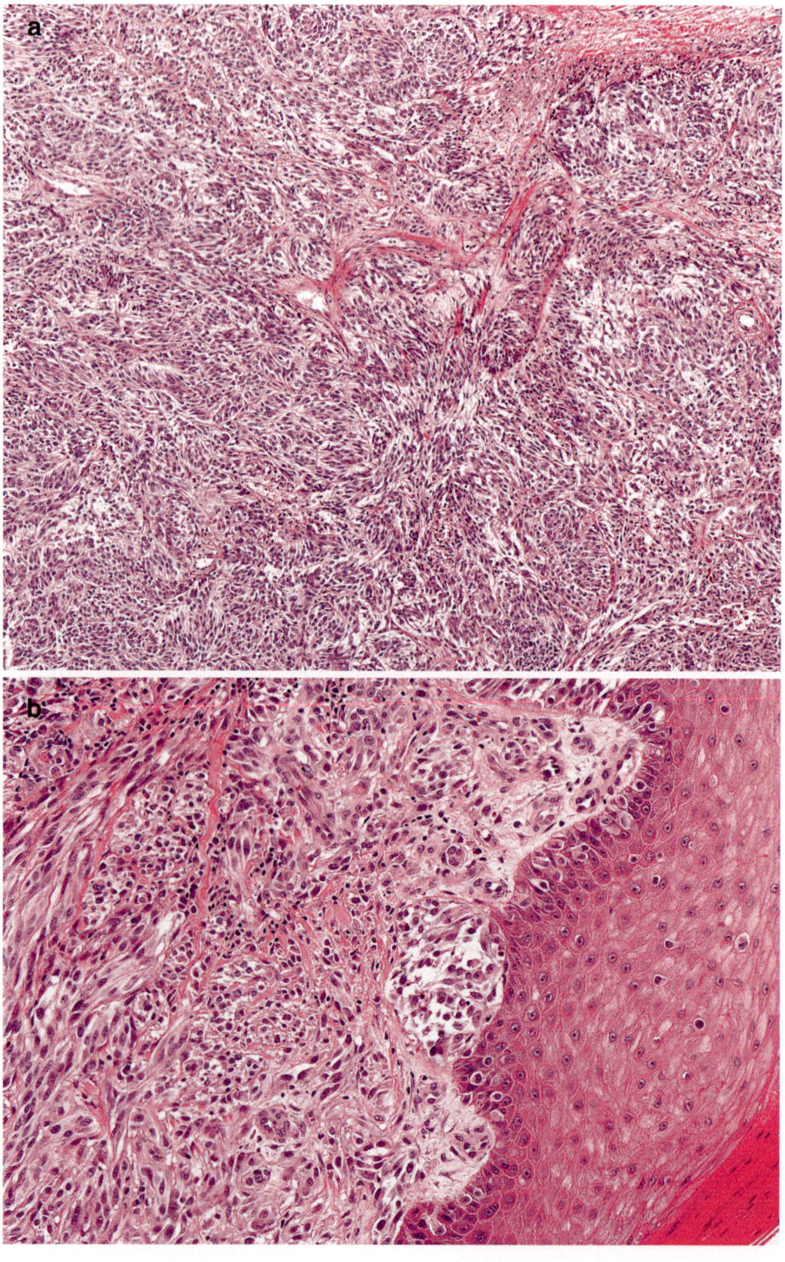

Fig. 12.7 Clear cell sarcoma. (**a**) Nests of spindle to fusiform cells separated by fibrous septa. (**b**) Junctional component and intraepidermal spread mimicking malignant melanoma

nocytic markers Melan-A, HMB45, SOX10, MiTF, and NKI/C3. Synaptophysin, CD57, EMA, CD34, and CD117 (c-KIT) expressions have been observed in a minority of cases. Cytokeratins, desmin, and SMA are usually negative. The hallmark of clear cell sarcoma is a balanced t(12;22) (q13;q12) translocation resulting in fusion of *EWSR1* with the cAMP-regulated transcription factor *ATF1* (27–31). Four types of *EWSR1/ATF1* chimeric transcripts have been identified, without prognostic significance. A less common t(2;22) (q34;q12) rearrangement with *EWSR1/CREB1* fusion, primarily found in gastrointestinal CCS, has also been found in soft tissue and cutaneous examples. The downstream effect of the *EWSR/ATF1* fusion in clear cell sarcoma is constitutive activation of the melanocyte-specific MITF (MITF-M) promoter, resulting in

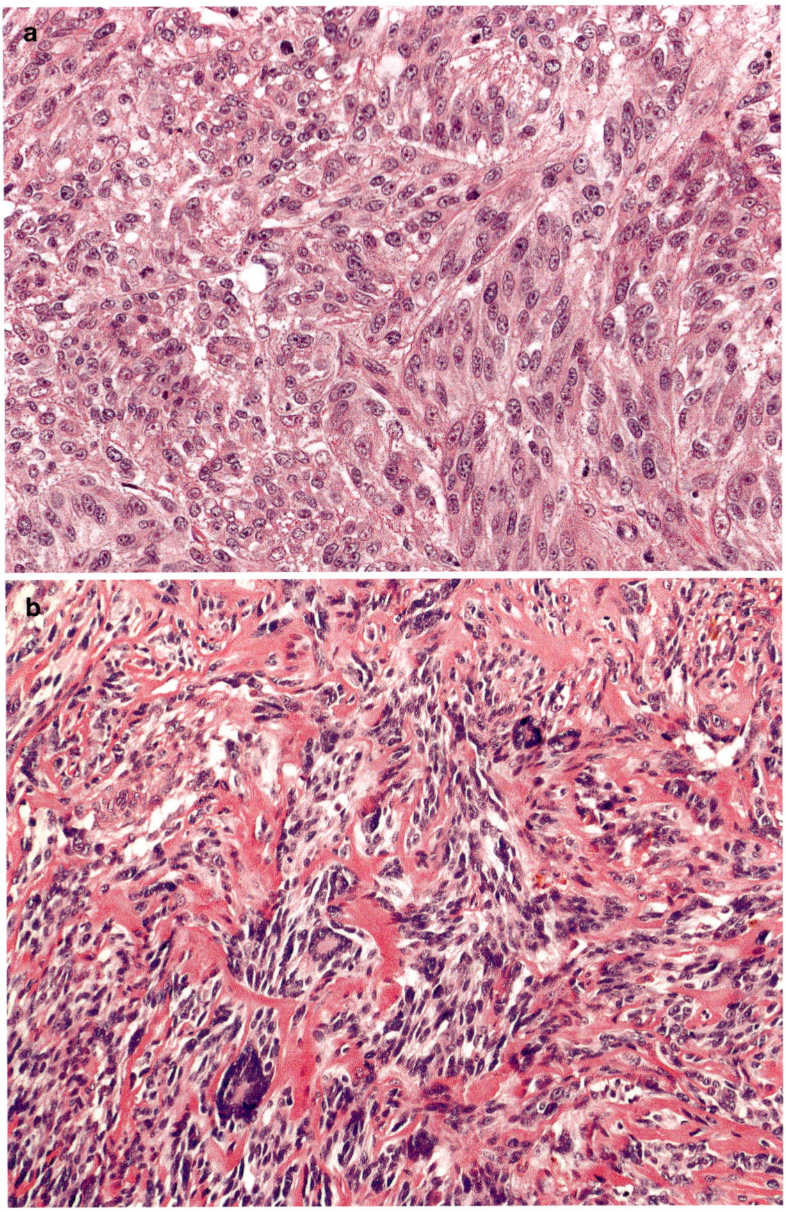

Fig. 12.8 Clear cell sarcoma. (**a**) Atypical spindle cells with eosinophilic granular cytoplasm, vesicular nuclei, and prominent nucleoli. (**b**) Wreath-like multinucleated tumor giant cells are characteristic

aberrant MITF expression that drives the melanocytic phenotype and c-Met oncogenic signaling. RT-PCR for the above fusion transcripts and fluorescence in situ hybridization (FISH) testing for the *EWSR1* gene rearrangement are very helpful ancillary diagnostic tests for CCS (Table 12.2).

Differential Diagnosis

It is essential to distinguish CCS from other neoplasms with melanocytic differentiation. The most problematic tumor in this regard is cutaneous or metastatic spindle cell melanoma, which can be virtually identical in terms of its morphology and immunophenotype. The monotonous appearance of the tumor nests (in contrast to more heterogeneous appearance in spindle cell melanomas) and wreath-like giant cells favor CCS. A junctional or lentiginous component is more typical of melanoma. However, as mentioned, tumor nests at the dermal-epidermal junction, intraepidermal involvement and pagetoid spread have all been observed in primary cutaneous CCS. Melanomas are negative for *EWSR1* gene rearrangements and often harbor *BRAF* mutations, which are very rare in CCS.

Amelanotic cellular blue nevus can resemble clear cell sarcoma because of the increased cellularity, nested arrangement of uniform spindle cells surrounded by fibrous septa, and scattered multinucleated giant cells. Cutaneous examples of CCS that secondarily involve the subcutis can mimic the dumbbell-shaped extension seen in cellular blue nevi. Identification of a second population of slender dendritic melanocytes, like those seen in common blue nevi, helps to distinguish cellular blue nevus from CCS. Most cellular blue nevi also lack the cytologic atypia and mitotic activity of CCS. In addition, blue nevi, including malignant blue nevi, lack *EWSR1* rearrangements.

Table 12.2 Key pathologic features: clear cell sarcoma

Nests of uniform spindle to fusiform cells, separated by fibrous bands
Large vesicular nuclei and prominent nucleoli
Usually lacks involvement of the epidermal/dermal junction or epidermis
Multinucleated wreath-like tumor giant cells are very helpful when present
Positive for all melanocytic markers
EWSR1/ATF1 or *EWSR1/CREB1* rearrangements

Cutaneous CCS with predominantly clear cytoplasm may have to be distinguished from cutaneous PEComa (discussed below). The perivascular growth pattern and the delicate capillary vasculature seen in association with the nests of tumor cells in PEComas are not a characteristic of CSS. Cutaneous PEComas co-express markers of melanocytic and smooth muscle differentiation (SMA, desmin, and caldesmon), the latter of which are consistently negative in CCS and lack *EWSR1* rearrangements.

Cutaneous Perivascular Epithelioid Cell Tumor (PEComa)

Clinical Features

Perivascular epithelioid cell tumors (PEComas) are a diverse family of mesenchymal neoplasms characterized by the presence of epithelioid perivascular tumor cells that co-express smooth muscle and melanocytic markers. PEComas occur at various anatomic sites, including the skin, soft tissues, bone, viscera, and related structures such as pelvic ligaments. The PEComa family also includes distinctive visceral neoplasms such as lymphangioleiomyomatosis, renal angiomyolipoma, and clear cell "sugar" tumor of the lung and an association with tuberous sclerosis complex. Primary cutaneous PEComas account for approximately 8% of all PEComas and appear to be clinically and genetically distinct from their visceral and soft tissue counterparts (discussed below).

Primary cutaneous PEComa typically affects adults in the fourth decade, with a striking female predilection. Cutaneous tumors usually appear on the legs, arms, or trunk as firm, tan, or pink-colored small (<2 cm) cutaneous nodules or plaques and are clinically reminiscent of fibrous histiocytoma. They usually behave in a benign fashion and rarely recur, although examples with histologically malignant features and aggressive behavior may be seen. Large studies detailing the behavior of histologically malignant cutaneous PEComa are currently lacking. Regardless, complete excision is recommended.

Pathologic Features

Cutaneous PEComas are centered in the dermis (Fig. 12.9) and are composed of irregular dermal nests, sheets, or cords of epithelioid to spindle cells with abundant clear or granular eosinophilic cytoplasm surrounding delicate capillary vessels. The cells have round, vesicular nuclei with small but very distinct nucleoli (Fig. 12.10a, b). The cells at the periphery intermingle with dermal collagen in a pattern reminiscent of benign fibrous histiocytoma (Fig. 12.11). The overlying epidermis is usually intact, and the subcutis can be involved with either a pushing or infiltrative margin. A mild degree of cellular pleomorphism and multinucleated wreath-like giant cells with peripherally located nuclei can be seen. The mitotic count is typically very low (<1/10 HPF).

The proposed histologic criteria for malignancy in deep soft tissue PEComas include size >5 cm, an infiltrative growth pattern, high nuclear grade, mitotic activity >1/50 HPF, necrosis, and vascular invasion. PEComas lacking any of these features are classified as benign, those with two or more features as malignant, and those with only nuclear pleomorphism/giant cells (so-called "symplastic PEComas") or size >5 cm as having uncertain malignant potential. It is uncertain if this classification scheme is equally applicable to cutaneous PEComas, which usually behave in a benign fashion, but it should probably be utilized until there is evidence to the contrary.

PEComas demonstrate variable co-expression of melanocytic markers (MITF, NKI/C3, HMB45, Melan-A, and S100) and markers of smooth muscle differentiation (desmin, SMA, caldesmon, and calponin) and express cathepsin K. HMB45 and MITF are the most sensitive melanocytic markers in cutaneous PEComas, whereas focal S100 protein expression is seen in a minority of cases. Of the muscle markers, desmin appears to be the most sensitive, but SMA expression in the absence of desmin can be observed. Cytokeratins and EMA are negative in PEComas (Table 12.3).

Visceral and soft tissue PEComas may be associated with *TSC1/TSC2* mutations and tuberous sclerosis complex with downstream activa-

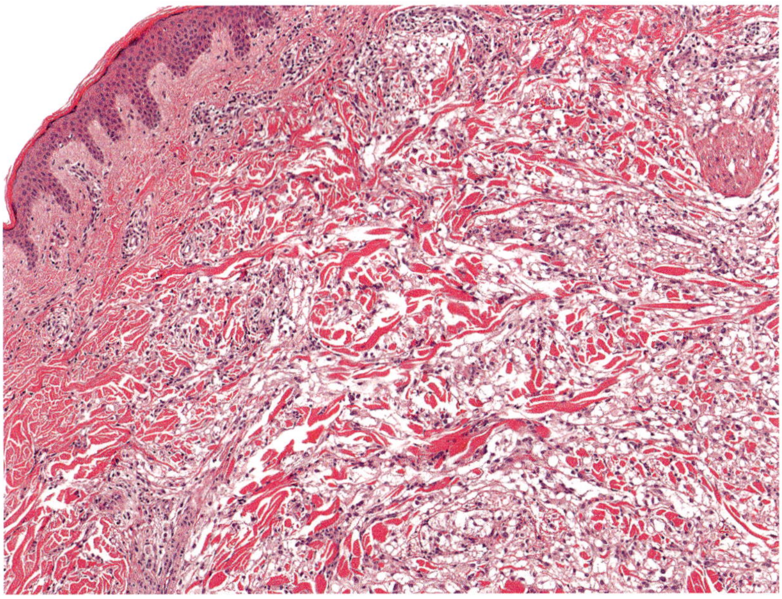

Fig. 12.9 Cutaneous perivascular epithelioid cell tumor (PEComa). The tumor is centered in the dermis with minimal subcutaneous involvement

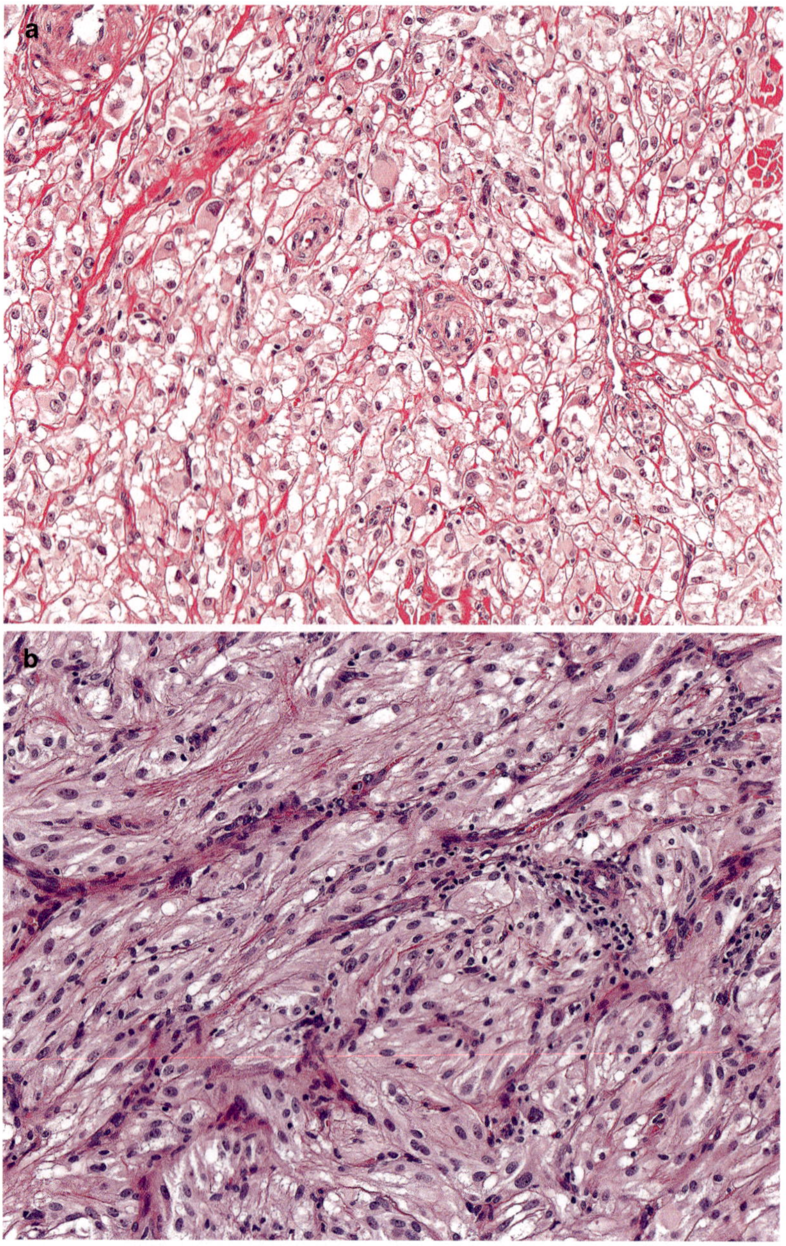

Fig. 12.10 Cutaneous PEComa. (**a**, **b**) Nests of epithelioid or spindle cells with abundant clear or eosinophilic granular cytoplasm and round nuclei with small prominent nucleoli. The nests are seen in association with a delicate capillary vasculature

tion of the mammalian target of rapamycin (mTOR) pathway. A subset of PEComas show transcription factor E3 (*TFE3*) gene rearrangements, which may drive the myomelanocytic phenotype in these tumors. Reported primary cutaneous PEComas do not appear to be associated with either *TSC* mutations or *TFE3* rearrangements. However, expression of 4E-binding protein 1 (4EBP1), a downstream target in the mTOR pathway, has been observed in cutaneous PEComas.

Differential Diagnosis

Cutaneous PEComas need to be distinguished from a variety of cutaneous tumors with clear or granular cytoplasm. Benign fibrous histiocytoma

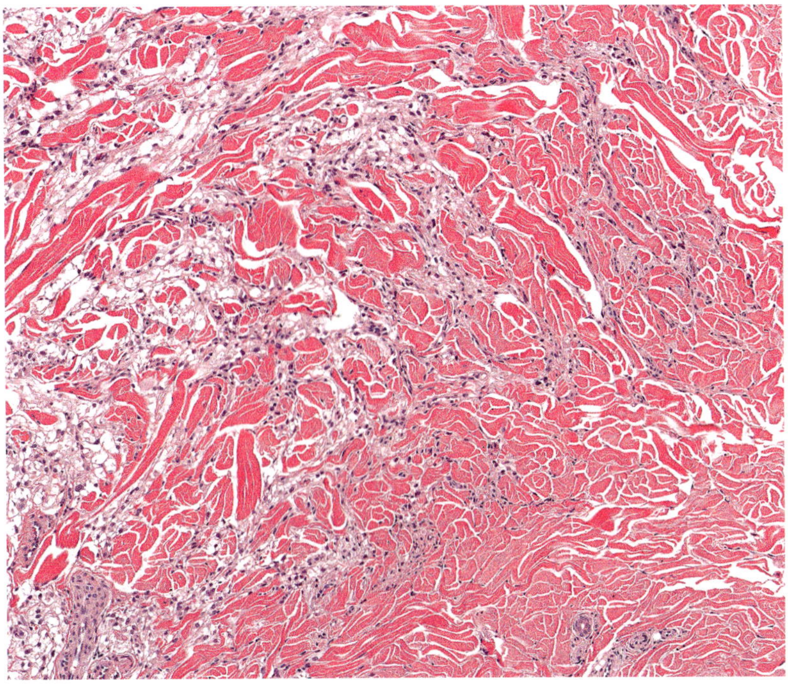

Fig. 12.11 Cutaneous PEComa. Interface with the dermis in cutaneous PEComa is reminiscent of collagen trapping seen in fibrous histiocytomas

Table 12.3 Key pathologic features: cutaneous PEComa

Nests of clear to eosinophilic epithelioid or spindle cells separated by delicate vascular septa, with perivascular condensation
Round, vesicular nuclei with small distinct nucleoli and mild cellular pleomorphism; mitotic count is very low (<1/10HPF)
Multinucleated giant cells with peripherally located nuclei
Co-express melanocytic and smooth muscle markers
Rare histologically malignant examples

(dermatofibroma) with clear cell change, also referred to as clear cell fibrous histiocytoma, can be confused with PEComa. Fibrous histiocytoma differs from PEComa by the presence of overlying epidermal hyperplasia, a conventional "fibrohistiocytic" spindle cell component with irregular bland nuclei, peripheral collagen trapping, the lack of a distinctive well-defined capillary vasculature, and the absence of melanocytic differentiation. Unlike cutaneous PEComa, granular cell tumor demonstrates a more syncytial arrangement of constituent cells, absence of a prominent vasculature, and lack of nucleoli. That being said, an uncommon clear cell variant of granular cell tumor can be more difficult to distinguish from PEComa, because it has very similar cytologic characteristics. However, both conventional and clear cell granular cell tumors are negative for HMB45, Melan-A, desmin, and SMA and are uniformly strongly positive for S100 protein and SOX10. Cutaneous myoepitheliomas with clear cell morphology have somewhat of an overlapping immunophenotype because markers of myoepithelial differentiation S100, SOX10, SMA, and calponin can also be expressed in cutaneous PEComas. However, myoepithelial tumors can be readily distinguished from PEComas by co-expression of cytokeratins and EMA and lack of HMB45 or MiTF immunoreactivity.

Of the malignant tumors with clear cytoplasm, cutaneous metastases and melanoma with balloon cell change are the most important differential diagnostic considerations. Metastatic renal cell and hepatocellular carcinoma can be separated from PEComa based on cytokeratin and EMA immunoreactivity and lack of melanocytic and smooth muscle marker expression. Helpful features to distinguish balloon cell nevi and melanoma from PEComa include the presence of a junctional melanocytic component or intraepidermal pagetoid spread, peripheral inflammatory infiltrates, and lack of a distinctive vasculature. Balloon cell nevi and melanoma diffusely express S100 protein and lack expression of smooth muscle markers. The differential diagnosis with clear cell sarcoma is discussed above.

Ossifying Fibromyxoid Tumor

Clinical Features

Ossifying fibromyxoid tumor (OFMT) occurs in middle-aged adults without a gender predilection. Most are solitary, well-circumscribed painless masses involving the superficial tissues of the lower limbs, but OFMTs may present anywhere including the upper limbs, trunk, head, and neck and in unusual locations like the skeletal muscle, mediastinum, retroperitoneum, thyroid gland, and breast. The average size is 3–4 cm.

Most OFMTs behave in a benign fashion with a small but definite risk of local recurrence (~20%) and low risk of systemic metastasis (<5%). However, a small proportion of cases, particularly those with atypical histologic features, have higher rates of local recurrence and potential for metastasis (up to 60%). The risk for metastasis can be assessed using the three-tier system developed by Folpe and Weiss (described below) and validated in several other retrospective series. Reported metastatic sites include the lungs, adrenal glands, and soft tissue. The treatment of choice for OFMTs is complete surgical excision.

Pathologic Features

OFMT is circumscribed and possesses a fibrous pseudocapsule. The mass typically involves the subcutis, with only rare dermal involvement. Focal infiltrative growth and microscopic satellite nodules may be seen. The classic histologic feature of OFMT is a peripheral shell of mature lamellar bone (Fig. 12.12a); however, this feature is variably present (40–85% of cases). The remaining examples represent the so-called non-ossifying variant of OFMT (Fig. 12.12b). Both variants are variably cellular and are composed of epithelioid or spindle cells arranged in corded, nested, trabecular, or sheet-like patterns; the stroma shows variable proportions of myxoid, fibrous, densely hyalinized, and chondroid zones (Figs. 12.13, 12.14 and 12.15) and may show deposits of woven bone. Many cases show prominent arcuate vessels. Microcystic changes, spindle cell areas with or without fascicle formation, and rhabdoid-like morphology may also occur. This morphologic diversity may occasionally be present within a single case. Irrespective of the growth pattern, all OFMTs show strikingly similar, uniform oval nuclei with fine chromatin and delicate pinpoint nucleoli (Fig. 12.16). These nuclear features are one of the most helpful clues for identifying OFMT. In most cases, the nuclei are banal, and there is virtually no mitotic activity.

More worrisome histologic features including nuclear atypia, high cellularity, necrosis, or increased mitotic activity can be associated with aggressive behavior. Folpe and Weiss proposed an outcome-based risk stratification system dividing OFMTs into typical, atypical, and malignant forms. Malignant OFMT is defined as having high nuclear grade (Fig. 12.17a) or a combination of high cellularity and a mitotic count of >2/50 HPF (Fig. 12.17b). Cases having at least one atypical feature such as mitotic count >2/50 HPF alone or high cellularity or moderate nuclear atypia with a mitotic count ≤2/50 HPF are considered atypical OFMTs. Although some malignant OFMTs arise de novo, areas suggestive of benign OFMT are usually focally present in most malignant OFMTs.

OFMTs express S100 protein in approximately 70–90% of cases, but expression can be focal. Desmin is expressed in 10–40% of cases. OFMTs show inconsistent immunoreactivity for SMA, p63, GFAP, and CD10. EMA and cytokeratins may show focal expression, although

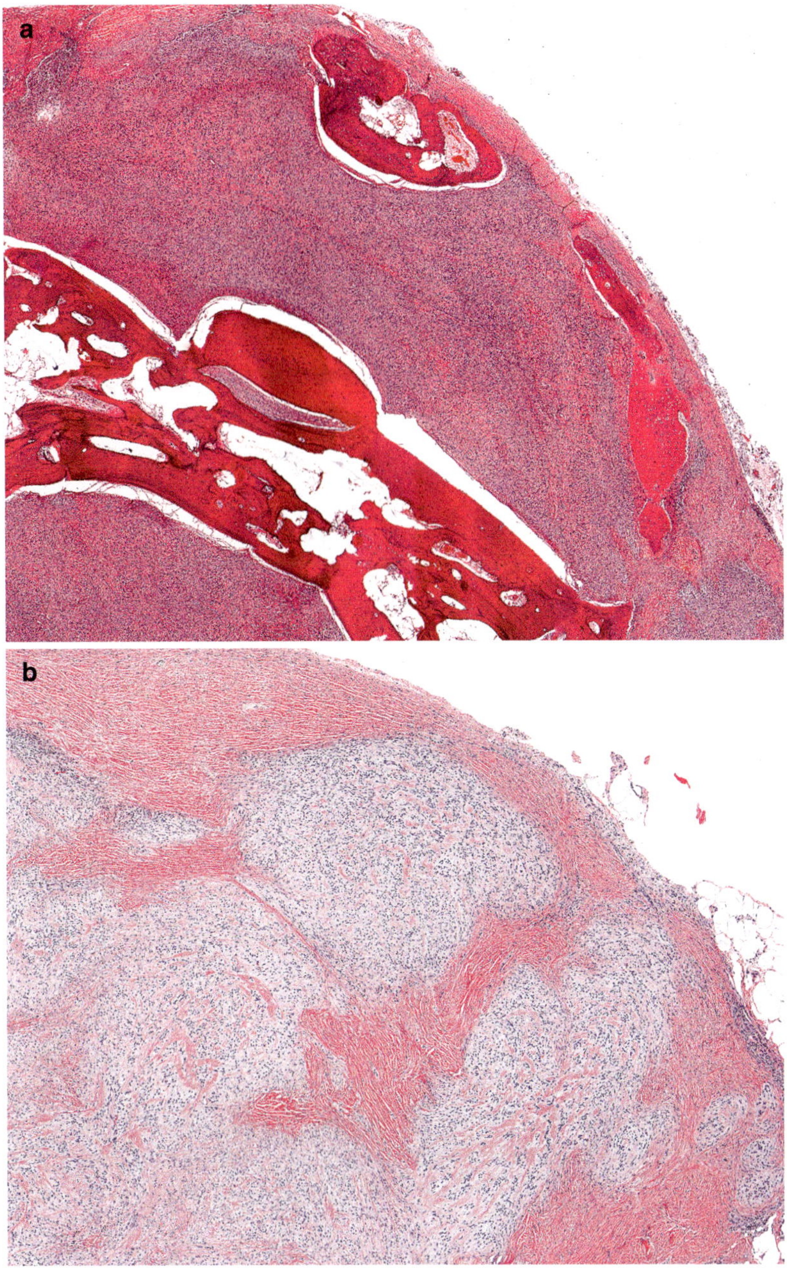

Fig. 12.12 Ossifying fibromyxoid tumor. (**a**) A well-circumscribed ovoid cellular mass with a shell of lamellar bone at the periphery. (**b**) Many tumors lack ossification and are surrounded by a dense fibrous pseudocapsule

only in a minority of cases and more often in malignant OFMT. OFMTs are negative for melanocytic markers, CD34 and CD31. Approximately a quarter of cases express MUC4.

More than 80% of OFMTs (including typical, atypical, and malignant cases) have recurrent gene rearrangements, most commonly involving *PHF1* on 6p21 with fusion partners including *EP400*, *MEAF6*, and *EPC1*. Novel variant fusions that may be seen include *ZC3H7B-BCOR*, *CREBBP-BCOR1*, and *KDMA2-WWTR1*. Most of the above genes participate in epigenetic regulation and histone modification, but no association with the clinical behavior has been found. FISH to detect

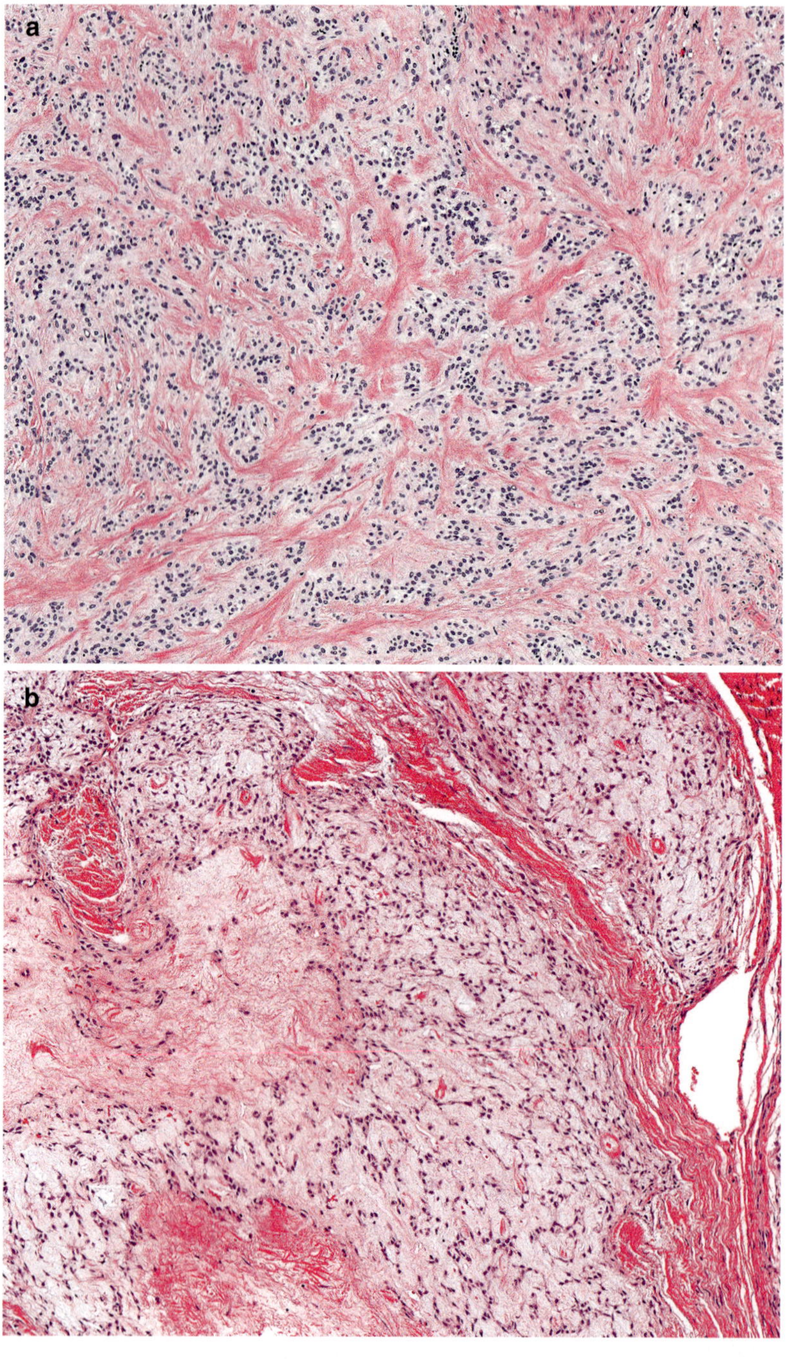

Fig. 12.13 Growth patterns in ossifying fibromyxoid tumor: (**a**) Nested pattern in a collagenous stroma and (**b**) reticular pattern in a myxoid background

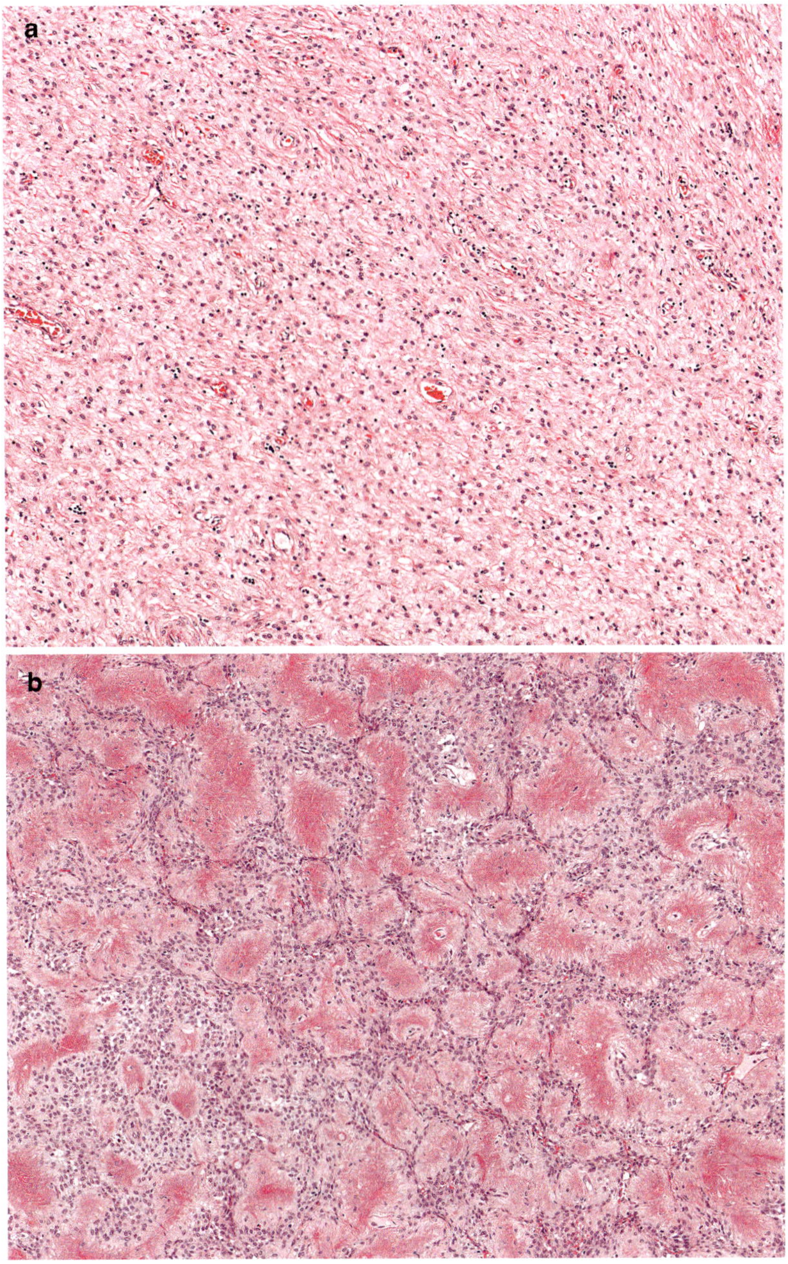

Fig. 12.14 Growth patterns in ossifying fibromyxoid tumor: (**a**) Lace-like pattern and (**b**) sheet-like pattern in a heavily collagenized background

PHF1 rearrangements is a useful ancillary diagnostic technique in difficult cases (Table 12.4).

Differential Diagnosis

Given the variety of growth patterns and the lack of a peripheral shell of bone in many cases, it is not surprising that OFMTs often are mistaken for other cutaneous mesenchymal neoplasms. The most difficult differential diagnosis in our opinion is with cutaneous myoepithelioma and myoepithelial carcinoma. Like OFMT, cutaneous myoepithelioma consists of epithelioid or spindle cells arranged in various combinations of reticular, trabecular, and nested patterns, within a fibro-

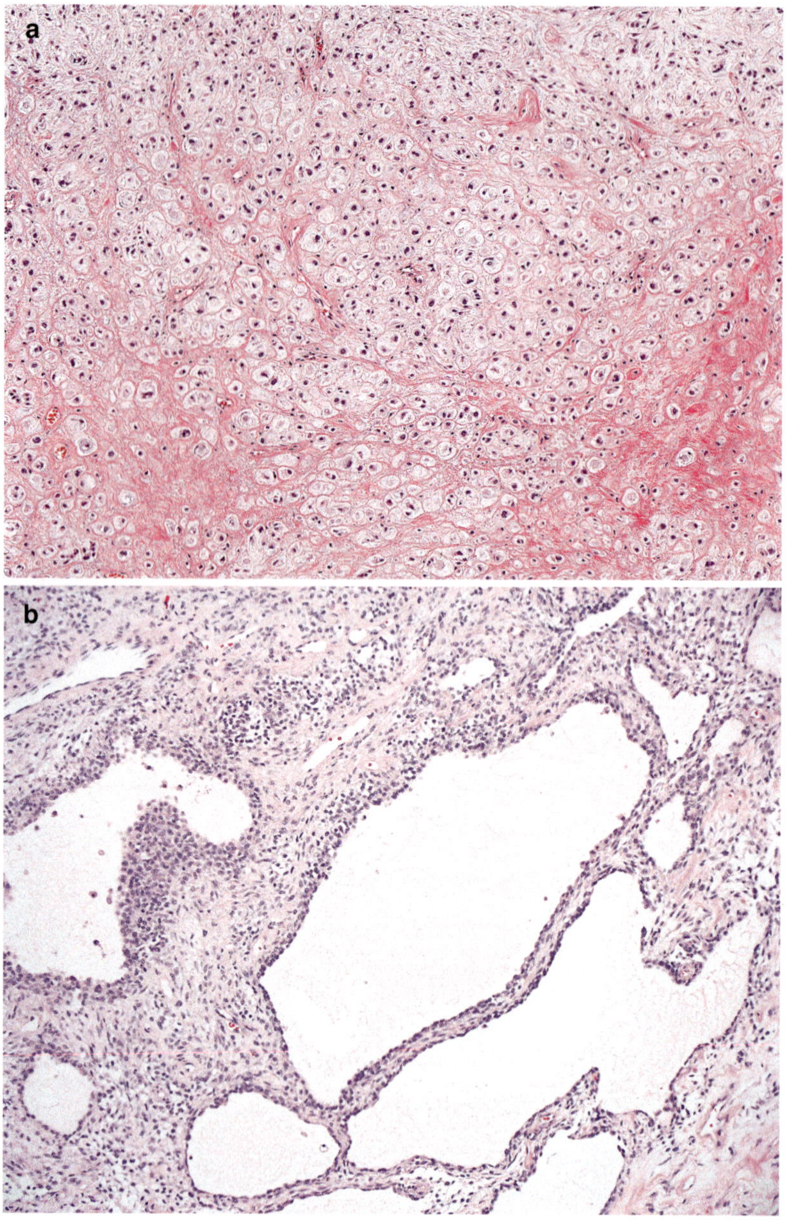

Fig. 12.15 Growth patterns in ossifying fibromyxoid tumor: (**a**) Chondroid pattern and (**b**) microcystic change

myxoid stroma. Cartilaginous and osseous differentiation may occur in myoepithelial tumors, although it rarely takes the form of a peripheral rim of mature lamellar bone as seen in OFMT. Markers of myoepithelial differentiation such as p63, SMA, and particularly S100 protein are of limited value, because they are also expressed in OFMT. However, strong diffuse expression of keratins and EMA would favor a myoepithelial tumor since these markers are expressed in only a small percentage of OFMT and usually only focally. *PHF1* gene rearrangement has not been observed in myoepithelial tumors, which, in contrast, may demonstrate rearrangements of either *EWSR1* (~50% of cases) or *PLAG1*.

Epithelioid schwannomas resemble OFMT, because they are also composed of epithelioid

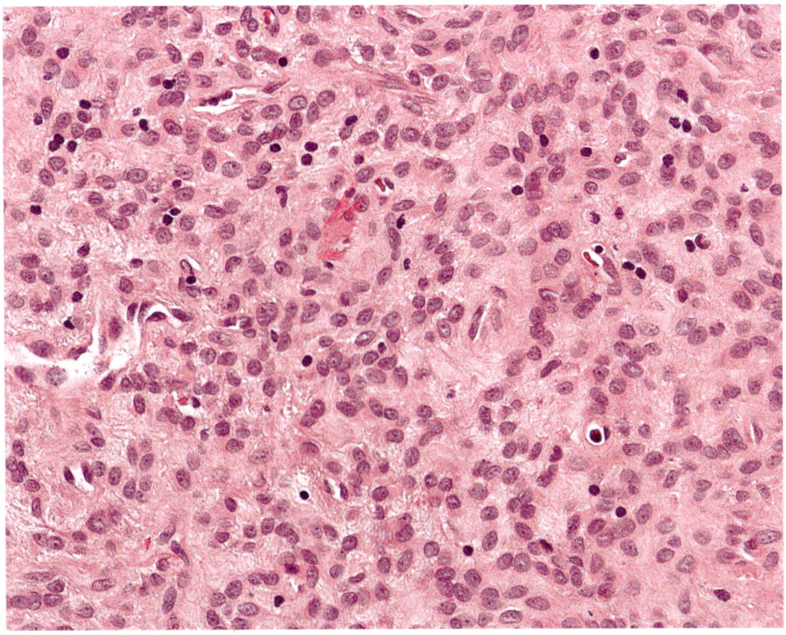

Fig. 12.16 Very uniform oval low-grade nuclei with delicate pinpoint nucleoli present in all typical OFMTs irrespective of the growth pattern

cells arranged in a nested or trabecular pattern, have hyalinized or myxoid stroma and often lack Antoni A areas. The nuclei in epithelioid schwannomas are more irregular and reniform in appearance. The presence of a conventional schwannoma component, a true capsule with EMA or GLUT1-positive perineurial cells and very strong, diffuse immunoreactivity for SOX10 favor epithelioid schwannoma. Malignant OFMT may be confused with epithelioid MPNST. Although separating these two entities might be virtually impossible in some cases without ancillary testing, epithelioid MPNSTs are typically deep-seated soft tissue tumors, lack desmin immunoreactivity, and show strong and diffuse S100 expression. SMARCB1/INI loss is a characteristic of epithelioid MPNSTs, while INI1 is usually retained or only focally lost in a mosaic pattern in OFMT.

OFMTs with a prominent spindle cell component may resemble low-grade fibromyxoid sarcoma (LGFMS). A prominent whorled/storiform arrangement of constitutive tumor cells and characteristic arcades of vessels in myxoid zones favor a diagnosis of LGFMS. OFMTs with particularly densely hyalinized stroma and cord-like arrangement of lesional cells can be confused with sclerosing epithelioid fibrosarcoma (SEF). By immunohistochemistry, both LGFMS and SEF are more often positive for EMA and negative for S100. MUC4, a sensitive and specific marker of both LGFMS and SEF, can be positive in 20–30% of OFMT, although the staining is usually focal. Diagnostically challenging cases can be resolved by application of FISH testing for *FUS* and *EWSR1* (rearranged in both LGFMS and SEF) and/or *PFH1* rearrangements. See Chap. 6 for a detailed discussion of low-grade fibromyxoid sarcoma.

Although the hallmark feature of OFMT is a well-formed shell of lamellar bone at the tumor periphery, some cases show a more diffuse, lace-like, or random pattern of woven bone deposition. If coupled with atypical or malignant cytology, such cases may be mistaken for extraskeletal osteosarcoma. Marked atypia and nuclear pleomorphism would favor osteosarcoma as these features are not typical of OFMT, even in malignant cases. Clinical history is also very helpful as almost all cutaneous/subcutaneous osteosarcomas occur in the setting of metastatic disease.

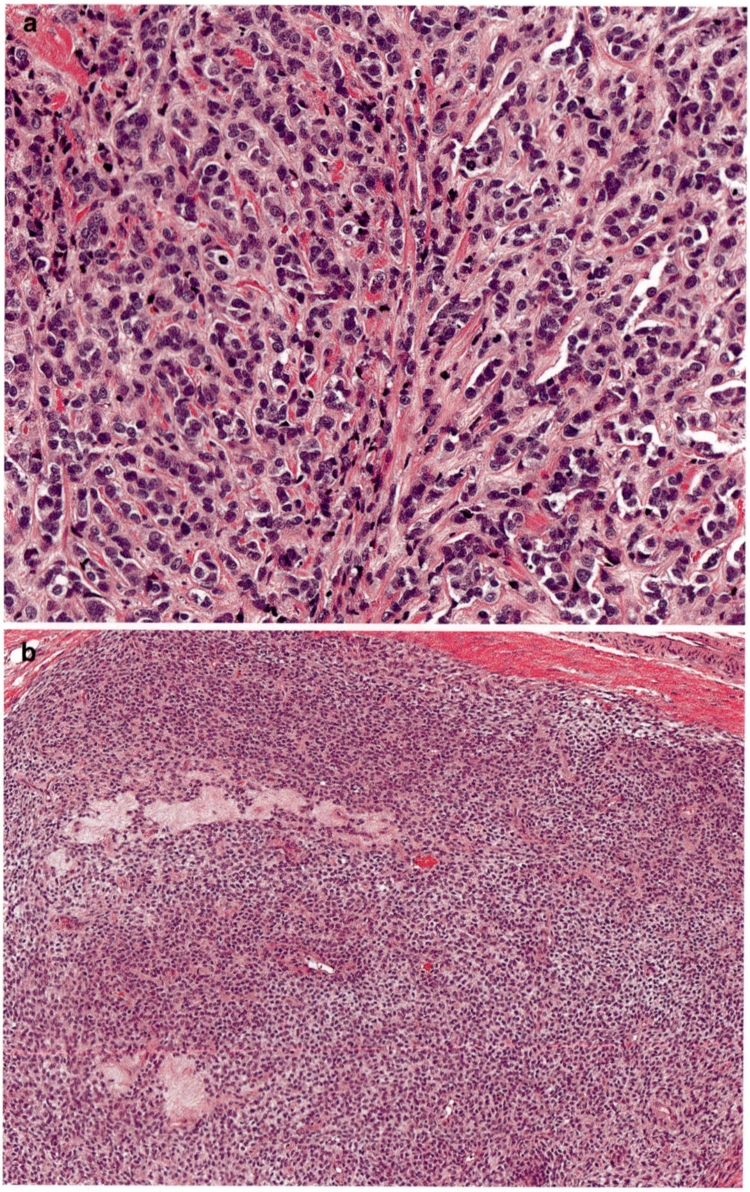

Fig. 12.17 Malignant ossifying fibromyxoid tumor. (**a**) High-grade nuclear atypia and mitotic activity and (**b**) increased cellularity and mitotic activity >2/50 high-power fields

Table 12.4 Key pathologic features: ossifying fibromyxoid tumor

Well-circumscribed subcutaneous lesion with fibrous pseudocapsule and occasional satellite nodules
A rim of mature lamellar bone is characteristic, but present in only 40–85% of cases
Many architectural patterns, but all have uniform, oval nuclei with fine chromatin, and pinpoint nucleoli; exceptions are atypical and malignant cases, which may be classified by the system developed by Folpe and Weiss
Rearrangements involving *PHF1*

Pleomorphic Hyalinizing Angiectatic Tumor and Hemosiderotic Fibrolipomatous Tumor

Clinical Features

Pleomorphic hyalinizing angiectatic tumor (PHAT) and hemosiderotic fibrolipomatous tumor (HFLT) are distinctive subcutaneous neoplasms of adults with potential for local recurrence and, in rare cases, progression to a higher-grade sarcoma. Although morphologically these tumors may be distinct, cases with combined features of both have been described, and the tumors are therefore discussed together.

PHAT is a low-grade, slow-growing subcutaneous neoplasm of middle-aged adults, which has a predilection for the lower extremities but can also occur at other sites such as the arm, thigh, buttocks, or trunk. The median size of a typical lesion is approximately 6 cm. Because ectatic, hyalinized vessels are a prominent feature, PHAT may be clinically mistaken for a hematoma, vascular neoplasm, or schwannoma. HFLT was initially thought to represent a reactive process possibly related to trauma but was subsequently recognized as a true neoplasm. HFLT manifests as a slowly growing subcutaneous mass or plaque, with a female predilection and a tendency to affect the dorsal surface of the ankle, foot, or hand, although other sites may be involved. Because of their infiltrative nature, both PHAT and HFLT are associated with a significant (30–50%) risk of local recurrence and therefore are considered to represent tumors of intermediate malignant potential. Limited studies indicate that HFLT and PHAT may undergo transformation to a higher-grade sarcoma and acquire metastatic potential. The optimal treatment option for both lesions is a complete surgical excision with tumor-free margins.

Pathologic Features

PHAT is a vaguely circumscribed mass composed of spindle or pleomorphic cells surrounding clusters of thin-walled, hyalinized, ectatic vessels with subendothelial and intraluminal

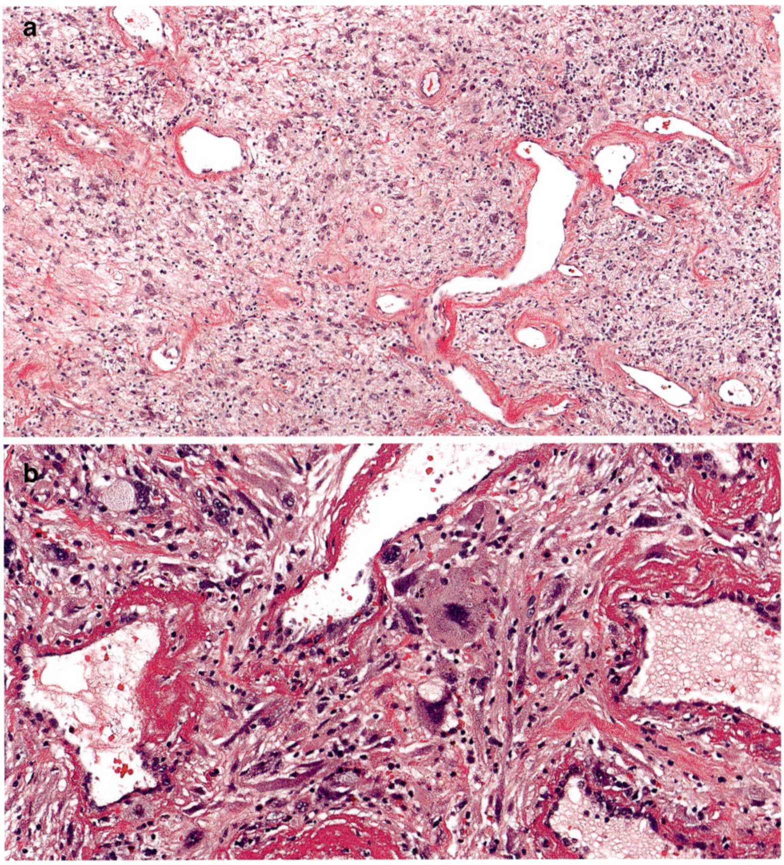

Fig. 12.18 Pleomorphic hyalinizing angiectatic tumor. (**a** and **b**) Pleomorphic tumor cells with clusters of hyalinized ectatic vessels with subendothelial and intraluminal fibrin deposits

fibrin deposits (Fig. 12.18a, b). Although PHAT may seem circumscribed at low power, the margin is usually infiltrative. Constituent tumor cells range from hyperchromatic and spindle to strikingly pleomorphic and may show frequent intranuclear inclusions (Fig. 12.19a). Mitotic activity in PHAT is low (<1/50 HPF). Hemosiderin deposits can be seen in macrophages or in the cytoplasm of the lesional cells (Fig. 12.19b). Scattered inflammatory cells are usually present.

HFLTs are ill-defined fascicular proliferations of bland fibroblastic cells that percolate through adipose tissue in a streaming, whirling, nodular, or more diffuse, honeycomb-like pattern reminiscent of dermatofibrosarcoma protuberans (Fig. 12.20a, b). A prominent feature of

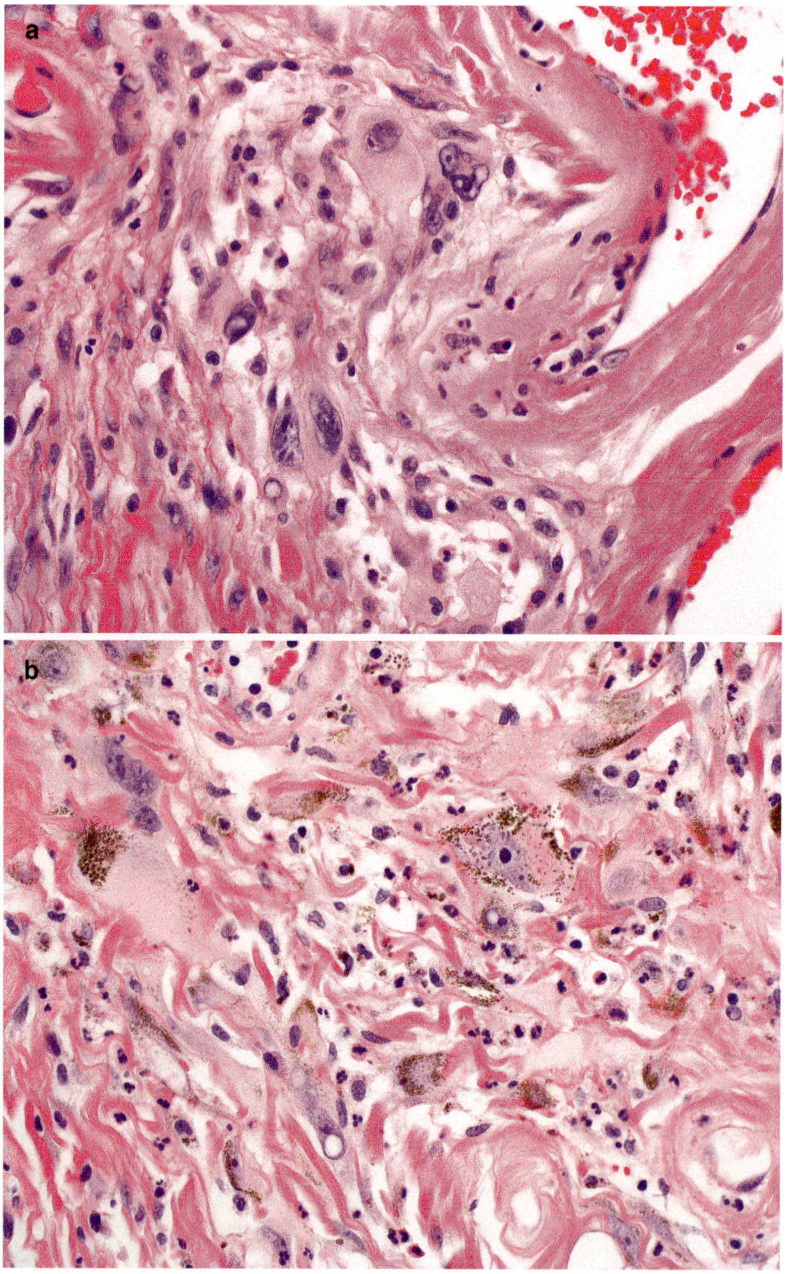

Fig. 12.19 Pleomorphic hyalinizing angiectatic tumor. (**a**) The lesional cells are hyperchromatic and spindle to markedly pleomorphic with frequent intranuclear inclusions. Mitotic figures are not seen. (**b**) Hemosiderin deposits can be found in the stroma and in the cytoplasm of constituent cells

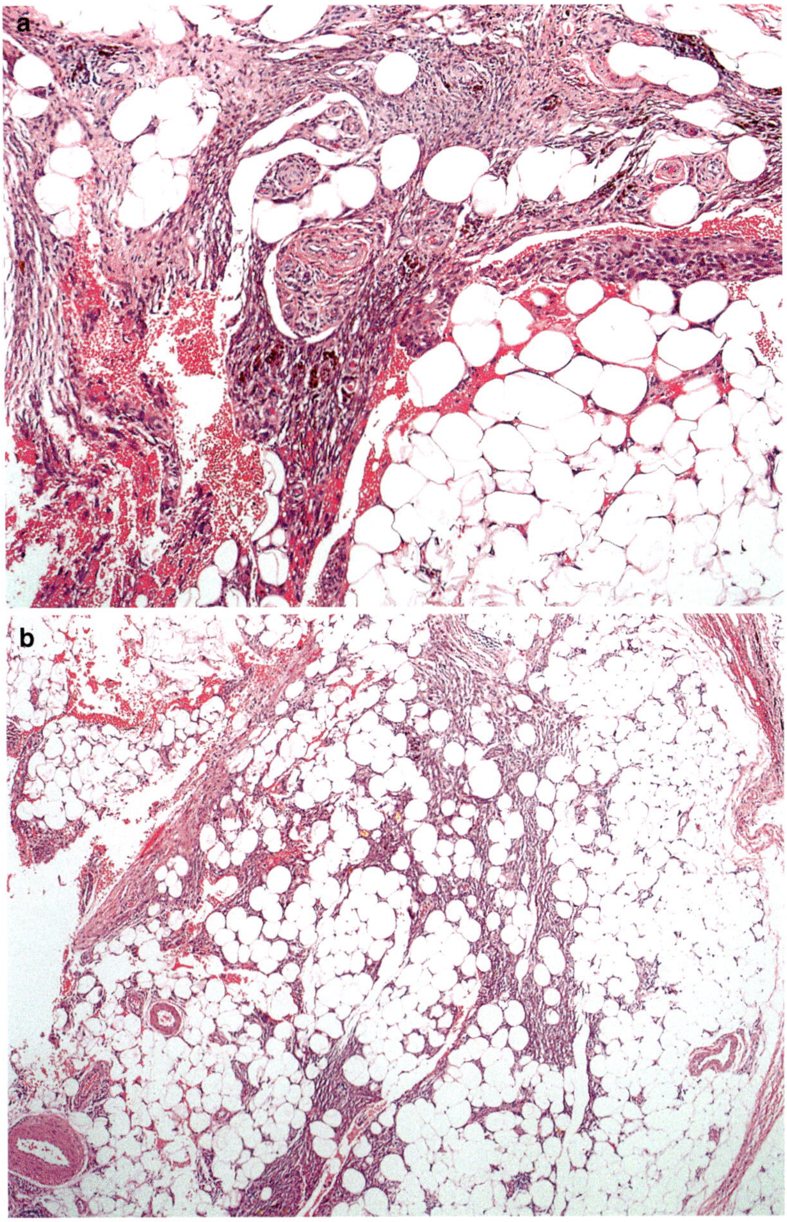

Fig. 12.20 Hemosiderotic fibrolipomatous tumor. Fascicles of spindle cells infiltrating adipose tissue in a streaming, nodular (**a**), or diffuse (**b**) pattern reminiscent of dermatofibrosarcoma protuberans (Photomicrographs courtesy of Dr. Karen Fritchie, Mayo Clinic)

HFLT is hemosiderin that can be found in the stroma, in macrophages and in the cytoplasm of the spindle cells. Myxoid stroma is focally present, and usually there is a prominent inflammatory component. Cytologically, HFLT is composed of bland fibroblastic cells without significant mitotic activity (Fig. 12.21a, b). Small ectatic vessels with mural hyalinization or fibrinous thrombi and scattered osteoclast-type giant cells may be present. HFLT-like areas can be found at the periphery or admixed with otherwise typical examples of PHAT. This observation led to a hypothesis that HFLT might be a precursor lesion of PHAT.

Rarely, PHAT and HFLT may progress to a sarcoma of higher histologic grade, especially in the setting of local recurrence. The sarcomatous components associated with PHAT and HFLT often have myxoid stroma and a prominent inflammatory infiltrate and can show a striking

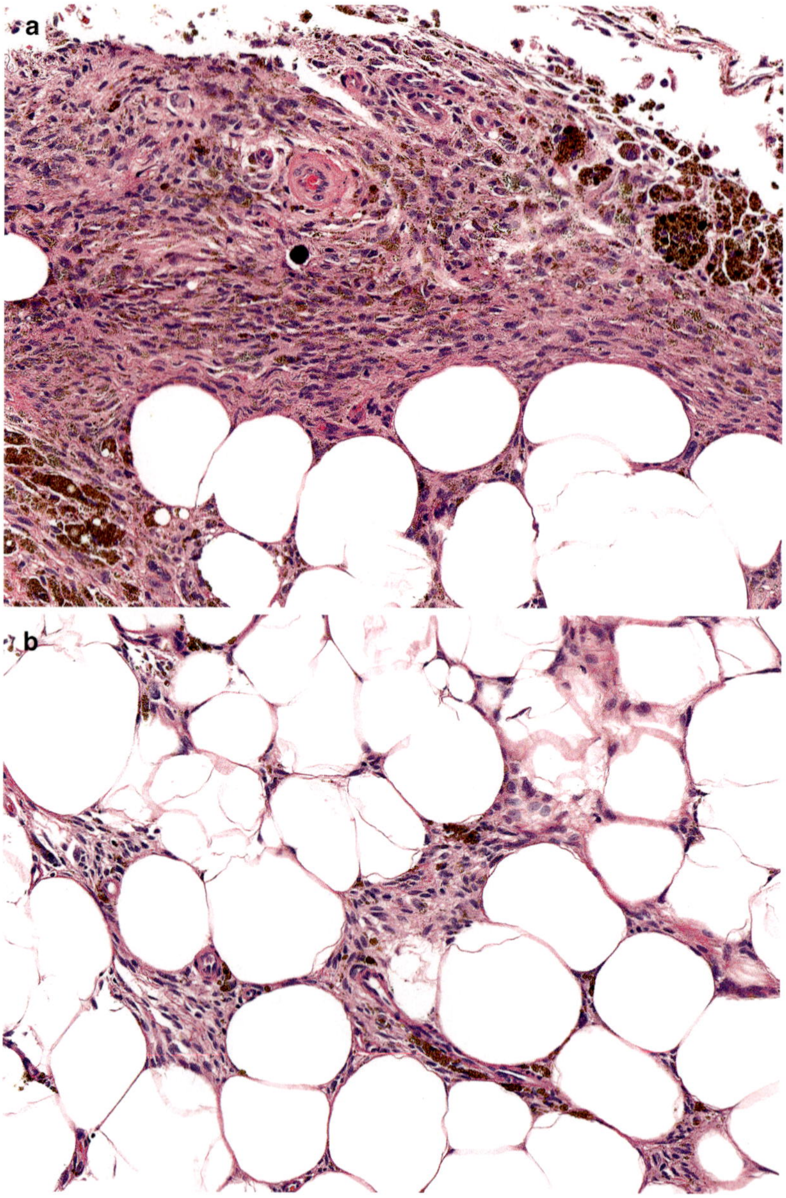

Fig. 12.21 Hemosiderotic fibrolipomatous tumor. (**a**) Cytologically bland fibroblastic cells without mitotic activity. Stromal and intracytoplasmic hemosiderin deposits are characteristic. (**b**) Diffusely infiltrative pattern can mimic dermatofibrosarcoma protuberans or lipofibromatosis

resemblance to myxoinflammatory fibroblastic sarcoma (MIFS). Solid, undifferentiated spindle cell sarcoma-like morphology can also occur (Fig. 12.22a, b).

Most PHATs and HFLTs are positive for CD34 and negative for S100 protein, SMA, and desmin. HFLT harbors a recurrent t(1;10)(p22;q24) rearrangement involving the *TGFBR3* and *MGEA5* genes. *TGFBR3* and *MGEA5* gene rearrangements have also been found in tumors showing mixed features of HFLT and PHAT and, less consistently, in classic PHAT, findings that further support the view that PHAT and HFLT may be related. FISH for *TGFBR3* and *MGEA5* rearrangements can be used in diagnostically challenging cases (Table 12.5).

More controversial is the relationship of HFLT and PHAT to myxoinflammatory fibroblastic sarcoma (MIFS), a distinctive low-grade sarcoma that affects distal extremities of middle-aged adults and morphologically resembles myxoid sarcomas evolving from HFLT and PHAT.

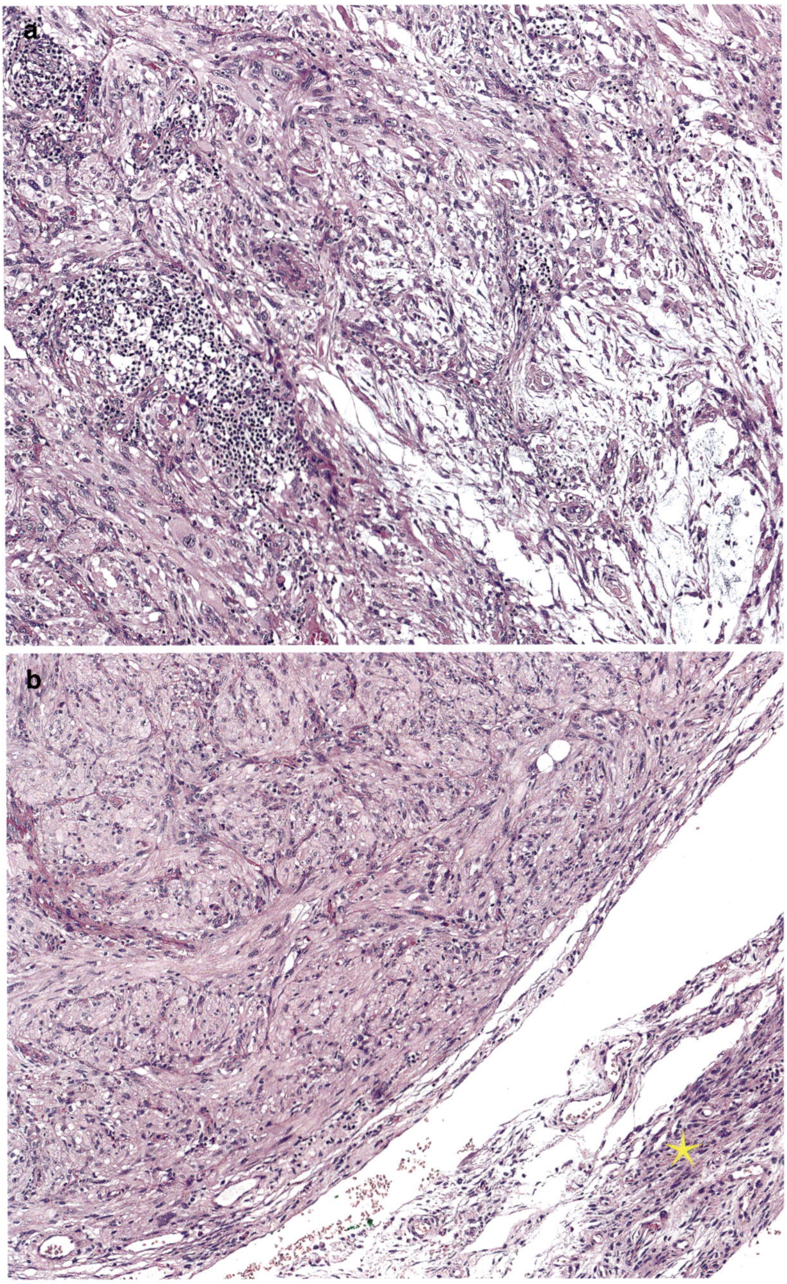

Fig. 12.22 Malignancy in hemosiderotic fibrolipomatous tumor. (**a**) HFLT with progression to a more cellular spindle cell neoplasm with myxoid stroma and a prominent inflammatory component reminiscent of myxoinflammatory fibroblastic sarcoma. (**b**) Solid, undifferentiated spindle cell sarcoma-like morphology adjacent to an area of HFLT (asterisk)

Although earlier genetic and molecular studies showed that some MIFS also harbor *TGFBR3* and *MGEA5* rearrangements suggesting that HFLT, PHAT, and MIFS may represent a morphologic spectrum of related lesions, most recent evidence argues against this. It has been shown that *TGFBR3* and *MGEA5* rearrangements are common only to so-called "hybrid" HFLT/MIFS tumors (tumors with features of both entities) but are quite unusual in pure MIFS that morphologically lack a HFLT component. Also, some of the myxoid sarcomas associated with HFLT are histologically high-grade tumors (uncommon in classic examples of MIFS) and

Table 12.5 Key pathologic features: PHAT and HFLT

PHAT
- Slow-growing subcutaneous neoplasm with infiltrative border, most common in lower extremities (leg, ankle, and foot) - Spindle to ovoid cells with frequent intranuclear inclusions surrounding hyalinized, thin-walled ectatic vessels with fibrin deposition - Hemosiderin (in lesional cells or macrophages) and scattered inflammatory cells - Marked nuclear atypia and pleomorphism, but low mitotic activity (<1/50 HPF)
HFLT
- Slow-growing subcutaneous mass on the dorsal surface of the ankle, foot, or hand - Ill-defined lesions with fascicular/whirling/honeycomb patterned growth of bland spindle cells percolating through adipose tissue - Hemosiderin pigment is prominent as are inflammatory cells - Mitotic activity is very low/absent - May occur at periphery of PHAT
- Most positive for CD34 and negative for S100, SMA, and desmin - Rearrangements in *TGFBR3* and *MGEA5* genes present in HFLT, in mixed HFLT/PHAT, and, less commonly, in classic PHAT

lack the typical stromal hyalinization and virocyte-like (Reed-Sternberg-like) cells that epitomize MIFS. Thus, it appears that myxoid sarcomas that occur in association with HFLT are likely unrelated to MIFS but may rather represent a form of sarcomatous progression in HFLT. The possibility of a pathogenetic link between these entities continues to be investigated (Table 12.5).

Differential Diagnosis

PHAT can closely mimic schwannoma with degenerative ("ancient") change, which often contains clusters of hyalinized vessels, inflammatory aggregates, and pleomorphic Schwann cells. In contrast to PHAT, schwannomas are well-circumscribed and encapsulated lesions without a HFLT-like component at the periphery. S100 protein is diffusely expressed in schwannomas and is consistently negative in PHAT. Owing to the striking degree of nuclear atypia and pleomorphism often seen in PHAT, it can be misdiagnosed as undifferentiated pleomorphic sarcoma; however, a lack of conspicuous mitotic activity would favor the former over the latter. By contrast, identification of a bona fide spindle cell sarcoma with myxoid stroma in association with a classic PHAT may indicate sarcomatous progression.

Important mimickers of HFLT include dermatofibrosarcoma protuberans (DFSP), plexiform fibrohistiocytic tumor, atypical lipomatous tumor (ALT), and lipofibromatosis. Separating DFSP and HFLT can be difficult, especially in a small biopsy. DFSP has a more uniform appearance than HFLT and lacks hemosiderin deposits and ectatic hyalinized vessels. FISH for the characteristic *PDGFB* rearrangement of DFSP can be employed in difficult cases. Like HFLT, plexiform fibrohistiocytic tumor is a slow-growing, infiltrative subcutaneous neoplasm with similarly bland fibroblastic cells arranged in fascicles. In plexiform fibrohistiocytic tumor fascicles of fibroblastic cells connect nodules of epithelioid histiocytic cells admixed with osteoclast-type giant cells, while HFLT has a more monotonous appearance. The spindle cell component of plexiform fibrohistiocytic tumor expresses SMA in keeping with its myofibroblastic phenotype; SMA is typically negative in HFLT. In both DFSP and plexiform fibrohistiocytic tumor, fatty infiltration occurs at the edge of the tumor, whereas in HFLT the adipocytic component is more intimately admixed with the lesional cells and may dominate the histologic picture. ALT rarely occurs in superficial locations and can be distinguished from HFLT by the presence of atypical, hyperchromatic stromal cells within expanded interlobular septa and lack of hemosiderin deposits. In the pediatric population, lipofibromatosis may appear similar to HFLT and can be distinguished based on the more monotonous appearance of the constituent spindle cells and collections of small univacuolated cells at the interface between the adipocytic and spindle cell components. Giant cells and hemosiderin deposits are not typical of lipofibromatosis.

Solitary Fibrous Tumor

Clinical Features

Solitary fibrous tumor (SFTs), originally described in the pleura, may be found in any location. The use of a historic term "hemangiopericytoma" is no longer recommended as these tumors are now incorporated into the SFT category. SFTs most often affect middle-aged or older adults of both sexes and have a predilection for body cavities, viscera, head and neck, deep soft tissues of the trunk and extremities, and intracranial locations. Superficial SFTs arising in the subcutis and dermis are rare, with fewer than 50 cases reported to date. They are more common in women and typically involve the head, especially the scalp, but also the trunk and extremities, and average 3 cm in size.

The behavior of SFTs has been extensively studied over the years. Most extracranial SFTs with typical morphologic features tend to behave in an indolent fashion with a small risk of systemic metastasis, leading to the classification as a tumor of intermediate malignant potential. A small subset of SFTs undergoes dedifferentiation into a high-grade sarcoma, and these tumors behave comparably to other soft tissue sarcomas. However, the ability to predict behavior in ordinary SFTs that lack overt sarcomatoid or anaplastic features is limited. Traditional histologic criteria for malignancy in SFTs like cytologic atypia, nuclear pleomorphism, necrosis, hypercellularity, and mitotic activity >4/10 HPF have been variably associated with adverse outcome, but even seemingly, the most banal-looking SFTs have been shown to metastasize. Recently, a more rigorously studied four-variable model of risk assessment for the development of metastasis in extracranial SFTs was put forth by Demicco et al. In this model, a score is assigned based on the patient's age, tumor size, mitotic count, and presence of necrosis, and the overall risk (low, intermediate, or high) is calculated based on the total score. Cutaneous SFTs appear to behave in an indolent fashion, since all but one reported case showed no local recurrence or metastasis. Whether the above risk assessment system is applicable to cutaneous SFTs requires further study. In the largest series of cutaneous SFT to date, 23/23 tumors were assigned low-risk and showed no evidence of recurrence or metastasis at 24-month follow-up. Treatment of cutaneous SFTs is usually complete local excision with tumor-free margins.

Table 12.6 Key pathologic features: solitary fibrous tumor

Well-circumscribed dermal or subcutaneous lesion with alternating cellular and hypocellular fibrous zones
Short spindle cells with uniform oval nuclei arranged in a "patternless" pattern around prominent branching staghorn-like vessels
Variants include myxoid, fat-forming, giant cell-rich (so-called giant cell angiofibroma), and dedifferentiated SFT
Nuclear expression of STAT6 is a very sensitive and specific diagnostic marker
Patient age, tumor size, mitotic activity, and tumor cell necrosis are the most robust predictors of malignant behavior based on the proposed risk stratification model by Demicco et al.

Pathologic Features

SFTs have a broad spectrum of histologic features. Cutaneous tumors are generally circumscribed and unencapsulated and arise in the subcutis and/or dermis (Fig. 12.23a) and show variable proportions of more cellular and less cellular fibrous or myxoid zones, usually in a somewhat alternating configuration (Fig. 12.23b). The cellular zones contain monotonous short spindle cells arranged in a vaguely fascicular pattern commonly referred to as a "patternless pattern" with minimal intervening collagenous stroma. There are typically numerous branching staghorn-like vessels (Fig. 12.24a). The cells contain uniform round to oval nuclei with vesicular chromatin and usually have inconspicuous nucleoli and amphophilic or basophilic cytoplasm (Fig. 12.24b). In the fibrous zones, the cells are separated by a large amount of collagenous stroma, which may contain keloidal- or ropey-type collagen fibers (Fig. 12.25a, b). The vessels in the less cellular zones are larger and more

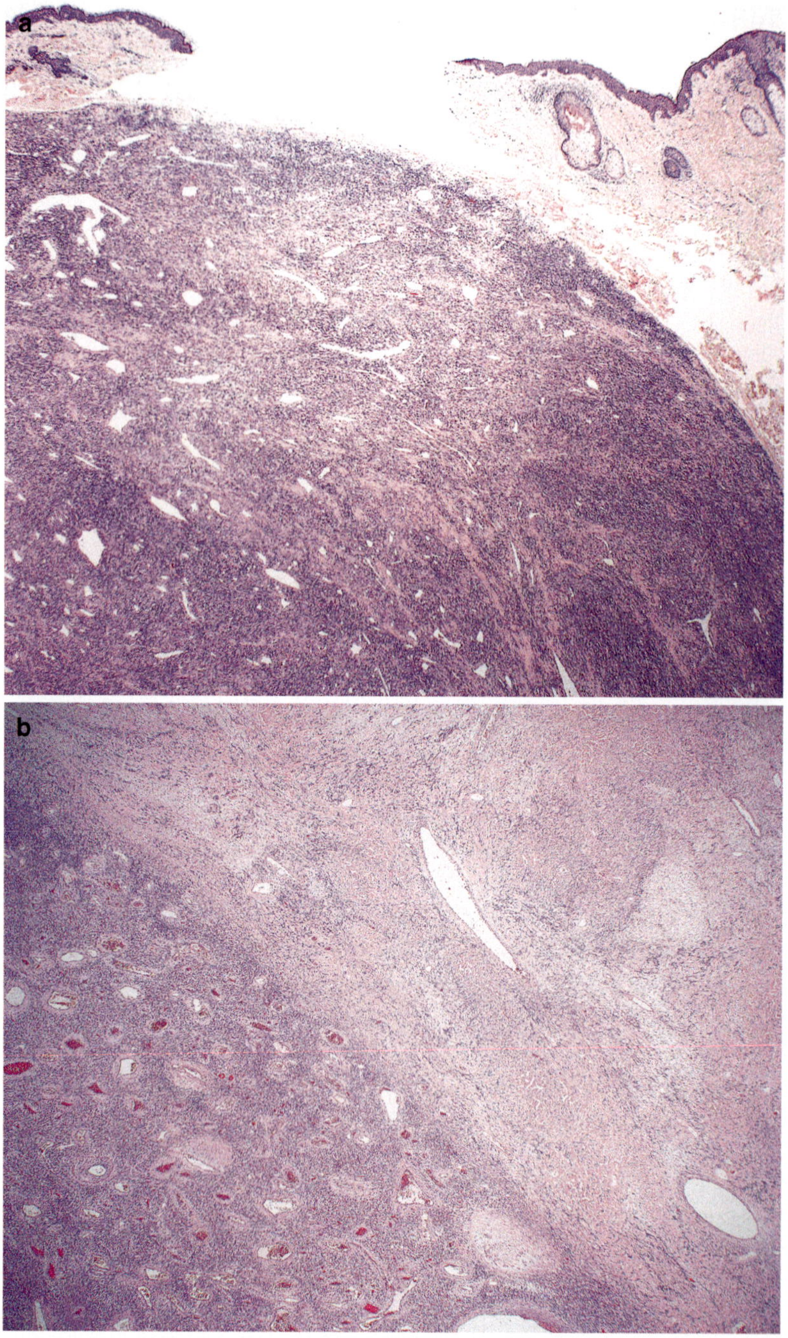

Fig. 12.23 Superficial solitary fibrous tumor. (**a**) Circumscribed unencapsulated mass with alternating more cellular and less cellular areas. (**b**) Another example with sharply demarcated cellular and hypocellular fibrous areas

dilated, often with hyalinized walls or intraluminal fibrin. Microcystic changes, stromal hyalinization, myxoid changes, inflammatory and mast cells, clear cell changes, and pseudovascular or "angiectoid" spaces can be present. The latter are most prevalent in a giant cell-rich variant of SFT (formerly referred to as giant cell angiofibroma), which contains distinctive multinucleated giant cells often lining these spaces (Fig. 12.26). Other well-characterized variants of SFT include those with predominantly myxoid stroma (Fig. 12.27a) and a lipomatous or fat-forming variant

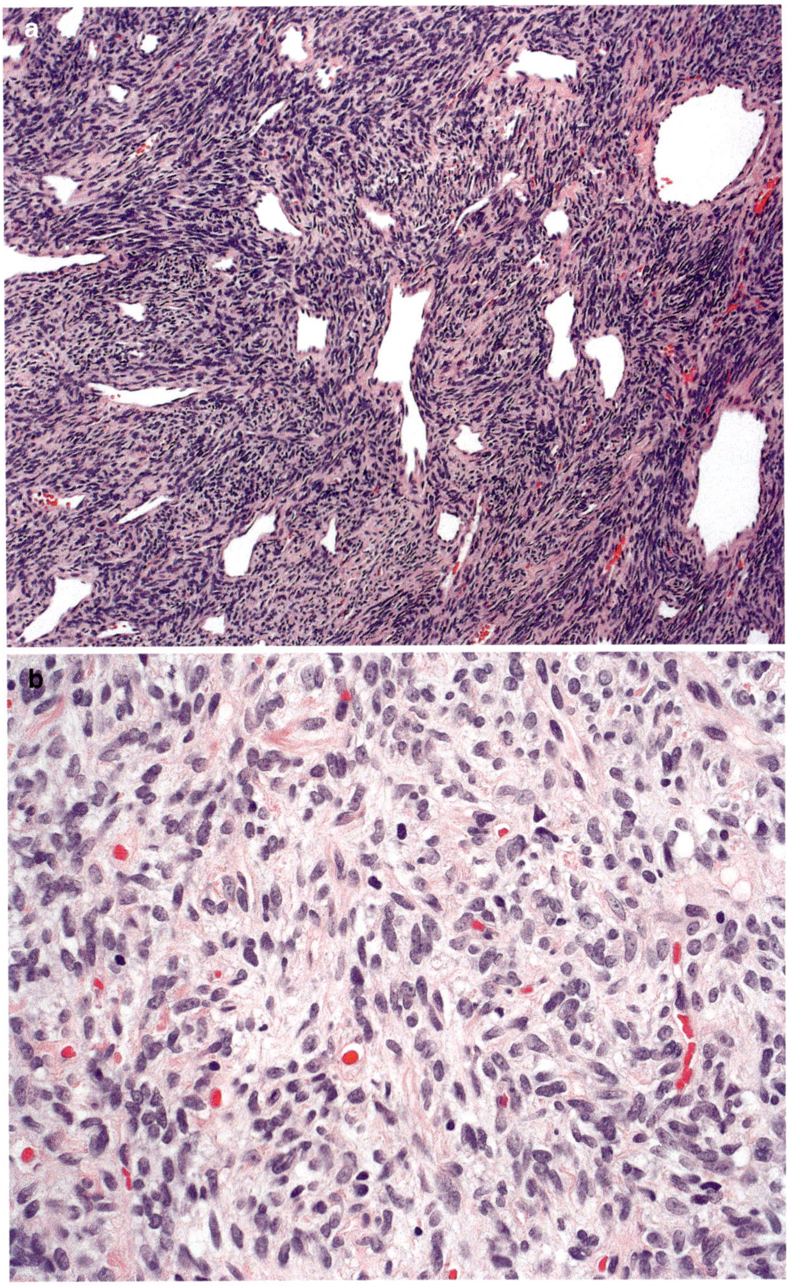

Fig. 12.24 Superficial solitary fibrous tumor. (**a**) Monotonous short spindle cells arranged in a vaguely fascicular (or "patternless") pattern with minimal intervening stroma. Prominent branching staghorn-like vessels are present. (**b**) Uniform oval nuclei with little atypia or mitotic activity

(Fig. 12.27b). These all have been observed in cutaneous examples of SFT. As discussed above, hypercellularity, cytologic atypia, necrosis, and increased mitotic activity within a conventional SFT (Fig. 12.28) warrant closer assessment, although the most robust predictors of malignant behavior in SFTs are size, mitotic activity, and necrosis. Dedifferentiated SFTs usually show areas of anaplasia or an abrupt transition to a high-grade spindle cell or pleomorphic sarcoma, but dedifferentiation toward other lineages, such as rhabdomyosarcoma and osteosarcoma, has been reported. This phenomenon has not yet been described in cutaneous SFTs.

Strong diffuse expression of CD34 is seen in most classic SFTs and in the abovementioned

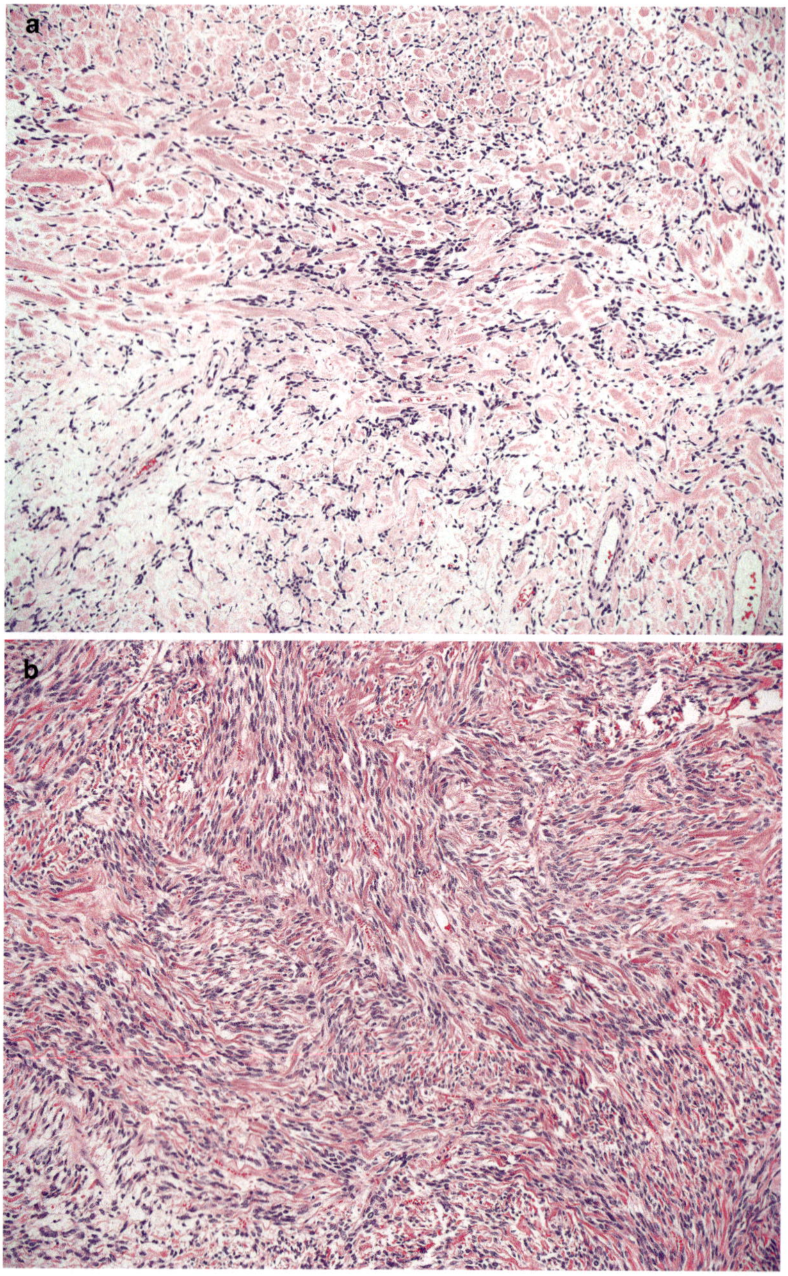

Fig. 12.25 Fibrous areas in solitary fibrous tumor may contain keloidal (**a**) or ropey (**b**) collagen fibers reminiscent of spindle cell lipoma

variants, but this marker lacks specificity and may be lost in approximately 10% of cases, especially in histologically malignant examples. Most SFTs also express CD99, a highly non-specific finding in the context of mesenchymal neoplasms, and show variable expression of SMA, EMA, beta-catenin, and GFAP. A huge advance occurred with the identification of the *NAB2-STAT6* gene fusion and subsequent detection of nuclear STAT6 expression by immunohistochemistry in SFTs from all sites. The latter has been found to be a highly sensitive diagnostic test. The specificity of STAT6 IHC to differentiate SFTs from histologic mimics varies somewhat with the antibody clone utilized, with a near 100% specificity being achieved using a rabbit monoclonal

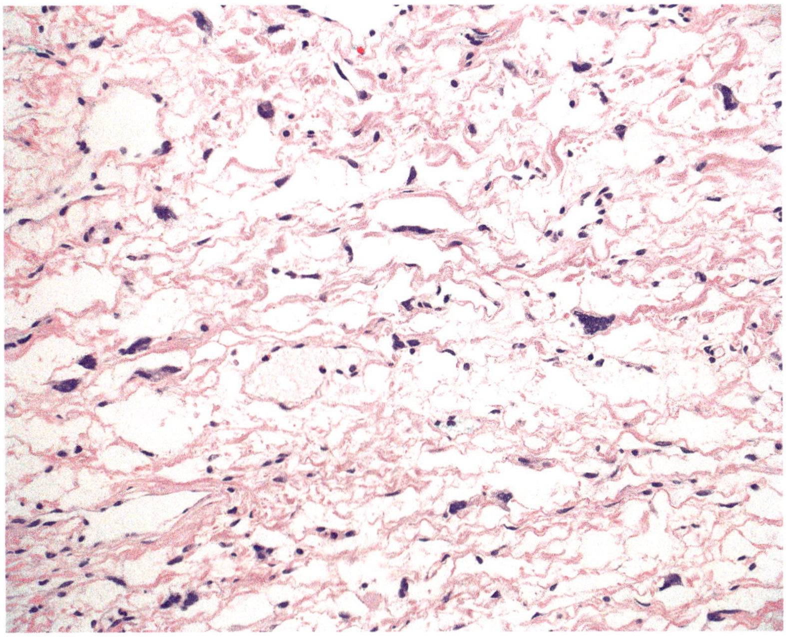

Fig. 12.26 Superficial solitary fibrous tumor. Giant cell-rich solitary fibrous tumor forming "angiectoid" cleft-like spaces lined by multinucleated giant cells

antibody. STAT6 expression may be lost in dedifferentiated SFTs. GRIA2 IHC has also emerged as a potentially useful marker of SFTs, although it lags in sensitivity compared to STAT6 (80%) and can be expressed in important diagnostic mimics of SFT like dermatofibrosarcoma protuberans and synovial sarcoma (Table 12.6).

Differential Diagnosis

The most important diagnostic pitfall are the CD34-positive mesenchymal tumors common in superficial locations. Spindle cell lipoma, cellular angiofibroma, and mammary-type myofibroblastoma and related entities characterized by *RB1* deletion on 13q are especially similar to SFT, being composed of short and bland CD34-positive spindle cells in a whorled or vaguely fascicular pattern in a fibrous background containing mast cells and hyalinized vessels. However, the classic dilated staghorn-like vascular pattern is not a typical feature. STAT6 is not expressed in these tumors, and conversely, the loss of Rb expression does not occur in SFTs. Another important diagnostic mimic, particularly in younger patients, is dermatofibrosarcoma protuberans (DFSP), which enters the differential diagnosis based on the whorled arrangement of the monotonous short spindle cells with bland nuclei and diffuse CD34 expression. The juvenile counterpart of DFSP, giant cell fibroblastoma, can closely mimic giant cell-rich SFT. Diffuse myxoid stroma can also occur in both lesions. In general, keloidal collagen fibers and ectatic hyalinized staghorn vessels of SFTs are not typical of DFSP, but the most reliable features to exclude the latter are diffuse infiltration of the subcutis in a "honeycomb" pattern and entrapment of adnexal structures. DFSPs and giant cell fibroblastomas are negative for STAT6 expression and may be confirmed by FISH for *PDGFB* rearrangement, which is not seen in SFTs.

Within the spectrum of fibrous histiocytomas (FH), superficial SFT can be confused with deep FH. This is because deep FH is a well-circumscribed, predominantly subcutaneous tumor, which lacks typical peripheral collagen trapping and contains a relatively monotonous population of spindle, histiocytic cells arranged in a whorled pattern. Prominent branching staghorn-like vessels are very common in deep FH (40%), and up to 40% are CD34-positive. Thus, this diagnostic confusion is not surprising.

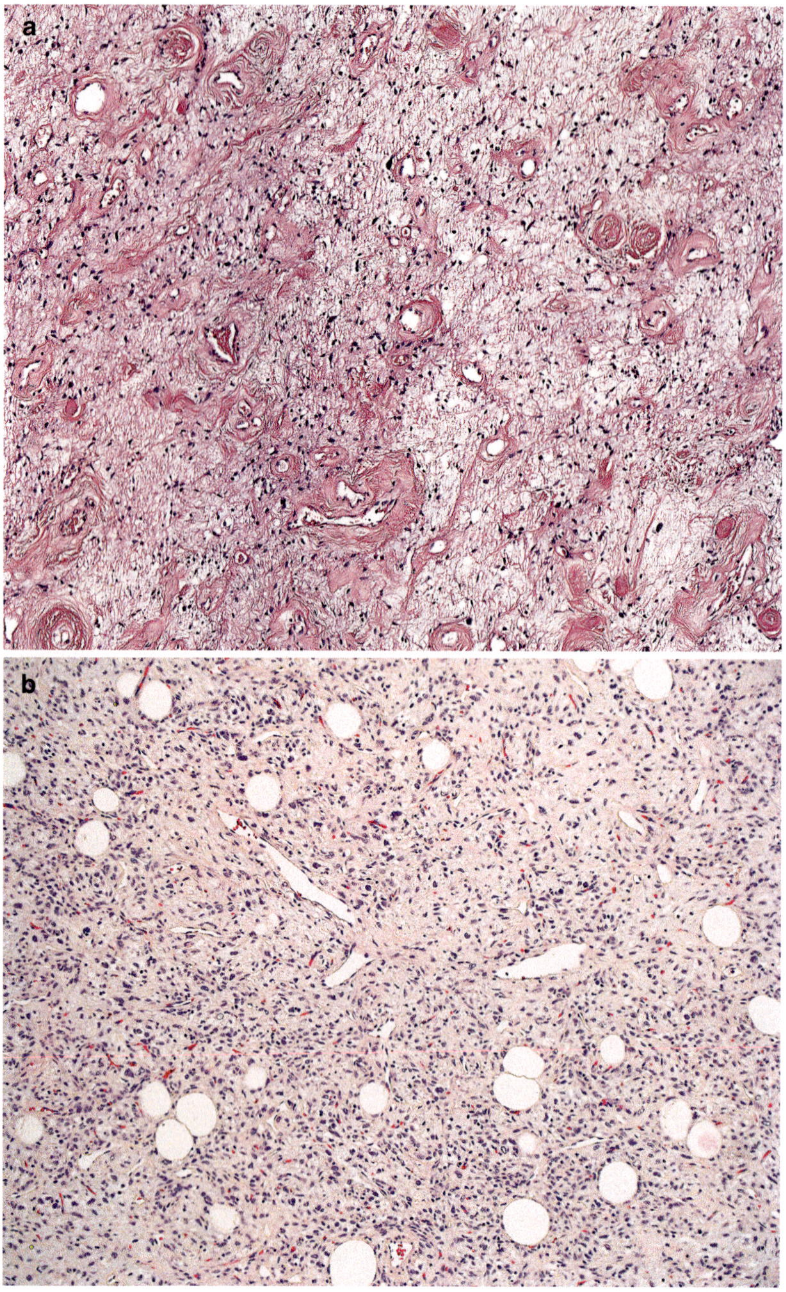

Fig. 12.27 Myxoid (**a**) and lipomatous or fat-forming (**b**) variants of solitary fibrous tumor

Of note, characterization of deep FH as an entity predates the discovery of *NAB2-STAT6* fusion, and it is possible that some cases described within the spectrum of deep FH are in fact, superficial SFTs. The cytologic features of deep FH are somewhat different from those seen in SFT, with plump eosinophilic granular cytoplasm, in keeping with histiocytic differentiation, and a somewhat heterogeneous composition that includes an admixture of secondary elements such as foamy histiocytes, hemosiderin deposits, osteoclast-type giant cells, and inflammatory cells. Deep FHs are negative for STAT6 expression.

Soft tissue perineuriomas and hybrid schwannomas/perineuriomas are well-circumscribed, often subcutaneous tumors composed of

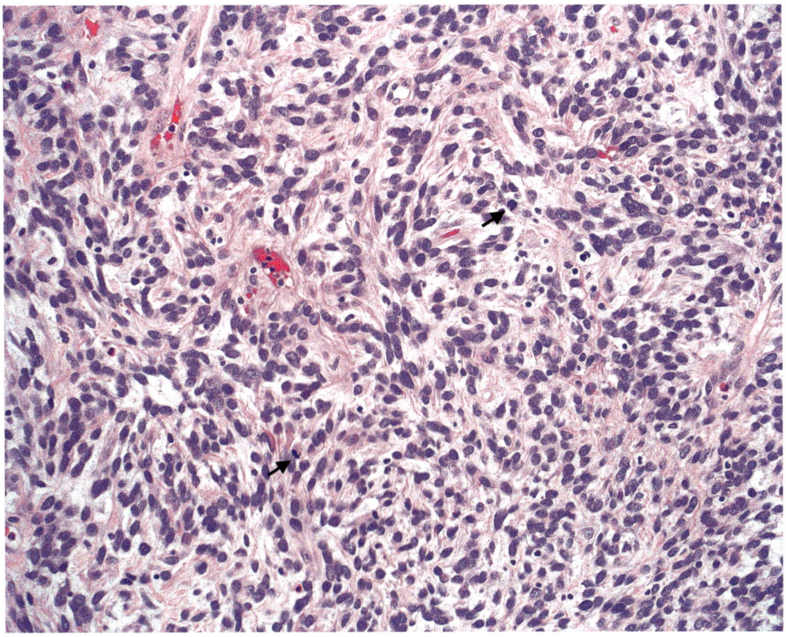

Fig. 12.28 Increased cytologic atypia and frequent mitotic figures (arrows) in malignant solitary fibrous tumor

cytologically bland spindle cells with slender bipolar processes arranged in a whorled growth pattern in a collagenous background, and are often CD34-positive. These tumors can resemble cellular SFTs, although they typically lack the distinctive staghorn vessels and perivascular hyalinization. The slender bipolar processes that typify perineurial cells are not seen in SFTs, although this feature may be difficult to appreciate in perineuriomas as well, without special stains. A helpful IHC combination in this context would include EMA and/or GLUT1 to highlight the bipolar processes in perineurioma and STAT6, which would be positive in SFTs but negative in perineuriomas.

Finally, cellular SFTs with fascicular architecture as well as hypercellular and cytologically atypical SFTs may resemble monophasic synovial sarcoma and fibrosarcomatous DFSP. This differential diagnosis is discussed below.

Synovial Sarcoma

Clinical Features

Synovial sarcoma (SS) is an uncommon translocation-associated malignant mesenchymal neoplasm with partial epithelial differentiation. The typical presentation is an extremity-based periarticular soft tissue tumor in children, adolescents, or young adults, but SS may occur at virtually any anatomic site and affect a broad age range. Dermatopathologists may encounter synovial sarcomas in smaller soft tissue biopsies and excisions from the hands and feet or head and neck area, and rarely, as primary cutaneous tumors or cutaneous metastases. Radiographically, they often have calcifications.

SS may have a protracted clinical course but ultimately behaves aggressively with late local recurrences and systemic metastases, most commonly to lungs, lymph nodes, and bones. SS has an overall approximately 60% 5-year survival. Adverse clinical parameters include large tumor size (>5 cm), visceral location, and poorly differentiated tumor morphology, while the most favorable outcomes are observed in small fibrous and extensively calcified SS of hands and feet, as they are amenable to complete excision. For localized disease, surgical excision is the treatment of choice, while a multimodal approach, utilizing tyrosine kinase inhibitors (imatinib, pazopanib) or immunotherapy targeting NY-ESO-1 and other biomarkers, can be used for locally advanced and metastatic disease.

Pathologic Features

Histologically, SS are broadly divided into three main subtypes: biphasic (spindle cell and epithelial features), monophasic (pure spindle cell), and poorly differentiated subtype with round cell morphology. The monophasic spindle cell variant predominates and is composed of monotonous fascicles of basophilic spindle cells arranged in a so-called "herringbone" pattern (Fig. 12.29a). The spindle cells show uniform elongated vesicular nuclei with evenly distributed chromatin, scant cytoplasm, and indistinct cell borders (Fig. 12.29b). Nuclear pleomorphism is not a characteristic of treatment-naïve SS. The stroma usually demonstrates delicate wiry collagen fibers or little intervening collagen, but in other examples, the stroma can be markedly fibrous,

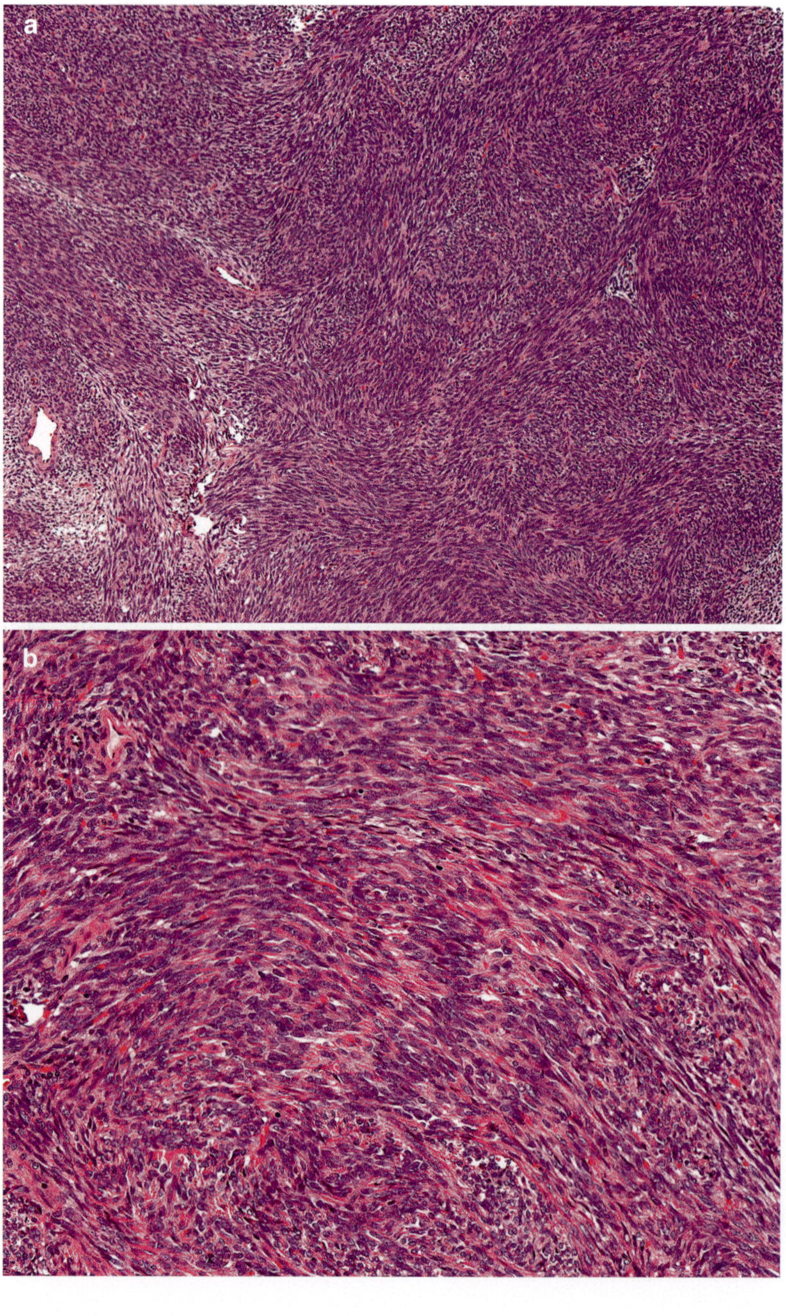

Fig. 12.29 Monophasic synovial sarcoma. (**a**) Sweeping fascicles of monotonous basophilic spindle cells. (**b**) Uniform elongated nuclei with evenly distributed chromatin and scant basophilic cytoplasm separated by delicate wiry collagen fibers

hyalinized, or myxoid (Fig. 12.30a, b). Cystic changes, areas of hemorrhage, and mast cells are common (Fig. 12.31a). Many spindle cell SS have prominent branching staghorn-like vessels like those seen in SFTs (Fig. 12.31b).

Biphasic SS is composed of an admixture of a monotonous spindle cell component and epithelial cells forming elaborate glandular structures and papillary projections lined by cuboidal or columnar cells (Fig. 12.32a). The epithelial cells have uniform round to oval nuclei and evenly distributed chromatin, somewhat resembling the nuclei in the spindle cell component. Rarely, biphasic synovial sarcoma may show focal squamous differentiation (Fig. 12.32b). Pure monophasic epithelial tumors are rare. Calcifications

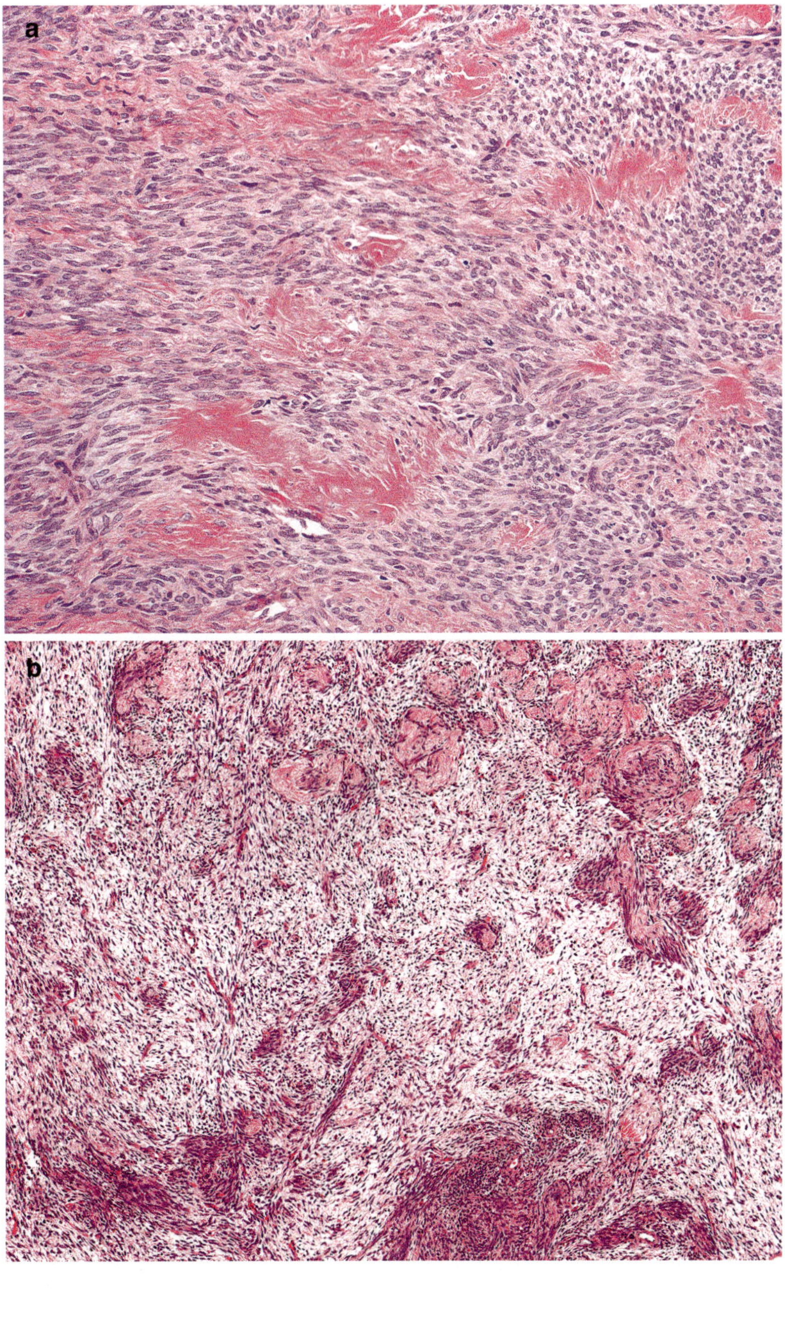

Fig. 12.30 Monophasic synovial sarcoma with fibrous (**a**) and myxoid (**b**) stroma

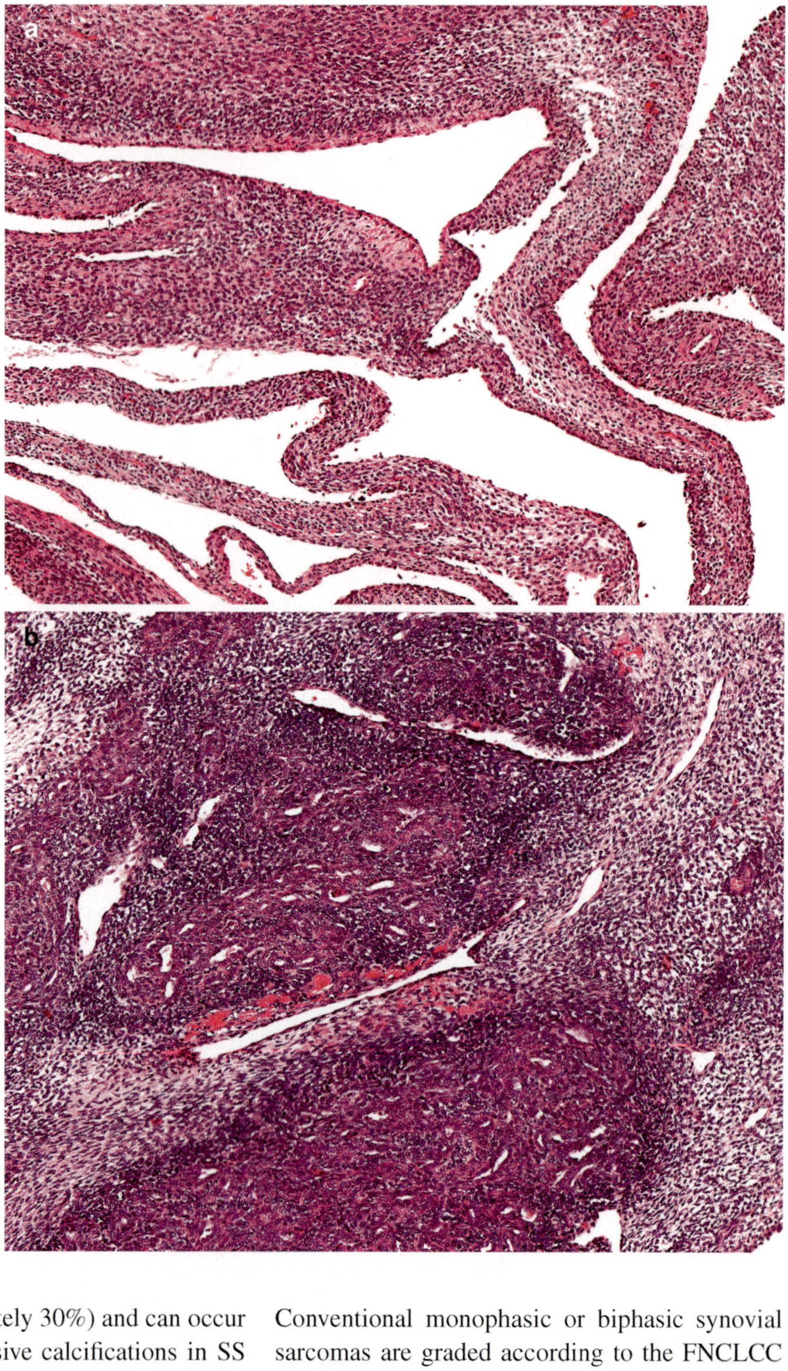

Fig. 12.31 Monophasic synovial sarcoma with cystic change (**a**) and prominent staghorn-like vessels resembling solitary fibrous tumor (**b**)

are common (approximately 30%) and can occur in both subtypes. Extensive calcifications in SS replacing glandular structures or associated with hyalinized fibrous stroma and cytologically low-grade spindle cells are referred to as calcifying SS (Fig. 12.33a). This variant can be associated with improved outcome. Less common features include ossification, rhabdoid features, granular cell change, and primary intraneural location. Conventional monophasic or biphasic synovial sarcomas are graded according to the FNCLCC grading system.

Poorly differentiated areas are identified in 20–30% of conventional monophasic or biphasic SS. This subtype is referred to as poorly differentiated SS. The latter is composed of sheets of ovoid cells with rounded atypical nuclei, scant cytoplasm, variably prominent nucleoli, frequent

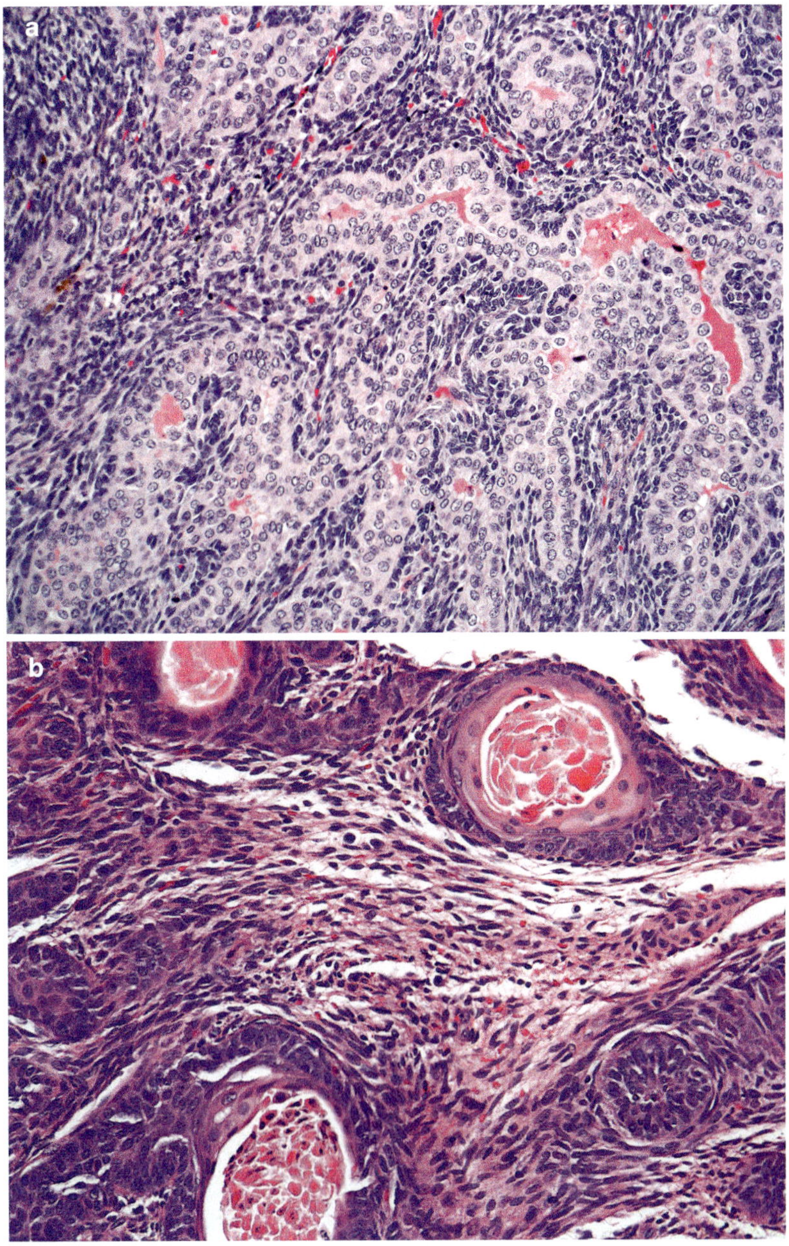

Fig. 12.32 (**a**) Biphasic synovial sarcoma forming elaborate glandular structures lined by uniform columnar to cuboidal epithelioid cells in a background of spindle tumor cells. (**b**) Rarely, the epithelial elements demonstrate squamous differentiation

mitotic figures, and areas of necrosis resembling an undifferentiated round cell sarcoma (Fig. 12.33b). SS with rhabdoid morphology are also best considered as poorly differentiated.

Both monophasic and biphasic SS express variable combinations of epithelial markers including cytokeratins and EMA, but these markers may be only focally expressed. CD34 is negative. CD99 is seen in approximately 70% of SS emphasizing the poor specificity of this marker in the context of mesenchymal spindle cell neoplasms. A third of cases may express S100. Nuclear expression of TLE1 has excellent sensitivity for the diagnosis of synovial sarcoma; however, this antibody is used with variable success due to difficulties with optimization and reduced specificity.

SS are defined by a reciprocal t(X;18)(p11.2;q11.2), with pathognomonic *SS18-SSX1*,

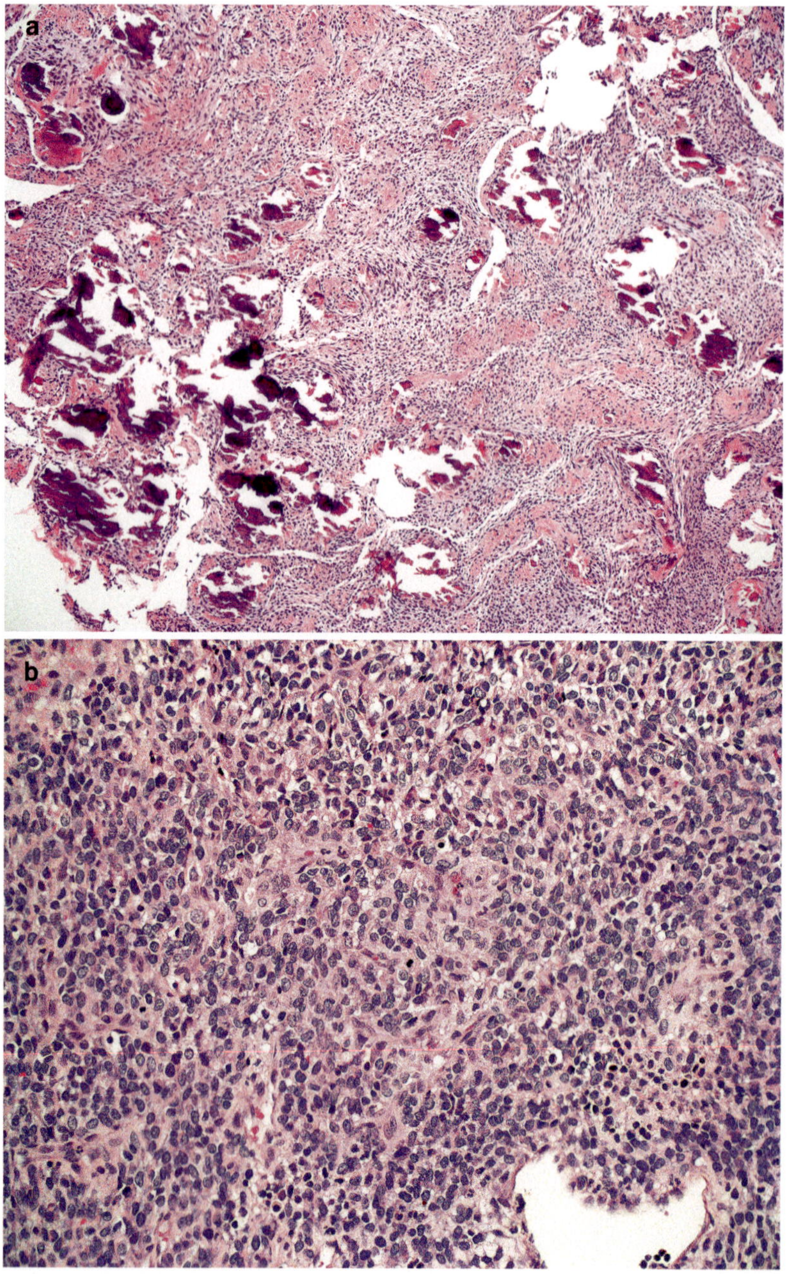

Fig. 12.33 (**a**) Calcifying synovial sarcoma showing numerous stromal calcifications associated with cytologically low-grade spindle cells. (**b**) Poorly differentiated synovial sarcoma composed of atypical mitotically active round cells resembling undifferentiated round cell sarcoma

SS18-SSX2, or, rarely, *SS18-SSX4* or other cryptic gene fusions. FISH for *SS18* gene rearrangement or RT-PCR for SS fusion transcripts, which has greater sensitivity compared to FISH, are the most useful and practical diagnostic tests to confirm the diagnosis. There is no prognostic correlation with the monophasic vs. biphasic histology or the type of fusion transcript (Table 12.7).

Differential Diagnosis

In the skin and subcutis, the most important diagnostic considerations include spindle cell melanoma, fibrosarcomatous DFSP, conventional MPNST, and cutaneous SFT. Spindle cell melanoma affects an older patient population and morphologically may display a focally nested

Table 12.7 Key pathologic features: synovial sarcoma

Three broad subtypes: monophasic, biphasic, and poorly differentiated
Monophasic spindle cell SS: fascicles of monotonous basophilic spindle cells arranged in a so-called "herringbone" pattern
Biphasic SS: an admixture of monotonous spindle cell component admixed with glandular structures and papillary projections lined by cuboidal or columnar cells with uniform nuclear features
Variably prominent stromal collagen, branching staghorn-like vessels, hemorrhage, cystic changes, and myxoid stroma
Calcifications are common and may be extensive
Poorly differentiated SS resembles undifferentiated round cell sarcoma
FISH for *SS18* gene rearrangement or RT-PCR for SS fusion transcripts are useful diagnostic tests

growth pattern and a junctional component. S100 protein can be positive in both tumors and therefore is of limited value in this context, although strong, diffuse expression would favor spindle cell melanoma. SOX10 is a very helpful marker because it is positive in most melanomas, including the spindle cell subtypes, and is usually negative in SS, being observed only in primary intraneural examples of this entity. The fascicular and monotonous growth pattern of fibrosarcomatous DFSP can mimic SS. The most helpful histologic clue is the identification of a conventional DFSP component. CD34 can serve as a quick screening tool as it is variably positive in fibrosarcomatous DFSP but consistently negative in SS. SS with prominent collagenous stroma and staghorn vessels can be mistaken for SFT, but the latter typically lacks a fascicular growth pattern and the elongated overlapping nuclei of SS (although they may be seen in atypical and malignant examples). STAT6 expression can readily distinguish SFT from SS. MPNSTs and SS may be virtually identical histologically, especially in poorly differentiated tumors, and can express S100. Unlike SS, MPNSTs are positive for SOX10 (approximately 70%) and about one-half of cases show loss of H3K27me3 by immunohistochemistry. The glandular structures in SS can mimic adenocarcinoma, but display less cytologic pleomorphism, and the intervening stroma consists of the spindle tumor cells in contrast to the reactive fibroblasts seen in adenocarcinomas. In all of these scenarios, FISH and RT-PCR for SS gene fusions are extremely helpful, as these tests are universally negative in the histologic mimics of SS.

Alveolar Soft Part Sarcoma

Clinical Features

Alveolar soft part sarcoma (ASPS) is a rare, distinctive mesenchymal neoplasm that usually presents as a deep-seated, extremity-based mass in teenagers and young adults or as an orbital or tongue tumor in children. Rarely, ASPS may affect the female genital tract, bladder, or other visceral organs and body cavities. Because of the aggressive vascular invasion, ASPS tends to metastasize early to the brain, lungs, bone, and a variety of other sites, including the skin. With extraordinarily rare exceptions, ASPS does not occur as a primary cutaneous malignancy. However, heightened diagnostic awareness for this entity by dermatopathologists is of importance because metastatic ASPS can be mistaken for cutaneous PEComa, granular cell tumor, or metastatic renal cell carcinoma. Treatment includes surgical excision for localized disease, variably effective combined strategies for the tumors presenting with metastases, and targeted inhibition of *MET* signaling cascade, which is a downstream pathway of *ASPSCR1-TFE3* gene fusion.

Pathologic Features

Histologically, ASPS is quite distinctive. The tumor is composed of large epithelioid polygonal cells arranged in nests surrounded by delicate capillary vessels (Fig. 12.34a). The prototypical pseudoalveolar pattern of this neoplasm is often present due to loss of cellular cohesion in the center of tumor nests (Fig. 12.34b). Tongue tumors in children tend to have a more solid, sheet-like growth pattern (Fig. 12.35a). Cytologically, the epithelioid cells are rather

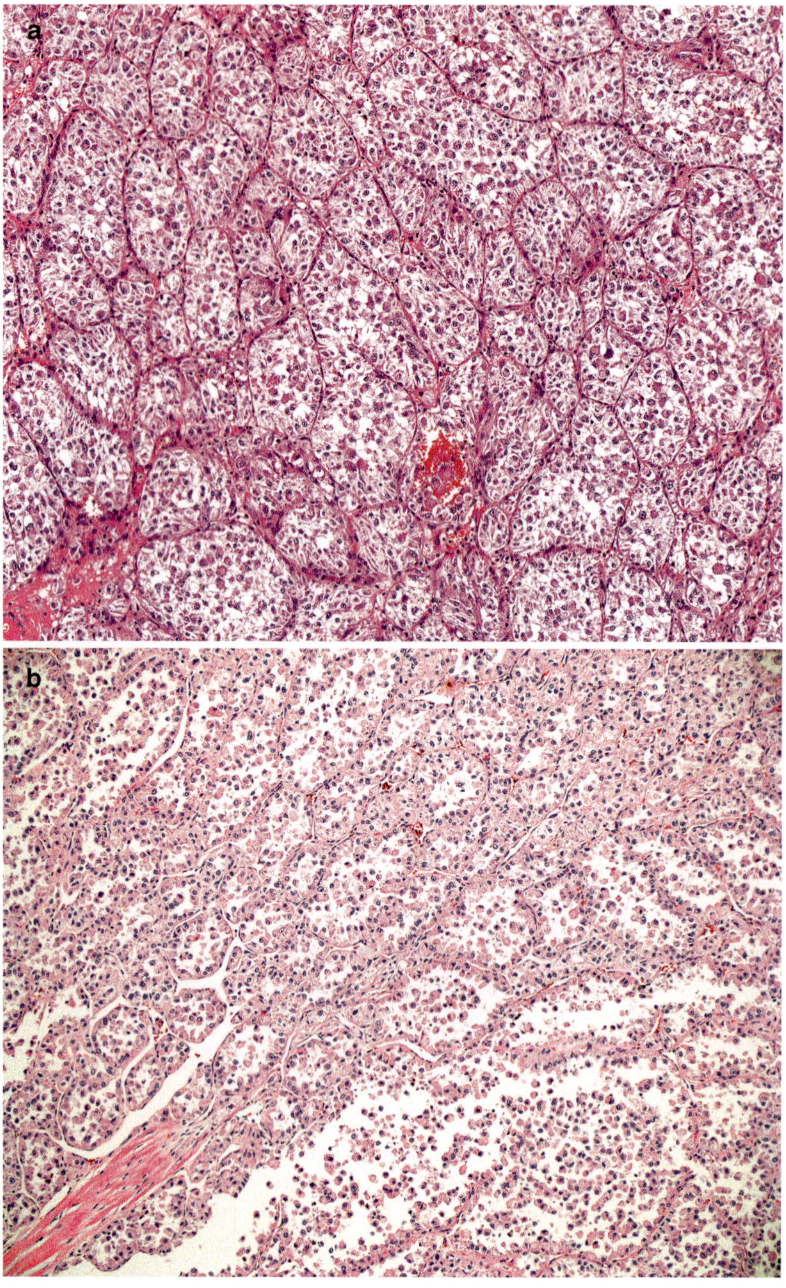

Fig. 12.34 Alveolar soft part sarcoma. (**a**) Large polygonal epithelioid cells in a nested configuration surrounded by delicate capillary vessels. (**b**) Loss of cellular cohesion resulting in a pseudoalveolar pattern

monotonous, with a large round nucleus, prominent nucleolus, and voluminous eosinophilic or sometimes clear cytoplasm, which often contains PAS-positive diastase-resistant rod- or rhomboid-shaped crystals (Fig. 12.35b) composed of monocarboxylate transporter 1 (MCT1) protein. Other examples contain rounded precursor granules (so-called crystal-deficient ASPS); one such case has been reported as a primary ASPS in the subcutis. Mitotic figures are rare, but vascular invasion is a consistent finding.

ASPS is characterized by an unbalanced translocation, der (17)t(X;17)(p11;q25), which results in a *ASPSCR1-TFE3* gene fusion, which can be detected by FISH or immunohistochemistry looking for nuclear expression of TFE3 protein.

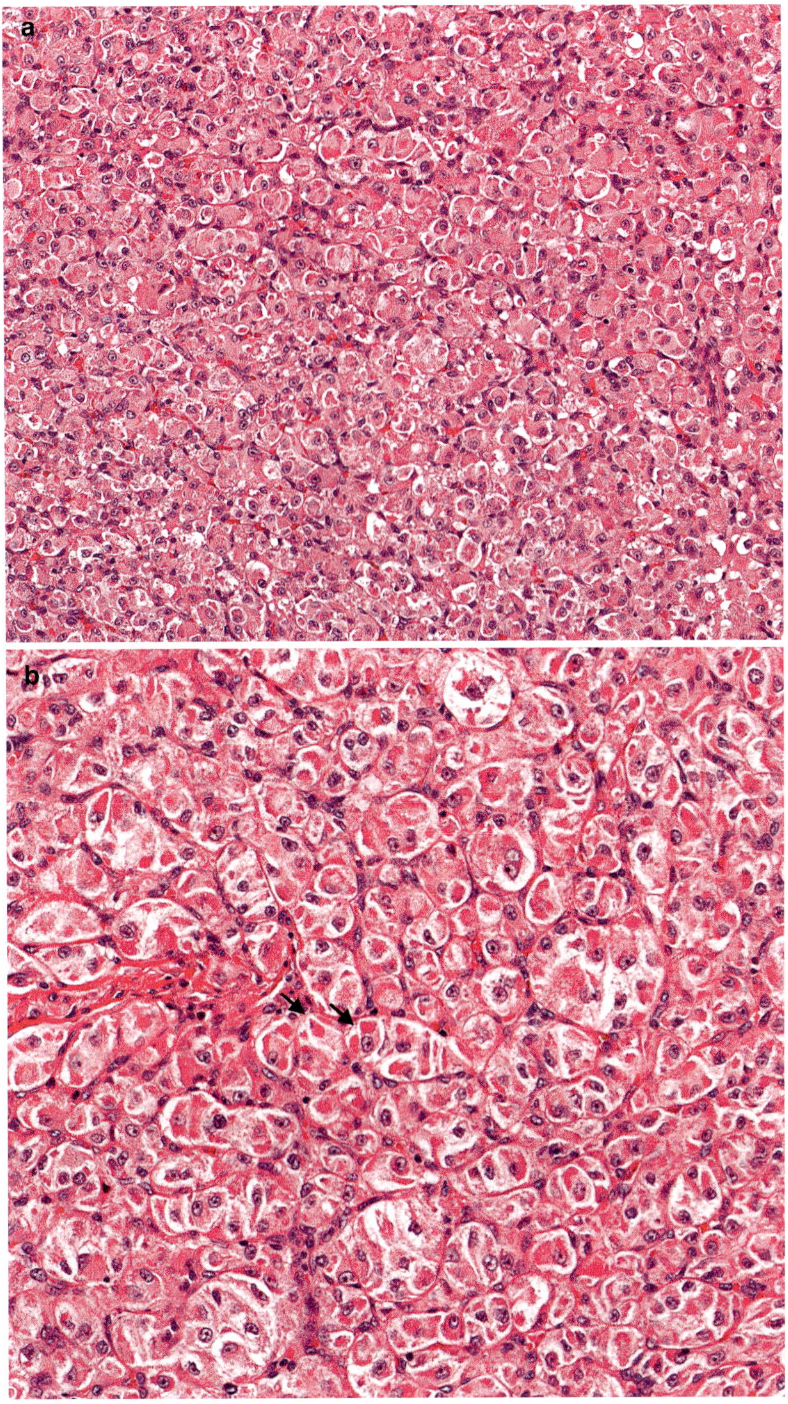

Fig. 12.35 Alveolar soft part sarcoma. (**a**) Solid sheet-like growth pattern. (**b**) The cells have large nuclei, prominent nucleoli, and voluminous eosinophilic cytoplasm often containing rhomboid- or rod-like crystals or granular material (arrow)

The immunoprofile of ASPS is otherwise nonspecific. Occasional expression of myogenic markers and S100 protein may occur, but other melanocytic markers are usually negative, as are markers of epithelial and neuroendocrine differentiation (Table 12.8).

Table 12.8 Key pathologic features: alveolar soft part sarcoma

Large epithelioid polygonal cells in a nested or pseudoalveolar pattern with central discohesion, surrounded by delicate capillary vessels
Tongue and orbital tumors in children have predominantly solid architecture
Round nuclei with prominent nucleoli and ample eosinophilic cytoplasm containing PAS-D-positive rod-like or rhomboid crystals or rounded precursor granules
Vascular invasion
ASPSCR1-TFE3 fusion with nuclear TFE3 expression

Differential Diagnosis

Metastatic renal cell carcinoma with eosinophilic or granular cytoplasm is the primary diagnostic consideration. Both tumors can look strikingly similar. This diagnostic dilemma may be resolved by the application of cytokeratin Cam5.2, EMA, CAIX, or PAX8 immunostains, which are usually negative in ASPS. TFE3 immunostaining can help confirm ASPS, but caution must be exercised in younger patients since some Xp11-associated pediatric renal cell carcinomas lack expression of various cytokeratins and/or EMA and have the same *ASPSCR1-TFE3* gene fusion and will express TFE3 by immunohistochemistry. In contradistinction to ASPS, this translocation is balanced. Granular cell tumors (GCT) have overlapping morphologic features with ASPS, being composed of large polygonal cells with granular cytoplasm and, like ASPS, are often positive for TFE3 by IHC. GCTs typically lack alveolar architecture and PAS-D-positive crystals (although granular material may be observed) and are usually strongly, diffusely positive for S100 protein and inhibin, unlike ASPS. Cutaneous PEComas (discussed earlier in this chapter) can closely resemble ASPS and may contain PAS-D positive cytoplasmic material. Unlike ASPS, cutaneous PEComas co-express melanocytic and muscle markers, such as desmin and SMA, and most do not appear to have *TFE3* gene rearrangements by FISH or TFE3 expression by immunohistochemistry.

Rosai-Dorfman Disease

Clinical Features

Rosai-Dorfman disease (RDD) is a multicentric histiocytic disorder of uncertain etiology characterized as a distinctive entity by Rosai and Dorfman in 1969. The nodal form of RDD is also known as sinus histiocytosis with massive lymphadenopathy, a name that aptly reflects the clinical presentation of painless, bulky, usually cervical lymphadenopathy associated with fever, weight loss, anemia, and other systemic inflammatory symptoms, in children and young adults. The extranodal form (40% of cases) manifests as a mass lesion with or without associated lymphadenopathy, most often involving the skin, subcutis, head and neck region, bone, and CNS. Unusual locations like the testes or breast may also be involved. In the skin, RDD presents as nodules, patches, or plaques, with predilection for middle-aged female adults. Subcutaneous or soft tissue involvement is usually in the form of a slowly growing mass.

The etiology of RDD remains uncertain but is likely related to immune dysregulation, which leads to a reactive non-Langerhans histiocytosis. Recently, recurrent *KRAS* and *MAP2K1* mutations have been identified in approximately one-third of sporadic RDD cases suggesting that at least a subset of these lesions represent clonal proliferations. Based on the various clinicopathologic associations, RDD is now classified into sporadic classical (nodal), extranodal, familial, neoplasia-associated, and immune disorder-associated forms. The presence of IgG4(+) plasma cells in RDD led to a suggestion that it might fall within the spectrum of IgG4-related sclerosing disease, but this association has proven to be inconsistent. Nonetheless, the recommendation by the Histiocyte Society is to evaluate the IgG4-positive plasma cell infiltrate in all cases of RDD.

Extranodal RDD, especially in cutaneous locations, follows an indolent course. Up to a third of cases regress spontaneously, while the remaining patients have chronic but stable disease. Approximately 10% of patients develop progressive disease or succumb to the mass effects of the tumor or infectious complications.

None of the conventional treatment modalities offer complete cure, with surgery remaining the treatment of choice for mass effect or cosmetic reasons. Identification of mutation in signaling pathways may open avenues for targeted therapies in the future.

Pathologic Features

The lesions are composed of broad syncytial layers of large pale histiocytes in association with an intervening lymphoplasmacytic infiltrate. This pattern is best appreciated at scanning magnification, as alternating pale and dark areas (Fig. 12.36). In the lymph nodes, these histiocytes massively expand the sinuses. In cutaneous and subcutaneous RDD cases, the margins are usually ill-defined. The histiocytes have round or oval vesicular nuclei with distinct nucleoli and palely eosinophilic voluminous, granular to wispy cytoplasm. The hallmark feature of RDD is *emperipolesis*—a passage of intact inflammatory cells through the cytoplasm of the histiocytes (Fig. 12.37a). The lymphoplasmacytic infiltrate is a mixture of lymphocytes, mature plasma cells, and, less often, neutrophils. Eosinophils may be present but are less common. There is no significant nuclear atypia, pleomorphism, or mitotic activity. Histiocytes in RDD strongly and diffusely express S100 protein, which also helps to highlight engulfed inflammatory cells (Fig. 12.37b). As mentioned, the plasma cell infiltrate in RDD is prominent and may contain a population of IGg4-positive plasma cells (Fig. 12.38 and Table 12.9).

Differential Diagnosis

Once the distinctive sheet-like arrangement of S100-positive histiocytes with emperipolesis is recognized, the diagnosis is usually straightforward. In limited samples, RDD must be distinguished from several mimics: histiocytic proliferations including Langerhans cell histiocytosis (LCH), juvenile xanthogranuloma and reticulohistiocytoma, inflammatory panniculitides, and cutaneous lymphoma. Similar to RDD, the inflammatory infiltrate in LCH often includes prominent eosinophils. The histiocytes

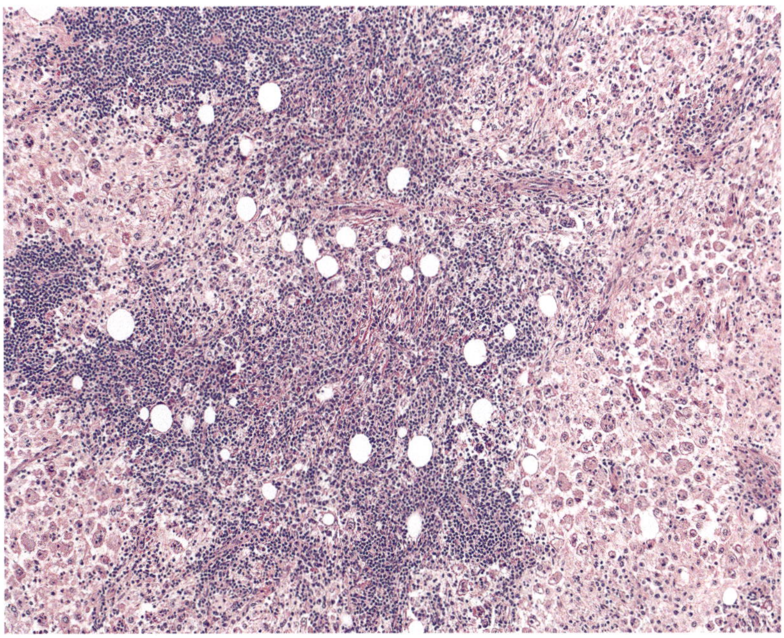

Fig. 12.36 Rosai-Dorfman disease. Ill-defined sheets of pale histiocytes with an intervening inflammatory infiltrate imparting an alternating light and dark pattern at scanning magnification

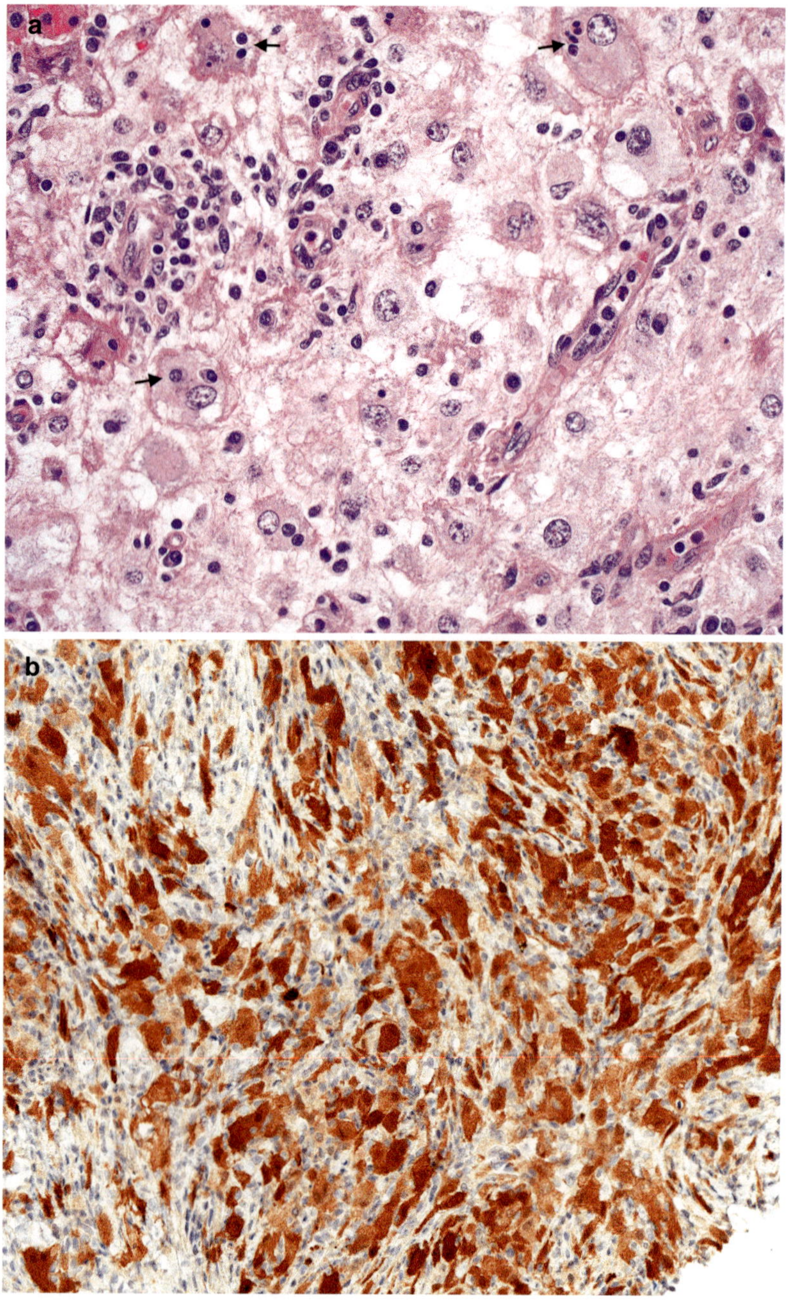

Fig. 12.37 Rosai-Dorfman disease. (**a**) Large histiocytes with mildly atypical vesicular nuclei and pale voluminous cytoplasm containing intact inflammatory cells, a finding known as emperipolesis (arrows). (**b**) The histiocytes are positive for S100 protein, which helps to highlight engulfed inflammatory cells, and are negative for CD1a and langerin

in LCH are also S100-positive; however, morphologically, LCH shows irregular, crinkled, or grooved nuclei that are eccentrically placed and, unlike RDD, are positive for CD1a and langerin. Juvenile xanthogranuloma presents as a sharply demarcated superficial papule and contains a polymorphous histiocytic population including Touton-type giant cells, which are usually not seen in RDD. Reticulohistiocytomas also tend to present as a more defined lesion composed of epithelioid histiocytes with distinctive glassy cytoplasm. Emperipolesis, a prominent plasma cell component (especially, IgG4-positive plasma cells), and S100 protein expression are

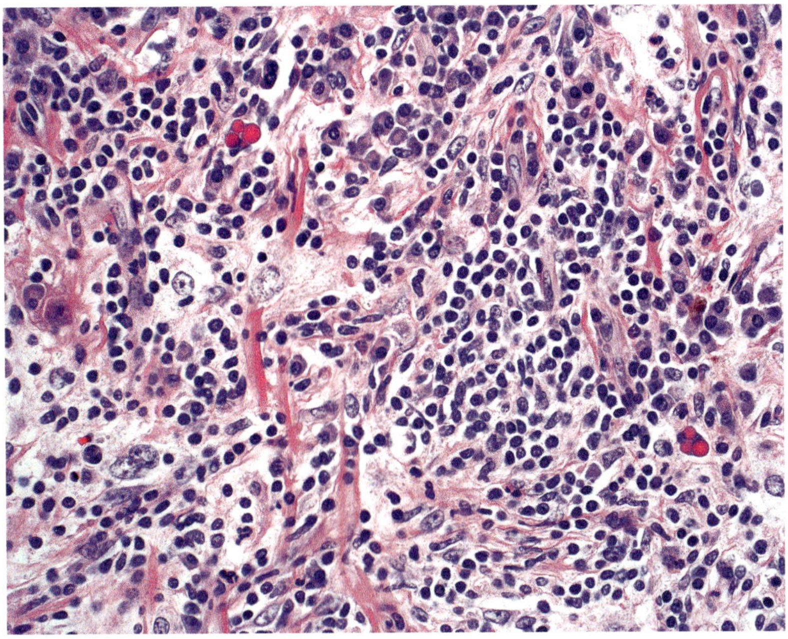

Fig. 12.38 Rosai-Dorfman disease. The inflammatory infiltrate is rich in plasma cells that can be IgG4-positive

Table 12.9 Key pathologic features: Rosai-Dorfman disease

Sheet-like proliferation of large pale histiocytes with intervening lymphoplasmacytic infiltrate and ill-defined margins, imparting an alternating light and dark appearance at low power
Round or oval vesicular nuclei with distinct nucleoli and palely eosinophilic voluminous cytoplasm containing intact inflammatory cells (emperipolesis)
The histiocytes are S100 protein-positive and negative for CD1a and langerin

not seen in juvenile xanthogranuloma or reticulohistiocytoma. Panniculitides have a predilection for either septal or lobular inflammation and are often associated with vasculitis, granulomatous inflammation, and predominance of neutrophilic infiltrates. The histiocytes in panniculitides are smaller, with bland oval nuclei, and lack a syncytial arrangement, emperipolesis, and S100 immunoreactivity. RDD with a prominent inflammatory infiltrate can mimic cutaneous lymphomas, especially those with a polymorphous background, such as T cell, anaplastic large cell, or Hodgkin lymphoma. These tumors invariably demonstrate cytologic atypia in the constituent lymphoid cells and, while they are often histiocyte-rich, large pale S100-positive histiocytes with emperipolesis are not identified. A prominent plasma cell component is also not a characteristic. In difficult cases, a questionable atypical lymphoid population can be delineated by appropriate lymphoid markers and clonality studies. Finally, distally located RDD may resemble myxoinflammatory fibroblastic sarcoma (MIFS) due to the infiltrative growth pattern and prominent inflammatory infiltrate. However, the constituent cell in MIFS is an atypical spindle to stellate fibroblast with striking inclusion-like (virocyte-like) macronucleoli, while the characteristic S100-positive histiocytes of RDD are not seen in MIFS.

Cutaneous Myoepithelial Tumors

Myoepithelial neoplasms represent a morphologically and genetically diverse family of tumors characterized by histologic, immunophenotypic, and ultrastructural features of myoepithelial differentiation. Myoepithelial tumors have a broad anatomic distribution including the skin, soft tissue, viscera, salivary glands, breast, and bone. Several types of myoepithelial neoplasms occur in the skin. Cutaneous mixed tumors (chondroid syringomas) are defined by at least focal tubuloductal differentiation and are histologically analogous to the mixed tumors (pleomorphic adenomas) of the salivary gland; these often show *PLAG1* gene rearrangements. On the other end of the morphologic spectrum are cutaneous myoepitheliomas and myoepithelial carcinomas composed only of epithelioid or spindle myoepithelial cells without ductal differentiation. Cutaneous myoepitheliomas fall into two categories: tumors with classic morphology representing the superficial/subcutaneous counterparts of primary myoepithelial tumors arising in the deep soft tissue, salivary gland, and visceral locations and cutaneous syncytial myoepithelioma.

Syncytial myoepithelioma is a newly described variant with a predilection for intraepidermal growth and a distinctive appearance and immunophenotype, which set it apart from other myoepithelial tumors. Awareness of this variant is especially important to dermatopathologists as it can be confused with histiocytic and melanocytic neoplasms and epithelioid sarcoma.

Clinical Features

Cutaneous mixed tumors (chondroid syringomas) occur in the skin and subcutis of the extremities or head and neck region, usually as small (<5 cm), firm, and painless nodules or papules. These tumors usually affect adults, without gender predilection. Malignant cutaneous mixed tumors are exceptionally rare. Myoepitheliomas and myoepithelial carcinomas occur over a broad age range without sex predilection and are relatively common in pediatric patients. Nearly half of the pediatric myoepithelial tumors are malignant. Cutaneous myoepitheliomas usually present as slowly growing, non-tender cutaneous, or subcutaneous palpable masses in the limbs, limb girdles, or head and neck area. The vast majority of these cutaneous mixed tumors and cutaneous myoepitheliomas behave in an indolent fashion but, much like their salivary gland counterparts, may recur locally in approximately 20% of cases. When cutaneous myoepitheliomas recur, it is usually in the setting of incomplete excision. Because of this, both cutaneous mixed tumors and cutaneous myoepitheliomas are best treated by complete local excision. Myoepithelial carcinomas of soft tissue behave more aggressively, with a recurrence rate of approximately 40% and a risk of systemic metastasis ranging from 30% to 50%, and are best treated by a multidisciplinary sarcoma team. Cutaneous myoepithelial carcinomas tend to have better prognosis compared to their deep soft tissue and visceral counterparts. Surgical resection remains the mainstay of therapy of myoepithelial carcinoma, but responses to chemotherapy have been documented. Metastatic sites include lungs, lymph nodes, and soft tissues. Histologically, myoepithelial carcinomas are defined based on the presence of cytologic atypia (discussed below). Syncytial myoepitheliomas usually arise in the extremities as small (median, 0.8 cm), painless polypoid nodules, and are slightly more common in males. Syncytial myoepitheliomas are benign and only rarely recur if incompletely excised. Simple conservative excision is usually curative in most cases. To date, metastatic examples have not been reported.

Pathologic Features

Cutaneous mixed tumors are well-circumscribed, typically unencapsulated nodules. Like their salivary gland counterparts, cutaneous mixed tumors may have an infiltrative growth pattern and satellite nodules. These are biphasic tumors composed of epithelioid to spindle to plasmacytoid cells arranged in sheets, cords, or nests dispersed in myxoid or hyaline stroma. By definition, tubuloductal differentiation, of either apocrine or eccrine type, is at least focally present in cutaneous mixed tumors (Fig. 12.39a). Cytologically, the cells have bland oval nuclei, inconspicuous nucleoli, and eosinophilic, amphophilic, or clear cytoplasm (Fig. 12.39b). Cytologic atypia and pleomorphism are usually not seen in cutaneous mixed tumors. Heterologous differentiation is often present, usually in the form of hyaline cartilage or bone. Squamous metaplasia and folliculosebaceous differentiation may occur (Figs. 12.39 and 12.40).

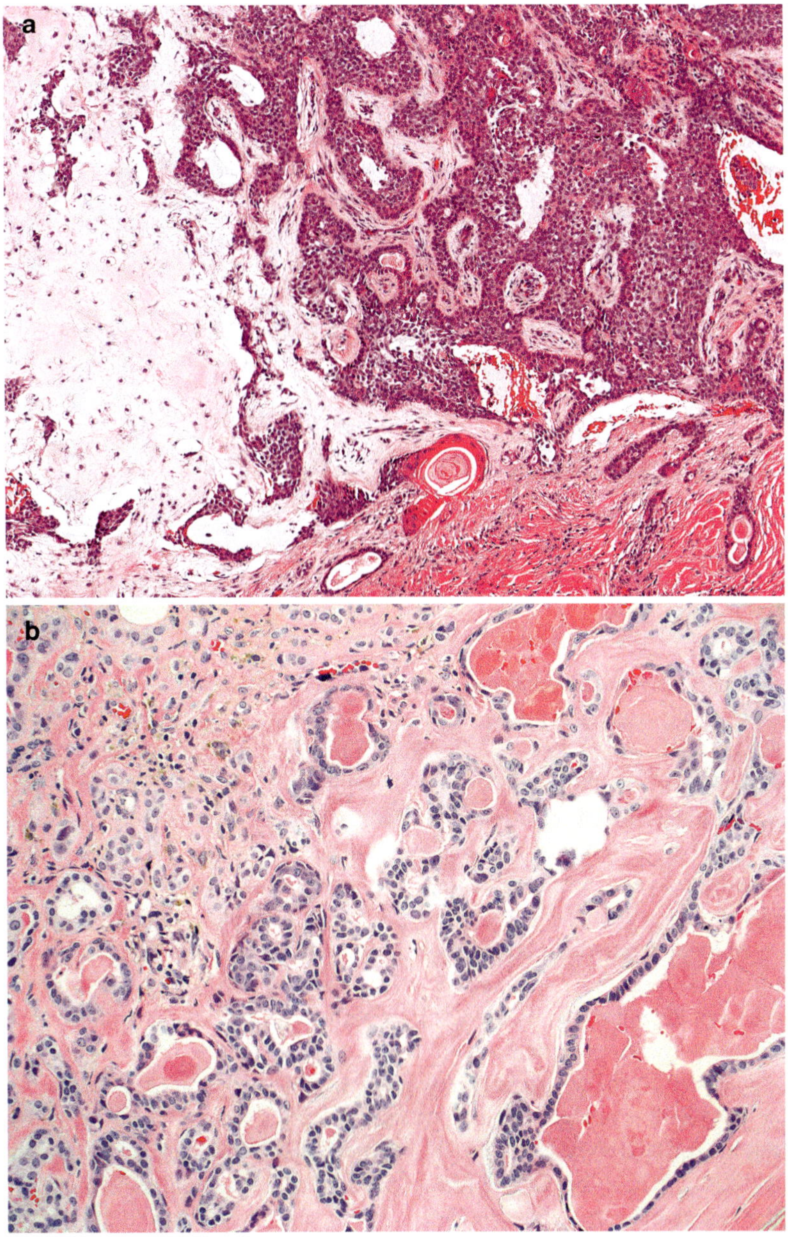

Fig. 12.39 Cutaneous mixed tumor (chondroid syringoma). (**a**) An architecturally complex lesion composed of sheets and nests of myoepithelial cells in a chondromyxoid stroma showing focal tubuloductal differentiation. (**b**) The ducts are lined by single or multiple layers of cuboidal to columnar cells with uniform bland nuclei, inconspicuous nucleoli, and eosinophilic cytoplasm. This example shows a hyalinized stroma and hemosiderin deposits

Myoepitheliomas and myoepithelial carcinomas are multilobulated, often infiltrative masses, which are morphologically very heterogeneous. They are typically composed of epithelioid to plasmacytoid to spindle cells arranged in a variety of growth patterns including reticular, trabecular, nested, corded, fascicular, or solid patterns (Figs. 12.41, 12.42, and 12.43). The stroma is myxoid, collagenous/hyalinized, or chondroid (Fig. 12.44). Multiple growth patterns are often seen within the same tumor, but in some cases, a single pattern predominates. Heterologous differentiation in the form of cartilage, bone, squamous, or adipocytic metaplasia is also often seen in myoepitheliomas, but ductal differentiation is absent. Cytologically,

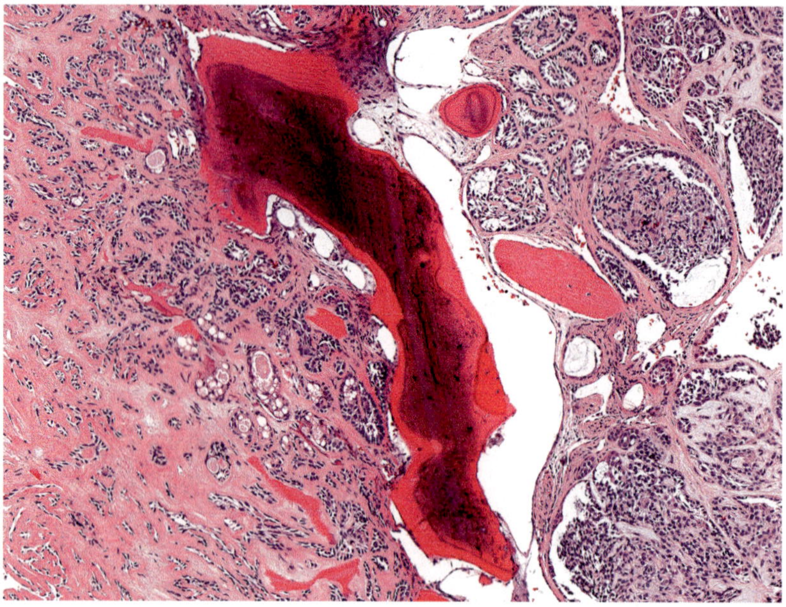

Fig. 12.40 Cutaneous mixed tumor (chondroid syringoma) showing glandular component and heterologous osseous differentiation

the cells have eosinophilic to amphophilic to clear cytoplasm and round to ovoid, uniform nuclei with inconspicuous or small nucleoli. Cases showing voluminous cytoplasm with vacuolization used to be referred to as "parachordomas." Myoepitheliomas do not have significant cytologic atypia. Normal mitotic figures may be observed.

Myoepithelial carcinomas have cytoarchitectural features similar to those of myoepitheliomas but demonstrate morphologic features of malignancy, including moderate to severe nuclear atypia with coarse or vesicular chromatin, prominent nucleoli or nuclear pleomorphism, increased mitotic activity, atypical mitotic figures, necrosis, and vascular invasion. Of all of these, myoepithelial carcinomas are defined largely by their significant nuclear atypia, as this feature most strongly correlates with aggressive behavior (Figs. 12.45, 12.46, and 12.47). Necrosis and increased mitotic activity alone are not used as criteria for malignancy.

Syncytial myoepitheliomas are relatively well-circumscribed, unencapsulated nodules usually centered in the dermis and abutting the overlying epidermis, and may show subcutaneous extension. They are composed of solid sheets of spindle, epithelioid, or histiocytoid cells with oval nuclei and eosinophilic cytoplasm without distinct cell borders, imparting a distinctive syncytial appearance at low power (Fig. 12.48a). There is no tubuloductal differentiation. At high power, the cells have cytologically banal oval nuclei with vesicular chromatin and a slightly granular quality to the cytoplasm, imparting an appearance similar to histiocytes (Fig. 12.48b). Multinucleated cells can be noted focally. Mitotic figures are uncommon, and there is no necrosis or vascular invasion. In contrast to classic myoepitheliomas that often have a prominent myxohyaline stroma, syncytial myoepitheliomas have very little or no associated stroma. Wispy collagen fibers and small myxoid islands can be seen, and a third of cases show chondro-osseous or adipocytic metaplasia (Fig. 12.49a). Some cases show entrapped epithelial structures (Fig. 12.49b). Recognition of adipocytic metaplasia and epithelial entrapment in these tumors is important, as these features can be misinterpreted as infiltrative growth, giving the impression of a more aggressive neoplasm. Prominent lymphoid aggregates may be seen, usually at the tumor periphery (Fig. 12.50).

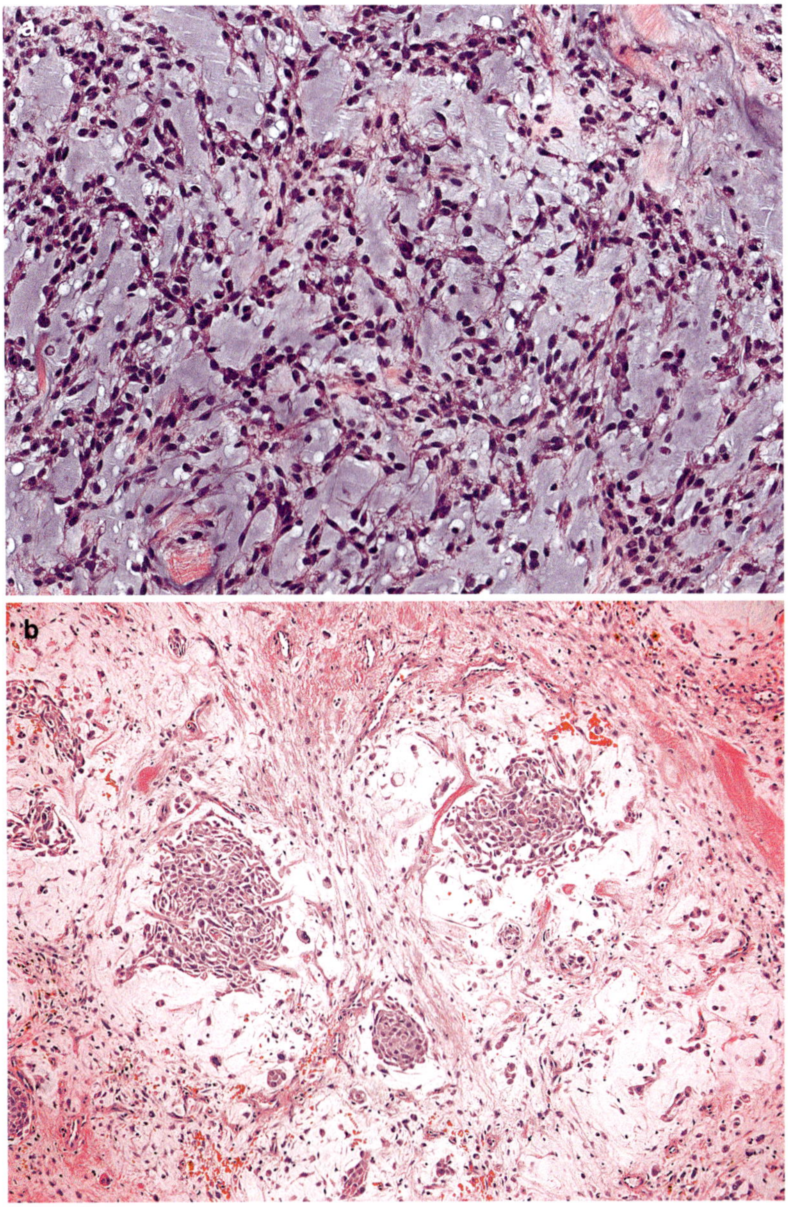

Fig. 12.41 Classic myoepithelioma. (**a**) Uniform myoepithelial cells arranged in a reticular pattern in a uniformly myxoid background. (**b**) Example of a nested growth pattern in a myxohyaline stroma containing prominent vessels

By immunohistochemistry, cutaneous mixed tumors, classic myoepitheliomas, and myoepithelial carcinomas consistently co-express cytokeratins, EMA, and S100 protein. SOX10, another robust marker of myoepithelial differentiation, can be seen in approximately 80% of mixed tumors and myoepitheliomas, but only in 30% of myoepithelial carcinomas. Expression of other myoepithelial markers such as p63, SMA, GFAP, and calponin is variable. SMARCB1/INI1 loss has been identified by immunohistochemistry in approximately 50% of myoepithelial carcinomas, especially in pediatric myoepithelial carcinomas with rhabdoid morphology. The immunoprofile of syncytial myoepitheliomas is somewhat different. These tumors frequently express EMA, usually diffusely, and S100 protein, which can be either diffuse or focal. Other myoepithelial markers like SOX10, p63, GFAP, and calponin are variably positive. In contrast to other myoepithelial tumors,

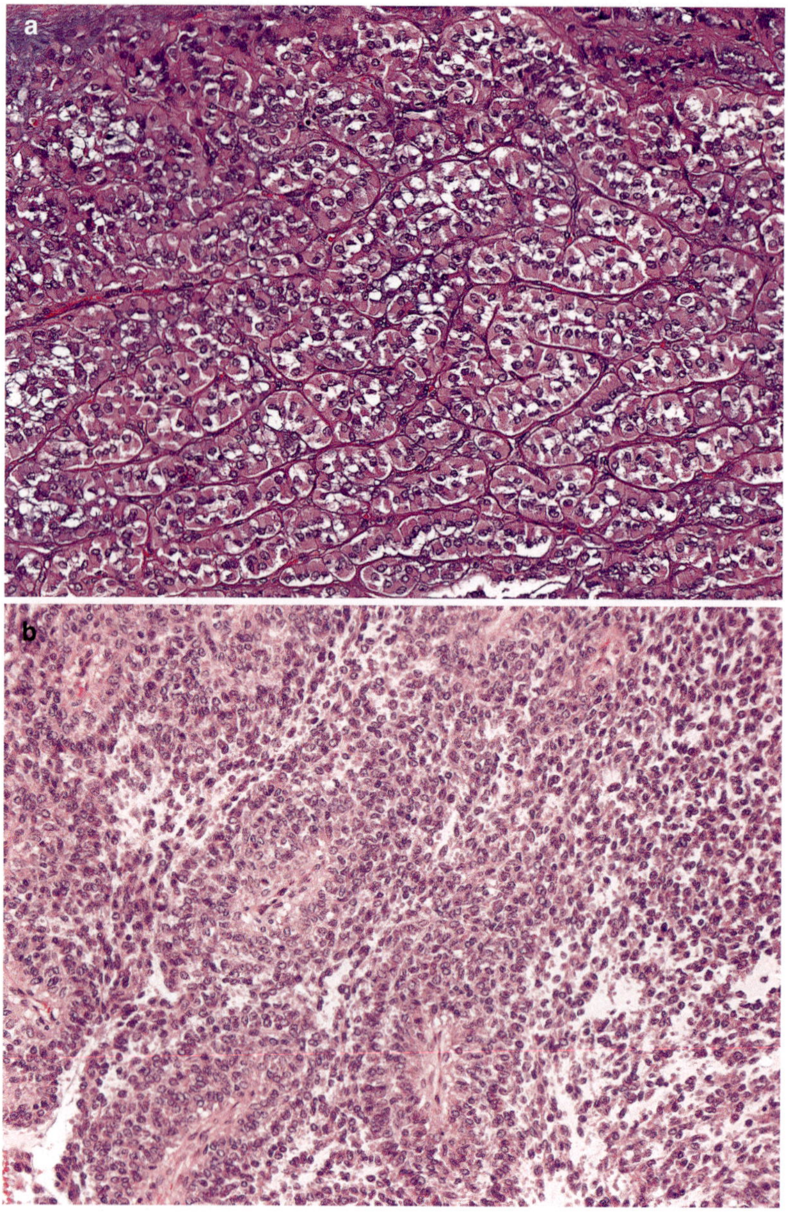

Fig. 12.42 Classic myoepithelioma. (**a**) Strikingly nested pattern composed of plasmacytoid myoepithelial cells with dense brightly eosinophilic cytoplasm (so-called hyaline cells). (**b**) In this example, the tumor cells are arranged in cords and perivascular rosettes

keratin expression is uncommon (approximately 10%) and is rarely diffuse. The INI1 expression pattern is uncertain (Table 12.10). Cutaneous mixed tumors often have *PLAG1* gene rearrangements analogous to the mixed tumors of the salivary gland and can show nuclear staining for PLAG1 by immunohistochemistry. Genetic findings in cutaneous myoepithelial tumors overlap with those found in myoepithelial tumors of soft tissue. *EWSR1* and, rarely, *FUS* gene rearrangements are found in approximately 50% of myoepithelial tumors of soft tissue and are more common in myoepithelial carcinomas. *PLAG1* gene rearrangements are usually negative in myoepithelial tumors that lack ductal differentiation, and it appears that *PLAG1*, *EWSR1*, and *FUS* rearrangements are mutually exclusive. A variety of fusion partners have been identified in *EWSR1*-

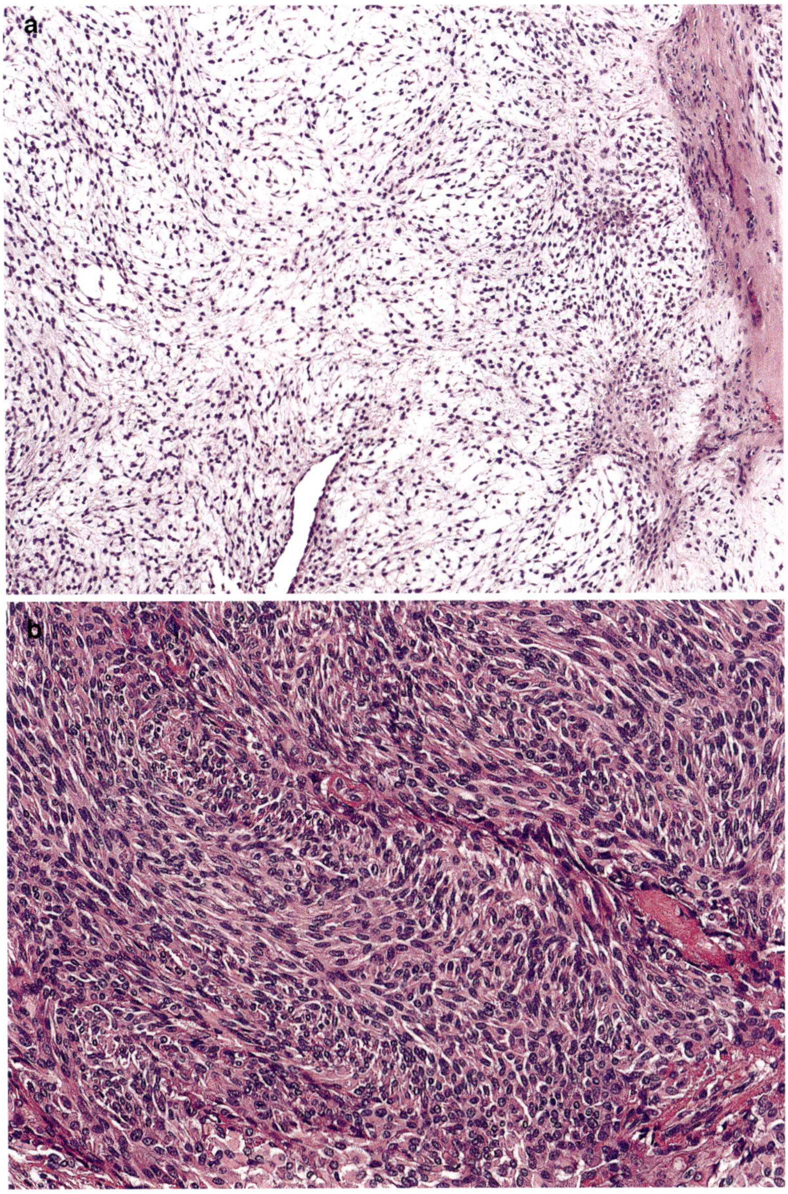

Fig. 12.43 Classic myoepithelioma. (**a**) Predominantly spindle cell tumor composed of short spindle cells uniformly distributed in a myxoid stroma. (**b**) An example of spindle cell myoepithelioma with fascicular growth which can mimic spindle cell sarcomas, fibroblastic neoplasms, and cellular schwannoma

rearranged myoepithelial tumors including *PBX1*, *POU5F1* (most common), *PBX3*, *ZNF444*, *ATF1*, and *KLF-17*. The latter can also be seen in *FUS*-rearranged cases. *EWSR1-POU5F1* fusion in deep soft tissue myoepithelial tumors is associated with young patient age and a distinctive clear cell morphology, whereas *PBX1* and *PBX3* translocations are seen in predominantly spindle cell examples, and *FUS-KLF17* fusions are observed in tumors with trabecular growth, bland epithelioid cells, and a hyalinized stroma. *EWSR1* gene rearrangement is less frequent in classic cutaneous myoepitheliomas (approximately 20–25%, with reported rates up to 44%) but is the most common rearrangement in syncytial myoepitheliomas (82% based on the largest series of 38 cases). The fusion gene partners in this subtype are yet to be completely defined. *FUS* gene rearrangement has not been observed in syncytial myoepitheliomas.

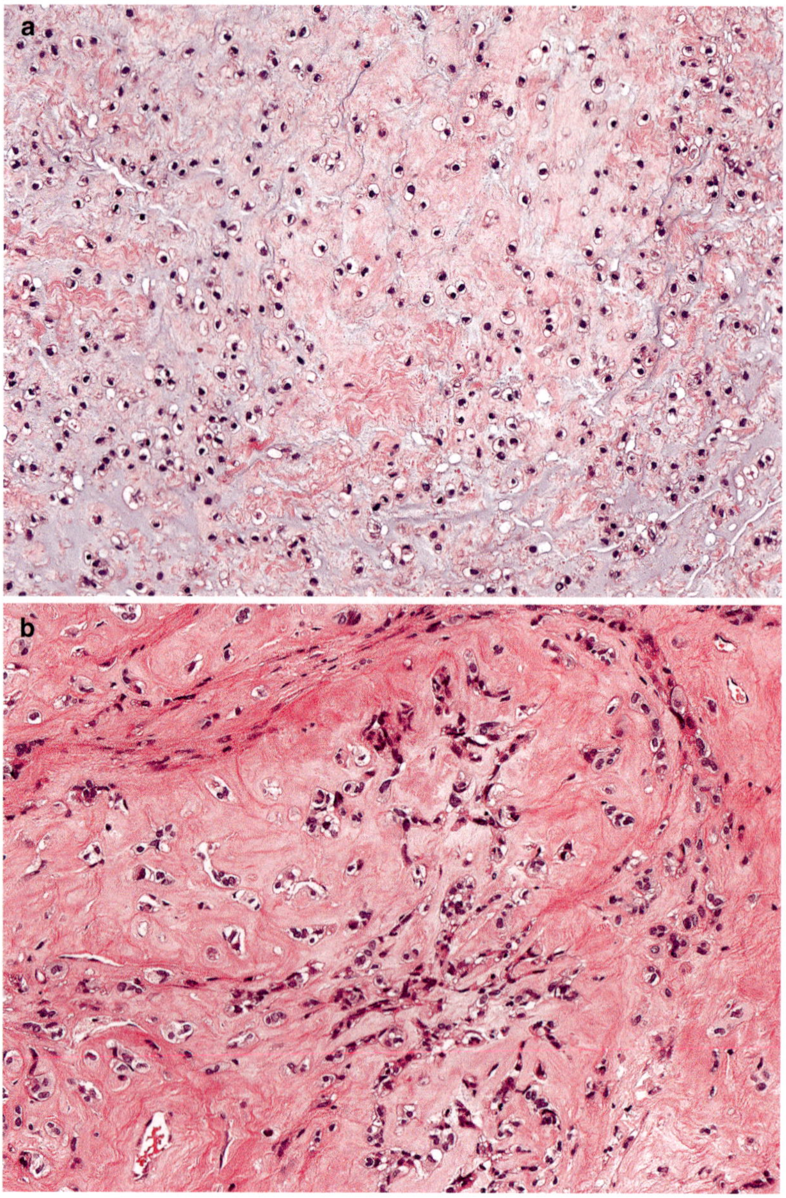

Fig. 12.44 Classic myoepithelioma. (**a**) Epithelioid myoepithelial cells with clear cytoplasm dispersed singly in a chondromyxoid stroma. (**b**) Corded growth pattern in a hyalinized stroma

Differential Diagnosis

Cutaneous mixed tumors rarely pose a diagnostic challenge once the presence of tubuloductal differentiation is recognized and the possibility of metastasis from mixed tumor of the salivary gland has been ruled out clinically. Glomus tumors with myxoid stroma can be confused with cutaneous mixed tumors based on the presence of their shared features of monomorphic epithelioid cells with bland nuclear features arranged in nests and sheets. However, glomus tumors do not form ducts but instead are characteristically arranged around prominent, often hyalinized vessels. A simple cytokeratin stain can resolve this dilemma in more challenging cases.

The differential diagnosis of classic cutaneous myoepitheliomas and myoepithelial carcinomas is dependent on the predominant histologic pattern. Tumors with epithelioid morphology and myxoid or myxohyaline stroma need to be distin-

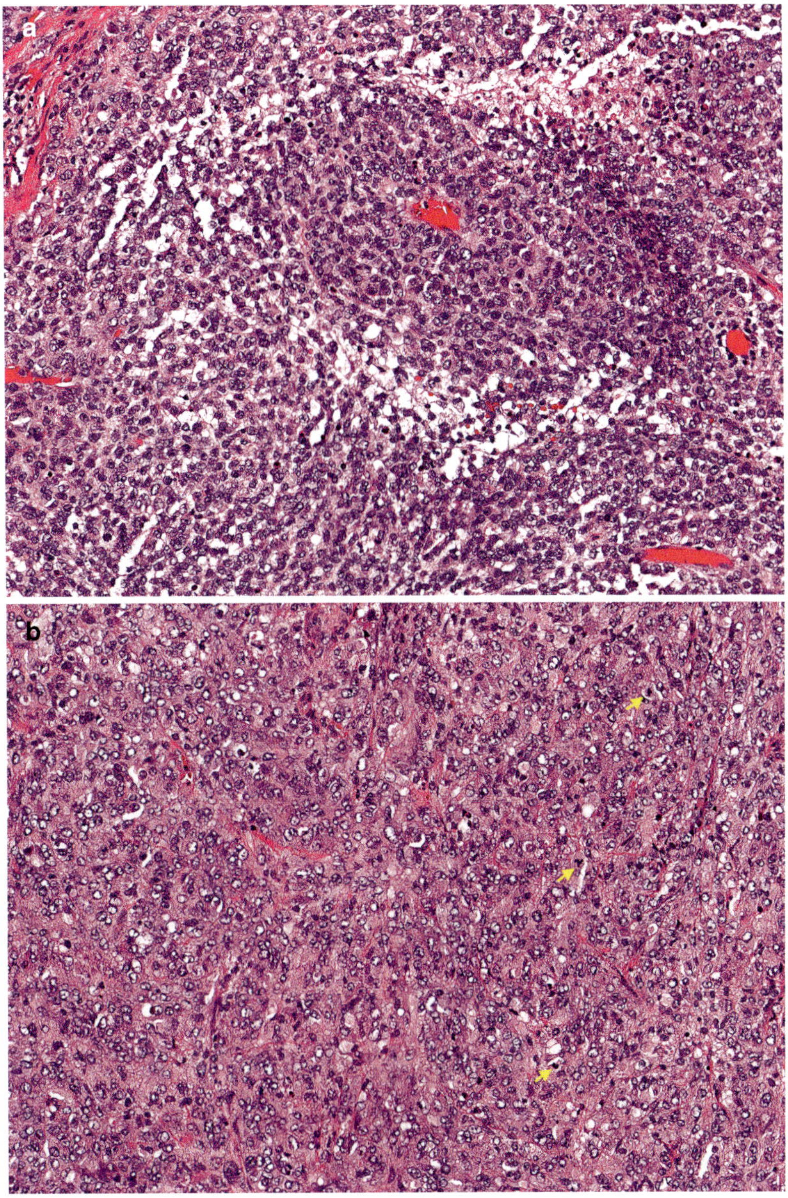

Fig. 12.45 Myoepithelial carcinoma. (**a**) The tumor shows increased cellularity and solid architectural arrangement. (**b**) Moderate-to-severe nuclear atypia with vesicular chromatin, prominent nucleoli, and frequent mitotic figures (arrows)

guished from ossifying fibromyxoid tumor, from epithelioid schwannoma, and, in malignant cases, from metastatic carcinomas, malignant melanoma, malignant ossifying fibromyxoid tumor, proximal-type epithelioid sarcoma, and epithelioid malignant peripheral nerve sheath tumor. Areas of heterologous osseous or cartilaginous differentiation may be confused with primary osseous and cartilaginous tumors of the skin and soft tissue, especially in limited biopsy material. Predominantly spindle cell myoepithelial tumors can be mistaken for fascicular neoplasms including nerve sheath tumors, synovial sarcoma, or fibrosarcomatous dermatofibrosarcoma protuberans. A very helpful morphologic clue is that classic myoepithelial tumors, irrespective of anatomic site, are quite heterogeneous in appearance, with a variety of cytoarchitectural patterns within the same neoplasm and the presence of at least focal myxoid stroma, in contrast to the above mimics. A notable exception is ossifying fibromyxoid tumor (discussed above), which might be virtu-

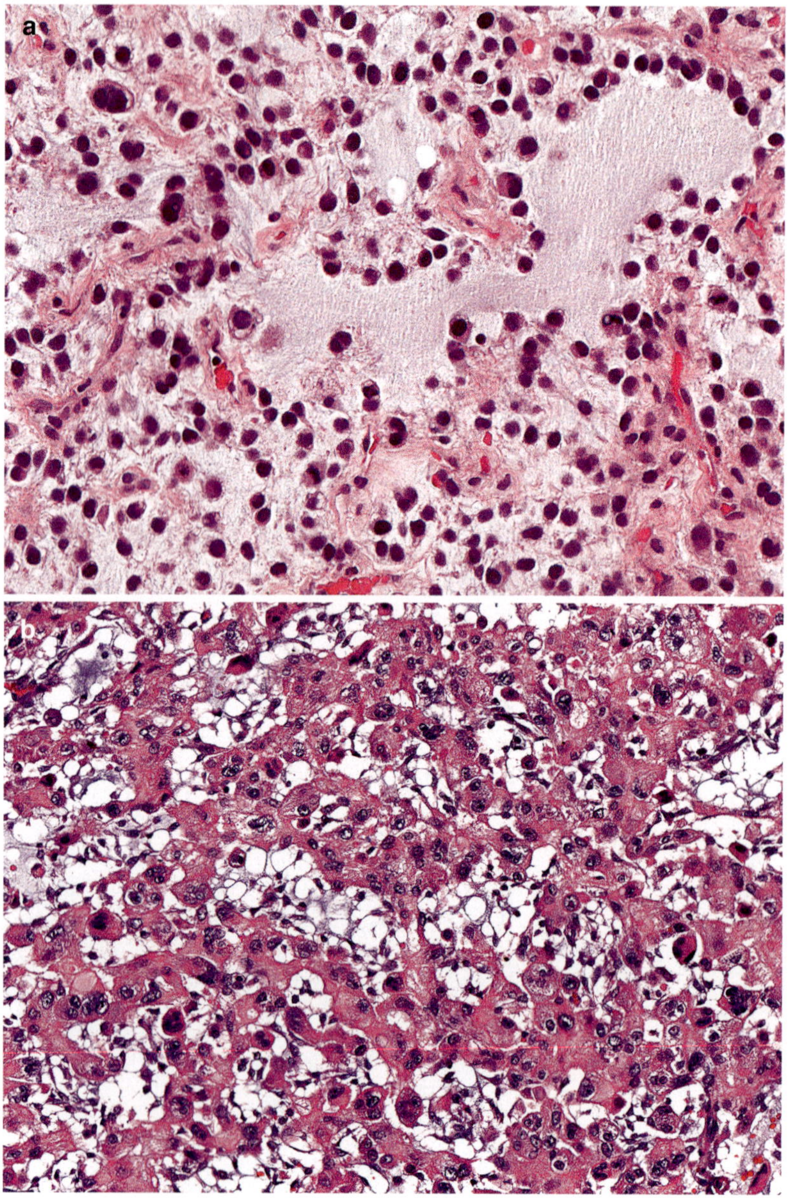

Fig. 12.46 Myoepithelial carcinoma. These examples show corded arrangement in a myxoid background with moderate (**a**) and severe (**b**) nuclear atypia and frequent mitotic figures

ally impossible to separate from myoepithelial tumors on morphologic grounds as it also consists of cytologically bland epithelioid or spindle cells arranged in various combinations of reticular, trabecular and nested patterns, within a fibromyxoid stroma. Cartilaginous and osseous differentiations are not uncommon in ossifying fibromyxoid tumor, although the latter usually takes the form of a peripheral rim of mature lamellar bone. Markers of myoepithelial differentiation such as p63, SMA, and particularly S100 protein are of limited value, because they are also expressed in ossifying fibromyxoid tumor. However, strong diffuse expression of keratins and EMA and SOX10 expression would favor a myoepithelial tumor, since these markers are expressed in only a small percentage of OFMTs and usually only focally. *PHF1* gene rearrangement characteristic of ossifying fibromyxoid tumor has not been described in myoepithelial tumors, which, in contrast, may demonstrate rearrangements of either *EWSR1* or

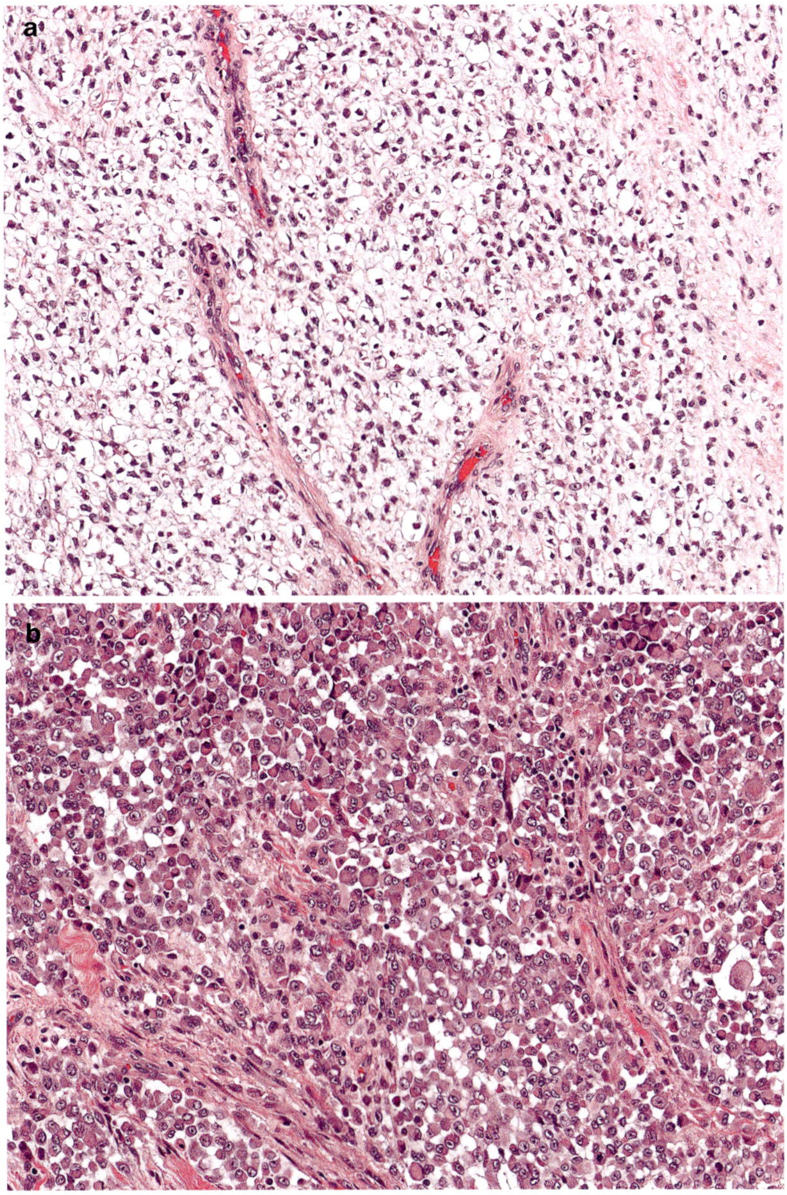

Fig. 12.47 Myoepithelial carcinoma. A nested arrangement of cells with abundant clear cell cytoplasm (**a**) and rhabdoid morphology showing globoid perinuclear eosinophilic inclusion (**b**)

PLAG1. Epithelioid schwannoma is also composed of epithelioid cells arranged in a nested or trabecular pattern in myxoid or collagenous stroma. Like myoepithelial tumors, epithelioid schwannomas express S100 protein and SOX10 and may show a loss of INI1 expression. The presence of a conventional schwannoma component, lack of cytokeratin expression, and a true capsule with EMA- or GLUT1-positive perineurial cells help to distinguish epithelioid schwannoma from myoepithelial tumors. With regard to the potential mimics of myoepithelial carcinoma, epithelioid malignant peripheral nerve sheath tumor is strongly and diffusely positive for S100 protein and variably positive for SOX10 and is usually negative for cytokeratins and other myoepithelial markers. INI1 IHC is not helpful as approximately 70% of epithelioid malignant peripheral nerve sheath tumors and 50% of myoepithelial carcinomas have loss of INI1

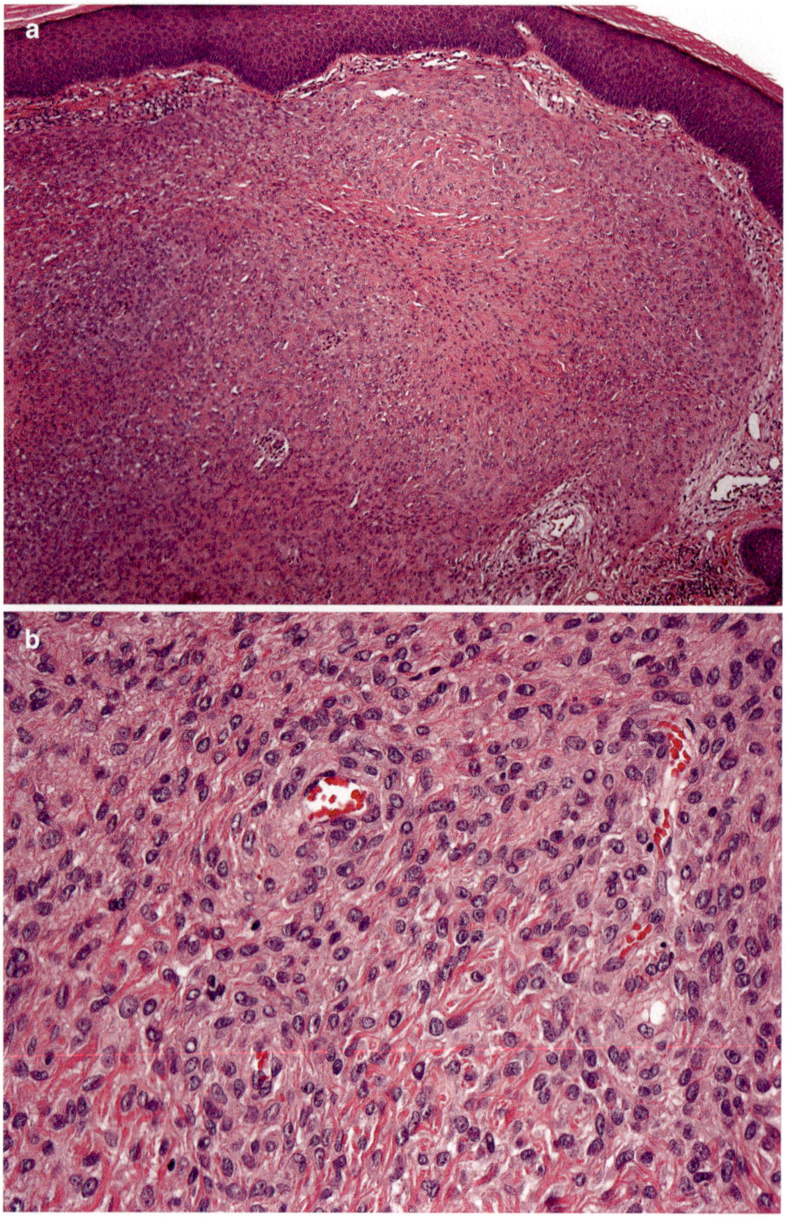

Fig. 12.48 Syncytial myoepithelioma. (**a**) Somewhat polypoid intradermal neoplasm with syncytial growth pattern abutting the overlying epidermis. (**b**) Sheets of benign epithelioid, spindle, or histiocytoid cells with banal oval nuclei, inconspicuous nucleoli, and eosinophilic, slightly granular cytoplasm with indistinct cytoplasmic borders (Photomicrographs courtesy of Dr. Vickie Jo, Brigham and Women's Hospital, Boston, MA)

expression. The differential diagnosis with proximal-type epithelioid sarcoma is discussed earlier in this chapter. Diffusely myxoid stroma as often seen in myoepithelial carcinomas is not a feature of either malignant peripheral nerve sheath tumor or epithelioid sarcoma.

Spindle cell predominant myoepithelial tumors can be confused with synovial sarcoma because of the biphasic growth pattern; monotonous nuclear features, especially in the lower-grade tumors; and expression of cytokeratins, EMA, and S100 protein. FISH testing for *SS18* gene rearrangement or RT-PCR for synovial sarcoma fusion products can readily distinguish synovial sarcoma from myoepithelial tumors. SOX10 expression, when present, is also quite helpful as this marker is not expressed in synovial sarcomas. Another potential mimic is cellular schwannoma,

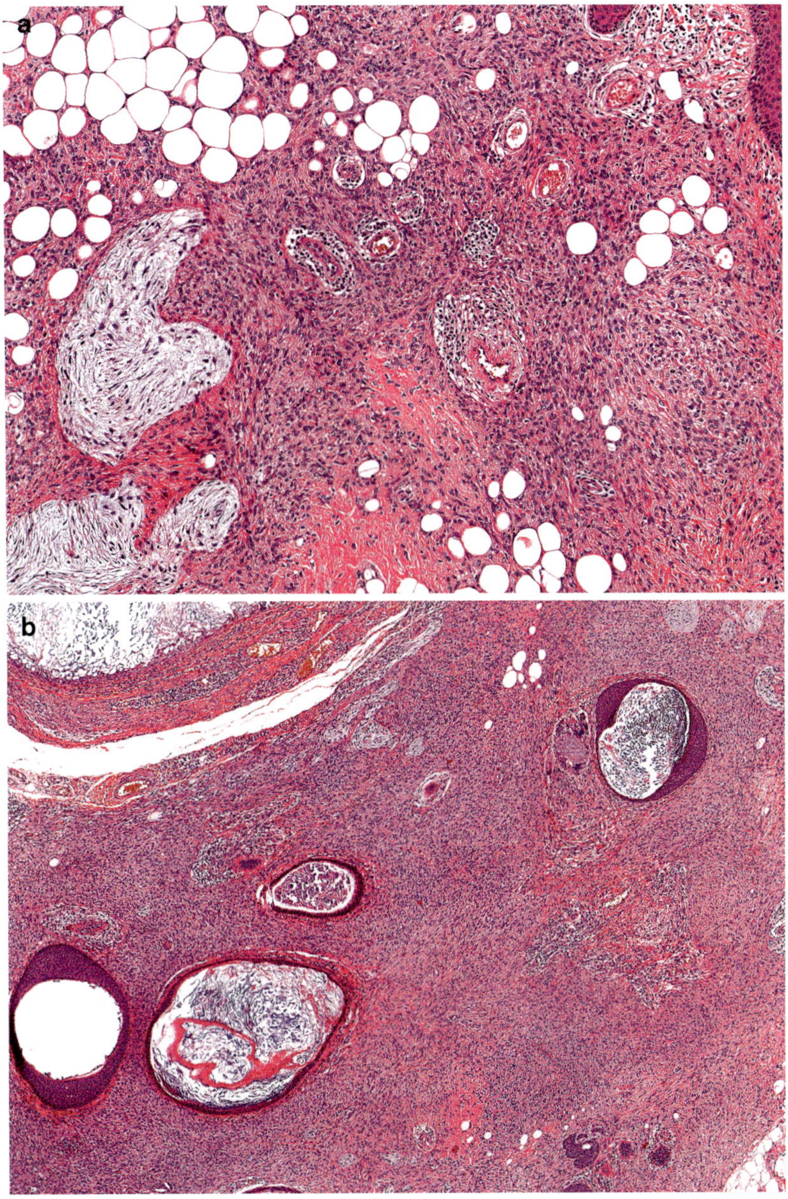

Fig. 12.49 Syncytial myoepithelioma. (**a**) In this example, small myxoid islands and prominent adipocytic metaplasia are noted. The latter may be mistaken for more infiltrative growth. (**b**) Entrapment of epithelial structures can be seen

which similarly expresses S100 protein and SOX10 proteins, but in contrast to myoepithelial tumors, it is negative for cytokeratins, EMA (which should be limited to the perineurial cells within the capsule), and other myoepithelial markers. Cutaneous fibroblastic neoplasms like fibrosarcomatous dermatofibrosarcoma protuberans lack expression of cytokeratins and myoepithelial markers. Distinction from metastatic carcinomas and malignant melanoma can be accomplished by select panel of immunohistochemical stains including cytokeratins (negative

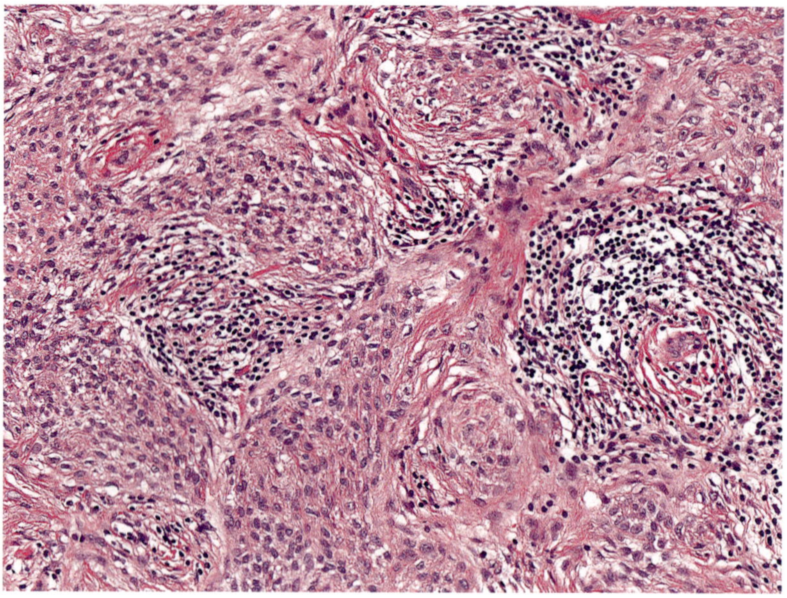

Fig. 12.50 Syncytial myoepithelioma. In this example, prominent lymphoid aggregates surround the sheets of myoepithelial cells

Table 12.10 Key pathologic features: cutaneous myoepithelial tumors

Cutaneous mixed tumor (chondroid syringoma) Defined by tubuloductal differentiation Analogous to the mixed tumors of salivary gland (pleomorphic adenoma) *PLAG1* gene rearrangement and nuclear PLAG1 expression by IHC
Classic myoepitheliomas Epithelioid, plasmacytoid, spindle, or clear myoepithelial cells arranged in reticular, trabecular, nested, corded, fascicular, or solid patterns Myxoid, myxohyaline, collagenous, or chondroid stroma Heterologous osseous, cartilaginous or squamous metaplasia Bland oval nuclei with open chromatin and inconspicuous nucleoli
Myoepithelial carcinomas The same architectural patterns as in classic myoepitheliomas Defined solely by the presence of moderate-to-severe nuclear atypia Necrosis and increased mitotic activity are often present but do not correlate well with aggressive behavior Rhabdoid or clear cell features may occur, especially in pediatric tumors
Chondroid syringomas and classic myoepithelial tumors co-express cytokeratins, EMA, and markers of myoepithelial differentiation: S100, SOX10, SMA, GFAP, p63
Syncytial myoepithelioma Distinctive intradermal variant with solid, syncytial growth of epithelioid, spindle, or histiocytoid myoepithelial cells Usually no intervening stroma except rare myxoid islands or wisps of collagen Bland oval nuclei with open chromatin and inconspicuous nucleoli; pale eosinophilic, slightly granular cytoplasm with indistinct borders; low mitotic activity Osteocartilaginous or adipocytic metaplasia; the latter can impart an infiltrative growth pattern Unique IHC pattern: co-expression of EMA and S100 (focal or diffuse) but infrequent (approximately 10%) expression of cytokeratins, usually only focally
EWSR1 gene rearrangement in up to 20% of cutaneous myoepitheliomas/myoepithelial carcinomas with classic morphology and in 80% of syncytial myoepitheliomas

in melanoma) and myoepithelial markers like S100 protein, SOX10, or SMA, typically not expressed in most carcinomas, with notable exception of S100 protein and SOX10 expression in carcinomas of the breast. FISH for *EWSR1* gene rearrangement or *PLAG1* immunohistochemistry can be attempted when the distinction between carcinoma and a mixed or myoepithelial tumor is problematic.

Syncytial myoepitheliomas may pose a diagnostic challenge as they differ morphologically and immunophenotypically from classic cutaneous myoepithelial tumors. The most clinically important lesions to distinguish syncytial myoepitheliomas from are melanocytic neoplasms like nevoid melanomas, especially when S100 expression is present. An immunohistochemical panel including other melanocytic markers, EMA, cytokeratins, and, in difficult cases, FISH for *EWSR1* gene rearrangement are helpful in excluding melanocytic neoplasms. Distal-type epithelioid sarcoma (discussed above) can demonstrate morphologic and immunohistochemical overlap with syncytial myoepithelioma as well. The constituent cells of epithelioid sarcoma are usually only mildly atypical and can look similar to those seen in syncytial myoepithelioma, and they variably co-express EMA and cytokeratins. However, the geographic necrosis, and nuclear palisading that characterizes distal-type epithelioid sarcoma, is not typical of syncytial myoepithelioma. Distal-type epithelioid sarcoma is usually negative for myoepithelial markers and expresses CD34 in 50% of cases. CD34 is negative in syncytial myoepithelioma, which also retains nuclear INI1 expression.

On the benign end of the spectrum, fibrohistiocytic tumors with epithelioid morphology like epithelioid fibrous histiocytoma (EFH), cellular neurothekeoma, and juvenile xanthogranuloma can resemble syncytial myoepithelioma. EFH usually presents as a well-circumscribed dermal nodule with an epidermal collarette, is composed of cytologically bland epithelioid or plasmacytoid cells with frequent binucleation, and can be positive for EMA. However, EFH lacks a distinctive syncytial growth pattern; rather, the cells are dispersed in prominent collagenous stroma containing variable vessels. Adipocytic metaplasia is not a characteristic of EFH. Immunohistochemistry is helpful as most EFHs show strong diffuse staining with Factor XIIIa and ALK and are consistently negative for S100 protein and other myoepithelial markers. Cellular neurothekeoma has histiocytoid cells that are arranged in a distinctive nodular or plexiform growth pattern separated by fibrous bands rather than forming syncytia. Cellular neurothekeoma lacks S100 protein, EMA, and other myoepithelial marker expression and does not have an *EWSR1* gene rearrangement. Juvenile xanthogranulomas might arguably resemble syncytial myoepithelioma if they lack Touton-type giant cells and foamy histiocytes, but these tumors are usually more polymorphous in appearance compared to syncytial myoepithelioma and frequently contain inflammatory cells, such as eosinophils. They are negative for S100 protein, EMA, and myoepithelial markers.

Selected References

1. Achtman JC, Pavlidakey PG, Zhang PJ, Elenitsas R, Gutman AB. Synovial sarcoma with cutaneous metastasis. J Cutan Pathol. 2016;43(1):85.
2. Alomari AK, Brown N, Andea AA, Betz BL, Patel RM. Cutaneous syncytial myoepithelioma: a recently described neoplasm which may mimic nevoid melanoma and epithelioid sarcoma. J Cutan Pathol. 2017;44(10):892.
3. Amin MB, Patel RM, Oliveira P, Cabrera R, Carneiro V, Preto M, Balzer B, Folpe AL. Alveolar soft-part sarcoma of the urinary bladder with urethral recurrence: a unique case with emphasis on differential diagnoses and diagnostic utility of an immunohistochemical panel including TFE3. Am J Surg Pathol. 2006 Oct;30(10):1322–5.
4. Antonescu CR, Tschernyavsky SJ, Woodruff JM, Jungbluth AA, Brennan MF, Ladanyi M. Molecular diagnosis of clear cell sarcoma: detection of EWS-ATF1 and MITF-M transcripts and histopathological and ultrastructural analysis of 12 cases. J Mol Diagn. 2002;4(1):44.
5. Antonescu CR, Zhang L, Chang NE, et al. EWSR1-POU5F1 fusion in soft tissue myoepithelial tumors. A molecular analysis of sixty-six cases, including soft tissue, bone, and visceral lesions, showing common involvement of the EWSR1 gene. Genes Chromosomes Cancer. 2010;49(12):1114.
6. Antonescu CR, Zhang L, Nielsen GP, Rosenberg AE, Dal Cin P, Fletcher CD. Consistent t(1;10) with

rearrangements of TGFBR3 and MGEA5 in both myxoinflammatory fibroblastic sarcoma and hemosiderotic fibrolipomatous tumor. Genes Chromosomes Cancer. 2011;50(10):757.
7. Antonescu CR, Zhang L, Shao SY, et al. Frequent PLAG1 gene rearrangements in skin and soft tissue myoepithelioma with ductal differentiation. Genes Chromosomes Cancer. 2013;52(7):675.
8. Antonescu CR, Sung YS, Chen CL, et al. Novel ZC3H7B-BCOR, MEAF6-PHF1, and EPC1-PHF1 fusions in ossifying fibromyxoid tumors – molecular characterization shows genetic overlap with endometrial stromal sarcoma. Genes Chromosomes Cancer. 2014;53(2):183.
9. Atanaskova Mesinkovska N, Buehler D, McClain CM, Rubin BP, Goldblum JR, Billings SD. Ossifying fibromyxoid tumor: a clinicopathologic analysis of 26 subcutaneous tumors with emphasis on differential diagnosis and prognostic factors. J Cutan Pathol. 2015;42(9):622.
10. Bahrami A, Dalton JD, Krane JF, Fletcher CD. A subset of cutaneous and soft tissue mixed tumors are genetically linked to their salivary gland counterpart. Genes Chromosomes Cancer. 2012;51(2):140.
11. Boland JM, Folpe AL. Hemosiderotic fibrolipomatous tumor, pleomorphic hyalinizing angiectatic tumor, and myxoinflammatory fibroblastic sarcoma: related or not? Adv Anat Pathol. 2017;24(5):268.
12. Browne TJ, Fletcher CD. Haemosiderotic fibrolipomatous tumour (so-called haemosiderotic fibrohistiocytic lipomatous tumour): analysis of 13 new cases in support of a distinct entity. Histopathology. 2006;48(4):453.
13. Calder KB, Schlauder S, Morgan MB. Malignant perivascular epithelioid cell tumor ('PEComa'): a case report and literature review of cutaneous/subcutaneous presentations. J Cutan Pathol. 2008;35(5):499.
14. Carter JM, Sukov WR, Montgomery E, et al. TGFBR3 and MGEA5 rearrangements in pleomorphic hyalinizing angiectatic tumors and the spectrum of related neoplasms. Am J Surg Pathol. 2014;38(9):1182.
15. Charli-Joseph Y, Saggini A, Vemula S, Weier J, Mirza S, LeBoit PE. Primary cutaneous perivascular epithelioid cell tumor: a clinicopathological and molecular reappraisal. J Am Acad Dermatol. 2014;71(6):1127.
16. Chase DR, Enzinger FM. Epithelioid sarcoma. Diagnosis, prognostic indicators, and treatment. Am J Surg Pathol. 1985;9(4):241.
17. Chbani L, Guillou L, Terrier P, et al. Epithelioid sarcoma: a clinicopathologic and immunohistochemical analysis of 106 cases from the French sarcoma group. Am J Clin Pathol. 2009;131(2):222.
18. Cheah AL, Billings SD, Goldblum JR, Carver P, Tanas MZ, Rubin BP. STAT6 rabbit monoclonal antibody is a robust diagnostic tool for the distinction of solitary fibrous tumor from its mimics. Pathology. 2014;46(5):389.
19. Chung EB, Enzinger FM. Malignant melanoma of soft parts. A reassessment of clear cell sarcoma. Am J Surg Pathol. 1983;7(5):405.
20. Demicco EG, Harms PW, Patel RM, et al. Extensive survey of STAT6 expression in a large series of mesenchymal tumors. Am J Clin Pathol. 2015;143(5):672.
21. Demicco EG, Wagner MJ, Maki RG, et al. Risk assessment in solitary fibrous tumors: validation and refinement of a risk stratification model. Mod Pathol. 2017;30(10):1433.
22. Doyle LA, Vivero M, Fletcher CD, Mertens F, Hornick JL. Nuclear expression of STAT6 distinguishes solitary fibrous tumor from histologic mimics. Mod Pathol. 2014;27(3):390.
23. El Beaino M, Araujo DM, Lazar AJ, Lin PP. Synovial sarcoma: advances in diagnosis and treatment identification of new biologic targets to improve multimodal therapy. Ann Surg Oncol. 2017;24(8):2145.
24. Emile JF, Abla O, Fraitag S, et al. Revised classification of histiocytoses and neoplasms of the macrophage-dendritic cell lineages. Blood. 2016;127(22):2672.
25. Enzinger FM, Weiss SW, Liang CY. Ossifying fibromyxoid tumor of soft parts. A clinicopathological analysis of 59 cases. Am J Surg Pathol. 1989;13(10):817.
26. Falconieri G, Bacchi CE, Luzar B. Cutaneous clear cell sarcoma: report of three cases of a potentially underestimated mimicker of spindle cell melanoma. Am J Dermatopathol. 2012;34(6):619.
27. Feasel PC, Cheah AL, Fritchie K, Winn B, Piliang M, Billings SD. Primary clear cell sarcoma of the head and neck: a case series with review of the literature. J Cutan Pathol. 2016;43(10):838.
28. Feasel P, Al-Ibraheemi A, Fritchie K, et al. Superficial solitary fibrous tumor: a series of 26 cases. Am J Surg Pathol. 2018;42(6):778–85.
29. Flieder DB, Moran CA. Primary cutaneous synovial sarcoma: a case report. Am J Dermatopathol. 1998;20(5):509.
30. Flucke U, Palmedo G, Blankenhorn N, Slootweg PJ, Kutzner H, Mentzel T. EWSR1 gene rearrangement occurs in a subset of cutaneous myoepithelial tumors: a study of 18 cases. Mod Pathol. 2011;24(11):1444.
31. Folpe AL, Deyrup AT. Alveolar soft-part sarcoma: a review and update. J Clin Pathol. 2006;59(11):1127.
32. Folpe AL, Kwiatkowski DJ. Perivascular epithelioid cell neoplasms: pathology and pathogenesis. Hum Pathol. 2010;41(1):1.
33. Folpe AL, Weiss SW. Ossifying fibromyxoid tumor of soft parts: a clinicopathologic study of 70 cases with emphasis on atypical and malignant variants. Am J Surg Pathol. 2003;27(4):421.
34. Folpe AL, Weiss SW. Pleomorphic hyalinizing angiectatic tumor: analysis of 41 cases supporting evolution from a distinctive precursor lesion. Am J Surg Pathol. 2004;28(11):1417.
35. Folpe AL, Mentzel T, Lehr HA, Fisher C, Balzer BL, Weiss SW. Perivascular epithelioid cell neoplasms of soft tissue and gynecologic origin: a clinicopathologic study of 26 cases and review of the literature. Am J Surg Pathol. 2005;29(12):1558.
36. Foo WC, Cruise MW, Wick MR, Hornick JL. Immunohistochemical staining for TLE1

distinguishes synovial sarcoma from histologic mimics. Am J Clin Pathol. 2011;135(6):839.
37. Foucar E, Rosai J, Dorfman R. Sinus histiocytosis with massive lymphadenopathy (Rosai-Dorfman disease): review of the entity. Semin Diagn Pathol. 1990;7(1):19.
38. Garces S, Medeiros LJ, Patel KP, et al. Mutually exclusive recurrent KRAS and MAP 2K1 mutations in Rosai-Dorfman disease. Mod Pathol. 2017;30(10):1367.
39. Gebre-Medhin S, Nord KH, Moller E, et al. Recurrent rearrangement of the PHF1 gene in ossifying fibromyxoid tumors. Am J Pathol. 2012;181(3):1069.
40. Graham RP, Weiss SW, Sukov WR, et al. PHF1 rearrangements in ossifying fibromyxoid tumors of soft parts: A fluorescence in situ hybridization study of 41 cases with emphasis on the malignant variant. Am J Surg Pathol. 2013;37(11):1751.
41. Guillou L, Wadden C, Coindre JM, Krausz T, Fletcher CD. "Proximal-type" epithelioid sarcoma, a distinctive aggressive neoplasm showing rhabdoid features. Clinicopathologic, immunohistochemical, and ultrastructural study of a series. Am J Surg Pathol. 1997;21(2):130.
42. Guillou L, Gebhard S, Coindre JM. Lipomatous hemangiopericytoma: a fat-containing variant of solitary fibrous tumor? Clinicopathologic, immunohistochemical, and ultrastructural analysis of a series in favor of a unifying concept. Hum Pathol. 2000a;31(9):1108.
43. Guillou L, Gebhard S, Coindre JM. Orbital and extraorbital giant cell angiofibroma: a giant cell-rich variant of solitary fibrous tumor? Clinicopathologic and immunohistochemical analysis of a series in favor of a unifying concept. Am J Surg Pathol. 2000b;24(7):971.
44. Hallor KH, Sciot R, Staaf J, et al. Two genetic pathways, t(1,10) and amplification of 3p11-12, in myxoinflammatory fibroblastic sarcoma, haemosiderotic fibrolipomatous tumour, and morphologically similar lesions. J Pathol. 2009;217(5):716.
45. Hantschke M, Mentzel T, Rutten A, et al. Cutaneous clear cell sarcoma: a clinicopathologic, immunohistochemical, and molecular analysis of 12 cases emphasizing its distinction from dermal melanoma. Am J Surg Pathol. 2010;34(2):216.
46. Hisaoka M, Ishida T, Kuo TT, et al. Clear cell sarcoma of soft tissue: a clinicopathologic, immunohistochemical, and molecular analysis of 33 cases. Am J Surg Pathol. 2008;32(3):452.
47. Hornick JL, Fletcher CD. Myoepithelial tumors of soft tissue: a clinicopathologic and immunohistochemical study of 101 cases with evaluation of prognostic parameters. Am J Surg Pathol. 2003;27(9):1183.
48. Hornick JL, Fletcher CD. Cutaneous myoepithelioma: a clinicopathologic and immunohistochemical study of 14 cases. Hum Pathol. 2004;35(1):14.
49. Hornick JL, Dal Cin P, Fletcher CD. Loss of INI1 expression is characteristic of both conventional and proximal-type epithelioid sarcoma. Am J Surg Pathol. 2009;33(4):542.
50. Huang SC, Chen HW, Zhang L, et al. Novel FUS-KLF17 and EWSR1-KLF17 fusions in myoepithelial tumors. Genes Chromosomes Cancer. 2015;54(5):267.
51. Jo VY, Antonescu CR, Zhang L, Dal Cin P, Hornick JL, Fletcher CD. Cutaneous syncytial myoepithelioma: clinicopathologic characterization in a series of 38 cases. Am J Surg Pathol. 2013;37(5):710.
52. Kacerovska D, Michal M, Nemcova J, et al. Crystal-deficient alveolar soft-part sarcoma with cutaneous involvement: a case report. Am J Dermatopathol. 2009;31(3):272.
53. Kao YC, Sung YS, Zhang L, Chen CL, Huang SC, Antonescu CR. Expanding the molecular signature of ossifying fibromyxoid tumors with two novel gene fusions: CREBBP-BCORL1 and KDM2A-WWTR1. Genes Chromosomes Cancer. 2017;56(1):42.
54. Kilpatrick SE, Hitchcock MG, Kraus MD, Calonje E, Fletcher CD. Mixed tumors and myoepitheliomas of soft tissue: a clinicopathologic study of 19 cases with a unifying concept. Am J Surg Pathol. 1997;21(1):13.
55. Kosemehmetoglu K, Vrana JA, Folpe AL. TLE1 expression is not specific for synovial sarcoma: a whole section study of 163 soft tissue and bone neoplasms. Mod Pathol. 2009;22(7):872.
56. Kroft SH. Rosai-Dorfman disease: familiar yet enigmatic. Semin Diagn Pathol. 2016;33(5):244.
57. Kutzner H, Mentzel T, Kaddu S, Soares LM, Sangueza OP, Requena L. Cutaneous myoepithelioma: an under-recognized cutaneous neoplasm composed of myoepithelial cells. Am J Surg Pathol. 2001;25(3):348.
58. Ladanyi M, Antonescu CR, Drobnjak M, et al. The precrystalline cytoplasmic granules of alveolar soft part sarcoma contain monocarboxylate transporter 1 and CD147. Am J Pathol. 2002;160(4):1215.
59. Lieberman PH, Brennan MF, Kimmel M, Erlandson RA, Garin-Chesa P, Flehinger BY. Alveolar soft-part sarcoma. A clinico-pathologic study of half a century. Cancer. 1989;63(1):1.
60. Liegl B, Hornick JL, Fletcher CD. Primary cutaneous PEComa: distinctive clear cell lesions of skin. Am J Surg Pathol. 2008;32(4):608.
61. Lin L, Skacel M, Sigel JE, et al. Epithelioid sarcoma: an immunohistochemical analysis evaluating the utility of cytokeratin 5/6 in distinguishing superficial epithelioid sarcoma from spindled squamous cell carcinoma. J Cutan Pathol. 2003;30(2):114.
62. Liu L, Perry AM, Cao W, et al. Relationship between Rosai-Dorfman disease and IgG4-related disease: study of 32 cases. Am J Clin Pathol. 2013;140(3):395.
63. Llamas-Velasco M, Mentzel T, Requena L, Palmedo G, Kasten R, Kutzner H. Cutaneous PEComa does not harbour TFE3 gene fusions: immunohistochemical and molecular study of 17 cases. Histopathology. 2013;63(1):122.
64. Mantilla JG, Goldberg-Stein S, Wang Y. Extranodal Rosai-Dorfman disease: clinicopathologic series of 10 patients with radiologic correlation and review of the literature. Am J Clin Pathol. 2016;145(2):211.

65. Marshall-Taylor C, Fanburg-Smith JC. Hemosiderotic fibrohistiocytic lipomatous lesion: ten cases of a previously undescribed fatty lesion of the foot/ankle. Mod Pathol. 2000;13(11):1192.
66. Menon MP, Evbuomwan MO, Rosai J, Jaffe ES, Pittaluga S. A subset of Rosai-Dorfman disease cases show increased IgG4-positive plasma cells: another red herring or a true association with IgG4-related disease? Histopathology. 2014;64(3):455.
67. Mentzel T, Requena L, Kaddu S, Soares de Aleida LM, Sangueza OP, Kutzner H. Cutaneous myoepithelial neoplasms: clinicopathologic and immunohistochemical study of 20 cases suggesting a continuous spectrum ranging from benign mixed tumor of the skin to cutaneous myoepithelioma and myoepithelial carcinoma. J Cutan Pathol. 2003;30(5):294.
68. Mentzel T, Reisshauer S, Rutten A, Hantschke M, Soares de Almeida LM, Kutzner H. Cutaneous clear cell myomelanocytic tumour: a new member of the growing family of perivascular epithelioid cell tumours (PEComas). Clinicopathological and immunohistochemical analysis of seven cases. Histopathology. 2005;46(5):498.
69. Miettinen M, Fanburg-Smith JC, Virolainen M, Shmookler BM, Fetsch JF. Epithelioid sarcoma: an immunohistochemical analysis of 112 classical and variant cases and a discussion of the differential diagnosis. Hum Pathol. 1999;30(8):934.
70. Miettinen M, Finnell V, Fetsch JF. Ossifying fibromyxoid tumor of soft parts – a clinicopathologic and immunohistochemical study of 104 cases with long-term follow-up and a critical review of the literature. Am J Surg Pathol. 2008;32(7):996.
71. Miettinen M, McCue PA, Sarlomo-Rikala M, et al. Sox10 – a marker for not only schwannian and melanocytic neoplasms but also myoepithelial cell tumors of soft tissue: a systematic analysis of 5134 tumors. Am J Surg Pathol. 2015;39(6):826.
72. Mosquera JM, Fletcher CD. Expanding the spectrum of malignant progression in solitary fibrous tumors: a study of 8 cases with a discrete anaplastic component – is this dedifferentiated SFT? Am J Surg Pathol. 2009;33(9):1314.
73. Moyano S, Aguilera P, Petit A, et al. Alveolar soft part sarcoma presenting with cutaneous metastases: report of a case with immunohistochemical and molecular characterization. J Am Acad Dermatol. 2009;61(1):117.
74. Naujokas A, Charli-Joseph Y, Ruben BS, et al. SOX-10 expression in cutaneous myoepitheliomas and mixed tumors. J Cutan Pathol. 2014;41(4):353.
75. Panagopoulos I, Mertens F, Isaksson M, Mandahl N. Absence of mutations of the BRAF gene in malignant melanoma of soft parts (clear cell sarcoma of tendons and aponeuroses). Cancer Genet Cytogenet. 2005;156(1):74.
76. Patel RM, Downs-Kelly E, Weiss SW, Folpe AL, Tubbs RR, Tuthill RJ, Goldblum JR, Skacel M. Dual-color, break-apart fluorescence in situ hybridization for EWS gene rearrangement distinguishes clear cell sarcoma of soft tissue from malignant melanoma. Mod Pathol. 2005 Dec;18(12):1585–90.
77. Portera CA Jr, Ho V, Patel SR, et al. Alveolar soft part sarcoma: clinical course and patterns of metastasis in 70 patients treated at a single institution. Cancer. 2001;91(3):585.
78. Robinson DR, Wu YM, Kalyana-Sundaram S, et al. Identification of recurrent NAB2-STAT6 gene fusions in solitary fibrous tumor by integrative sequencing. Nat Genet. 2013;45(2):180.
79. Schofield JB, Krausz T, Stamp GW, Fletcher CD, Fisher C, Azzopardi JG. Ossifying fibromyxoid tumour of soft parts: immunohistochemical and ultrastructural analysis. Histopathology. 1993;22(2):101.
80. Smith ME, Fisher C, Weiss SW. Pleomorphic hyalinizing angiectatic tumor of soft parts. A low-grade neoplasm resembling neurilemoma. Am J Surg Pathol. 1996;20(1):21.
81. Solomon DA, Antonescu CR, Link TM, O'Donnell RJ, Folpe AL, Horvai AE. Hemosiderotic fibrolipomatous tumor, not an entirely benign entity. Am J Surg Pathol. 2013;37(10):1627.
82. Thway K, Fisher C. Synovial sarcoma: defining features and diagnostic evolution. Ann Diagn Pathol. 2014;18(6):369.
83. Thway K, Fisher C. PEComa: morphology and genetics of a complex tumor family. Ann Diagn Pathol. 2015;19(5):359.
84. Varela-Duran J, Enzinger FM. Calcifying synovial sarcoma. Cancer. 1982;50(2):345.
85. Wang WL, Mayordomo E, Zhang W, et al. Detection and characterization of EWSR1/ATF1 and EWSR1/CREB1 chimeric transcripts in clear cell sarcoma (melanoma of soft parts). Mod Pathol. 2009;22(9):1201.
86. Williams A, Bartle G, Sumathi VP, et al. Detection of ASPL/TFE3 fusion transcripts and the TFE3 antigen in formalin-fixed, paraffin-embedded tissue in a series of 18 cases of alveolar soft part sarcoma: useful diagnostic tools in cases with unusual histological features. Virchows Arch. 2011;458(3):291.
87. Zreik RT, Carter JM, Sukov WR, et al. TGFBR3 and MGEA5 rearrangements are much more common in "hybrid" hemosiderotic fibrolipomatous tumor-myxoinflammatory fibroblastic sarcomas than in classical myxoinflammatory fibroblastic sarcomas: a morphological and fluorescence in situ hybridization study. Hum Pathol. 2016;53:14.

13 Miscellaneous Mesenchymal Tumors: Smooth Muscle, Skeletal Muscle, Cartilaginous, and Osseous Tumors

Steven D. Billings and Rajiv M. Patel

Abstract

This chapter will cover a variety of cutaneous mesenchymal tumors including those with smooth muscle, skeletal muscle, and cartilaginous and osseous differentiation. Entities covered include leiomyoma, angioleiomyoma, smooth muscle hamartoma, leiomyosarcoma, rhabdomyomatous mesenchymal hamartoma, rhabdomyosarcoma, soft tissue chondroma, extraskeletal myxoid chondrosarcoma, osteoma cutis, fibro-osseous pseudotumor, and extraskeletal osteosarcoma.

Leiomyoma

Clinical Features

Cutaneous leiomyomas may be sporadic or hereditary and typically arise in young to middle-aged adults. Sporadic leiomyomas may be solitary or multiple and usually present as painful papules or nodules on the extensor surface, head and neck, or trunk. A second subset of leiomyomas arises in the genital skin or the nipple. In contrast to leiomyomas arising at most cutaneous sites, tumors in these locations tend to be painless. Genital tumors are discussed in more detail in Chap. 11. Heritable forms present as multiple lesions and are associated with hereditary leiomyomatosis and renal cell cancer (HLRCC) syndrome, also known as multiple cutaneous and uterine leiomyomatosis syndrome (Reed syndrome), which is an autosomal dominant disorder related to mutations of the fumarate hydratase gene. Almost all affected women with this disorder have uterine leiomyomas, and close to 80% of patients have cutaneous manifestations. Between 10% and 34% of patients have renal cell carcinoma, typically papillary type 2 renal cell carcinoma. The renal tumors usually present in middle age and have a 70% mortality rate. Other tumors associated with the syndrome include urothelial carcinoma, prostate carcinoma, gastrointestinal stromal tumor, pheochromocytoma, testicular Leydig cell tumor, adrenal adenoma, ovarian cystadenoma, and benign renal cysts. Cutaneous leiomyomas are frequently the presenting sign of the syndrome. The presence of cutaneous leiomyomas should prompt investigation of the patient's clinical history to determine if additional testing to rule out HLRCC syndrome is warranted. Cutaneous leiomyomas are benign and may be cured by simple excision if it is clinically practical to excise in the case of multiple lesions.

S. D. Billings (✉)
Department of Pathology, Cleveland Clinic, Cleveland, OH, USA
e-mail: billins@ccf.org

R. M. Patel
Department of Pathology, University of Michigan Medical School, Ann Arbor, MI, USA

S. D. Billings et al. (eds.), *Soft Tissue Tumors of the Skin*,
https://doi.org/10.1007/978-1-4939-8812-9_13

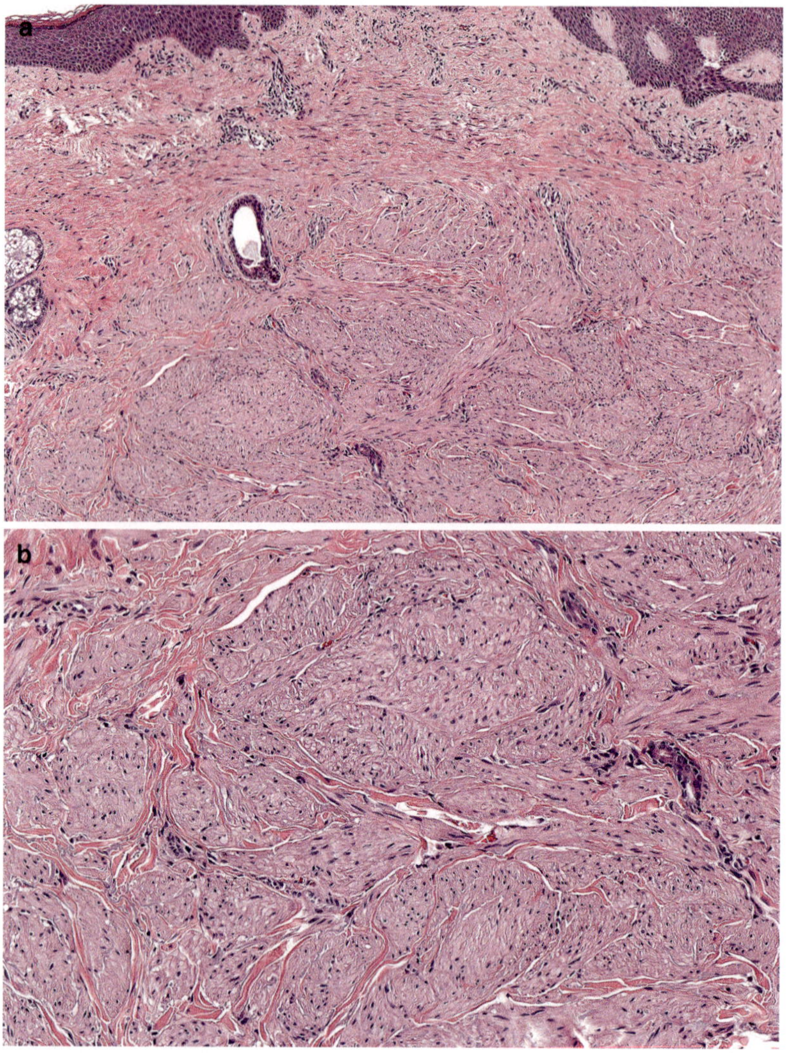

Fig. 13.1 Leiomyoma. (**a**) Poorly circumscribed proliferation of smooth muscle bundles in the dermis. (**b**) Higher-power image demonstrating intersecting fascicles and bland nuclear features

Pathologic Features

Cutaneous leiomyomas may be comprised of pilar or genital/nipple smooth muscle. The pilar leiomyomas are composed of a poorly circumscribed proliferation of haphazard intersecting fascicles of histologically bland smooth muscle tissue in the reticular dermis (Fig. 13.1a). The tumor cells are spindle shaped and have elongated blunt-ended (cigar-shaped) nuclei with abundant eosinophilic cytoplasm (Fig. 13.1b). Occasional tumor cells may show perinuclear cytoplasmic vacuoles. Genital and nipple leiomyomas are similar in appearance. Genital tumors are discussed in more detail in Chap. 11.

There is no reliable way to morphologically distinguish sporadic leiomyomas from those associated with HLRCC syndrome. However, the latter tend to have slightly increased nuclear atypia (Fig. 13.2a), but this is not a reliable discriminator. The uterine leiomyomas associated with HLRCC often have prominent nucleoli, unlike non-HLRCC-associated uterine leiomyomas. While genetic testing is the gold standard, immunostains for fumarate hydratase may be utilized, with HLRCC-associated tumors lacking expression in comparison to sporadic tumors (Fig. 13.2b). The sensitivity and specificity of immunohistochemical stains for fumarate hydratase are approximately 83% and 75%,

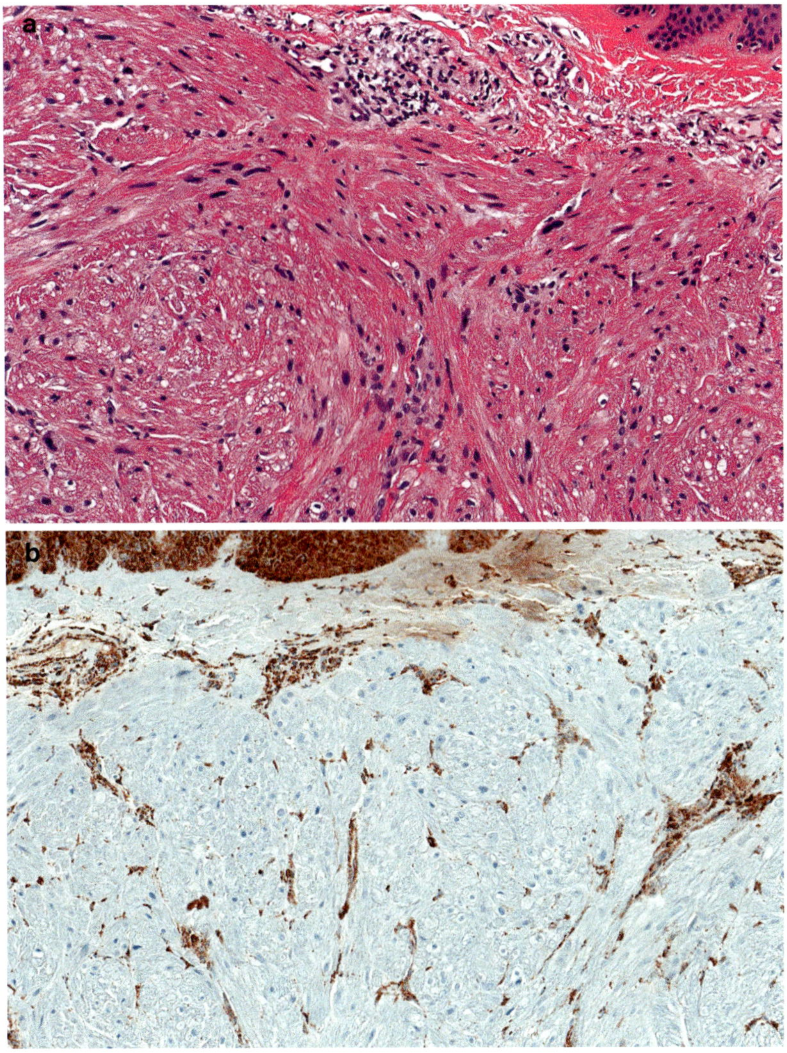

Fig. 13.2 Leiomyoma associated with HLRCC syndrome. (**a**) Leiomyomas with this syndrome tend to have increased nuclear atypia compared with sporadic leiomyomas. (**b**) Immunostains for fumarate hydratase are typically negative in the neoplastic cells

Table 13.1 Key pathologic features: leiomyoma

Intersecting fascicles
Bland spindled cells with elongated nuclei and eosinophilic cytoplasm
Pilar and nipple tumors poorly circumscribed
Genital tumors well-circumscribed
SMA and desmin positive

respectively. Both sporadic leiomyomas and HLRCC-associated leiomyomas are positive for SMA, desmin, and H-caldesmon. Rare cases may be positive for cytokeratin, but these lesions are consistently negative for S100 protein, SOX10, and CD34 (Table 13.1).

Differential Diagnosis

The primary differential diagnosis is with cutaneous leiomyosarcoma (see below). Leiomyosarcomas have more atypia and mitotic activity than leiomyomas. It should be stated that rare (≤1 per 10 HPF) mitotic figures may be seen in cutaneous leiomyomas. Leiomyomas may have degenerative atypia, leading to designation as so-called symplastic leiomyomas. Diagnostic criteria for cutaneous symplastic leiomyomas are not well established. It is our recommendation that this diagnosis be approached with caution. Any significant atypia should warrant conservative but complete excision.

Dermatomyofibroma (see Chap. 4) has horizontally oriented fascicles of myofibroblasts rather than an intersecting growth pattern. The tumor cells of dermatomyofibroma are usually desmin negative.

Congenital Smooth Muscle Hamartoma

Clinical Features

Congenital smooth muscle hamartoma most commonly presents in the lumbosacral region or proximal extremities of infants, as an indurated plaque with perifollicular papules. Coarse hairs may be present.

Pathologic Features

Microscopically, these lesions resemble pilar leiomyomas, being composed of poorly circumscribed, haphazardly arranged fascicles of bland smooth muscle cells (Fig. 13.3a, b). There is sometimes overlying epidermal change consisting of hyperkeratosis, acanthosis, and hyperpigmentation (Table 13.2).

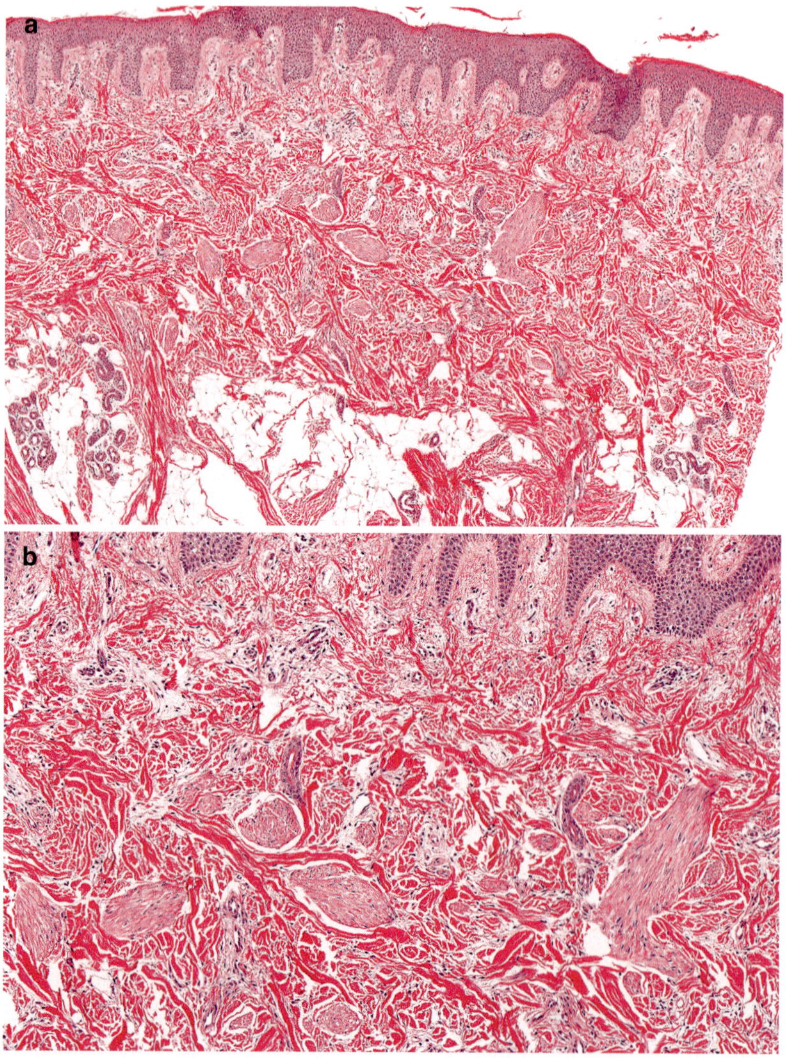

Fig. 13.3 Smooth muscle hamartoma. (**a**, **b**) Composed of smooth muscle bundles haphazardly arranged in the dermis

Table 13.2 Key pathologic features: congenital smooth muscle hamartoma

Presentation in infancy
Usually lumbosacral location
Haphazardly arranged fascicles of bland smooth muscle

Differential Diagnosis

Clinical presentation in infancy readily allows distinction from pilar leiomyoma. Congenital smooth muscle hamartoma also shares features with Becker nevus, but this entity also presents later in life and has more prominent epidermal change.

Epstein-Barr Virus-Associated Smooth Muscle Tumors

Clinical Features

Epstein-Barr virus (EBV)-associated smooth muscle tumors occur in the setting of immunosuppression, usually in the setting of AIDS and organ transplantation. Typically, they are deep soft tissue tumors, but rare presentation in the skin can occur. HIV-infected children may be particularly at risk. These lesions were formerly divided into benign and malignant tumors based on morphologic features, such as mitotic activity. It is now recognized that they are clinically indolent, provided that the underlying immunosuppression can be adequately addressed. There are rare reports of metastasis in the setting of HIV infection, but it is likely that these so-called metastatic lesions reflect multiple infectious events analogous to Kaposi sarcoma.

Pathologic Features

Histopathologically, Epstein-Barr virus (EBV)-associated smooth muscle tumors most commonly resemble angioleiomyoma (Fig. 13.4), but they may also resemble leiomyoma or leiomyosarcoma. Intratumoral lymphocytes are sometimes present. By immunohistochemistry, they are positive for smooth muscle markers. EBV RNA in situ hybridization (EBER-CISH) can be utilized to confirm the diagnosis (Table 13.3).

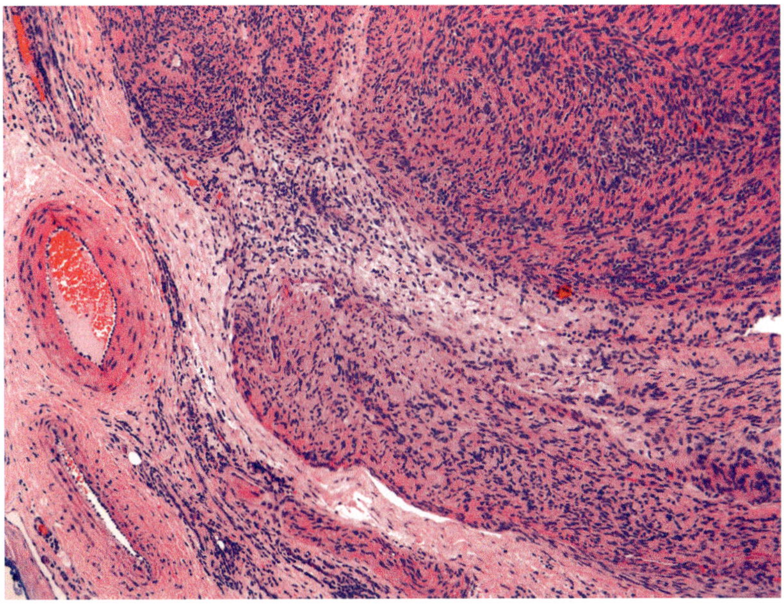

Fig. 13.4 EBV-associated smooth muscle tumor resembling angioleiomyoma. Note the intratumoral lymphocytes. (Courtesy of Dr. Wayne Grayson, Ampath National Laboratories, Johannesburg, South Africa)

Table 13.3 Key pathologic features: EBV-associated smooth muscle tumors

Occurs in immunosuppressed patients, especially in the setting of AIDS or transplantation
Frequently resembles angioleiomyoma and rarely leiomyosarcoma
EBER-CISH positive

Differential Diagnosis

The differential diagnosis depends on the predominant histologic features but generally includes angioleiomyoma, leiomyoma, and leiomyosarcoma. Knowledge of the clinical setting of immunosuppression should prompt consideration of EBER-CISH as a confirmatory test. The other entities in the differential diagnosis are not EBER-positive.

Leiomyosarcoma

Clinical Features

Superficial leiomyosarcomas are separated into those arising in the dermis and those arising in the subcutis. Those arising in the dermis are also called cutaneous leiomyosarcoma. These tumors usually arise in young adults in the extremities. They may be painful like pilar leiomyomas. The tumors arising in the subcutis present in older patients as subcutaneous masses, again most often involving the extremities. Metastatic leiomyosarcoma from deep soft tissue or uterine primary tumors has also been described.

The behavior of these lesions differs markedly depending on the anatomic location. Cutaneous leiomyosarcomas confined to the dermis have a risk of local recurrence, but essentially no risk of metastasis. For this reason some authors have proposed classifying them as "pleomorphic dermal smooth muscle tumors." However, there are rare reports of cutaneous leiomyosarcomas that have metastasized, typically those that show infiltration into the subcutis. We therefore prefer nomenclature that retains the term leiomyosarcoma. When reporting such cases, we comment on the low risk of aggressive behavior and recommend conservative but complete excision with clinical follow-up.

Leiomyosarcomas arising in the subcutis, however, behave in a distinctly different fashion. They arise from vascular smooth muscle and often demonstrate aggressive behavior with a mortality rate up to 50%.

Pathologic Features

The pathologic features depend on where the tumor arises. Cutaneous leiomyosarcomas somewhat resemble pilar leiomyomas. They are poorly circumscribed and usually composed of intersecting fascicles of tapered spindled cells with eosinophilic cytoplasm. They have increased nuclear atypia and mitotic activity, but necrosis and marked atypia are uncommon (Fig. 13.5). Tumors arising in the subcutis are variably infiltrative, and origin from a vessel wall is evident in some cases (Fig. 13.6). They often, though not invariably, have more pleomorphism and mitotic activity than their dermal counterparts. Rare cases have an epithelioid morphology (Table 13.4).

Metastatic leiomyosarcoma may involve the dermis or subcutis. Dermal metastases tend to be more circumscribed and have more pleomorphism than primary cutaneous leiomyosarcomas (Fig. 13.7).

Differential Diagnosis

Cutaneous leiomyomas with focal atypia need to be distinguished from cutaneous leiomyosarcoma. The latter has more diffuse atypia and greater mitotic activity. Atypical fibroxanthomas have a more random storiform to fascicular growth pattern rather than intersecting fascicles and a different clinical presentation. It should be noted that atypical fibroxanthoma is commonly positive for SMA, typically in a myofibroblastic "tram-track" pattern, but usually negative, or only focally positive, for desmin. Similarly, spindle cell squamous cell carcinomas may express

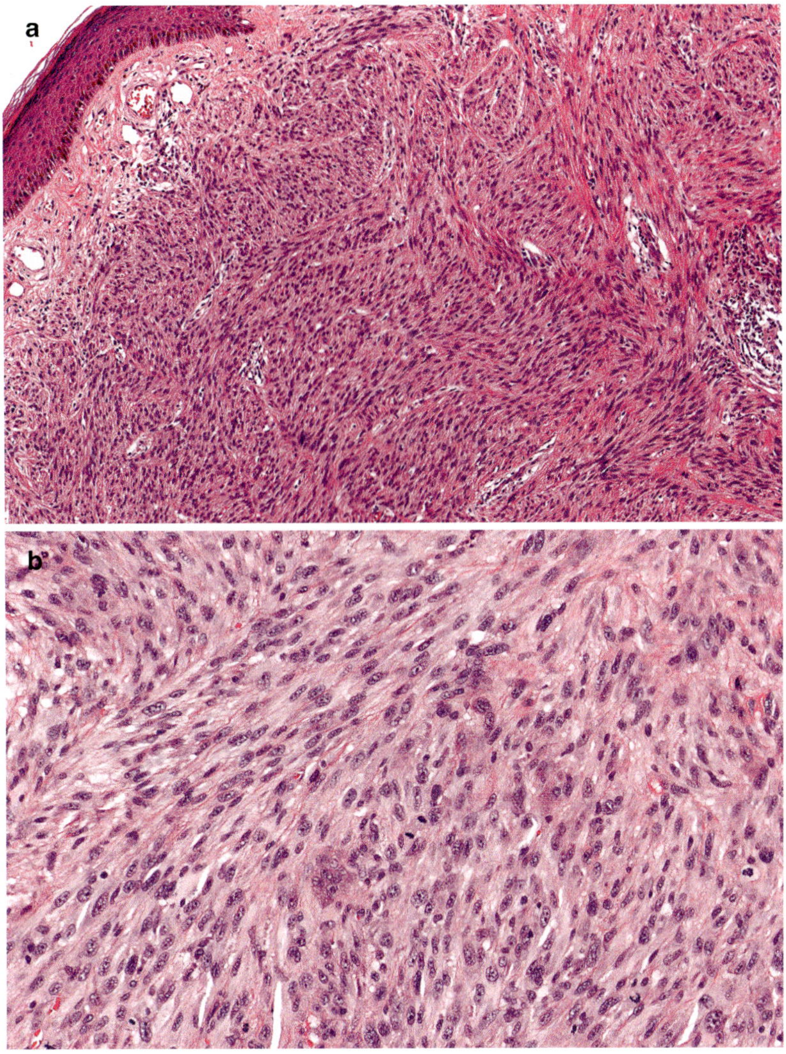

Fig. 13.5 Cutaneous leiomyosarcoma. (**a**) Intersecting fascicles of atypical smooth muscle with enlarged hyperchromatic nuclei. (**b**) Mitotic figures are typically conspicuous

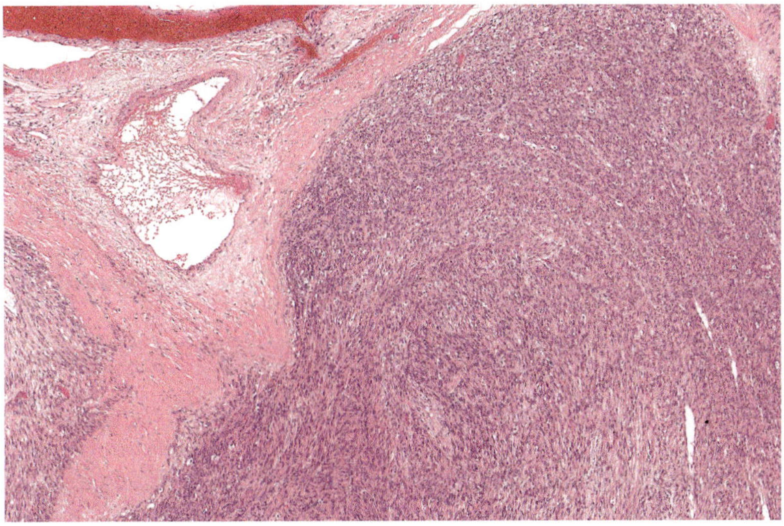

Fig. 13.6 Leiomyosarcoma arising within a vessel in subcutaneous tissue

Table 13.4 Key pathologic features: leiomyosarcoma

Intersecting fascicles of atypical spindled cells with eosinophilic cytoplasm
Nuclear atypia and mitotic activity
SMA and desmin positive
Tumors confined to the dermis have essentially no risk of metastasis
Tumors arising in the subcutis are aggressive with high rates of metastasis and mortality

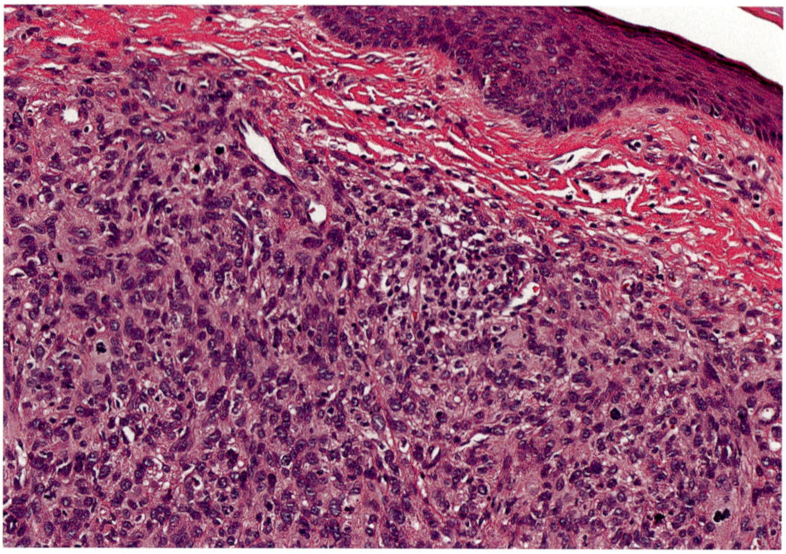

Fig. 13.7 Metastatic leiomyosarcoma. Metastatic tumors often show more atypia and are more circumscribed compared with primary cutaneous leiomyosarcomas

SMA in this pattern but are typically desmin negative. Also, spindle cell squamous cell carcinomas do not have the intersecting fascicular pattern typical of cutaneous leiomyosarcoma. It should be pointed out that rare cases of leiomyosarcoma can be focally keratin positive. Spindle cell melanomas are positive for S100 protein and SOX10. The tumor cells of cellular fibrous histiocytoma are less eosinophilic and negative for desmin. Peripheral collagen trapping, seen in cellular fibrous histiocytoma, is not seen in cutaneous leiomyosarcoma.

Subcutaneous leiomyosarcomas should be differentiated from undifferentiated pleomorphic sarcoma, soft tissue leiomyoma, and nodular fasciitis. Undifferentiated pleomorphic sarcoma usually has more diffuse pleomorphism and lacks an intersecting fascicular growth pattern. In certain cases immunostains may be required. Immunoreactivity for both SMA and desmin helps identify leiomyosarcoma. Soft tissue leiomyomas are quite rare. Any atypia and mitotic activity in a deep soft tissue smooth muscle tumor suggests the possibility of leiomyosarcoma, with perhaps pediatric tumors being the lone exception. Deep soft tissue leiomyomas may have rare mitotic figures. Nodular fasciitis sometimes is confused with leiomyosarcoma due to increased mitotic activity and immunoreactivity for SMA (usually in a myofibroblastic tram-track pattern). Nodular fasciitis has a loose storiform growth pattern with hemorrhage, myxoid stroma, and cystic breakdown, features not typical of leiomyosarcoma. The tumor cells of nodular fasciitis have more delicate, amphophilic cytoplasm and do not have nuclear atypia.

Rhabdomyoma

Clinical Features

Most rhabdomyomas present in deep soft tissue or the heart. The extra-cardiac cases are subdivided into adult and fetal types. Both types usually involve the head and neck and are more common in males. In the adult type, the tumors most commonly involve the salivary glands and oral cavity. The fetal type tends to present around the ear or orbit. These are benign tumors cured by simple excision.

Pathologic Features

The adult type is composed of large, polygonal cells with small nuclei and abundant eosinophilic cytoplasm with evident cross striations (Fig. 13.8). The fetal type is composed of variable amounts of immature round to spindled rhabdomyoblasts set in a myxoid stroma (Fig. 13.9a, b). They are immunoreactive for desmin, myoglobin, and muscle-specific actin. They may also be focally positive for SMA and S100 protein (Table 13.5).

Differential Diagnosis

Adult rhabdomyoma could potentially be confused with granular cell tumor. The granular nature of the cytoplasm of the latter and immunoreactivity for SOX10 easily allow distinction. Pleomorphic rhabdomyosarcoma has more nuclear atypia and mitotic activity. The lack of nuclear pleomorphism and mitotic activity also distinguishes fetal-type rhabdomyoma from embryonal rhabdomyosarcoma.

Rhabdomyomatous Mesenchymal Hamartoma

Clinical Features

This is a rare congenital lesion that presents on the head and neck in neonates and infants as a polyp resembling an acrochordon. Most present on the central face, but rare lesions involving the digits, vagina, and sternoclavicular area have been reported.

Pathologic Features

The tumor is composed of mature skeletal muscle with variable admixed adipose and fibrous tissue in the reticular dermis (Fig. 13.10) (Table 13.6).

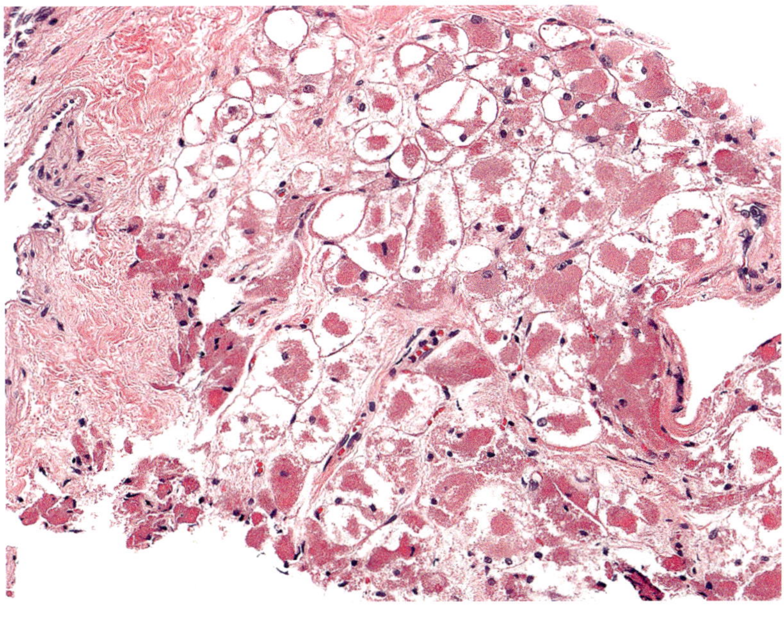

Fig. 13.8 Adult rhabdomyoma characterized by large, polygonal cells with abundant eosinophilic cytoplasm

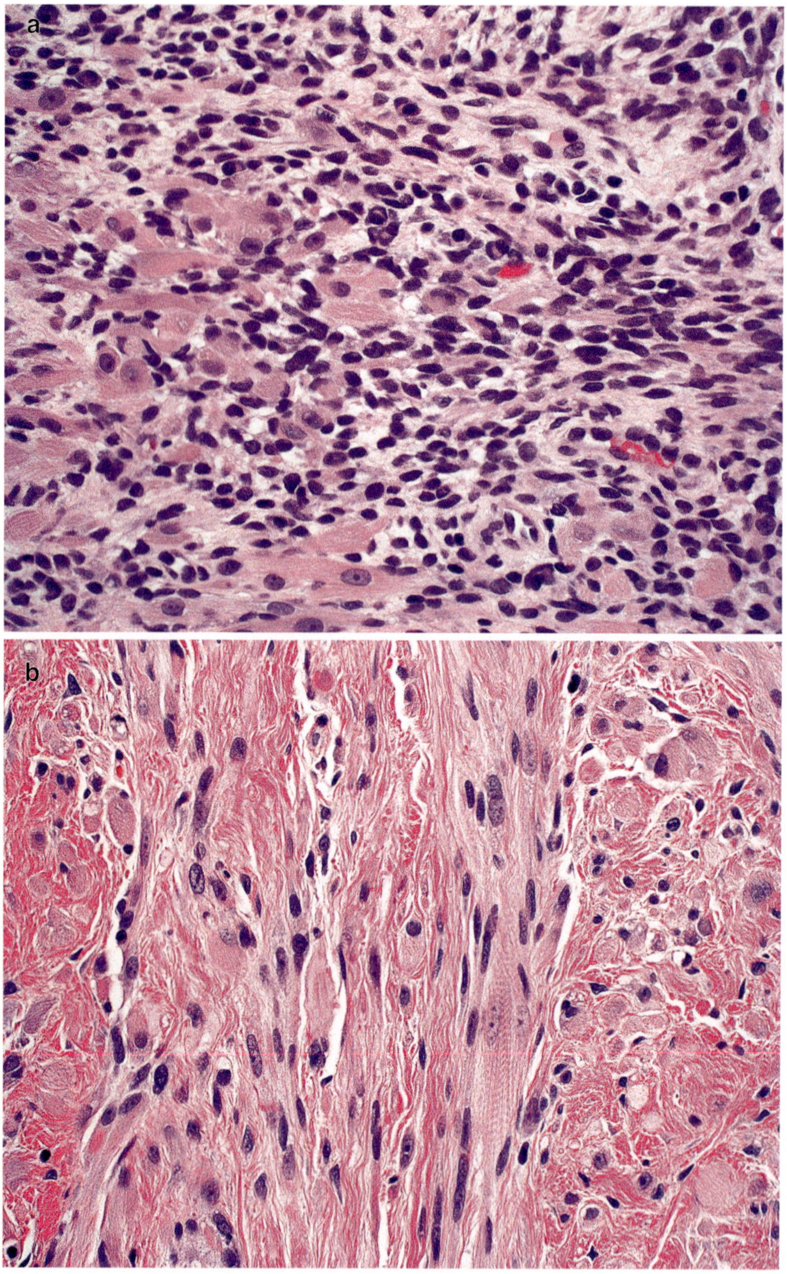

Fig. 13.9 Fetal rhabdomyoma. (**a**) Fetal rhabdomyoma predominantly composed of primitive, round rhabdomyoblasts. (**b**) Example of fetal rhabdomyoma composed predominantly of spindled rhabdomyoblasts

Table 13.5 Rhabdomyoma: key pathologic features

Adult-type rhabdomyoma Head and neck, especially the oral cavity and salivary glands Large polygonal cells with abundant eosinophilic cytoplasm Desmin+
Fetal-type rhabdomyoma Head and neck, especially around the ear and orbit Mixture of round to spindled rhabdomyoblasts in myxoid stroma No atypia or mitotic activity Desmin+

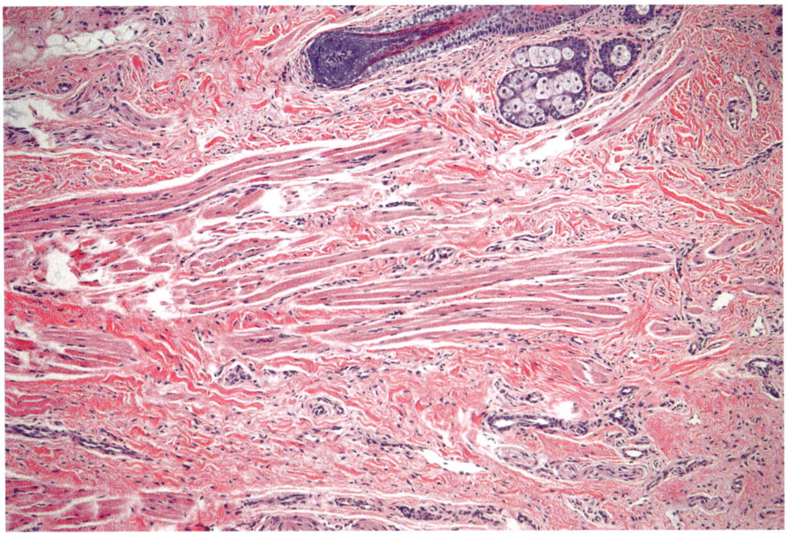

Fig. 13.10 Rhabdomyomatous mesenchymal hamartoma composed of elongated mature skeletal muscle fibers in the reticular dermis. (Courtesy of Dr. Cheryl Coffin, Vanderbilt University)

Table 13.6 Key pathologic features: rhabdomyomatous mesenchymal hamartoma

Polypoid cutaneous tumor of neonates and infants
Mature skeletal muscle admixed with adipocytes and fibrous tissue in the dermis

Differential Diagnosis

Rhabdomyomas may be considered in the differential diagnosis, as these tumors also most commonly present in the head and neck. However, they tend to be more deeply situated and do not present as cutaneous polypoid lesions. Adult-type rhabdomyomas have more polygonal cells, and fetal-type rhabdomyomas have immature spindled rhabdomyoblasts rather than the mature skeletal muscle of rhabdomyomatous mesenchymal hamartoma.

Cutaneous Rhabdomyosarcoma

Clinical Features

Primary cutaneous rhabdomyosarcoma is rare, and it is critical to exclude a metastasis before establishing this diagnosis. Like its deep soft tissue counterpart, there is a bimodal age distribution, with young patients and the elderly mainly being affected. Embryonal and alveolar rhabdomyosarcomas affect infants to teenaged children. Cutaneous embryonal rhabdomyosarcomas most commonly involve the head and neck, whereas the alveolar subtype usually arises in the extremities. Both subtypes may present in other cutaneous locations as well. In adults, the most common subtype reported is pleomorphic rhabdomyosarcoma, which often involves the head and neck and extremities. Only rare cases of cutaneous epithelioid rhabdomyosarcoma have been described. In our experience, they are more common in the head and neck. With the exception of the botryoid forms of embryonal rhabdomyosarcoma, the clinical presentation is not distinctive, with most lesions presenting as a cutaneous nodule or mass. While it is difficult to compare behavior of cutaneous rhabdomyosarcoma with deep soft tissue rhabdomyosarcoma due to their rarity, they appear to behave aggressively, with metastasis and/or significant mortality reported for all subtypes.

Pathologic Features

The histologic features are dependent on the subtype. Embryonal rhabdomyosarcoma is composed of uniform round to spindled cells with scant cytoplasm with alternating cellular and myxoid zones (Fig. 13.11a, b). Rhabdomyoblasts characterized by polygonal or spindled tumor cells with abundant eosinophilic cytoplasm may be present or entirely absent. Alveolar rhabdomyosarcoma is typically composed of aggregates of tumor cells separated by fibrous septa (Fig. 13.12). At the periphery of the aggregates, the tumor cells adhere to the surrounding stroma but are dyshesive centrally, resulting in the characteristic alveolar pattern. In some cases this pattern is absent or only focally present. The individual tumor cells have round to oval nuclei, which are somewhat larger and more atypical than the nuclei seen in embryonal rhabdomyosarcoma. Multinucleated tumor cells are also common and are a helpful diagnostic feature when present. Rhabdomyoblasts may be seen but are absent in the majority of cases. Pleomorphic rhabdomyosarcoma is composed of sheets of pleomorphic cells with abundant eosinophilic cytoplasm (pleomorphic rhabdomyoblasts) (Fig. 13.13). Epithelioid rhabdomyosarcoma is characterized by a sheetlike growth pattern of

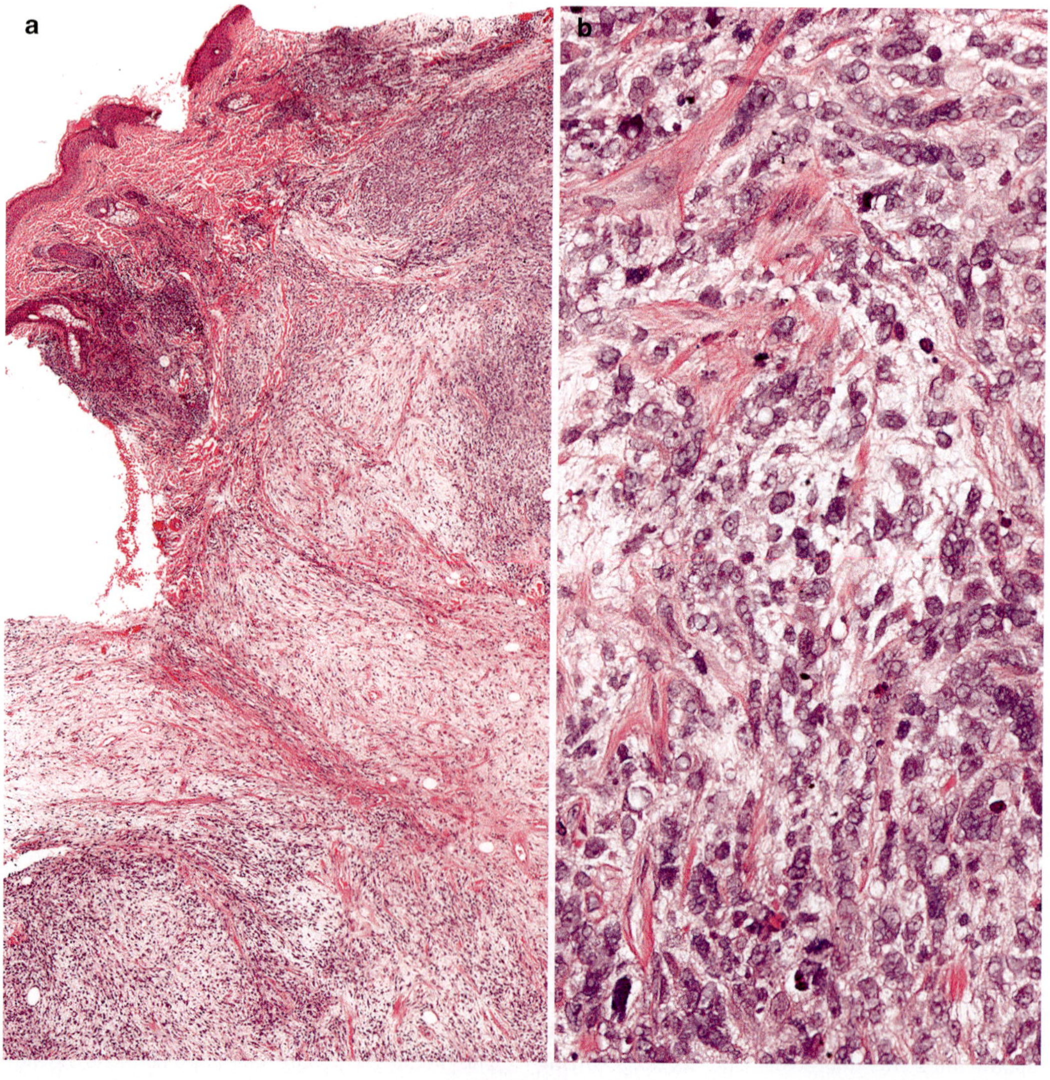

Fig. 13.11 Embryonal rhabdomyosarcoma (**a**) Low-power image demonstrating tumor cells in myxoid stroma involving the dermis. (**b**) High-power image demonstrating small relatively uniform round rhabdomyoblasts in myxoid stroma

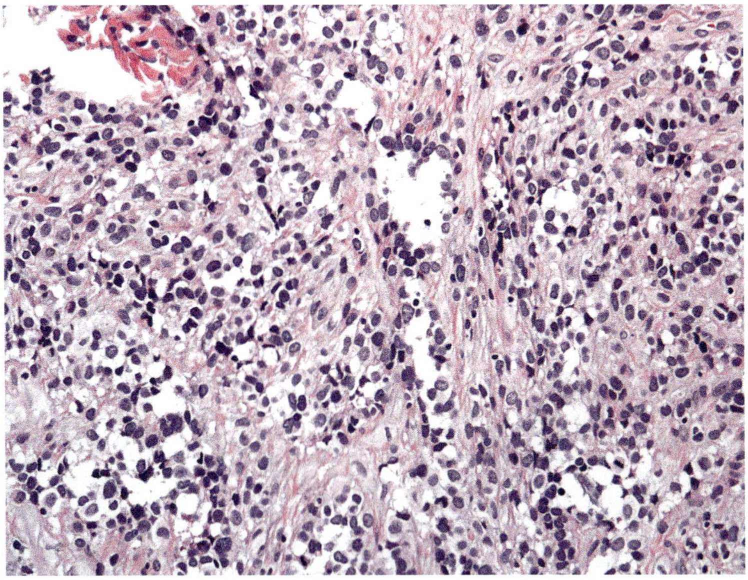

Fig. 13.12 Alveolar rhabdomyosarcoma characterized by dyshesive nests of tumor cells in an alveolar pattern

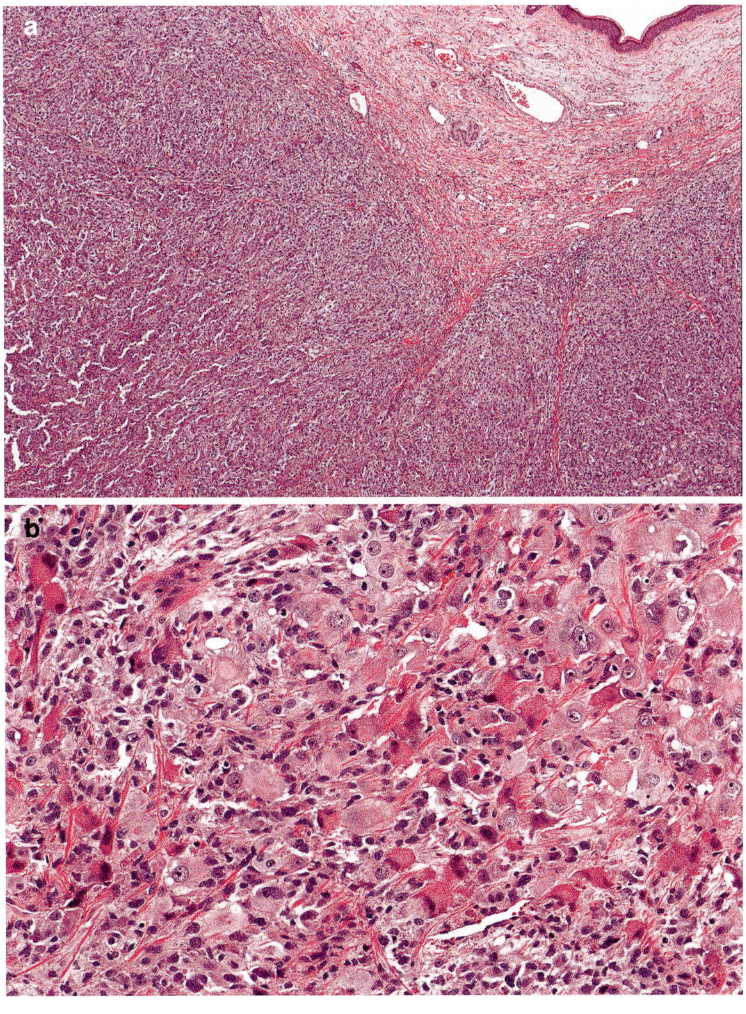

Fig. 13.13 Pleomorphic rhabdomyosarcoma. (**a**) Sheetlike growth pattern of tumor cells in the dermis. (**b**) High-power image demonstrating pleomorphic rhabdomyoblasts with abundant eosinophilic cytoplasm

uniform but atypical epithelioid tumor cells with vesicular nuclei, prominent nucleoli, and relatively abundant amphophilic to eosinophilic cytoplasm (Fig. 13.14) (Table 13.7).

By immunohistochemistry, all forms of rhabdomyosarcoma are positive for desmin and at least one specific skeletal muscle marker, myogenin and/or MYOD1. It should be noted that immunoreactivity for myogenin and MYOD1 is often patchy. Rhabdomyosarcomas are frequently positive for muscle-specific actin and variably positive for myoglobin as well. As a caveat, immunoreactivity for SMA, cytokeratin, neuroendocrine markers, CD99, and S100 protein may also be seen. When present, immunoreactivity for S100 protein and cytokeratin tends to be focal.

Most alveolar rhabdomyosarcomas have a recurrent t(2;13)(q35;q14) translocation resulting in a *PAX3-FOXO1* fusion. A variant t(1;13)(p36;q14) with a *PAX7-FOXO1* fusion is seen in a subset. Using break-apart FISH probes to detect the translocation can help confirm the diagnosis of alveolar rhabdomyosarcoma. However, cases morphologically consistent with the alveolar subtype may lack the translocation. In this setting the diagnosis should be based on the morphologic and immunohistochemical features. The other rhabdomyosarcoma subtypes lack recurring translocations.

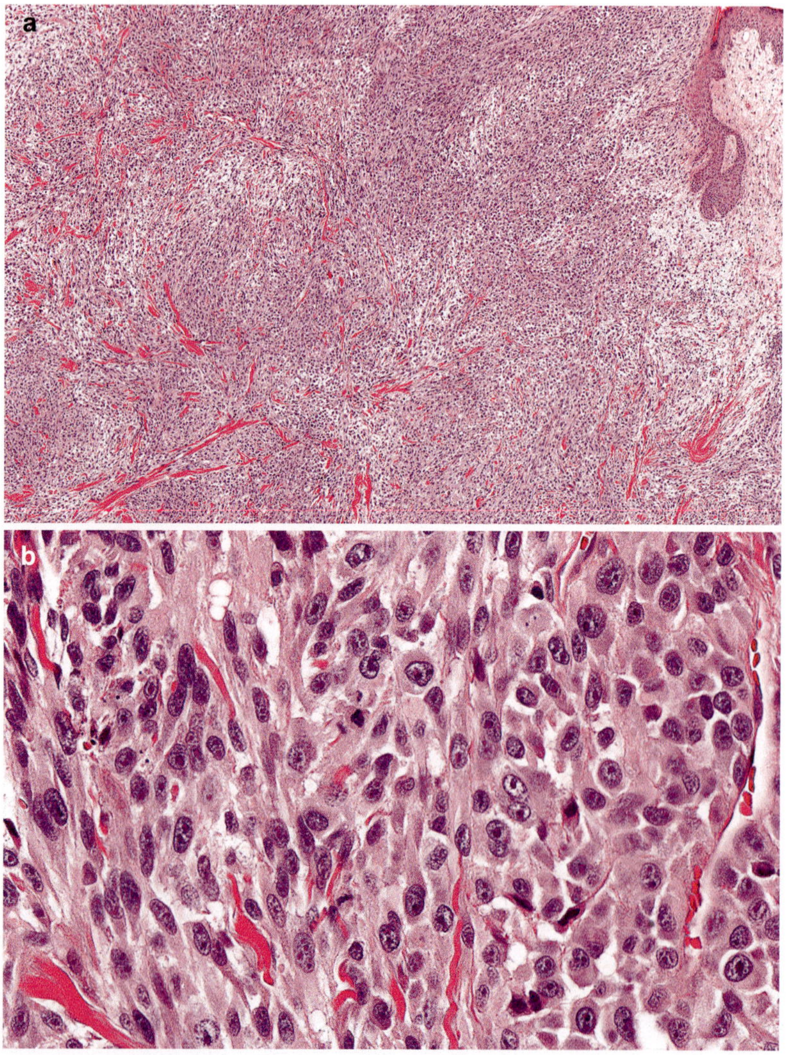

Fig. 13.14 Epithelioid rhabdomyosarcoma. (**a**) Low-power image demonstrating sheetlike proliferation of epithelioid tumor cells in the dermis. (**b**) High-power image demonstrating epithelioid to spindled tumor cells with uniform nuclei that have prominent nucleoli

Table 13.7 Key pathologic features: cutaneous rhabdomyosarcoma

Embryonal rhabdomyosarcoma Infants and children Uniform round tumor cells with or without rhabdomyoblasts Varying cellularity with myxoid stroma
Alveolar rhabdomyosarcoma Dyshesive aggregates of round to oval tumor cells separated by fibrous septa (alveolar pattern) Multinucleated tumor cells frequent *PAX3-FOXO1* or *PAX7-FOXO1* fusion
Pleomorphic rhabdomyosarcoma Elderly patients, often on the head and neck Pleomorphic rhabdomyoblasts
Epithelioid rhabdomyosarcoma Sheets of atypical epithelioid cells with vesicular nuclei and prominent nucleoli Absent or focal immunoreactivity for cytokeratin Diffuse immunoreactivity for desmin

Differential Diagnosis

The differential diagnosis is dependent on the subtype. Embryonal and alveolar rhabdomyosarcoma needs to be distinguished from other small round blue cell tumors, especially Ewing sarcoma. Ewing sarcoma is diffusely positive for CD99 in a membranous pattern and typically negative for desmin. While desmin immunoreactivity has been reported in Ewing sarcoma, it is uncommon and, when present, usually only focal. Ewing sarcoma is negative for skeletal muscle-specific markers and also has rearrangement of *EWSR1*, which can be detected by FISH or RT-PCR.

Pleomorphic and epithelioid rhabdomyosarcomas primarily need to be distinguished from sarcomatoid carcinoma and melanoma. This can be complicated by focal cytokeratin immunoreactivity seen in rhabdomyosarcoma. It is important to always consider the possibility of pleomorphic rhabdomyosarcoma if pleomorphic tumor cells with abundant eosinophilic cytoplasm are present. In that situation, we recommend adding a desmin stain to screen for the possibility of rhabdomyosarcoma, followed by stains for myogenin and/or MYOD1 if there is strong desmin positivity.

The differential diagnosis of epithelioid rhabdomyosarcoma is more difficult. Carcinomas or melanomas with morphology resembling epithelioid rhabdomyosarcoma would be expected to have more diffuse immunoreactivity for cytokeratins and expression of melanocyte-specific markers, respectively. In the absence of expected results of immunohistochemical stains in an epithelioid malignancy, addition of a desmin stain may prove useful. Rare cases of true rhabdomyo sarcomatous/rhabdomyoblastic differentiation have been reported in melanocytic nevi, Merkel cell carcinoma, and other cutaneous carcinomas. It is therefore imperative to identify the precursor lesion for accurate diagnosis.

Soft Tissue Chondroma

Clinical Features

Soft tissue chondromas usually occur in the hands and feet of middle-aged adults. They are benign lesions, but local recurrence has been reported.

Pathologic Features

Soft tissue chondromas are well-circumscribed tumors arising in the dermis or subcutis. They are composed of mature hyaline cartilage, but hypercellularity and focal nuclear atypia, including binucleated chondrocytes, are commonly present (Fig. 13.15a, b). These features are not indicative of malignancy in this clinical setting. Calcification and ossification are also commonly seen. By immunohistochemistry, they are positive for S100 protein and ERG. They are negative for cytokeratins, desmin, and SMA (Table 13.8).

Differential Diagnosis

Diagnosis of soft tissue chondroma is typically straightforward. Knowledge that atypia and hypercellularity may be seen helps avoid the

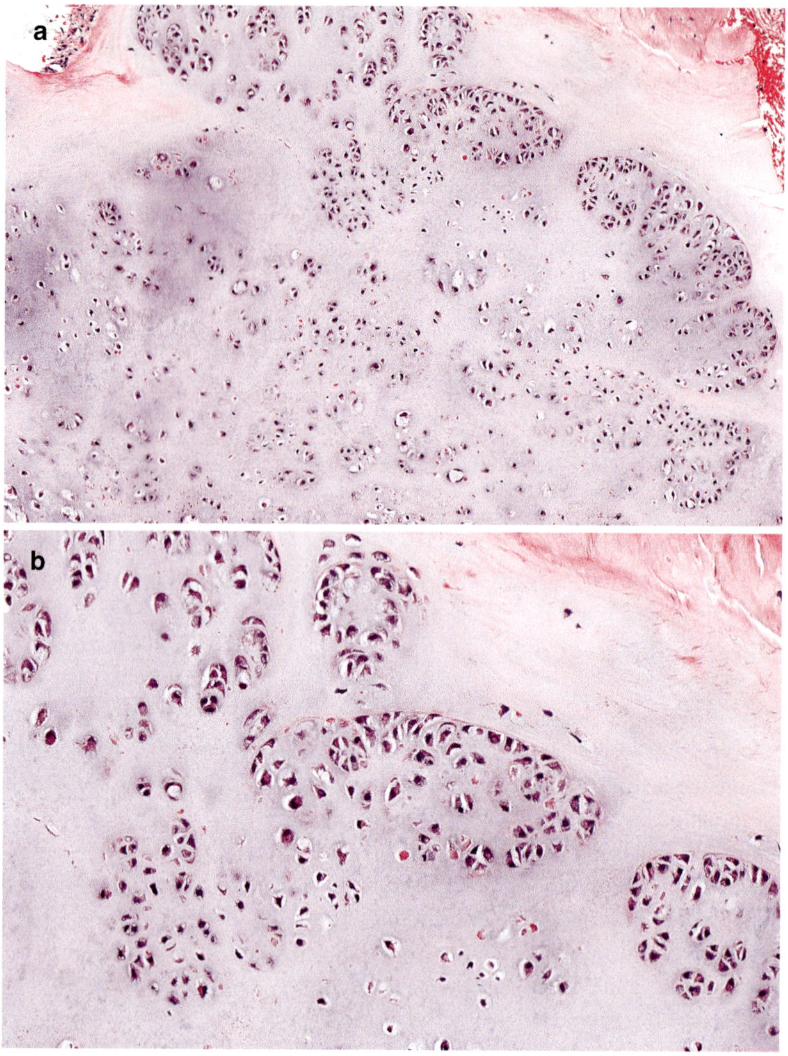

Fig. 13.15 Chondroma. (**a**) Chondromas are characterized by a lobular proliferation of chondrocytes. (**b**) Some atypia is a common finding in chondromas and is not indicative of malignancy

Table 13.8 Key pathologic features: soft tissue chondroma

Usually acral sites
Well circumscribed
May have cytologic atypia

erroneous diagnosis of chondrosarcoma. Chondrosarcomas do not present as small nodules in the hands and feet. Myoepitheliomas and cutaneous mixed tumors may have a chondroid matrix, but generally have evidence of epithelial differentiation either by morphology or immunohistochemistry.

Extraskeletal Myxoid Chondrosarcoma

Clinical Features

Extraskeletal myxoid chondrosarcoma usually arises in the deep soft tissue of the proximal extremities/limb girdles in adults, but occasional cases may arise in the subcutis. The M:F ratio is 2:1. Local recurrence is common, as is late (>5 years post-diagnosis) metastasis. For this reason, patients need lifelong follow-up.

Pathologic Features

The tumor has a lobular growth pattern and is composed of cords and nests of uniform epithelioid cells arranged in an abundant myxoid stroma (Fig. 13.16a, b). The tumor cells have uniform round to slightly spindled nuclei and eosinophilic cytoplasm. Intratumoral hemorrhage is commonly present (Fig. 13.16c). The mitotic rate is typically low.

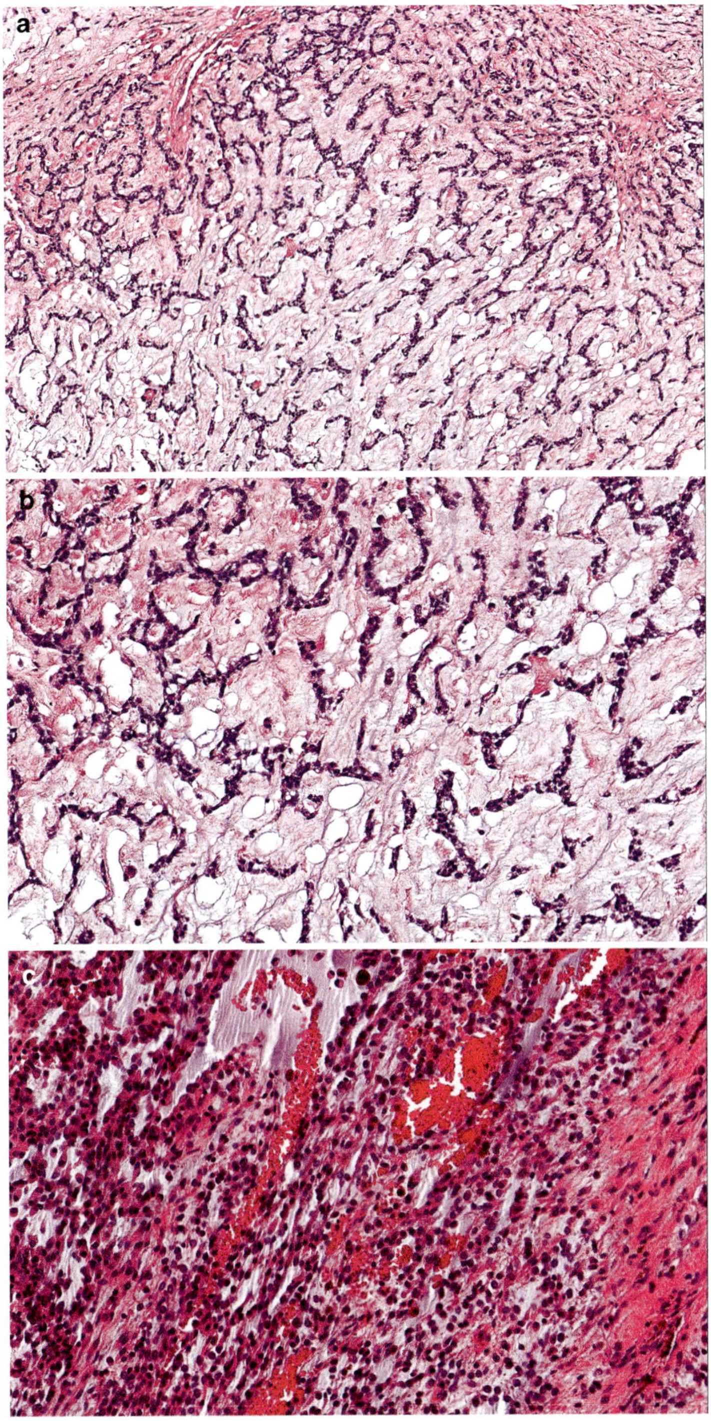

Fig. 13.16 Extraskeletal myxoid chondrosarcoma (**a**) The tumor cells are typically arranged in cords and nests in a myxoid stroma. (**b**) The tumor is composed of uniform round to oval tumor cells with eosinophilic cytoplasm. (**c**) Intratumoral hemorrhage is a common finding

Table 13.9 Key pathologic features: extraskeletal myxoid chondrosarcoma

Cords and nests of uniform tumor cells in myxoid stroma
Tumor cells with round to spindled nuclei and eosinophilic cytoplasm
Intratumoral hemorrhage common
NR4A3-EWSR1 or *NR4A3-TAF2N* gene fusions

Immunohistochemistry plays little to no role in the diagnosis. Less than 20% of cases show focal immunoreactivity for S100 protein or EMA. Occasional cases may show immunoreactivity for neuroendocrine markers. The only consistently positive marker is vimentin, which is entirely nonspecific and generally of no diagnostic utility.

About 70% of extraskeletal myxoid chondrosarcomas have a recurring t(9;22)(q22;q12) most commonly resulting in a *NR4A3-EWSR1* fusion. A minority of cases have a t(9;17)(q22;q11) with a *NR4A3-TAF2N* fusion. Molecular studies to detect rearrangement of *NR4A3* are useful in confirming the diagnosis (Table 13.9).

Differential Diagnosis

The primary differential diagnosis is soft tissue myoepithelioma and myxoid liposarcoma. Myoepitheliomas are typically positive for S100 protein and cytokeratin or EMA and are variably positive for SMA and p63. Most extraskeletal myxoid chondrosarcomas are negative for these markers. Myoepitheliomas do not have rearrangement of *NR4A3*, but it should be remembered that they may have rearrangement of *EWSR1*. Myxoid liposarcoma only exceptionally presents as a superficial mass and typically has a uniform plexiform vasculature and lipoblasts, which are not seen in extraskeletal myxoid chondrosarcoma. Myxoid liposarcoma also demonstrates rearrangement of *DDIT3*, which is not found in extraskeletal myxoid chondrosarcoma.

Osteoma Cutis

Clinical Features

Osteoma cutis is not strictly a neoplasm but a reactive process. It can be seen in a variety of settings. It is a frequent finding in facial skin in patients with a history of acne. If multiple lesions are encountered in young children, the possibility of underlying Albright hereditary osteodystrophy should be considered.

Pathologic Features

Osteoma cutis consists of nodules of mature lamellar bone. Some may contain marrow spaces (Fig. 13.17) (Table 13.10).

Differential Diagnosis

Osteoma cutis can be mistaken for dystrophic calcification if the presence of bone is not recognized.

Extraskeletal Osteosarcoma

Clinical Features

Although usually a deep soft tissue tumor, cutaneous extraskeletal osteosarcoma has been reported. It usually occurs in older adults; presentation in younger patients should prompt consideration of metastasis from an underlying bone tumor. Some cutaneous tumors represent metastasis from deep soft tissue or bone primaries. Roughly 10% of cases arise in the setting of prior radiotherapy, and cases associated with scars have been described. This is a potentially aggressive tumor. Although data are lacking regarding behavior of cutaneous examples, extraskeletal osteosarcoma has an overall mortality rate of approximately 75%.

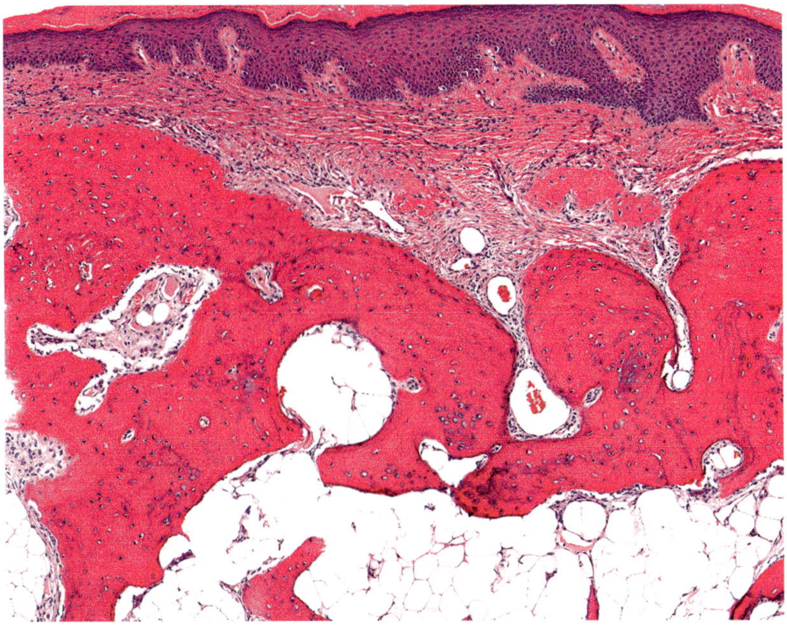

Fig. 13.17 Osteoma cutis composed of fragments of mature bone that sometimes has marrow elements, as in this case

Table 13.10 Key pathologic features: osteoma cutis

Small nodules of mature bone
Present at sites of prior inflammation or scarring
Presentation in young children prompts consideration of Albright hereditary osteodystrophy

Pathologic Features

Extraskeletal osteosarcoma is composed of atypical spindled to ovoid pleomorphic cells and is associated with malignant osteoid formation (Fig. 13.18a, b). Occasional cases may also show chondroid matrix production (chondroblastic osteosarcoma). Osteoclasts may be present in variable numbers and numerous in rare cases. The tumor cells are positive for SATB2 (Table 13.11).

Differential Diagnosis

The primary differential diagnosis is undifferentiated pleomorphic sarcoma. Recognition of malignant osteoid excludes this diagnosis. Cutaneous carcinosarcoma, defined as a distinctly biphasic tumor composed of carcinoma (especially basal cell carcinoma) and sarcoma components, may show osteosarcomatous differentiation. Recognition of the carcinoma component is the key to the correct diagnosis. Distinction is not trivial as carcinosarcoma is less aggressive than extraskeletal osteosarcoma. Other bone-forming tumors can also be considered in the differential diagnosis. Ossifying fibromyxoid tumor, including malignant variants, usually does not display the degree of cytologic atypia seen in extraskeletal osteosarcoma. Also, the bone formation tends to be at the periphery of the lesion. Similarly, giant cell tumor of soft tissue has less atypia with peripheral bone rather than malignant osteoid. Fibro-osseous pseudotumor presents on the digits and lacks the atypia and pleomorphism of extraskeletal osteosarcoma.

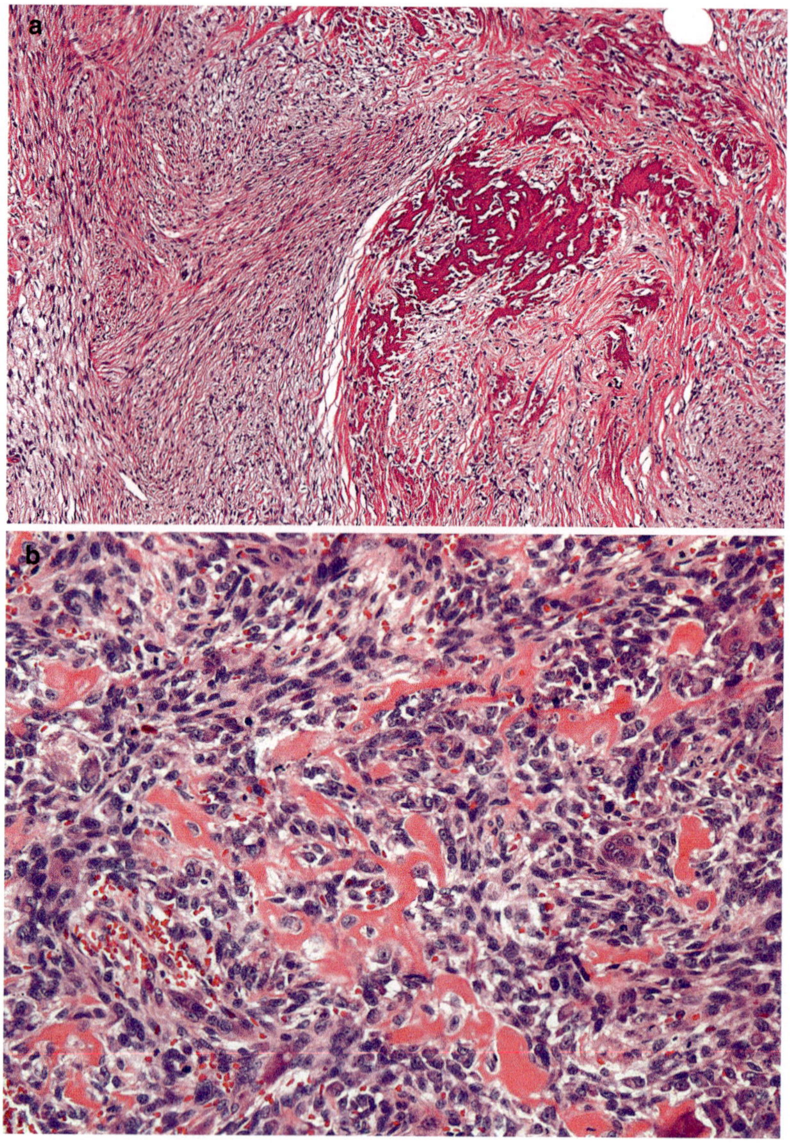

Fig. 13.18 Extraskeletal osteosarcoma (**a**) Hyperchromatic spindled cells admixed with malignant osteoid. (**b**) High-power image of a different case with hyperchromatic to spindled cells with lacelike osteoid

Table 13.11 Key pathologic features: extraskeletal osteosarcoma

Nuclear atypia and pleomorphism
Malignant osteoid formation
Rare cases with chondroid matrix
Tumor cells SATB2 positive

Selected References

1. Adhikari LA, McCalmont TH, Folpe AL. Merkel cell carcinoma with heterologous rhabdomyoblastic differentiation: the role of immunohistochemistry for Merkel cell polyomavirus large T-antigen in confirmation. J Cutan Pathol. 2012;39(1):47–51.
2. Alam NA, Olpin S, Leigh IM. Fumarate hydratase mutations and predisposition to cutaneous leiomyomas, uterine leiomyomas and renal cancer. Br J Dermatol. 2005;153(1):11–7.
3. Batalla A, Suh-Oh HJ, Pardavila R, de la Torre C. True cutaneous chondroma: a case report. J Cutan Pathol. 2015;42(9):657–9.
4. Benini S, Cocchi S, Gamberi G, Magagnoli G, Vogel D, Ghinelli C, Righi A, Picci P, Alberghini M, Gambarotti M. Diagnostic utility of molecular investigation in extraskeletal myxoid chondrosarcoma. J Mol Diagn. 2014;16(3):314–23.

5. Berger TG, Levin MW. Congenital smooth muscle hamartoma. J Am Acad Dermatol. 1984;11(4 Pt 2):709–12.
6. Chabra IS, Obagi S. Evaluation and management of multiple miliary osteoma cutis: case series of 11 patients and literature review. Dermatol Surg. 2014;40(1):66–8.
7. Chang Y, Dehner LP, Egbert B. Primary cutaneous rhabdomyosarcoma. Am J Surg Pathol. 1990;14(10):977–82.
8. Cook DL, Pugliano-Mauro MA, Schultz ZL. Atypical pilar leiomyomatosis: an unusual presentation of multiple atypical cutaneous leiomyomas. J Cutan Pathol. 2013;40(6):564–8.
9. Deyrup AT, Lee VK, Hill CE, Cheuk W, Toh HC, Kesavan S, Chan EW, Weiss SW. Epstein-Barr virus-associated smooth muscle tumors are distinctive mesenchymal tumors reflecting multiple infection events: a clinicopathologic and molecular analysis of 29 tumors from 19 patients. Am J Surg Pathol. 2006;30(1):75–82.
10. Falconieri G, Cataldi P, Kavalar R, Štitič V, Luzar B. Cutaneous osteoblastic osteosarcoma: report of 2 new cases integrated with SATB2 immunohistochemistry and review of the literature. Am J Dermatopathol. 2016;38(11):824–31.
11. Farshid G, Pradhan M, Goldblum J, Weiss SW. Leiomyosarcoma of somatic soft tissues: a tumor of vascular origin with multivariate analysis of outcome in 42cases. Am J Surg Pathol. 2002;26(1):14–24.
12. Fletcher CD, Powell G, McKee PH. Extraskeletal myxoid chondrosarcoma: a histochemical and immunohistochemical study. Histopathology. 1986;10(5):489–99.
13. Hammond MI, Miner AG, Piliang MP. Acral and digital angioleiomyomata: 14-year experience at the Cleveland Clinic and review of the literature. J Cutan Pathol. 2017;44(4):342–5.
14. Hayes M, van der Westhuizen N. Congenital rhabdomyomatous mesenchymal hamartoma. Am J Dermatopathol. 1992;14(1):64–5.
15. Heffernan MP, Smoller BR, Kohler S. Cutaneous epithelioid angioleiomyoma. Am J Dermatopathol. 1998;20(2):213–7.
16. Hoang MP, Sinkre P, Albores-Saavedra J. Rhabdomyosarcoma arising in a congenital melanocytic nevus. Am J Dermatopathol. 2002;24(1):26–9.
17. Holst VA, Junkins-Hopkins JM, Elenitsas R. Cutaneous smooth muscle neoplasms: clinical features, histologic findings, and treatment options. J Am Acad Dermatol. 2002;46(4):477–90; quiz, 491–4.
18. Hsueh S, Santa Cruz DJ. Cartilaginous lesions of the skin and superficial soft tissue. J Cutan Pathol. 1982;9(6):405–16.
19. Jeong KH, Lew BL, Sim WY. Osteoma cutis as the presenting feature of Albright hereditary osteodystrophy associated with pseudopseudohypoparathyroidism. Ann Dermatol. 2009;21(2):154–8.
20. Kawagishi N, Kashiwagi T, Ibe M, Manabe A, Ishida-Yamamoto A, Hashimoto Y, Iizuka H. Pleomorphic angioleiomyoma. Am J Dermatopathol. 2000;22(3):268–71.
21. Kobos JW, Yu GH, Varadarajan S, Brooks JS. Primary cutaneous osteosarcoma. Am J Dermatopathol. 1995;17(1):53–7.
22. Kraft S, Fletcher CD. Atypical intradermal smooth muscle neoplasms: clinicopathologic analysis of 84 cases and a reappraisal of cutaneous "leiomyosarcoma". Am J Surg Pathol. 2011;35(4):599–607.
23. Llamas-Velasco M, Rütten A, Requena L, Mentzel T. Primary cutaneous osteosarcoma of the skin: a report of 2 cases with emphasis on the differential diagnoses. Am J Dermatopathol. 2013;35(6):e106–13.
24. Llamas-Velasco M, Requena L, Kutzner H, Schärer L, Rütten A, Hantschke M, Paredes BE, Mentzel T. Fumarate hydratase immunohistochemical staining may help to identify patients with multiple cutaneous and uterine leiomyomatosis (MCUL)and hereditary leiomyomatosis and renal cell cancer (HLRCC) syndrome. J Cutan Pathol. 2014;41(11):859–65.
25. MacDonald DM, Sanderson KV. Angioleiomyoma of the skin. Br J Dermatol. 1974;91(2):161–8.
26. Marburger TB, Gardner JM, Prieto VG, Billings SD. Primary cutaneous rhabdomyosarcoma: a clinicopathologic review of 11 cases. J Cutan Pathol. 2012;39(11):987–95.
27. Marco VS, Bosch SB, Almeida LV. Acral angioleiomyoma with tumoral calcinosis: a complication of the insertional Achilles tendinopathy. J Cutan Pathol. 2017; https://doi.org/10.1111/cup.12956. [Epub ahead of print].
28. Massi D, Franchi A, Alos L, Cook M, Di Palma S, Enguita AB, Ferrara G, Kazakov DV, Mentzel T, Michal M, Panelos J, Rodriguez-Peralto JL, Santucci M, Tragni G, Zioga A, Dei Tos AP. Primary cutaneous leiomyosarcoma: clinicopathological analysis of 36 cases. Histopathology. 2010;56(2):251–62.
29. Matthews JH, Pichardo RO, Hitchcock MG, Leshin B. Cutaneous leiomyoma with cytologic atypia, akin to uterine symplastic leiomyoma. Dermatol Surg. 2004;30(9):1249–51; discussion 1251.
30. McMenamin ME, Goh SG, Poblet E, Gostelow BE, Robson A, Calonje E. Sarcomatoid basal cell carcinoma-predilection for osteosarcomatous differentiation: a series of 11 cases. Am J Surg Pathol. 2006;30(10):1299–308.
31. Metzker A, Merlob P. Congenital smooth muscle hamartoma. J Am Acad Dermatol. 1986;14(4):691.
32. Miettinen M. Smooth muscle tumors of soft tissue and non-uterine viscera: biology and prognosis. Mod Pathol. 2014;27(Suppl 1):S17–29.
33. Mills AE. Rhabdomyomatous mesenchymal hamartoma of skin. Am J Dermatopathol. 1989;11(1):58–63.
34. Nascimento AG, Karas M, Rosen PP, Caron AG. Leiomyoma of the nipple. Am J Surg Pathol. 1979;3(2):151–4.
35. Newman PL, Fletcher CD. Smooth muscle tumours of the external genitalia: clinicopathological analysis of a series. Histopathology. 1991;18(6):523–9.

36. Petersson F, Huang J. Epstein-Barr virus-associated smooth muscle tumor mimicking cutaneous angioleiomyoma. Am J Dermatopathol. 2011;33(4):407–9.
37. Ramdial PK, Sing Y, Deonarain J, Hadley GP, Singh B. Dermal Epstein Barr virus-associated leiomyosarcoma: tocsin of acquired immunodeficiency syndrome in two children. Am J Dermatopathol. 2011;33(4):392–6.
38. Roth SI, Stowell RE, Helwig EB. Cutaneous ossification. Report of 120 cases and review of the literature. Arch Pathol. 1963;76:44–54.
39. Salamanca J, Dhimes P, Pinedo F, de la Fuente EG, Pérez Espejo G, Martínez-Tello FJ. Extraskeletal cutaneous chondroblastic osteosarcoma: a case report. J Cutan Pathol. 2008;35(2):231–5.
40. Slifman NR, Harrist TJ, Rhodes AR. Congenital arrector pili hamartoma. A case report and review of the spectrum of Becker's melanosis and pilar smooth-muscle hamartoma. Arch Dermatol. 1985;121(8):1034–7.
41. Tetzlaff MT, Nosek C, Kovarik CL. Epstein-Barr virus-associated leiomyosarcoma with cutaneous involvement in an African child with human immunodeficiency virus: a case report and review of the literature. J Cutan Pathol. 2011;38(9):731–9.
42. Winchester DS, Hocker TL, Brewer JD, Baum CL, Hochwalt PC, Arpey CJ, Otley CC, Roenigk RK. Leiomyosarcoma of the skin: clinical, histopathologic, and prognostic factors that influence outcomes. J Am Acad Dermatol. 2014;71(5):919–25.

Index

S. D. Billings et al. (eds.), *Soft Tissue Tumors of the Skin*,
https://doi.org/10.1007/978-1-4939-8812-9

D

H

I

J

N

Printed by Printforce, the Netherlands